ANNUAL REVIEW OF PUBLIC HEALTH

ANNUAL REVIEW OF PUBLIC HEALTH

VOLUME 23, 2002

JONATHAN E. FIELDING, *Editor*
University of California at Los Angeles

ROSS C. BROWNSON, *Associate Editor*
Saint Louis University

BARBARA STARFIELD, *Associate Editor*
Johns Hopkins University

www.annualreviews.org   science@annualreviews.org   650-493-4400

ANNUAL REVIEWS
4139 El Camino Way • P.O. BOX 10139 • Palo Alto, California 94303-0139

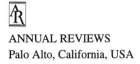

ANNUAL REVIEWS
Palo Alto, California, USA

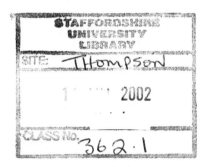
International Standard Serial Number: 0163-7525
International Standard Book Number: 0-8243-2723-3

Typeset by TechBooks, Fairfax, VA
Printed and Bound in the United States of America

PREFACE

The central role of public health practice in protecting the health of all was dramatically underscored by events in the fall of 2001. The anthrax exposures, cases, and deaths changed perceptions of bioterrorism from an intriguing but second tier concern to the center of the public safety and public health agenda.

For the first time in many years, public health infrastructure was viewed as critical by more than those of us in public health. Federal, state, and local elected political leaders started to ask questions about public health preparedness for bioterrorism and also chemical and radiological terrorism. Increased Federal funding has been appropriated for enhanced epidemiological surveillance, laboratory capacity, communications, and emergency response planning and systems.

The *Annual Review of Public Health* contributes to the science and policy analysis necessary to improve public protection from biological or other forms of terrorism. As we consider where and how much to invest to improve our preparedness to identify and respond to acts of biological, chemical, or radiological terrorism, cost-effectiveness is a critical consideration. In this volume is a review by Briggs et al. of improvements in analysis and presentation of uncertainty in cost-effectiveness studies. The World Trade Center bombing may have affected air quality and related health risks. Discussion by Morgenstern & Krupnick of the Clean Air Act and limitations in its evaluation helps us understand how to improve its regulation and better assess health effects of local disasters.

Measurement of public health capacity and program effectiveness is being considered by policymakers as more important than before because of the need to better assess our collective preparedness. The article in this volume by Derose et al. on public health quality measurement treats both the conceptual issues and challenges in developing systems to assess system and program quality.

One of the issues raised by the threat of biological terrorism is the potential need for quarantining patients and/or exposed groups. The most relevant recent experience in the United States is quarantining patents with multiple drug resistance tuberculosis, part of the discussion of the comprehensive review of tuberculosis by Tiruviluamala & Reichman.

Social environments are important determinants of both the likelihood and form of weapons of mass destruction and the vulnerability of the intended target population. The review by Evans & Kantrowitz thoughtfully considers socioeconomic conditions and disparities as a health determinant.

Finally, as the anthrax exposures and cases demonstrated, early recognition and treatment of those exposed is often the difference between life and death. Reducing medical errors from lack of early diagnosis or inappropriate treatment helps to improve preparedness for new or unaccustomed pathogens. The article in this volume on medical errors by Phillips & Bredder highlights the nature and extent of this large problem.

Improving public health infrastructure, capacity, and performance requires a broad and multi-faceted approach anchored in what we know from careful assessment of the literature. The contribution of the *Annual Review of Public Health* is to provide carefully crafted, analytic reviews so that all those in the field can know what the subject matter experts know. We help to bridge the gap between research and practice, and the stakes have never been higher.

Jonathan E. Fielding
Barbara Starfield
Ross C. Brownson

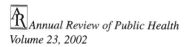*Annual Review of Public Health*
Volume 23, 2002

CONTENTS

ERRATA

An online log of corrections to *Annual Review of Public Health*
chapters (if any have yet been occasioned, 1997 to the present)
may be found at http://publhealth.annualreviews.org/

RELATED ARTICLES

Annu. Rev. Public Health 2002. 23:1–21

PUBLIC HEALTH QUALITY MEASUREMENT:
Concepts and Challenges[1]

Stephen F. Derose
Southern California Kaiser Permanente, Pasadena, California 91101;
e-mail: Stephen.F.Derose@kp.org

Mark A. Schuster
Departments of Pediatrics and Health Services, University of California, Los Angeles,
California 90095; RAND, Santa Monica, California 90407; e-mail: schuster@rand.org

Jonathan E. Fielding
Department of Health Services, University of California, Los Angeles; County of
Los Angeles Department of Health Services, Los Angeles, California 90012;
e-mail: jfielding@dhs.co.la.ca.gov

Steven M. Asch
Veterans Affairs Greater Los Angeles Healthcare System, Los Angeles; Department
of Medicine, University of California, Los Angeles, California 90095; RAND,
Santa Monica, California 90407; e-mail: sasch@rand.org

Key Words outcome and process assessment (health care), public health administration/indicator, quality/quality assurance, health care/public health practice

■ **Abstract** Public health agencies increasingly are recognizing the need to formally and quantitatively assess and improve the quality of their programs, information, and policies. Measuring quality can help organizations monitor their progress toward public health goals and become more accountable to both the populations they serve and policy makers. Yet quality assessment is a complex task that involves precise determination and specification of useful measures. We discuss a well-established conceptual framework for organizing quality assessment in the context of planning and delivery of programs and services by local health departments, and consider the strengths and limitations of this approach for guiding quality improvement. We review several past and present quality measurement–related initiatives designed for public health department use, and discuss current and future challenges in this evolving area of public health practice.

INTRODUCTION

The mission of the public health system in the United States is to promote and protect the nation's health. Historically, the public health system has achieved much success in pursuing this mission (2). However, future gains will likely depend upon the system's ability to continually transform services and programs to effectively meet evolving population health needs. A commitment to quality is one of the cornerstones of continued success in public health practice. As such, quality assessment tools can be used to measure and promote the quality of public health activities, which ultimately affect the public's health through programs, information, and policies aimed at individuals and population groups.

Many industries and institutions, other than public health departments, have recognized the value of utilizing quality assessment tools and quality improvement methods (20, 29, 39, 40), and comparable efforts are being implemented within the personal health care system (12, 18, 35, 41, 47, 60, 68, 69, 71). Similarly, many public health agencies have recognized the potential benefits of quality assessment and improvement, and efforts are under way to institute measurement-based assessments to monitor practice performance (11, 48, 59, 79). Although few evaluations have been undertaken to determine the effectiveness of quality assessment and improvement initiatives in public health, there is some qualitative, if not quantitative, evidence that these efforts are improving public health services. For example, both Texas and Illinois have reported positive experiences with initiatives measuring local health department (LHD) performance. In Texas, quality measurement within LHDs fostered team building, role clarification among individuals and programs, and communication with external audiences (28). Similarly, in Illinois, LHDs reported an increased understanding of internal strengths and weaknesses and of community health problems (79). Population-based quality measurement also can benefit state public health programs: for example, measures of participant satisfaction have informed quality improvement attempts in North Carolina's Women, Infants, and Children (WIC) Program (26).

Incorporating quality measurement into public health can be challenging. Part of the difficulty is the scarcity of background theory, research, evidence-based standards, and practical experience upon which public health professionals can draw to develop quality indicators (or measures) for public health practice. In this article, we attempt to fill this gap by discussing important concepts underlying quality measurement in public health, examining the range of activities that can be measured, providing an overview of existing quality measurement-related initiatives, and considering further steps to build and implement effective quality measurement systems. Our discussion focuses on the LHD because it has the primary responsibility for ensuring and improving the public's health; however, we also consider the broader public health system.

CONCEPTUAL OVERVIEW OF PUBLIC HEALTH QUALITY ASSESSMENT

The Terminology of Evaluation

The terms used in the literature to refer to quality and performance measurement often are not consistently applied, which can complicate the interpretation of measurement results and comparisons across locations (43). We summarize some of the terms commonly used to describe quality measurement. The Institute of Medicine (IOM) has defined *quality* of health care as "the degree to which health services for individuals and populations increase the likelihood of desired health outcomes and are consistent with current professional knowledge" (44). *Quality assessment* in public health is the measurement of achievement of population health objectives and practices by a particular organization or a group of individuals. *Performance assessment*, on the other hand, tracks progress towards organizational objectives and can include measures not only of quality, but also of cost/efficiency (e.g., the number of people a program serves, the cost per service). Despite this distinction, "quality assessment" and "performance measurement" often are used interchangeably in the literature. We use the term "quality assessment" here because our discussion does not extend to measuring costs or efficiency. Indicators are the basic unit of quantitative quality assessment. Public health *quality indicators* are quantitative statements about the capacity (structure), actions (processes), or results (outcomes) of public health practices.

Defining the Range of Public Health Assessment

A working description of the range of public health activities (i.e., programs, information, and policies), broadly outlined in terms of public health functions or services, is a prerequisite for defining the content and boundaries of public health quality assessments. However, there is a potential pitfall in defining public health for measurement purposes—a definition that simply, and empirically, mirrors current tasks in some LHDs may lack generalizability to other LHDs or may inadvertently help perpetuate outdated services. This can be a problem, especially since over the past century the U.S. public health system has sometimes experienced difficulties in adjusting to changing population health needs (e.g., the AIDS epidemic) and in adopting technological transformations (e.g., information technologies) (54, 77).

Instead, an ideal description should have a theoretical basis, such as the one described in the Institute of Medicine's (IOM) 1988 report, *The Future of Public Health*. This report recommended that the public health system change from its traditional service-oriented perspective to a broader conceptualization involving three fundamental "core functions" of public health: assessment, policy development, and assurance (38). The assessment function means that LHDs are expected to monitor and analyze the health of various populations. The policy development function involves formulating and promoting scientifically sound public health policies. The assurance function guarantees public health services (including personal healthcare) for everyone, by either encouraging or requiring another organization to perform the service or providing the service directly (24). When LHDs successfully carry out these core functions, the results are programs and services that meet the health needs of the local population.

In 1989, the Centers for Disease Control and Prevention, Public Health Practice Program Office (CDC-PHPPO) convened a workgroup to recast these somewhat abstract core functions into more measurable terms (24). The workgroup developed the "ten public health practices," which define each of the IOM's core functions in greater detail, by outlining key activities that an organization must perform to fulfill the three core functions of public health. Likewise, a similar detailed description of public health activities, termed the "ten essential services," emerged from the debate on health reform in the early part of the Clinton administration. The Office of the Assistant Secretary of Health began to form a consensus on public health activities in 1994; the Public Health Functions Working Group and Steering Committee (composed of U.S. Public Health Service agencies and other leading public health organizations) built on this work to develop the ten essential services (Table 1) (10, 63). As Table 1 shows, the range of public health activities described in the ten practices and the ten essential services differs only slightly. Unlike the ten practices, the ten essential services explicitly state the personal health responsibilities of public health agencies and recognize a role for research. Both sets describe key public health activities from a practical perspective, and thus can be used to guide measurement efforts (10).

Another useful conceptualization of public health activities, particularly as they are distinguished from primary care, divides the functions of public health agencies into primary, secondary, and tertiary prevention, and the target groups into average- and high-risk individuals and populations (72). In combining these categories, this taxonomy delineates the linkages between public and personal health functions. For example, secondary prevention by environmental monitoring of populations at average risk traditionally has been the purview of the public health system, whereas tertiary prevention in high-risk individuals conventionally has been that of the personal health system.

There are advantages and disadvantages to each of the conceptualizations of public health functions described in this section. The list of ten essential services is appealing because it is widely accepted and expresses the mission and goals of public health for a broad audience. Below we describe a framework for quality assessment designed to incorporate most models of public health functions.

Framework for Assessment

A conceptualization and working definition of public health functions or services drives the choice of domains for quality assessment, but in and of itself does not

TABLE 1   The ten public health practices and the ten essential public health services

Public health practices (24)	Essential public health services (10, 63)
Assessment	
• Assess the health needs of the community • Investigate the occurrence of adverse health effects and hazards • Analyze the determinants of health needs	• Monitor health status to identify and solve community health needs • Diagnose and investigate health problems and health hazards in the community
Policy Development	
• Advocate for public health, build constituencies, and identify resources in the community • Set priorities among health needs • Develop plans and policies to address priority health needs	• Mobilize community partnerships and action to solve health problems • Develop policies and plans that support individual and community health efforts
Assurance	
• Manage and coordinate resources and develop the public health system's organizational structure • Implement programs by ensuring or providing services • Evaluate programs and provide quality assurance • Inform and educate the public on health issues	• Assure a competent workforce—public health and personal health care • Enforce laws and regulations that protect health and assure safety • Link people to needed personal health services and assure the provision of health care when otherwise unavailable • Evaluate effectiveness, accessibility, and quality of personal and population-based health services • Inform, educate, and empower people about health issues • Research for new insights and innovative solutions to health problems

provide a framework (and method) for assessment. To find a measurement framework useful for organizing evaluations, we turn to the quality assessment work of Donabedian. Donabedian's framework divides quality into three dimensions: 1. *structural quality*, which assesses the organizational characteristics and resources of public health agencies (or the larger public health system); 2. *process quality*, which assesses what public health agencies do, although LHD functions can be difficult to measure; and 3. *outcome quality*, which assesses the influence of actions by public health agencies on the public's health (22, 62). In Figure 1, we adapt this framework for quality assessment of local public health systems and illustrate how structure, process, and outcome are related (50). Structural elements make processes possible, and processes, in turn, lead to short-term results (intermediate outcomes) and, ultimately, to community health outcomes. This framework can be used to evaluate the public health activities of both LHDs and

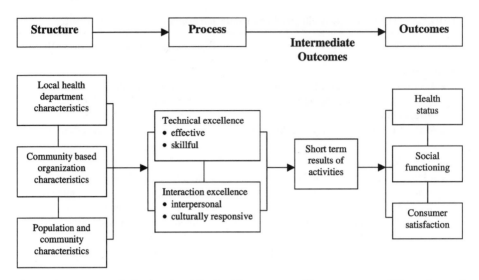

Figure 1   Framework for local public health system quality assessment. Dimensions of quality (*structure, process, outcome*) and aspects for assessment (*boxes*) are depicted. Characteristics of process quality (*bullets*) are listed within technical excellence and interaction excellence. The quality of both the planning and the delivery of programs and services may be assessed within this framework.

community-based organizations (CBOs, such as educational institutions, religious institutions, civic organizations, health providers, businesses), which together constitute the local public health system. Furthermore, it demonstrates the interconnectedness of various agencies' effects on public health outcomes and is consistent with a CDC-PHPPO framework that describes the function and infrastructure of the public health system (24).

In the columns of the figure, under each dimension of quality assessment—structure, process, and outcome—are boxes indicating aspects of public health *planning*, or decision-making, and the *delivery* of programs and services that can be measured using quality indicators. Structural aspects include population and community characteristics that can influence outcomes and that the local public health system may be able to affect, through lobbying or other means (e.g., the availability of government-sponsored health insurance among otherwise uninsured children, the tax on alcohol and tobacco products). Process quality may be evaluated on grounds of technical excellence, which applies to the execution of all activities, or interaction excellence, which refers to those programs and services that have contact with consumers of public health services (e.g., the public, other organizations). Intermediate outcomes are the short-term results of public health activities. The intermediate outcomes of planning are combinations of programs and services that aim to fulfill local health needs. Planning determines how resources (structure) will be used and how public health services will be delivered.

The intermediate outcomes of delivery are the direct, short-term results of these programs and services (e.g., immunization rates for vaccination programs). Ultimate community health outcomes include health status, social functioning, and consumer satisfaction.

The Donabedian framework aids in identifying quality measures within each core public health function or essential service. For example, if we chose the first essential service (see Table 1), "monitoring health status to identify and solve community health needs," we could conceive of structural measures [e.g., the presence of computerized tuberculosis (TB) tracking systems], process measures (e.g., the proportion of TB cases reported), and outcomes measures (e.g., rates of TB) for this domain. The following section describes in greater detail structure, process, and outcomes as they apply to public health.

The Dimensions of Quality Evaluation

STRUCTURE   Structural quality assesses those organizational elements and resources of an LHD or the larger local public health system that affect its ability to meet community health needs and to promote healthy lives. The structural aspects of quality are necessary, although not sufficient, to facilitate the processes that affect outcomes (e.g., computers are necessary, but not sufficient, to conduct most epidemiological analyses). Structural quality can be divided into 1. inputs, which include personnel (e.g., the number of epidemiologists on staff), physical resources (e.g., computerized information systems, workspace), and financial resources; and 2. organization, which includes how resources are arranged and managed (e.g., administrative policies, the decision-making hierarchy, the particular mix of inputs used) (22).

In deciding which specific structural features to measure, it is important to focus on factors that are amenable to change and that affect processes (and thus outcomes). For example, whether an LHD compiles a registry of CBOs and their activities might be a good structural feature to assess because the registry could be used to improve the timeliness and comprehensiveness of LHD-led community health planning and such planning could ultimately affect health outcomes. Structural measures are particularly useful for developing and strengthening the infrastructure of a local public health system when capacity is insufficient to meet local needs. However, once the necessary infrastructure has been developed (e.g., there are a sufficient number of experienced epidemiologists on staff), structural indicators have limited value. Moreover, since they are more remote from outcomes than are other measures, structural measures provide limited information about the day-to-day actions of an organization, and thus are less useful for guiding quality improvement efforts.

PROCESS   Process quality assesses what LHDs (or other agencies) do for or with population groups, organizations, and individuals, and how well they perform those actions. Process measures examine specific actions and provide timely information about activities that can be changed to improve outcomes. Examples of process quality measures include the proportion of provider organizations that report more than 90% of measles cases to the LHD, the proportion of active TB case contacts that are traced and appropriately treated, and the proportion of small water systems that are inspected as frequently as state law specifies. It is best to choose process indicators that have a clear, causal link to outcomes; however, determining whether a process measure relates to and affects an outcome can be difficult (49). Ideally, the link between a process measure and outcome should be established through scientific evidence, although the evidentiary base is not always sufficient to form such a connection (14). In practice, a consensus of expert opinion often is used, despite the potential for introducing bias (15). In addition, a causal link is sometimes assumed when there is a strong logical connection between an action and its result. Causal models, in the form of analytic or logic frameworks, are useful tools to depict and clarify the determinants of problems in public health (13, 21).

As noted above, process quality has two main aspects: technical excellence and interaction excellence. Technical excellence, which refers to the application of science and technology to public health practice, means that programs and services are effectively planned and skillfully delivered. For quality assessment purposes, effective planning indicates that the health benefits expected from a chosen course of action exceed benefits from alternative strategies. Skillful delivery means proficiency in performance by the individuals and organizations involved.

Interaction excellence, which pertains primarily to service delivery, concerns the human behavioral aspects of activities and includes both humane interpersonal conduct and cultural responsiveness: is a personal interaction during a public health intervention or collaboration respectful, ethical, and responsive to the individual or organization involved and is the program or service delivered in a manner respectful of and responsive to the preferences and special circumstances of population groups and individuals? One example is whether program information is provided in the primary languages of all recipients.

Although many people find the assessment of day-to-day organizational tasks (e.g., the delivery of a program) intuitive, public health planning is more difficult to assess. For LHDs, planning involves complex decision-making to establish a set of programs and services that best meets the health needs of the local population, especially under constrained resources. LHD planning includes 1. resource allocation, in which the LHD plans to maximize health-related social welfare through its distribution of resources; and 2. intervention selection and coordination, in which the LHD, often in concert with community partners, implements specific programs in a way that meets health objectives for targeted populations effectively.

An assessment of planning results (intermediate outcomes) is feasible, although difficult, whereas planning processes are currently more challenging to evaluate. For example, the quality of the results of decision-making for resource allocation might be measured by calculating the dollars spent per preventable disability-adjusted life years (DALYs) for the most common causes of morbidity and mortality in a local area (3, 55). However, an assessment of the planning process involves the much more complex evaluation of actions involved in public health decision-making, including, for example, whether goals and objectives are stated plainly, evidence-based community health interventions are identified systematically from the literature and the information is utilized, community input is elicited, competing interests are considered, available resources are identified, and the logic of the intervention strategy and its evaluation are defined clearly.

In addition, the process of public health planning is difficult to directly assess currently because of inadequate measurement methods and lack of general agreement on standards for community health interventions, although attempts to produce them are under way (76). Moreover, political and fiscal factors, such as constraints on the use of funds, necessarily influence planning decisions; therefore, for theoretical and practical reasons these factors are usually separated from evaluations of quality (22). Thus, although planning is an important LHD role and domain of assessment, the delivery of programs and services can be evaluated more readily. Furthermore, a successful program or policy suggests good planning, albeit indirectly.

OUTCOME   Outcome quality assesses the influence of public health activities on community health. Public health outcomes can be divided into ultimate, or true, population health outcomes, and intermediate outcomes. Ultimate outcomes, the effects of public health activities on the health of a defined population, fall into three categories: 1. health status, which assesses the physical and mental status of a population (e.g., rates of motor vehicle accident deaths, measles, or depression); 2. social functioning, which assesses the ability of a defined population to function in society (e.g., rates of persons with disabilities living independently); and 3. consumer satisfaction, which assesses the response to public health services from a population or other stakeholder (e.g., client satisfaction with tobacco cessation programs) (62). Stakeholders, such as citizens, high-risk groups, health care providers, government policy makers, and health department staff, may all contribute unique and valid perspectives on the quality of LHD services from their own experience.

Consumer satisfaction can be an important component in determining how often population-based programs provide services and can help improve quality by motivating health departments to meet consumer needs (45). However, consumer ratings may not be reliable indicators of quality, particularly for public health activities, because consumers are not always able to determine whether services are appropriate or technically good (4), and the ratings may not reflect the outcome for the entire population at risk (for instance, some patients isolated for TB or treated for addictions may dislike programs that are effective and beneficial to the public and themselves).

Intermediate outcomes indicate the effects of public health activities on risk factors associated with population health status (62). They assess changes in health risks that are demonstrated or assumed to be associated with the health status of the community (e.g., teenage smoking rates, the proportion of children with high lead levels, immunization rates, or measures of industrial toxins in the environment). Intermediate outcomes include the short-term results of programs and services, and they may, with appropriate caution, be used as proxy measures for true health outcomes (62). Intermediate outcomes can take many forms, reflecting the diversity of public health activities. For example, in health promotion programs, intermediate outcomes may include measures of change in knowledge (e.g., how HIV is transmitted), attitudes (e.g., toward condom use), and risk behavior (e.g., self-reported rates of condom use) (17, 27). Although the number of persons served by a program is generally not used as an indicator of quality, the proportion of a high-risk population served by an outreach program is often considered a feature of program quality (i.e., accessibility) and is thus used as an intermediate outcome.

Both process measures and intermediate outcomes are particularly useful in quality evaluation because 1. the lag between implementing public health services and changes in the rates of targeted health problems (such as cancers or heart disease) often extends to many years; 2. some important ultimate health outcomes occur infrequently (such as meningococcal meningitis outbreaks), whereas their associated processes and intermediate outcomes are more frequent; and 3. ultimate health status outcomes often are influenced by many factors outside the control of the public health system, whereas processes and intermediate outcomes are influenced more directly by the LHD and other public health organizations.

Outcomes can be used to evaluate the overall quality of a local public health system, agency, or intervention. However, to effectively use outcome indicators for quality assessment and improvement, the measures should be linked (e.g., using analytic or logic frameworks) to public health processes. If we do not know how our actions affect results, it is difficult to determine how to improve performance. In addition, external factors that affect outcomes must be taken into account in order to draw valid conclusions about the quality of outcomes. Other contributory factors (covariates or risk-adjustment variables) often affect outcomes but remain outside the control or influence of the LHD and the local public health system; these include both community and population characteristics (e.g., age and income distribution, school system quality, the number of liquor stores per capita, the price of tobacco products, and other social and economic factors), which make it difficult to determine the results of LHD activities. The effects of these covariates on health outcomes (e.g., the influence of age distribution on a community's most common causes of death) are important and, when possible, these variables should be measured in order to statistically adjust and compare outcomes over time or across LHD jurisdictions. Statistical adjustment involves predicting outcomes based on population characteristics and comparing the observed to the expected number of events. When adjusting outcomes for several variables simultaneously, regression models can be used in a manner that is analogous to the indirect standardization of mortality rates (16, 37). When adjustment for influential covariates is not possible, clearly stated caveats must accompany the interpretation of outcomes quality.

If an LHD has little or no control over an outcome measure, the LHD cannot be held fully accountable for that measure, and it is not a useful indicator of quality.

Nevertheless, an outcome indicator with low accountability can still be a useful measure of population health status. Measures of health status are used to inform the public and policy makers on issues in public health. Moreover, they can be used to define goals for public health, as has been done with *Healthy People 2000* and *Healthy People 2010* (82, 83).

OVERVIEW OF PUBLIC HEALTH MEASUREMENT INITIATIVES

Although many of the public health measurement systems described in this section have been widely used, they were not designed specifically for quality evaluation purposes. Nevertheless, a critical appraisal of their component measures and the way in which they fit into the theoretical framework described above can help guide future initiatives for quality measurement.

Early Initiatives

Initiatives designed to measure public health practice in the United States were first introduced in the early part of the twentieth century. The American Public Health Association (APHA) developed two important measurement tools: the APHA *Appraisal Form* and subsequently the APHA *Evaluation Schedule*. Both tools focused primarily on the services that LHDs and other agencies provided and were used to rate and compare LHD performance (77). The *Appraisal Form* is a means of voluntary self-evaluation that was developed in 1925 to formally assess citywide public health practices (8, 9). Used until the early 1940s, this tool gathered data and rated LHDs and other community health agencies on the type of activities (e.g., creating geographic maps of diseases) and the quantity of activities (e.g., the number of vaccinations given) that they provided. Also tracked were health department resources and regional mortality rates; however, this information was not used to compare LHD performance because it was considered to be too dependent on local circumstances and unmeasured covariates (8). In 1943, the *Evaluation Schedule* was developed to replace the *Appraisal Form* (6). This self-evaluation tool, which was used into the 1950s, measured the immediate results (intermediate outcomes) as well as the activities of local public health systems (33). The *Evaluation Schedule* provided more detailed quality assessment of LHDs by using more outcomes and process indicators and by endeavoring to measure, as objectively as possible, how well resources were used to meet local health needs (5).

These early instruments were quite complex. Both tools, particularly the *Evaluation Schedule*, used a mixture of 1. structural measures (e.g., the number of persons in a region per physician), 2. process measures (e.g., the percentage of reported syphilis case contacts examined by a physician), 3. intermediate outcomes measures (e.g., the percentage of children under two years of age who had received a smallpox vaccine), and 4. true health status outcomes measures (e.g., the number of TB deaths per 100,000 people over a five-year period) (6). However, because both tools focus on the delivery of services, they did not examine whether LHD planning resulted in programs, information, and policies that appropriately met changing community health needs.

National Self-Assessment Tools

More recent measurement initiatives include self-assessment tools, which use performance measures to help LHDs evaluate their ability to perform public health functions, address local health needs, and guide community health planning efforts. The most widely used self-assessment tool is the *Assessment Protocol for Excellence in Public Health (APEX/PH)* (56). Developed by the National Association of County and City Health Officials (NACCHO), *APEX/PH* allows local health officials to assess the organizational management of their departments, provides a framework for working with the community and assessing its health status, and helps to promote the leadership of the LHD within the community (56). *APEX/PH* has multiple ready-made indicators designed to measure organizational capacity (structure) and also includes some process measures. (For example, a structural indicator for community health assessment is, "Does the health department annually compile or update a listing of health-related information systems and databases maintained by community organizations that operate within its jurisdiction?") The organization assesses the perceived importance of the indicator and the degree to which it currently is being met.

Building on lessons learned from the *APEX/PH* project, a new tool, *Mobilizing for Action through Planning and Partnerships (MAPP)*, is being developed under NACCHO's guidance (57). This tool is intended to help communities improve health and quality of life through partnership mobilization and strategic action. The instrument enables communities to assess important community problems and strengths, the local public health system (using the *Local Public Health System Performance Assessment Instrument*, which is described later), the health status of the community, and forces of change. Local public health system indicators include a set of predefined measures of structure, process, and outcomes, but the tool provides flexibility in that it allows use of additional measures depending on local needs.

Model Standards is another widely used means of self-assessment developed by the APHA that is used to link the *Healthy People* national objectives to local efforts at health improvement (7). The tool employs easy-to-use worksheets that allow communities and LHDs to establish health objectives, and to identify programs, policies, and ideas for actions that will help them to achieve these goals. The instrument also suggests indicators to track progress. (For example, if the objective is to reduce tobacco use, interventions to achieve this goal are suggested: "By [date] the community will be served by smoking education programs, including: a) health provider programs, b) nonsmokers' rights campaigns ... e) school curriculum programs." Suggested indicators for monitoring strategies to reduce tobacco use include whether interventions "a-e" listed above have been implemented, or whether surveys that assess people's knowledge of smoking risks are being conducted.) Although the indicators that *Model Standards* provides lack detail, the process the tool employs can be useful for identifying aspects of the local public health system that need to be assessed.

State and Regional Assessments

Like national self-assessment tools, state and regionally developed LHD performance assessment systems are designed to guide community health planning and improve the infrastructure of local public health systems; however, they also can be used to aid state-level planning and policy development, guide funding decisions, and facilitate program evaluations (48). In 1997, at least 35 states were developing or conducting LHD performance assessments using methods ranging from externally developed assessment tools (such as *APEX/PH*) to internally and independently developed systems, or blends of the two (48, 84, 85). Typically, these regional LHD performance assessment protocols emphasize measures of structure and process (including access to services) (48), although they will probably incorporate more outcomes measures in the future. For example, the New York City Department of Health has developed a set of quality indicators for internal use that covers health department activities and includes mostly process measures; it also uses a smaller set of indicators for external (public) use that incorporates more outcomes measures (M. Merlino, personal communication). In addition, Los Angeles County is undertaking a comprehensive effort to develop key performance indicators for all major activities, and these include both process and outcomes measures.

Performance measurement also is used in state-based accreditation programs to determine whether LHDs are maintaining a predefined standard of practice. LHD accreditation efforts are well under way in the United States and seem to be gaining momentum (64). Illinois and Michigan, in particular, have developed extensive accreditation evaluation forms and have collected a broad range of population health data, including outcomes. Illinois based its LHD performance indicators on *APEX/PH* and the CDC's ten public health practices. Michigan also borrowed from *APEX/PH* and developed its own set of seven "core capacities" that is similar to the ten practices and ten essential services (51, 64). Most of the performance indicators included in both of these accreditation programs focus on LHD structure.

Population Health Outcomes-Focused Assessments

A number of initiatives utilize population health outcomes to measure public health performance and indirectly assess the quality of the public health system at the regional, state, and national levels. For example, in 1991 the CDC and the National Center for Health Statistics developed a consensus set of 18 health status indicators, based on the health goals set forth in *Healthy People 2000*, to help communities assess their general health status (1). The measures are those commonly used in public health, for which data are readily available, such as the number of births to adolescents as a percentage of total live births or the race-/ethnicity-specific infant mortality rate. *Healthy People 2010* also includes a "core list of leading health indicators" (19, 61). These indicators, along with measures of access to care and health risks, form the basis of community health "report cards," which are expected to play a major role in local public health system planning in the future (23, 25). Many communities throughout the United States are developing community health report cards, often with LHD involvement. A recent national survey indicated that these report cards are at an early stage of development and use—only about half of the communities surveyed used pre-existing formats or the experience of others as a guide for development, and there were wide variations in quality and issues covered (25). Report cards, such as *Health Plan Employer Data and Information Set* (HEDIS), are used in a similar way to evaluate the quality of provider organizations in personal health care (36, 45, 58, 67).

Population health outcomes can be used to rate and compare the quality of local public health systems and LHDs over time if the appropriate evaluation methods are implemented. For example, an outcomes-focused appraisal method for LHDs and an outcomes-based method of assessing and comparing health status across communities have been developed for use in Florida (73, 74). The appraisal system collects data on 1. indicators of population health status (e.g., the infant mortality rate); 2. covariates, including community demographics (e.g., the age distribution), economic factors (e.g., the unemployment rate), and health resource characteristics (e.g., the number of primary care physicians); 3. indicators of LHD operating efficiency (e.g., costs per service and services per provider unit); and 4. "effectiveness" indicators, including community outcomes (e.g., incidence of measles) and measures of program impact (intermediate outcomes, such as immunization rates). Once collected, performance data can be adjusted to account for the effects of external variables and the results can be compared.

Although outcomes comparison systems assess both intermediate and ultimate outcomes, they often do not examine the process measures that describe in detail LHD activities. Thus, when a poor program result or health status outcome is found, it is hard to determine the source of the problem. In addition, when comparing outcomes, accurately estimating the LHD's influence versus that of the many external variables outside the LHD's control is very difficult, but important.

Function-Based Assessments

Other attempts to formulate measurement have concentrated on assessing the core functions of public health by focusing on key activities that indicate these functions have been achieved. *Healthy People 2000* made this shift toward assessment of core function explicit in Objective 8.14, which states that 90% of the U.S. population should be served by an LHD that is addressing effectively the three core functions of public health (82). Likewise, a similar emphasis continues in *Healthy People 2010* by ensuring that health agencies have the infrastructure to provide effectively the ten essential public health services (83). Several researchers have studied compliance with the objectives of *Healthy People 2000* by developing surveys to measure how well LHDs provide the core functions of public health (34, 52, 53, 65, 66, 70, 78, 80, 81). The results from these studies strongly suggest that the LHDs surveyed were not completely fulfilling the core public health functions. Moreover, they reveal the need for a measurement initiative that examines decision-making processes (planning) to evaluate whether the appropriate organizational activities are being performed.

Aided by these research findings, the CDC-PHPPO is developing the *Local Public Health System Performance Assessment Instrument*, which is organized around the ten essential public health services and incorporates several measures from research on core function assessment (59). The instrument is part of the National Public Health Performance Standards Program, which is led by the CDC and aims to improve local public health system quality and performance, increase accountability, and strengthen the science base of public health practice. The instrument evaluates the capacity and performance quality of local public health systems and LHDs by surveying LHD representatives to determine whether important structural elements and processes are in place. Since the instrument assesses whether the local public health system uses available resources to effectively meet public health needs, it also indirectly reflects the quality of public health planning. While this instrument certainly will play an important role in building the capacity of the public health system, it relies heavily on the respondents' judgment rather than objective data and does not directly assess whether an LHD's set of services is most appropriate or how well it is provided.

CHALLENGES OF PUBLIC HEALTH QUALITY ASSESSMENT

Although the public health system in the United States has begun to utilize quantitative methods to measure the quality of its practices, many challenges remain for the implementation of quality evaluation systems. Currently, LHDs lack measurement systems that fully address and evaluate the steps an LHD takes to achieve its health objectives. Moreover, many existing indicator sets were developed for other purposes and therefore lack detailed measures that reveal the reasons for good or poor performances. To effectively evaluate and improve the quality of an LHD and community organizations that influence local public health, comprehensive and detailed assessment systems are needed that evaluate how well they address local public health responsibilities—a goal of assessment since the APHA *Evaluation Schedule* in the 1940s (6).

Ideally, a comprehensive quality assessment system would evaluate the full range of LHD activities, which can be quite variable, as well as an LHD's success in achieving the public health mission for both the planning and the delivery of programs and services. An assessment of LHD planning should promote the ability of these organizations to identify, develop, and implement programs and services that appropriately address community health needs. Although objective, quantifiable indicators of LHD planning are currently limited, a research priority should be to investigate the methods and standards necessary to directly assess planning quality. On the other hand, measures of the delivery of public health programs and services can be created more easily. Detailed indicator sets for the delivery of programs and services can be developed locally and used to monitor and improve the quality of public health activities. Such monitoring should help ensure that LHDs are providing public health programs and services well.

Efforts are being made to improve public health performance measurement. For example, the IOM's *Assessment of Performance Measures for Public Health, Substance Abuse, and Mental Health* is designed to help states assess the performance of public health programs (62). This publication lists broadly applicable public health outcome measures and provides definitions, examples, and advice concerning structure and process performance measures. Nevertheless, barriers to creating, implementing, and benefiting from public health quality assessment systems remain.

First, an expanded public health evidence base is needed to provide more information about efficient and effective services. The U.S. Public Health Service is making a major effort to remedy this problem in its *Guide to Community Preventive Services*. The guide aims to fill this gap by summarizing current information about the effectiveness of strategies for community-based disease prevention and control (75, 76). It also provides recommendations on public health interventions and their delivery based on available evidence. Likewise, similar efforts to develop guidelines for community health interventions are under way in Canada (30). These resources will help guide public health practitioners in their decisions and should aid in the development of evidence-based public health quality indicators and assessment systems.

Public health quality assessment will be advanced by creating more concrete measures based on data. This will require better public health data collection systems, particularly at the local level. Primary data collection, though costly, provides invaluable information. For example, the Los Angeles County Health Survey records a wealth of public health data that are not available from other sources (46). Where possible, existing data sources should be used. The Behavioral Risk Factor Surveillance System is an example of a federal database that provides information relevant to population health (62); however, these data are often collected sufficiently only for larger LHD jurisdictions. Similarly, states often maintain databases that are updated periodically with information relevant to LHDs; however, these databases vary from state to state. Cooperative agreements with large provider groups such as managed care organizations could be another potential source of data, although such arrangements might be difficult to implement (31, 32, 42). Data tracking systems can be developed, or adapted, and applied locally to gather information for internal LHD activities. Access to these data should allow experienced local public health personnel and researchers with expertise in formulating systems for quantitative quality measurement to devise data-driven measures sensitive to local needs and that capitalize on these local information resources.

Finally, improvements in the public health system's capacity to fulfill essential public health services should continue. Quality assessments will result in few improvements without a strong infrastructure that can respond to and integrate the results of evaluations. This need is addressed in *Healthy People 2010*, which defines new national objectives to improve the public health system infrastructure and achieve performance standards for essential public health services (61).

Despite these barriers, ongoing refinements and redefinitions of public health indicators will allow for evaluation of an increasingly broad range of public health activities, particularly as standards become available for public health practices. National and locally developed systems for quality assessment now emerging can be combined to promote LHD quality. Indicator systems such as the CDC's *Local Public Health Performance Assessment Tool* can be used to compare quality across LHD jurisdictions nationally, while specific LHD activities can be assessed by local systems. Experience from diverse industries including personal health services validates the utility of measurement systems in improving quality. The pursuit of quality assessment within the public health system holds equal promise of improved outcomes for public health.

ACKNOWLEDGMENTS

This research was supported by the Los Angeles County Department of Health Services—Public Health Programs and Services, and the Centers for Disease Control and Prevention (U48/CCU915773). In addition, Dr. Asch is the recipient of a Career Development Award from the VA Health Services and Research Development Service. We graciously thank Rena Hasenfeld for her extremely valuable assistance with this manuscript, and the many staff at Public Health Programs and Services who provided their time, knowledge, and expertise.

Visit the Annual Reviews home page at www.annualreviews.org

LITERATURE CITED

1. Consensus set of health status indicators for the general assessment of community health status–United States. 1991. *MMWR* 40:449–51

2. From the Centers for Disease Control and Prevention. 1999. Ten great public health achievements—United States, 1900–1999. *JAMA* 281:1481

3. L.A. uses new statistical method to chart health. 2000. *The Nation's Health*, p. 7. Washington, DC

4. Aharony L, Strasser S. 1993. Patient satisfaction: What we know about and what we still need to explore. *Med. Care Rev.* 50:49–79

5. Am. Public Health Assoc. 1944. From health honor role to national reporting area. *Am. J. Public Health* 34:1099–102

6. Am. Public Health Assoc. 1947. *Evaluation Schedule for Use in the Study and Appraisal of Community Health Programs*. New York: APHA

7. Am. Public Health Assoc. 1991. *Healthy Communities 2000: Model Standards*. Washington, DC: APHA. 3rd ed.

8. Am. Public Health Assoc., Comm. Admin. Pract. 1926. Appraisal form for city health work. *Am. J. Public Health* 16:1–65

9. Am. Public Health Assoc., Comm. Admin. Pract. 1934. *Appraisal form for city health work*. New York: APHA

10. Baker EL, Melton RJ, Stange PV, Fields ML, Koplan JP, et al. 1994. Health reform and the health of the public. Forging community health partnerships. *JAMA* 272:1276–82

11. Beitsch LM, Grigg CM, Mason K, Brooks RG. 2000. Profiles in courage: evolution of Florida's quality improvement and performance measurement system. *J. Public Health Manag. Pract.* 6:31–41

12. Blumenthal D, Kilo CM. 1998. A report card on continuous quality improvement. *Milbank Q.* 76: 511, 625–48

13. Briss PA, Rodewald LE, Hinman AR, Shefer AM, Strikas RA, et al. *Guide to Community Preventive Services: Vaccine-Preventable Diseases*. http://www.thecommunityguide.org/home_f.html

14. Briss PA, Zaza S, Pappaioanou M, Fielding J, Wright-De Aguero L, et al. 2000. Developing an evidence-based Guide to Community Preventive Services–methods. The Task Force on Community Preventive Services. *Am. J. Prev. Med.* 18:35–43

15. Brook R, Chassin M, Fink A, Solomon DH, Kosecoff J, Park RE. 1986. A method for detailed assessment of the appropriateness of medical technologies. *Int. J. Technol. Assess. Health Care* 2:53–63

16. Brownson RC, Petitti DB. 1998. *Applied Epidemiology: Theory to Practice*. New York: Oxford Univ. Press

17. Brownson RC, Simoes EJ. 1999. Measuring the impact of prevention research on public health practice. *Am. J. Prev. Med.* 16:72–129

18. Chan YC, Ho SJ. 1997. Continuous quality improvement: a survey of American and Canadian healthcare executives. *Hosp. Health Serv. Admin.* 42:525–44

19. Comm. Leading Health Indicators for Healthy People 2010, Div. Health Promot. Dis. Prevent. Inst. Med. 1999. *Leading Health Indicators for Healthy People 2010: Second Interim Report*. Washington, DC: Natl. Acad. Press

20. Deming WE. 1986. *Out of the Crisis*. Cambridge, MA: MIT Press

21. Dever GEA. 1997. *Improving Outcomes in Public Health Practice: Strategy and Methods*. Gaithersburg, MD: Aspen

22. Donabedian A. 1980. Explorations in Quality Assessment and Monitoring. Vol. 1: The Definition of Quality and Approaches to its Assessment. Ann Arbor, MI: Health Admin. Press

23. Durch JS, Bailey LA, Stoto MA. 1997. *Improving Health in the Community: A Role for Performance Monitoring*. Washington, DC: Natl. Acad. Press

24. Dyal WW. 1995. Ten organizational practices of public health: a historical perspective. *Am. J. Prev. Med.* 11:6–8

25. Fielding JE, Sutherland CE, Halfon N. 1999. Community health report cards. Results of a national survey. *Am. J. Prev. Med.* 17:79–86

26. Green CG, Harrison M, Henderson K, Lenihan A. 1998. Total quality management in the delivery of public health services: a focus on North Carolina WIC programs. *J. Public Health Manag. Pract.* 4:72–81

27. Green LW, Kreuter MW. 1991. *Health Promotion Planning in Educational and Environmental Approach*. Mountain View, CA: Mayfield. 2nd ed.

28. Griffin SR, Welch P. 1995. Performance-based public health in Texas. *J. Public Health Manag. Pract.* 1:44–49

29. Groocock JM. 1986. *The Chain of Quality: Market Dominance through Product Superiority.* New York: Wiley
30. Gyorkos TW, Tannenbaum TN, Abrahamowicz M, Oxman AD, Scott EA, et al. 1994. An approach to the development of practice guidelines for community health interventions. *Can. J. Public Health* 85(Suppl. 1):S8–13
31. Halverson PK, Mays GP, Kaluzny AD. 2000. Working together? Organizational and market determinants of collaboration between public health and medical care providers. *Am. J. Public Health* 90:1913–16
32. Halverson PK, Mays GP, Kaluzny AD, Richards TB. 1997. Not-so-strange bedfellows: models of interaction between managed care plans and public health agencies. *Milbank Q.* 75:113–38
33. Halverson WL. 1945. A 25 year review of the work of the committee on administrative practice. *Am. J. Public Health* 35:1253–59
34. Handler AS, Turnock BJ, Hall W, Potsic S, Munson J, et al. 1995. A strategy for measuring local public health practice. *Am. J. Prev. Med.* 11:29–35
35. Hannan EL, Kilburn H Jr, Racz M, Shields E, Chassin MR. 1994. Improving the outcomes of coronary artery bypass surgery in New York State. *JAMA* 271:761–66
36. Harris JR, Caldwell B, Cahill K. 1998. Measuring the public's health in an era of accountability: lessons from HEDIS. *Am. J. Prev. Med.* 14:9–13
37. Iezzoni LI. 1997. *Risk Adjustment for Measuring Healthcare Outcomes.* Chicago, IL: Health Admin. Press. 2nd ed.
38. Inst. Med., Comm. Study Future Public Health, Div. Health Care Serv. 1988. *The Future of Public Health.* Washington, DC: Natl. Acad. Press
39. Juran JM. 1988. *Juran on Planning for Quality.* New York/London: Free Press/Collier Macmillan
40. Juran JM, Godfrey AB. 1999. *Juran's Quality Handbook.* New York: McGraw-Hill. 5th ed.
41. Kahn KL, Rogers WH, Rubenstein LV, Sherwood MJ, Reinisch EJ, et al. 1990. Measuring quality of care with explicit process criteria before and after implementation of the DRG-based prospective payment system. *JAMA* 264:1969–73
42. Koplan JP, Harris JR. 2000. Not-so-strange bedfellows: public health and managed care. *Am. J. Public Health* 90:1824–26
43. Lichiello P, Berkowitz B, Thompson J, Katz A, Perrin EB. 1998. *Enabling Performance Measurement Activities in the State and Communities.* Seattle, WA: Univ. Wash. School Public Health & Commun. Med.
44. Lohr KN. 1990. *Medicare: A Strategy for Quality Assurance.* Washington, DC: Natl. Acad. Press
45. Longo DR, Land G, Schramm W, Fraas J, Hoskins B, Howell V. 1997. Consumer reports in health care. Do they make a difference in patient care? *JAMA* 278:1579–84
46. Los Angeles Cty. Dep. Health Serv. 2000. *Los Angeles County Health Survey.* http://lapublichealth.org/ha/haprog.htm
47. Marciniak TA, Ellerbeck EF, Radford MJ, Kresowik TF, Gold JA, et al. 1998. Improving the quality of care for Medicare patients with acute myocardial infarction: results from the Cooperative Cardiovascular Project. *JAMA* 279:1351–57
48. Mays GP, Halverson PK, Miller CA. 1998. Assessing the performance of local public health systems: a survey of state health agency efforts. *J. Public Health Manag. Pract.* 4:63–78
49. McGlynn EA, Asch SM. 1998. Developing a clinical performance measure. *Am. J. Prev. Med.* 14:14–21
50. McGlynn EA, Brook RH. 1996. Ensuring quality of care. In *Changing the U.S. Health Care System: Key Issues in Health Services, Policy, and Management,* ed. RM Andersen, TH Rice, GF Kominski, pp. 142–79. San Francisco: Jossey-Bass
51. Mich. Dep. Community Health. 1988.

Michigan Local Health Department Accreditation Guidance Document. Michigan: Mich. Dep. Community Health

52. Miller CA, Moore KS, Richards TB, Monk JD. 1994. A proposed method for assessing the performance of local public health functions and practices. *Am. J. Public Health* 84:1743–49

53. Miller CA, Richards TB, Christenson GM, Koch GG. 1995. Creating and validating practical measures for assessing public health practices in local communities. *Am. J. Prev. Med.* 11:24–28

54. Mountin JW. 1952. The health department's dilemma. *Public Health Rep.* 67: 223–29

55. Murray CJ, Acharya AK. 1997. Understanding DALYs (disability-adjusted life years). *J. Health Econ.* 16:703–30

56. Natl. Assoc. Cty. City Health Off. 1991. *APEXPH: Assessment Protocol for Excellence in Public Health.* Washington, DC: NACCHO

57. Natl. Assoc. Cty. City Health Off. 2000. *MAPP—Mobilizing for Action through Planning and Partnerships.* http://www.naccho.org/

58. Natl. Comm. Qual. Assur. 1997. *HEDIS 3.0.* Washington, DC: Natl. Comm. Qual. Assur.

59. Natl. Public Health Perform. Standards Prog., Public Health Pract. Prog. Off., Cent. Dis. Control. 2000. *Local Public Health System Performance Assessment Instrument.* http://www.phppo.cdc.gov/dphs/nphpsp/

60. O'Connor GT, Plume SK, Olmstead EM, Morton JR, Maloney CT, et al. 1996. A regional intervention to improve the hospital mortality associated with coronary artery bypass graft surgery. *JAMA* 275:841–46

61. Off. Dis. Prev. Health Promot., US Dep. Health Hum. Serv. 1999. *Healthy People 2010.* http://www.health.gov/healthypeople/default.htm

62. Perrin EB, Koshel JJ. 1997. *Assessment of Performance Measures for Public Health, Substance Abuse, and Mental Health.* Washington, DC: Natl. Acad. Press

63. Public Health Funct. Proj. 1998. *Public Health Functions Project.* http://web.health.gov/phfunctions/activiti.htm

64. Richards TB. 1998. The accreditation of local health agencies. *J. Public Health Manag. Pract.* 4:1–53

65. Richards TB, Rogers JJ, Christenson GM, Miller CA, Taylor MS, Cooper AD. 1995. Evaluating local public health performance at a community level on a statewide basis. *J. Public Health Manag. Pract.* 1:70–83

66. Roher JE, Dominguez D, Weaver M, Atchinson CG, Merchant JA. 1997. Assessing public health performance in Iowa's counties. *J. Public Health Manag. Prac.* 3:10–15

67. Schauffler HH, Mordavsky JK. 2001. Consumer reports in health care: Do they make a difference? *Annu. Rev. Public Health* 22:69–89

68. Schuster MA, Asch SM, McGlynn EA, Kerr EA, Hardy AM, Gifford DS. 1997. Development of a quality of care measurement system for children and adolescents. Methodological considerations and comparisons with a system for adult women. *Arch. Pediatr. Adolesc. Med.* 151:1085–92

69. Schuster MA, McGlynn EA, Brook RH. 1998. How good is the quality of health care in the United States? *Milbank Q.* 76:509, 517–63

70. Scutchfield FD, Hiltabiddle SE, Rawding N, Violante T. 1997. Compliance with the recommendations of the Institute of Medicine report, The Future of Public Health: a survey of local health departments. *J. Public Health Policy* 18:155–66

71. Shortell SM, Bennett CL, Byck GR. 1998. Assessing the impact of continuous quality improvement on clinical practice: What it will take to accelerate progress. *Milbank Q.* 76:510, 593–624

72. Starfield B. 1996. Public health and primary care: a framework for proposed linkages. *Am. J. Public Health* 86:1365–69

73. Studnicki J. 1995. Evaluating the performance of public health agencies: information needs. *Am. J. Prev. Med.* 11:74–80

74. Studnicki J, Steverson B, Myers B, Hevner AR, Berndt DJ. 1997. A community health report card: comprehensive assessment for tracking community health (CATCH). *Best Pract. Benchmark. Healthc.* 2:196–207

75. Task Force Community Prev. Serv. *Guide to Community Preventive Services.* http://www.thecommunityguide.org

76. Truman BI, Smith-Akin CK, Hinman AR, Gebbie KM, Brownson R, et al. 2000. Developing the Guide to Community Preventive Services—overview and rationale. The Task Force on Community Preventive Services. *Am. J. Prev. Med.* 18:18–26

77. Turnock BJ, Handler AS. 1997. From measuring to improving public health practice. *Annu. Rev. Public Health* 18:261–82

78. Turnock BJ, Handler A, Dyal WW, Christenson G, Vaughn EH, et al. 1994. Implementing and assessing organizational practices in local health departments. *Public Health Rep.* 109:478–84

79. Turnock BJ, Handler A, Hall W, Lenihan DP, Vaughn E. 1995. Capacity-building influences on Illinois local health departments. *J. Public Health Manag. Pract.* 1:50–58

80. Turnock BJ, Handler AS, Miller CA. 1998. Core function-related local public health practice effectiveness. *J. Public Health Manag. Pract.* 4:26–32

81. Turnock BJ, Handler A, Hall W, Potsic S, Nalluri R, Vaughn EH. 1994. Local health department effectiveness in addressing the core functions of public health. *Public Health Rep.* 109:653–58

82. US Dep. Health Hum. Serv. 1991. *Healthy People 2000: National Health Promotion and Disease Prevention Objectives.* Washington, DC: Off. Assist. Sec. Health

83. US Dep. Health Hum. Serv. 2000. *Healthy People 2010*, Vols. 1, 2. Pittsburgh, PA: US GPO

84. US Dep. Health Hum. Serv., Off. Insp. Gen. 1997. *Results-Based Systems for Public Health Programs.* Vol. 1: *Lessons from State Initiatives.* Chicago, IL: Off. Insp. Gen.

85. US Dep. Health Hum. Serv., Off. Insp. Gen. 1997. *Results-Based Systems for Public Health Programs.* Vol. 2: *State Case Studies.* Chicago, IL: Off. Insp. Gen.

Annu. Rev. Public Health 2002. 23:23–44

CASCADE EFFECTS OF MEDICAL TECHNOLOGY

Richard A. Deyo

University of Washington, Center for Costs and Outcomes Research, 146 North Canal Street, Suite 300, Seattle, Washington 98103-8652; e-mail: Deyo@u.washington.edu

Key Words technology, adverse effects, quality-of-care, diagnostic tests

■ **Abstract** Cascade effect refers to a process that proceeds in stepwise fashion from an initiating event to a seemingly inevitable conclusion. With regard to medical technology, the term refers to a chain of events initiated by an unnecessary test, an unexpected result, or patient or physician anxiety, which results in ill-advised tests or treatments that may cause avoidable adverse effects and/or morbidity. Examples include discovery of endocrine incidentalomas on head and body scans; irrelevant abnormalities on spinal imaging; tampering with random fluctuations in clinical measures; and unwanted aggressive care at the end of life. Common triggers include failing to understand the likelihood of false-positive results; errors in data interpretation; overestimating benefits or underestimating risks; and low tolerance of ambiguity. Excess capacity and perverse financial incentives may contribute to cascade effects as well. Preventing cascade effects may require better education of physicians and patients; research on the natural history of mild diagnostic abnormalities; achieving optimal capacity in health care systems; and awareness that more is not the same as better.

CASCADE EFFECTS OF MEDICAL TECHNOLOGY

Health professionals and laypersons alike tend to equate new medical technology with better-quality health care, assuming that newer is better. Much of the scientific literature on diffusion of innovations focuses on the anticipated beneficial effects of new technology and methods to ensure its rapid adoption (53). However, many new medical technologies are introduced and disseminated with only modest evaluation of efficacy, optimal indications, or impact on practice. Unfortunately, their use in routine care sometimes proves futile or even harmful. The adverse effects and consequences of new technology are often unanticipated (53). One of these is the cascade effect.

The term cascade effect, in reference to medical technology, was apparently coined by Mold & Stein in a 1986 article in the *New England Journal of Medicine* (44). In biology, the term cascade refers to a process that proceeds in stepwise fashion from an initiating event to a seemingly inevitable conclusion. A molecular example is the blood clotting cascade, typically initiated by a cut in the skin. The

0163-7525/02/0510-0023$14.00

disruption of capillary blood vessels prompts aggregation of platelets in the blood to form an initial plug, which in turn triggers a cascade of protein interactions, ultimately resulting in the formation of a firm blood clot. Mold & Stein argued that health care may be subject to similar cascade effects, in which an initiating factor is followed by a series of events with increasing momentum, so that the further events progress, the more difficult they are to stop. These events often include unnecessary tests, procedures, and risks for patients. The initiating factor is often physician anxiety, which may result, for example, in a diagnostic test, an unexpected result, and a chain of subsequent events that are ultimately to the patient's disadvantage.

Mold & Stein offered the story of a patient admitted to the hospital for elective repair of an inguinal hernia. He had a history of coronary disease with very mild arterial narrowing on a previous cardiac catheterization. Anxious about his cardiac status, the surgeons requested a preoperative cardiology consultation. Perhaps uncertain about his own clinical judgment, the cardiologist suggested obtaining an exercise tolerance test. This was delayed for six hours while the patient waited outside the test room, during which time he became anxious, agitated, and angry, and had some mild chest discomfort. Because of the chest discomfort, the test was not done and the patient was transferred to a telemetry unit. There he became more anxious and agitated, was found to have some electrocardiogram changes, and received medications. He underwent another cardiac catheterization, which actually showed slight improvement since his previous test. At that point, the hernia repair could not be performed because of a full operating room schedule, and the primary physician was left to try to reassure the patient that he was in no danger. The procedure had to be delayed for two weeks. In this example, the chain of events seemed to be fueled by physician anxiety, and it snowballed with the addition of patient anxiety (44).

Physicians who are anxious about a patient's problem may be tempted to do nearly anything in order to reduce their own anxiety. The first step typically appears to be a benign action, such as ordering a diagnostic test; however, the discovery of an unexpected abnormality leads to progressively riskier and costlier interventions that seem simultaneously unnecessary and unavoidable. Ober likened this situation to the story of Br'er Rabbit and the tar baby. In this classic Uncle Remus tale, Br'er Fox creates a tar baby to trap Br'er Rabbit. Br'er Rabbit greets the tar baby and takes its failure to communicate as snobbery. He hits the tar baby to teach it a lesson and gets stuck. In an effort to make the tar baby let go, he hits it with the other hand, then kicks it. With each blow he becomes more ensnared, rather than closer to a solution (45). Similarly, as physicians try to explain each new ambiguous result, they become ensnared by their own actions.

Mold & Stein pointed out that in clinical care, cascade effects could be triggered inappropriately by incomplete data gathering; overinterpretation of an abnormal lab result; underestimation of the risks of a test or treatment; underestimation of the possibility of false-positive results; and intolerance of ambiguity by the physician (44). Examples of some of these problems follow.

EXAMPLES OF COMMON CASCADES RESULTING FROM DIAGNOSTIC TECHNOLOGY

The problem of cascade effects may be best understood by considering some common examples (Table 1). Some of these are now reasonably well documented, though others undoubtedly remain to be described.

Endocrine Incidentalomas

Benign tumors of the adrenal glands (adenomas) are quite common and have been reported in almost 9% of patients in autopsy. Adrenal carcinomas are extremely rare, in contrast, with an incidence of 0.0004% per year (45). Unfortunately, the radiographic appearance of carcinomas and benign adenomas is generally indistinguishable. Many incidental adrenal masses are discovered in patients for whom imaging such as computed tomography is performed for vague or nonspecific abdominal complaints (underestimating the possibility of false positive results) (12). Once an incidentaloma is discovered, both patient and physician may have such a level of anxiety that additional testing becomes inevitable. This was one of the first described problems of incidental imaging findings and has spawned a growing literature and recent reviews on the management of adrenal incidentalomas (1, 2, 11, 12). A recent recommendation for follow-up for these incidentalomas includes multiple blood tests, urinary hormone assays, and repeat imaging tests within six months of discovery and annually thereafter (2). Thus, incidental findings can precipitate lifelong cascades of clinical events.

Similarly, benign adenomas of the pituitary gland are common incidental findings. As with adrenal tumors, incidental findings are identified in up to 10% of patients having MRI of the head, and autopsy studies reveal a prevalence of 1.5% to 27% for small pituitary adenomas unidentified during life. In contrast, pituitary lesions that are symptomatic as a result of either hormone excess or mass effect are rare. Their prevalence is about 20 cases per 100,000 persons, and the incidence is approximately two per 100,000 per year. Fortunately, current recommendations for follow-up of these incidentalomas include only a simple screening blood

TABLE 1   Examples of oft-repeated cascades with a substantial risk of adverse outcomes

Initial test	Potential consequence
Head, body scans	Endocrine incidentalomas
Electronic fetal monitoring	Unnecessary Cesarean sections
Coronary angiography in low-risk patients	Unnecessary invasive coronary interventions
Spinal MRI in the absence of sciatica	Unnecessary spine surgery
Pulmonary artery catheters	Tampering with cardiac physiology
Persistent testing in persons near end of life	Unwanted aggressive interventions

test for abnormal hormone secretion among patients who are truly asymptomatic
(1, 11).

Electronic Fetal Monitoring

Electronic fetal monitoring for women in labor is another technology that may lead
to cascade effects. These devices monitor fetal heart rate, and certain patterns are
associated with a greater likelihood of fetal distress. However, the risks of the test
were not well considered before its adoption into routine care. Use of such monitors
requires the mother to be relatively inactive in bed and may increase anxiety levels.
The combination of inactivity and anxiety may slow labor and lead to interventions
to speed up labor (e.g., by artificial rupture of the membranes). When labor is
accelerated, the pain of contractions increases and pain medication or epidural
anesthesia may be requested by the patient. The loss of amniotic fluid may lead
to higher pressures inside the baby's skull, which could lead to more abnormal
readings on the fetal heart rate monitor. Use of epidural anesthesia may lower
maternal blood pressure, similarly leading to more abnormal readings. Perhaps
as a consequence of such events, Cesarean section rates are 40% higher when
electronic monitoring is used rather than simple auscultation of the fetal heart
rate. Unfortunately, randomized trials have shown that fetal monitoring does not
improve overall fetal outcomes except for a possible small reduction in neonatal
seizures (56, 60). Thus, much of the intervention and cost associated with its use
has little benefit and does pose potential risks.

Testing and Treatment for Coronary
Disease Among Low-Risk Patients

Twenty years ago, Graboys considered the likely consequences of screening for oc-
cult heart disease among prospective runners over age 35. Such screening by means
of exercise stress testing was a common recommendation at the time. Approximately 10% would be expected to have positive results. Because asymptomatic
persons have a low probability of disease and because exercise electrocardiogra-
phy has a substantial false-positive rate, only one fourth of patients with positive
tests would actually have multivessel coronary artery narrowing. Assuming low
rates of cardiac catheterization complications and operative mortality, as well as
low rates of perioperative heart attacks, Graboys estimated the following consequences of the routine screening strategy. If 20 million persons were screened,
2 million would have positive exercise studies. If all of these underwent coronary
catheterization, approximately 2000 would die. Of the half million persons who
would then undergo bypass surgery, 10,000 would die, and there would be 40,000
new heart attacks. A conservative estimate of the cost in 1979 was $13 billion (24).
This analysis describes a typical cascade effect that may result from an ill-advised
strategy of routine testing in otherwise healthy adults.

A more recent study examined the use of cardiac catheterization among Medicare patients following heart attacks. Experience was compared between New

York, with a low rate of testing, and Texas, where the rates of post–heart attack catheterization were 50% higher. Patients in the two states appeared to have approximately equal severity of coronary artery disease, but Texans with mild disease were much more likely to undergo angiography and to receive revascularization procedures. Paradoxically, after two years of follow-up, the Texas patients had lower exercise tolerance, more angina, and higher overall mortality (26).

A randomized trial compared the use of coronary angioplasty versus medical therapy for patients with angina. Most patients had relatively mild coronary artery disease. After two years, angioplasty had reduced symptoms in the group with severe angina, but the risk of a heart attack or death was almost twice that in the medical therapy group (52). There are now four randomized trials that are remarkably consistent in showing that routine cardiac catheterization and revascularization does not reduce the likelihood of repeat heart attacks or death compared with a more conservative approach following acute coronary syndromes (unstable angina and acute heart attacks) (38). In a study of patients with relatively small heart attacks, an aggressive strategy was actually associated with higher mortality both during hospitalization and at one-year follow-up (9). An editorialist noted that there is a strong relationship between the availability of angiography in a geographic area and the likelihood that the more aggressive diagnostic and treatment strategy would be chosen. Factors encouraging the use of aggressive therapy include the abundance of facilities for cardiac catheterization and revascularization in the United States, large numbers of physicians trained to perform the procedures, and generous insurance reimbursement (38).

Spinal MRI

Spinal MRI exemplifies the problem of discovering more and more abnormalities with most having no clinical relevance (15). There are now many studies of asymptomatic patients demonstrating that herniated discs, degenerative discs, and bulging discs are frequent incidental findings (8, 32, 33). Clinically, such findings lead to overdiagnosis, anxiety on the part of patients, and conviction about the presence of disease. Some authors have suggested that clinically irrelevant findings on MRI may lead to unnecessary back surgery with its occasional complications (8). An Institute of Medicine study concluded that lumbar spine surgery is overused and misused in the United States (46), and the wide use of imaging studies may be a driver of this excess use.

In a study of geographic variations in back surgery rates, Keller et al. found that where surgery rates were highest in the state of Maine, patients had the mildest preoperative disease and the worst postoperative outcomes. Conversely, where surgery rates were the lowest, patients had the most severe preoperative disease and the best postoperative outcomes (36). These findings support the notion that some back surgery is unnecessary and may lead to poor patient outcomes. We may speculate that some of the unnecessary surgery is driven by irrelevant imaging results.

Other Unnecessary Surgery

Back surgery may be just one example of a larger problem of unnecessary surgical intervention. International comparisons suggest that the United States has a much higher rate of many forms of surgery than other developed countries. In an early study of surgical second opinion programs, 17.6% of recommendations for surgery were not confirmed. Other studies have used explicit criteria to identify indications for surgery and have demonstrated high rates of unnecessary surgery for procedures such as coronary bypass operations, hysterectomy, pacemaker insertion, and tonsillectomy. Extrapolating from the second opinion study, a Congressional subcommittee concluded that perhaps 2.4 million unnecessary operations are performed annually in the United States, at a cost of $3.9 billion and 11,900 deaths. The number of operative complications would be substantially higher (39).

Adverse outcomes due to poor surgical technique have long been a target of quality review efforts, but Roos and colleagues proposed similar attention to adverse outcomes produced simply by high rates of interventions. In a review of coronary artery surgery rates, they focused on communities with unusually high surgery rates and high mortality rates. At least as many deaths could have been prevented by reducing surgical rates to the U.S. average as by improving the technical quality of surgery (54).

For many common operations, indications remain controversial, and diagnostic test results may often drive ill-advised surgery. Leape notes that uncertainty stemming from a lack of consensus about surgical indications may lead surgeons to recommend operations for patients who wish to have them but from which they will not benefit. From a patient perspective, the combination of risk and the potential for dramatic cure gives surgery an aura of excitement lacking in other forms of therapy (39).

Pulmonary Artery Catheterization

Pulmonary artery catheters are inserted into peripheral veins, floated through the right side of the heart, and into the pulmonary artery. In this position, the catheter allows measurement of pressures of the central veins and the pulmonary artery, mixed venous blood gasses, cardiac output, and pulmonary capillary wedge pressure (reflecting pressures on the left side of the heart). These devices are used in critically ill patients to assess the need for intravenous fluids or for treatments to improve cardiac output. Approximately 1.5 million catheters are sold in the United States annually, and these are most frequently used in cardiac surgery, cardiac catheterization laboratories, coronary care units, medical intensive care, and high risk surgery and trauma (4).

When the catheter was introduced in 1970, there were no prospective trials to evaluate its clinical impact. In 1996, an observational study suggested that the use of pulmonary artery catheters may not only be unhelpful in patient care, but may on balance do more harm than good (27). Negative consequences of the pulmonary catheter can result from serious complications (e.g., cardiac arrhythmias, thromboembolism, and sepsis), but also from operational problems, errors in data interpretation, or exaggerated or inappropriate treatment responses to catheter data. The observational studies have led to randomized trials that are currently under way for some indications, but definitive data are not yet available.

Although it remains uncertain whether pulmonary artery catheterization is, on average, truly harmful, the potential for it to cause harm is based partly on the possible cascade effects of measuring numerous physiologic parameters, then tampering to try to optimize these parameters. This device may also illustrate the problem of judging a technology's benefits from surrogate outcomes such as cardiac output. Such physiologic measures may be optimized by the technology, even though the end results (patient survival) are unaffected or adversely affected.

Unwanted Aggressive Care at the End of Life

This may be one of the most familiar cascade effects that has adverse consequences for patients. Many are familiar with the elderly parent who wants to die with dignity but gets drawn into a series of well-intentioned medical interventions, only to die in an intensive care unit with intravascular catheters, artificial ventilation, multiple medications to support circulation or treat infection, and perhaps even renal dialysis to support failing kidneys. It may only be in retrospect that the family and physicians recognize that the patient did not want interventions but was drawn into them by frequent diagnostic testing, monitoring of blood parameters, and efforts to identify reversible disease.

Physicians may fail to appreciate that because older patients have many competing risks for death, the absolute effect of a new diagnosis on life expectancy may be very small (64). Thus, the potential gain in survival even from perfect therapy may be small. Furthermore, risks of any therapy generally increase with age, so the high burden of competing risks and high rates of treatment complications may reduce the net benefit of many treatments.

COMMON TRIGGERS FOR THE CASCADE EFFECT

Because of the near inevitability of certain cascades once they are initiated, the best chance of preventing unnecessary adverse consequences may be to prevent the triggering event. A wide variety of likely triggers have been identified, relating to both psychological and cognitive factors, as well as cultural attitudes and perverse incentives.

Shotgun Testing

A nearly ubiquitous feature of modern medical practice is the panel of laboratory tests ordered as a cluster. For many biochemical tests of blood or urine, the normal range is simply defined as two standard deviations from the mean of a healthy population. By definition, therefore, about 5% of results on each test from normal

TABLE 2   Probability that a healthy person will have abnormal results in a biochemical profile[a]

Number of tests	Probability of at least one abnormal test, %[b]
1	5
6	26
12	46
20	64
100	99.4

[a]Adapted from references 10 and 66.
[b]Assuming that each test in the battery is independent of the others.

persons will be mislabeled as abnormal. Table 2 shows the probability that at least one test will be abnormal for various numbers of tests performed. For a panel of 12 tests (common in modern practice), there is a 46% chance that at least one test will be abnormal even in completely healthy persons (10, 66). This phenomenon has led to the cynical saying that "the only normal person is someone who hasn't had enough tests." Unfortunately, both patients and naive physicians may fail to appreciate the statistical basis for the normal ranges of chemical tests, underestimate the likelihood of false-positive results, and fail to recognize that many abnormalities will not represent disease (50).

Underestimating the Likelihood of False-Positive Results

This is closely related to the problem of shotgun testing. Many clinicians are unfamiliar with the concept of positive predictive value and fail to appreciate the high probability that positive results among patients with a low probability of disease are likely to be false positives. This occurs most frequently when a physician searches for an uncommon condition.

As a resident, one of my colleagues embarked on an evaluation for acute intermittent porphyria (AIP) in a patient with abdominal pain. Acute intermittent porphyria is a very rare disease, for which common screening tests have only moderate sensitivity and specificity. The prevalence of AIP is estimated to be one to two per 100,000 in Europe, where it is more common than in the United States (35). A widely used screening test for emergency situations is the Watson-Schwartz test for an abnormal urinary excretion product in these patients who have a metabolic abnormality. The screening test is estimated to be about 32% sensitive and 82% specific (13). Table 3 shows the consequences of screening a large number of patients with abdominal pain using the Watson-Schwartz test. The moderate specificity means that out of 9990 patients who do not have AIP, 8192 will have a negative test. Unfortunately, there are 1798 who will have a positive test but no disease. Of the ten patients who have AIP, four will have a positive test. Thus, the predictive value of a positive test, which is the probability of AIP given abdominal pain and a positive Watson-Schwartz test, is 0.002, or 2/10 of

TABLE 3   Positive predictive value of a screening test for Acute Intermittent Porphyria (AIP), a rare metabolic abnormality, among patients with abdominal pain. The Watson-Schwartz test has a sensitivity of 38% and specificity of 82%. This table assumes that the prevalence of AIP among patients with abdominal pain is 10/10,000, much higher than the general population prevalence of 2/100,000

| | **Actual diagnosis** | | |
	AIP	**Not AIP**	**Total**
Test Result			
Positive	4	1,798	1,802
Negative	6	8,192	8,198
Total	10	9,990	10,000

Probability of AIP given abdominal pain and a positive Watson-Schwartz test = 4/1802 = .002 (2 tenths of 1%).

1%. When my colleague discovered a positive Watson-Schwartz test, however, he was off and running with further tests. Certain that the patient had this rare condition, he embarked on a lengthy and expensive diagnostic evaluation that yielded some additional ambiguous results until more definitive testing proved repeatedly negative. Unfortunately, this was a predictable series of events.

Inappropriate Screening

Well-meaning clinicians are sometimes prompted to undertake screening tests in asymptomatic patients whom they perceive to have a high risk of a serious disease. A common example is the smoker for whom a physician has concerns about lung cancer. Although many physicians have been tempted to obtain periodic chest X-rays, even as frequently as every six months, randomized trials have failed to show any benefit for such aggressive lung cancer screening. In one trial, five-year survival was 23% for lung cancers diagnosed in the screening group and 0% for those diagnosed in the control group (6). However, the improvement was entirely attributable to lead time and length biases because overall mortality from lung cancer was actually higher in the screened group, which indicated that the aggressive screening and subsequent intervention was neutral or even harmful. Similar concerns may be raised regarding other common practices, such as the use of EKG to screen for heart disease or exercise testing to screen potential runners for heart disease (described above).

Errors in Data Interpretation

Misinterpretation of a diagnostic test may lead to unnecessary interventions and their potential complications. As one example, coronary angiograms (from cardiac catheterization) from 308 randomly selected patients were reviewed by a blinded panel of three experienced radiologists and compared with the original interpretations. Technical deficiencies were found in over half the cases. The panel readings showed less significant disease, less severe stenosis, and lower extent of disease than the original interpretations. The classification of subsequent coronary bypass surgery changed from necessary/appropriate to uncertain/inappropriate for 17% to 33% of cases when the panel readings were used. Using an expert set of appropriateness criteria, it appeared that some 17% of coronary bypass procedures and 10% of angioplasty procedures recommended on the basis of these films would have been inappropriate (40).

Overestimating Benefits or Underestimating Risks

An example of this problem comes from consideration of carotid endarterectomy. Clinical trials on the efficacy of carotid endarterectomy have shown that the benefit of surgery must be carefully weighed against complication rates in order to judge whether operative benefit outweighs the risk. In a study of academic medical centers, an expert panel rated the indications for performing endarterectomy, and the charts of 1160 randomly selected endarterectomy patients were abstracted. The expert panel defined acceptable operative risk for the patients under consideration to be less than 3% for death, stroke, or heart attack. Using that definition and the actual hospital mortality rates, only 33% of the 1160 procedures could be classified as appropriate. Even when a more liberal definition of 5% risk for bad outcomes was used, only 58% of the procedures would have been judged appropriate (42). Thus, clinicians recommending carotid endarterectomy in many of these institutions must have overestimated benefits and underestimated risks in making their decisions.

In assessing criteria for appropriateness, physicians' opinions vary. In a study of six different surgical procedures, 45 panelists rated the appropriateness of various indications both independently and after a two-day discussion. Performers of the surgical procedures had the lowest threshold for appropriateness, followed by physicians in related specialties, and trailed by primary care providers. Approximately one fifth of actual procedures were for indications rated less than appropriate by primary care physicians, but appropriate by performers of the procedures (34).

The problem of testing and treatment in elderly patients has previously been discussed. Because of competing risks from other comorbid conditions, the value of identifying and treating a new condition may be substantially less in older patients than in younger patients. Furthermore, the side effects of most procedures are higher in elderly patients than in younger patients, so the result is sometimes a dramatically different benefit-to-risk ratio than in younger adults (64).

In some cases, diagnostic tests themselves carry iatrogenic risks, regardless of subsequent treatments. Perforation of the colon during colonoscopy or fetal injury during amniocentesis are just two examples (66).

Defensive Medicine

Physicians sometimes request unnecessary tests or treatments in order to avoid medicolegal liability for a missed diagnosis or treatment opportunity. As the examples here suggest, however, poorly thought-out testing may sometimes lead to more patient harm than good, paradoxically increasing medicolegal risks.

Formal decision analysis produces the somewhat surprising result that defensive medicine necessarily reduces the overall quality of patient care. This finding contradicts arguments that defensive testing may further the interests of both doctor and patient. The reason is related to the problem of false-positive and false-negative tests. Decision analysis allows calculation of an optimal testing threshold: a pretest likelihood of disease that makes testing the preferred strategy over simply treating without a test or not treating at all. This threshold depends in part on the true- and false-positive rates of the test, and the consequences of those errors. If a physician widens the range of possibilities over which he or she prefers testing in order to reduce liability, then some patients who would be better left untreated will instead be tested and treated if the test is positive. Similarly, some patients who should be treated will instead be tested, and treatment withheld if the test is negative. The argument is theoretical, and actual practice may rarely conform to the optimal strategy in any event, for a number of reasons. Nonetheless, the analysis suggests that defensive medicine is not merely a problem of increased cost, but also one of reduced quality-of-care (14).

Patient Demand

Commenting on excessive use of coronary catheterization and revascularization, Lange & Hillis suggest that some patients and families may insist on aggressive management in the face of a heart attack. The term conservative management may convey an aura of obsolescence, inadequacy, or inferiority. In an era of managed care, it may even have the connotation of saving money at the expense of quality-of-care. Patients and families may paradoxically be more understanding and forgiving if an aggressive approach is pursued with a bad outcome, even if the management approach contributed to the adverse results (38).

In a study of women's understanding of the mammography screening debate (whether to begin screening at age 40 or age 50), 83% of women believed that mammography had proven benefit for women aged 40 to 49, and 38% believed that its benefit was proven even for women younger than 40 years. In response to an open-ended question about why mammography has been controversial, the most common response was that the debate was about saving money, rather than a question of benefit (65). Also, most women were unaware that screening can detect cancers that never progress (55). Such misunderstandings probably contribute to patient demand for screening and diagnostic tests. In some studies, inappropriate diagnostic tests were most likely to be done among patients with the strongest perception of need (18).

Patients seem willing to pay for diagnostic certainty even when it has no clinical benefit. For example, in one survey, patients were asked about willingness to pay for a test for peptic ulcer disease that would be risk-free, but for which establishing the diagnosis would not alter the course of symptoms. Patients were far more willing to pay for such information (84%) than were managed care executives (43%) or even physicians (61%) (31). Similarly, patients are very willing to pay for fetal ultrasound during normal pregnancy, even though no benefits have been scientifically established. In part, such demand is a result of technology being generally oversold by health care providers.

Low Tolerance of Ambiguity by Doctor or Patient

One of my own elderly patients once presented to an emergency room complaining of difficulty seeing. Because of his age, the emergency room physician considered a diagnosis of temporal arteritis, a rare disease but one that can result in permanent visual loss. There is no specific blood test for this condition, although one nonspecific test for inflammation of any sort (the erythrocyte sedimentation rate) usually is positive in this condition. The test was done and was normal; but even so, the clinician was so concerned about the possibility that the patient was started on high doses of prednisone, a cortisone-like drug. The patient then suffered the new onset of diabetes related to the use of prednisone, experienced severe metabolic complications, psychiatric complications, two hospitalizations, and a temporal artery biopsy. Although the temporal artery biopsy was negative for temporal arteritis, the pathologist qualified his interpretation by noting that because the patient had been on prednisone, it was possible that the true diagnosis was masked, and he could not rule out the condition. Thus, hospital physicians continued the medication. Finally, I stopped the prednisone in the outpatient clinic, which resulted in prompt resolution of the patient's diabetes and his psychiatric symptoms, and there were no further visual complaints. In retrospect, it appeared that the original visual complaint was related to presbyopia (difficulty focusing on close objects) and that the cascade of adverse events was precipitated by low tolerance of any ambiguity.

Desire to Legitimize Compensation Claims

Anecdotally, it appears that some patients are driven to obtain diagnostic tests by attorneys who want to help patients establish the legitimacy of disability compensation claims. In the case of MRI for the low back, as noted above, some abnormality is extremely likely, even in normal persons. In the context of returning patients to work, well-meaning clinicians feel obliged to respond to these abnormalities. Perhaps as a result, patients covered by the Workers' Compensation System receive both more invasive types of back surgery and substantially more repeat back surgery than patients covered by other forms of insurance (59). Repeat back surgery is frequently regarded as an indication of poor outcome from the initial operation.

FACTORS THAT FACILITATE TRIGGERING CASCADES

Though not direct triggers, several factors may facilitate the initiation of cascade effects. One such factor is excess capacity of technology and specialists who use it. For example, the United States has an abundance of facilities for coronary catheterization and revascularization and of physicians trained to perform the procedures, in comparison to Canada and Europe (38, 49, 61). Cardiologists who perform angiography are more likely to recommend cardiac catheterization than are cardiologists who do not perform the procedure, and these in turn are more likely to recommend it than general internists (34). This probably accounts in part for the wider use of catheterization and revascularization in the United States, despite evidence that the higher rates of utilization do not overall result in patient benefit (38, 49).

A related factor is physician ownership or proximity to diagnostic facilities. Physicians who work in hospitals with catheterization facilities are more likely to recommend cardiac catheterization than those without easy access to such a facility (19, 48). Convincing evidence suggests that ownership of imaging facilities leads to greater use of imaging (29, 30).

Other perverse financial incentives may result in additional forms of conflict of interest. Identifying more disease means more business. This may partly explain screening campaigns by hospitals or health care systems and the aggressive marketing of diagnostic tests. The concept of physician-induced demand is a longstanding principle of health services, which suggests that physicians can order return visits, perform diagnostic tests, or recommend procedures to some desired level, especially when indications are vague or controversial. The availability of insurance reimbursement also affects health care utilization, as demonstrated in the use of pulmonary artery catheters. In a study of 27 hospitals, private insurance coverage was associated with a 73% greater likelihood of receiving a pulmonary artery catheter (51).

Another factor facilitating cascade effects is the attitude that more information is always better. However, in considering a problem such as pancreatic cancer, which has a high mortality but also a high treatment-associated mortality, a decision analysis suggested that certain diagnostic test strategies could actually result in higher mortality rates than not performing a diagnostic test. This result was in part related to the limited positive predictive value of the tests. The authors advocated wider use of decision analysis to help understand when diagnostic testing was really likely to produce overall better outcomes for large groups of patients (57).

Overdependence on surrogate endpoints in clinical trials may also promote ill-advised clinical cascades. Surrogate endpoints are physiologic phenomena such as blood tests or imaging results, which are assumed to be markers of the ultimate outcomes of concern to the patient (such as death, loss of vision, or other severe disability). A now classic example of problems with surrogate markers was the use of the antiarrhythmic drugs encainide and flecainide to suppress premature heartbeats among patients who had suffered a heart attack. These drugs were highly effective

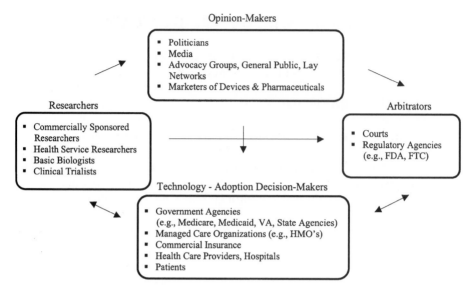

Figure 1   Influential parties in the adoption of new medical technology.

at suppressing extra beats, and such extra beats were known to be associated with higher mortality rates. Nonetheless, when the drugs were tested in a randomized trial, they resulted in approximately twice the mortality of placebo therapy, which indicated that the surrogate outcome of arrhythmia suppression was not an adequate marker of the outcome of interest (17). Several trials have suggested that shrinkage of malignant tumors is not an adequate marker for length of survival. In some trials, changes in CD4 cell counts have not accurately reflected changes in progression to AIDS or to death among HIV-positive patients (22). Such examples abound in medicine, and they indicate one of the ways in which test results can be overinterpreted.

Finally, a host of factors unrelated to scientific evidence may promote the use of new tests and treatments, often in the absence of strong evidence of their benefit. These factors include direct-to-consumer advertising, aggressive marketing to health care providers, media hype of new technology, political pressure from advocacy organizations, legal decisions, and even legislative action. Figure 1 is a diagram of the many factors that may influence the use of medical technology, sometimes in the face of limited evidence of benefit, or even evidence to the contrary.

CONSEQUENCES OF CASCADE PHENOMENA

Perhaps the most worrisome potential consequences of cascade phenomena are iatrogenic illness, morbidity, and mortality. For example, Starfield has summarized some of the evidence for adverse effects that occur because of iatrogenic injuries not associated with recognizable error. These include some 12,000 deaths a year from unnecessary surgery, 80,000 deaths per year from infections in hospitals, and 106,000 deaths per year from non–error-related adverse effects of medications (58). It is impossible to determine what fraction of these are related to cascade effects, but we may speculate that it is a substantial fraction. Data such as those from randomized trials of more aggressive or conservative management for acute coronary syndromes suggest that the aggressive strategy does not improve mortality, and its complications may increase mortality in some settings (38). Expert panels have judged that a substantial fraction of back surgery in the United States is unnecessary and exposes patients to unnecessary complications and even mortality (46). The abundance of technology and specialists in the United States, compared with most other developed countries, has not assured better public health: the United States ranks tenth or below for indicators such as low birth weight percentage, neonatal mortality, years of potential life lost, and life expectancy at age 1, age 15, and age 40 (58).

A less obvious consequence of cascade phenomena may be labeling effects for patients who have no disease. This problem has been demonstrated, for example, among children with benign heart murmurs, who experience greater restriction of physical activity than children without cardiac murmurs, despite having normal hearts (3). Anecdotal experience suggests that many patients who have spinal MRI tests attribute great importance to findings of bulging discs or other degenerative changes, despite evidence that these are as common in asymptomatic patients as among those with back pain. There is some evidence to suggest that simply attaching a diagnosis to patients who were previously unaware of having high blood pressure may result in greater work absenteeism, regardless of whether therapy is begun (28). Thus, labeling effects may be associated with unnecessary disability.

Unnecessary costs are an obvious consequence of cascade effects. The follow-up testing required for unexpected abnormalities, ongoing monitoring, and management of complications for unnecessary procedures are all examples of cost without benefit in the health care system.

One of the mechanisms by which treatment complications may occur is tampering with stable conditions. Tampering occurs when adjustments are made to correct deviations in a system that reflect random variation rather than systematic change. Intervening in response to random variations actually causes a system to become less stable and increases the likelihood of unnecessary treatment and adverse events (5, 21). Modern physicians are flooded with measurements as we monitor a host of physiologic phenomena. Multiple measures from the pulmonary artery catheter are examples in critically ill patients. Other examples include measuring prothrombin times and changing anticoagulant doses; measuring oxygen content of the blood and changing respirator settings; measuring fever and changing antibiotics; measuring blood pressure and changing antihypertensive therapy; measuring blood sugar and changing insulin doses; and a host of other common examples (5).

A false impression of high disease prevalence and great treatment efficacy are additional consequences of cascade effects and may in turn increase their likelihood. Newer diagnostic technology, which detects ever smaller or milder abnormalities, aggravates the problem. Many of the small abnormalities detected with new imaging techniques are clinically irrelevant. Even clinically important abnormalities are detected at much earlier stages than was previously possible. Because of this, their outcomes superficially appear to be improved, when in fact much of the improvement is due to lead time bias and length bias. Higher rates of detection create the impression of higher disease incidence and prevalence, which, along with seemingly improved treatment efficacy, lead to ever more frequent testing and treatment (6). This cycle affects both individual patients and large populations of patients for whom resources are unnecessarily wasted. Such interventions may also lead to unnecessary iatrogenic illness.

Good evidence for a misleading change in apparent disease outcome was described in a study of patients with lung cancer. In 1977, patients with every stage of lung cancer had better outcomes than in cohorts treated in 1953 or 1967 at the same institutions. On record review, it became apparent that this occurred because newer diagnostic techniques identified small metastases that formerly had been silent and unidentified, so that many patients who previously would have been classified in a good stage instead had migrated to a bad stage. The migration of patients out of the good stage meant that those remaining in the good stage had an even better outcome than would have previously occurred. Furthermore, because those who migrated into the bad stage represented the mildest and earliest form of disease in that stage, survival rates in the bad stage also improved. However, individual outcomes had not changed at all between time periods (20). When patients were classified according to symptoms in a fashion that would be unaffected by diagnostic tests, the two cohorts had similar survival rates. This observation was wryly named the "Will Rogers phenomenon," recalling a comment on the dustbowl era: "When the Okies left Oklahoma and moved to California, they raised the average intelligence level in both states" (20).

WHY IS THERE LITTLE AWARENESS OF CASCADE EFFECTS?

Many have commented that the United States is a culture that assumes more and newer technology must be superior to less and older technology. In a 1994 survey, 33% of Americans, 27% of Canadians, and 11% of Germans thought "modern medicine can cure any illness with access to advanced technology" (7). Furthermore, the use of technology promotes a wider patient expectation of its use. This was shown in a randomized trial in which low-risk patients with back pain were allocated to either early spine X-rays or a brief educational intervention. Baseline beliefs that "everyone with back pain should have an X-ray" were equivalent between the groups and remained stable in the education group, but increased in the group that received X-rays (16).

Patients often do not recognize unnecessary medical care, and patient requests for unnecessary care are common in day-to-day practice. Patients often equate laboratory testing and imaging with high-quality care and assume that the only reason for not performing such tests is financial. At least some fraction of unnecessary surgery appears to be driven by patient demand. Thus, physicians and patients may unwittingly conspire to perform unnecessary tests and therapeutic interventions. Both may perceive this to be in their best interests, and complications or costs are seen as the price of providing good medical care.

The marketing of new technology is designed to maximize demand, and this has reached its extreme expression in direct-to-consumer advertising of prescription pharmaceuticals. Many physicians report that patients request unnecessarily expensive drugs, or even unnecessary drugs, based on effective print or television advertisements.

Many of the factors that initiate cascades, including physician anxiety and fear of litigation, undoubtedly fuel cascades in progress. Many physicians are not well trained in the implications of false-positive and false-negative diagnostic tests and do not incorporate the concept of positive predictive value in making clinical decisions. Thus, from the physician perspective, many initiating events seem perfectly justified and appropriate. As a result, there is little recognition by either patients or physicians of undesirable cascade effects, except in extreme examples.

AVOIDING CASCADE EFFECTS

Because cascade effects are difficult to identify while they are in action, highly specific recommendations are likely to remain elusive. Nonetheless, certain efforts may help to reduce the likelihood of initiating events. In their seminal article, Mold & Stein suggested the importance of performing a complete patient history and physical examination in order to identify previously recognized conditions, diagnoses, abnormalities, or test results, and to avoid unnecessary duplication of tests. They also pointed out that a complete clinical evaluation is critical to providing an appropriate clinical suspicion (pretest probability) for any subsequent diagnostic testing (44). A related factor is continuity of care. A single primary care provider becomes more familiar with patients and can recognize true deviations from their usual health state in a more sensitive and specific fashion. A health care provider seeing a patient for the first time or only on a single occasion cannot have an equivalent understanding of the patient's usual health, usual responses to symptoms and illness, and style of using medical care.

Physicians should acquire a more complete understanding of the predictive value of diagnostic tests. While this is unlikely to result in highly quantitative calculations in routine clinical settings, it would help physicians to better understand the probability of false-positive tests, circumstances in which testing is unlikely to be beneficial, and the importance of understanding the performance characteristics

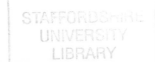

of the tests they order. In a similar vein, diagnostic testing should only be undertaken to answer very specific questions in order to avoid a shotgun approach. Highly selective approaches are more likely to avoid test complications, false-positive results, costs, and anxiety.

Involving patients more completely in clinical decisions may also be important. When patients are well informed of the benefits and risks of alternative approaches to clinical problems, they often have preferences that differ from their physicians'. For example, patients generally have higher thresholds for beginning antihypertensive therapy or anticoagulant therapy in many clinical circumstances (41, 43). In screening for prostate cancer, well-informed patients are more likely to decline tests than patients receiving routine care (23). Thus, when patients understand the stakes involved with clinical decisions, they may be helpful in averting unnecessary risks.

Researchers may help by better exposing the natural history of increasingly mild disorders detected by advanced technology. Better evaluation of the benefits and harms of treating such mild disease will also facilitate future screening and diagnostic decisions.

Clinicians should insist on proven benefits of therapy for the particular types of patients being considered for treatment. They should be increasingly aware of complication rates in their own hands and in their own facilities. The example of balancing risks and benefits of carotid endarterectomy provides an instructive example (42).

It is important to study the impact of system capacity with regard to tests and interventions. For example, lower capacity for invasive cardiac interventions in Canada reduces their use without apparent detriment to overall health. More deliberate deployment and dissemination of new technology and regionalizing some procedures may have similar benefits. Concentrating high-risk procedures in the hands of centers and physicians with a high clinical volume appears likely to improve outcomes and reduce complication rates (25, 47, 37).

Clinical guidelines, now promoted in many quarters, may help to reduce the unnecessary use of new technology and offer health benefits as well. Decision aids based on clinical guidelines, such as computer-based decision support systems, appear to help reduce the use of unnecessary tests (62).

While the use of second opinions in planning surgical procedures has become fairly common, it is less common to seek second opinions in test interpretation. Nonetheless, second opinions in the interpretation of complex diagnostic tests such as coronary angiograms and pathologic specimens may be warranted in certain situations where the consequences of those interpretations have major implications for both patient benefit and risk.

Physicians and patients alike must recognize that newer and more is not the same as better. Innovators, researchers, and early adopters of new technology should be alert to unanticipated adverse effects. For new medications, premarketing evaluation is quite rigorous, but this is less true of devices and procedures. For all of these new technologies, postmarketing surveillance has been relatively informal and poorly organized, and better surveillance (e.g., with disease or treatment registries) may help to identify problems at an earlier stage of technology dissemination. Registries for new devices, for example, may serve to identify unexpected complications or a high rate of complications sooner than unmonitored routine practice.

ACKNOWLEDGMENT

Thanks to Dr. Linda Pinsky and Dr. Scott Ramsey for critical reviews of an earlier draft. Pam Hillman provided expert clerical support. Supported in part by grant #042251 from the Robert Wood Johnson Foundation's Investigator Awards in Health Policy Research Program.

Visit the Annual Reviews home page at www.annualreviews.org

LITERATURE CITED

1. Aron DC, Howlett TA. 2000. Pituitary incidentalomas. *Endocrinol. Metab. Clin. North Am.* 29(1):205–21
2. Barzon L, Boscaro M. 2000. Diagnosis and management of adrenal incidentalomas. *J. Urol.* 163:398–407
3. Bergman AB, Stamm SJ. 1967. The morbidity of cardiac nondisease in school children. *N. Engl. J. Med.* 275:1008–13
4. Bernard GR, Sopko G, Cerra F, Demling R, Edmunds H, et al. 2000. Pulmonary artery catheterization and clinical outcomes: National Heart Lung and Blood Institute and Food and Drug Administration Workshop Report. *JAMA* 283:2568–72
5. Berwick DM. 1991. Controlling variation in health care: a consultation from Walter Shewhart. *Medical Care* 29:1212–25
6. Black WC, Welch HG. 1993. Advances in diagnostic imaging and overestimation of disease prevalence and the benefits of therapy. *N. Engl. J. Med.* 328:1237–43
7. Blendon RJ, Benson J, Donelan K, Leitman R, Taylor H, et al. Who has the best health care system? *Health Affairs* Winter 1995:221–30
8. Boden SD, Davis DO, Dina TS, Patronas NJ, Wiesel SW. 1990. Abnormal magnetic resonance scans of the lumbar spine in asymptomatic subjects. A prospective investigation. *J. Bone Joint Surg. [AM].* 72:403–8
9. Boden WE, O'Rourke RA, Crawford MH, Blaustein AS, Deedwania PK, et al. 1998. Outcomes in patients with acute non-Q wave myocardial infarction randomly assigned to an invasive as compared with a conservative management strategy. *N. Engl. J. Med.* 338:1785–92
10. Cebul RD, Beck JR. 1987. Biochemical profiles: application in ambulatory screening and preadmission testing of adults. *Ann. Intern. Med.* 106:403–13
11. Chidiac RM, Aron DC. 1997. Incidentalomas. A disease of modern technology. *Endocrinol. Metab. Clin. North Am.* 26:233–53
12. Copeland PM. 1983. The incidentally discovered adrenal mass. *Ann. Intern. Med.* 98:940–45
13. Deacon AC, Peters TJ. Identification of acute porphyria: evaluation of a commercial screening test for urinary porphobilinogen. *Ann. Clin. Biochem.* 35:726–32
14. Dekay ML, Asch DA. 1998. Is the defensive use of diagnostic tests good for patients, or bad? *Med. Decis. Making* 18:19–28

15. Deyo RA. 1994. Magnetic resonance imaging of the lumbar spine: terrific test or tar baby? *N. Engl. J. Med.* 331:115–16

16. Deyo RA, Diehl AK, Rosenthal M. 1987. Reducing roentgenography use. Can patient expectations be altered? *Arch. Intern. Med.* 147:141–45

17. Echt DS, Liebson PR, Mitchell LB, Peters RW, Obias-Manno D, et al. 1991. Mortality and morbidity in patients receiving encainide, flecainide, or placebo. The Cardiac Arrhythmia Suppression Trial. *N. Engl. J. Med.* 324:781–88

18. Espeland A, Baerheim A, Albrektsen G, Korsbrekke K, Larsen JL. 2001. Patients' views on importance and usefulness of plain radiography for low back pain. *Spine* 2626:1356–63

19. Every NR, Larson EB, Litwin PE, Maynard C, Fihn SD, et al. 1993. The association between on-site cardiac catheterization facilities and the use of coronary angiography after acute myocardial infarction. *N. Engl. J. Med.* 329:546–51

20. Feinstein AR, Sosin DM, Wells CK. 1985. The Will Rogers phenomenon. Stage migration and new diagnostic techniques as a source of misleading statistics for survival in cancer. *N. Engl. J. Med.* 312:1604–8

21. Fisher ES, Welch HG. 1999. Avoiding the unintended consequences of growth in medical care. How might more be worse? *JAMA* 281:446–53

22. Fleming TR, DeMets DL. 1996. Surrogate endpoints in clinical trials: Are we being mislead? *Ann. Intern. Med.* 125:605–13

23. Flood AB, Wennberg JE, Nease RF, Fowler FJ, Ding J, et al. 1996. The importance of patient preference in the decision to screen for prostate cancer. Prostate patient outcomes research team. *J. Gen. Intern. Med.* 11:342–49

24. Graboys TB. 1979. The economics of screening joggers. *N. Engl. J. Med.* 301:1067

25. Grumbach K, Anderson GM, Luft HS, Roos LL, Brook R. 1995. Regionalization of cardiac surgery in the United States and Canada. Geographic access, choice, and outcomes. *JAMA* 274:1282–88

26. Guadagnoli E, Haupman PJ, Ayanian JZ, Pashos CL, McNeil BJ, et al. 1995. Variation in the use of cardiac procedures after acute myocardial infarction. *N. Engl. J. Med.* 333:573–78

27. Hall JB. 2000. Use of the pulmonary artery catheter in critically ill patients: Was invention the mother of necessity? *JAMA* 283:2577–78

28. Haynes RB, Sackett DL, Taylor DW, Gibson ES, Johnson AL. 1978. Increased absenteeism from work after detection and labeling of hypertensive patients. *N. Engl. J. Med.* 299:741–44

29. Hillman BJ, Olson GT, Griffith PE, Sunshine JH, Joseph CA. 1992. Physicians' utilization and charges for outpatient diagnostic imaging in a Medicare population. *JAMA* 268:2050–54

30. Hillman BJ, Joseph CA, Mabry MR, Sunshine JH, Kennedy SD, et al. 1990. Frequency and costs of diagnostic imaging in office practice—comparison of self-referring and radiologist-referring physicians. *N. Engl. J. Med.* 323:1604–8

31. Hirth RA, Bloom BS, Chernew ME, Fendrick AM. 1999. Willingness to pay for diagnostic certainty: comparing patients, physicians, and managed care executives. *J. Gen. Intern. Med.* 14:193–95

32. Jarvik JG, Deyo RA. 2000. Imaging of lumbar intervertebral disc degeneration and aging, excluding disc herniations. *Radiol. Clin. North Am.* 38:1265–66

33. Jensen MC, Brant-Zawadzki MN, Obuchowski N, Modic MT, Malkasian D, et al. 1994. Magnetic resonance imaging of the lumbar spine in people without back pain. *N. Engl. J. Med.* 331:69–73

34. Kahan JP, Park RE, Leape LL, Bernstein SJ, Hilborne LH, et al. 1996. Variations by specialty in physician ratings of the appropriateness and necessity of indications for procedures. *Medical Care* 34:512–23

35. Kappas A, Sassa S, Galbraith RA, Nordmann Y. 1995. The porphyrias. In *The*

Metabolic and Molecular Basis of Inherited Disease, ed. CR Scriver, AL Beaudet, WS Sly. New York: McGraw-Hill, 2103 pp.

36. Keller RB, Atlas SJ, Soule DN, Singer DE, Deyo RA. 1999. Relationship between rates and outcomes of operative treatment for lumbar disc herniation and spinal stenosis. *J. Bone Joint Surg.* 81A:752–62

37. Kreder HJ, Deyo RA, Koepsell T, Swiontkowski MF, Kreyter W. 1997. Relationship between the volume of total hip replacements performed by providers and the rates of postoperative complications in the state of Washington. *J. Bone Joint Surg. Am.* 79:485–94

38. Lange RA, Hillis LD. 1998. Use and overuse of angiography and revascularization for acute coronary syndromes. *N. Engl. J. Med.* 338:1838–39

39. Leape LL. 1992. Unnecessary surgery. *Ann. Rev. Public Health* 13:363–83

40. Leape LL, Park RE, Bashore TM, Harrison JK, Davidson CJ, Brook RH. 2000. Effect of variability in the interpretation of coronary angiograms on the appropriateness of use of coronary revascularization procedures. *Am. Heart J.* 139:106–13

41. Man-Son-Hing M, Laupacis A, O'Connor AM, Biggs J, Drake E, et al. 1999. A patient decision aid regarding antithrombotic therapy for stroke prevention in atrial fibrillation: a randomized controlled trial. *JAMA* 282:737–43

42. Matchar DB, Oddone EZ, McCrory DC, Goldstein LB, Landsman PB, et al. 1997. Influence of projected complication rates on estimated appropriate use rates for carotid endarterectomy. Appropriateness project investigators. Acad. Med. Ctr. Consortium. *Health Serv. Res.* 32:325–42

43. McAlister FA, O'Connor AM, Wells G, Grover SA, Laupacis A. 2000. When should hypertension be treated? The different perspectives of Canadian Family physicians and patients. *Can. Med. Assoc. J.* 163:403–8

44. Mold JW, Stein HF. 1986. The cascade

effect in the clinical care of patients. *N. Engl. J. Med.* 314:512–14

45. Ober KT. 1987. Uncle Remus and the cascade effect in clinical medicine: Br'er Rabbit kicks the tar baby. *Am. J. Med.* 82:1009–13

46. Osterweis M, Kleinman A, Mechanic D, eds. 1951. *Pain and Disability: Clinical, Behavioral and Public Policy Perspectives.* Washington, DC: Natl. Academy, 204 pp.

47. Phillips KA, Luft HS, Ritchie JL. 1995. The association of hospital volumes of percutaneous transluminal coronary angioplasty with adverse outcomes, length of stay and charges in California. *Medical Care* 33:502–14

48. Pilote L, Miller DP, Califf RM, Rao JS, Weaver WD, et al. 1996. Determinants of the use of coronary angiography and revascularization after thrombolysis for acute myocardial infarction. *N. Engl. J. Med.* 335:1198–205

49. Pilote L, Granger C, Armstrong PW, Mark DB, Haltky MA. 1995. Differences in the treatment of myocardial infarction between the United States and Canada: a survey of physicians in the GUSTO trial. *Medical Care* 33:598–610

50. Rang M. 1972. The Ulysses syndrome. *Can. Med. Assoc. J.* 106:122–23

51. Rapoport J, Teres D, Steingrub J, Higgins T, McGee W, Lemeshow S. 2000. Patient characteristics and ICU organizational factors that influence frequency of pulmonary artery catheterization. *JAMA* 283:2559–66

52. RITA-2 Trial Participants. 1997. Coronary angioplasty versus medical therapy for angina: the second Randomized Intervention Treatment of Angina (RITA-2) Trial. *Lancet* 350:461–68

53. Rogers EM. 1995. *Diffusion of Innovations.* New York: Free Press. 4th ed.

54. Roos NP, Black CD, Roos LL, Tate RB, Carriere KC. 1995. A population-based approach to monitoring adverse outcomes of medical care. *Medical Care* 33:127–38

55. Schwartz LM, Woloshin S, Sox HC,

Fischoll B, Welch HG. 2000. U.S. women's attitudes to false positive mammography results and the detection of ductal carcinoma in-situ: cross-sectional survey. *Br. Med. J.* 320:1635–40

56. Shy KK, Larson EB, Luthy DA. 1987. Evaluating a new technology: the effectiveness of electronic fetal monitoring. *Annu. Rev. Public Health* 8:165–90

57. Sisson JC, Schoomaker EB, Ross JC. 1976. Clinical decision analysis: the hazard of using additional data. *JAMA* 236:1259–63

58. Starfield BA. 2000. Is U.S. healthcare really the best in the world? *JAMA* 284:483–85

59. Taylor VM, Deyo RA, Ciol M, Kreuter M. 1996. Surgical treatment of patients with back problems covered by workers compensation versus those with other sources of payment. *Spine* 21:2255–59

60. Thacker SB, Stroup D, Chang M. 2001. Continuous electronic heart rate monitoring for fetal assessment during labor (Cochrane Review). In *The Cochrane Library*, Issue 2

61. Tu JV, Pashos CL, Naylor D, Chen E, Normand S-L. 1997. Use of cardiac procedures and outcomes in elderly patients with myocardial infarction in the United States and Canada. *N. Engl. J. Med.* 536:1500–5

62. Van Wijk MAM, Van der Lei J, Mosseveld M, Bohnen AM, Van Bremmel JH. 2001. Assessment of decision support for blood test ordering in primary care: a randomized trial. *Ann. Intern. Med.* 134:274–81

63. Verrilli D, Welch HG. 1996. The impact of diagnostic testing on therapeutic interventions. *JAMA* 275:1189–91

64. Welch HG, Albertsen PC, Nease RF, Bubolz TA, Wasson JH. 1996. Estimating treatment benefits for the elderly: the effect of competing risks. *Ann. Intern. Med.* 124:577–84

65. Woloshin S, Schwartz LM, Byram SJ, Sox HC, Fischoff B, Welch HG. 2000. Women's understanding of the mammography screening debate. *Arch. Intern. Med.* 160:1434–40

66. Woolf SH, Kamerow DB. 1990. Testing for uncommon conditions: the heroic search for positive test results. *Arch. Intern. Med.* 150:2451–58

Annu. Rev. Public Health 2002. 23:45–71

THE EFFECTIVENESS OF STATE-LEVEL TOBACCO CONTROL INTERVENTIONS: A Review of Program Implementation and Behavioral Outcomes

Michael Siegel

Social and Behavioral Sciences Department, Boston University School of Public Health, Boston, Massachusetts 02118; e-mail: mbsiegel@bu.edu

Key Words   adolescent behavior, mass media, program evaluation, smoking, tobacco smoke pollution

■ **Abstract**   In 2001, nearly one billion dollars will be spent on statewide tobacco control programs, including those in California, Massachusetts, Arizona, and Oregon, funded by cigarette tax revenues, and the program in Florida, funded by the state's settlement with the tobacco industry. With such large expenditures, it is imperative to find out whether these programs are working. This paper reviews the effectiveness of the statewide tobacco control programs in California, Massachusetts, Arizona, Oregon, and Florida. It focuses on two aspects of process evaluation—the funding and implementation of the programs and the tobacco industry's response, and four elements of outcome evaluation—the programs' effects on cigarette consumption, adult and youth smoking prevalence, and protection of the public from secondhand smoke. The paper formulates general lessons learned from these existing programs and generates recommendations to improve and inform the development and implementation of these and future programs.

INTRODUCTION

In 1989, California became the first state in the nation to establish a comprehensive, statewide tobacco control program funded by dedicated revenues from an increase in the state cigarette excise tax (10). This approach was soon followed by Massachusetts (in 1993), Arizona (in 1995), and Oregon (in 1997) (19, 22, 39, 42, 51). In 1998, Florida established a comprehensive statewide tobacco control program using dedicated funds from the state's settlement of its Medicaid fraud lawsuit against the tobacco industry (34). More recently, several states have established comprehensive statewide tobacco control programs using funds allocated from their share of the national $206 billion tobacco settlement or their own settlements with the tobacco industry (28). Tobacco control activity at the state level has increased strikingly from a decade ago, when Novotny et al. (57b), in an *Annual Review of Public Health* summary of the state of tobacco control, reported the

0163-7525/02/0510-0045$14.00

existence of only one comprehensive statewide program (California) but correctly predicted that California's success would encourage other states to fund similar programs.

Because public health practitioners in several states are now using cigarette tax revenues and tobacco settlement funds to establish tobacco control as part of the public health infrastructure, more money is being spent on state tobacco control programs than ever before in the nation's history. In fiscal year 2001, nearly $1 billion will be spent on statewide tobacco prevention and cessation programs (30). It is therefore imperative to find out whether these programs are working, how well they are working, and what changes can be made to improve their effectiveness.

This paper reviews the effectiveness of the statewide comprehensive tobacco control programs in California, Massachusetts, Arizona, Oregon, and Florida. It considers both process evaluation (assessment of the faithfulness of program implementation) and outcome evaluation (assessment of desired knowledge, attitudinal, behavior, or disease outcomes of a program). This paper focuses on two elements of process evaluation—the funding and implementation of the programs and the tobacco industry's response—and four elements of outcome evaluation— the programs' effects on cigarette consumption, adult smoking prevalence, youth smoking prevalence, and protection of the public from secondhand smoke. The objective of the review is not only to determine whether these programs are working, but to generate recommendations to improve these programs and inform the development and implementation of similar programs in the future.

The process evaluation is critical because unless one considers whether the programs are being implemented faithfully, it is impossible to accurately assess whether any failure to observe a program's effect is due to flawed design or simply to inadequate implementation. This paper focuses on the two aspects of program implementation that are most likely to have a bearing on program effectiveness: the amount of funds being expended for the programs and the scope and nature of the specific activities funded.

The outcome evaluation is critical as well, because changes in smoking behavior (and ultimately disease incidence and mortality) are the stated goals of each state program. In most cases, the programs have not been in place long enough to assess disease outcomes, and smoking behavior is used as a preliminary measure of effectiveness. In one case (California), the program has been in operation long enough to evaluate effects on disease outcome (heart disease mortality) as well as smoking behavior. Several programs are so new that even analyses to determine behavioral outcomes are insufficient; in these cases, data are presented only to give a preliminary indication of program effectiveness. In addition to reviewing the effects on smoking behavior of the overall statewide tobacco control programs, this paper attempts, where possible, to review the specific effects of the anti-smoking media campaigns, because these are a central element of the tobacco control programs in each of the five states.

Outstanding general reviews of the effectiveness of comprehensive state tobacco control programs (50, 83, 84) and of state anti-smoking media campaigns

(61, 62) have been published previously. It is hoped that this review will expand upon the existing literature by (*a*) including more recent data that allow a fuller evaluation of the effects of more recently established programs; (*b*) focusing more on program funding and implementation to generate lessons that can be applied both to existing and future programs; and (*c*) emphasizing distal outcomes (including disease outcomes) and the specific weight of various program elements (including media campaigns and clean indoor air policies) to better inform the improvement of existing programs and the development of new ones.

PROCESS EVALUATION

California

PROGRAM FUNDING AND IMPLEMENTATION   Proposition 99, passed by California voters in 1988, increased the state cigarette excise tax by 25 cents per pack and allocated 20% of the revenues for tobacco prevention and cessation programs (10). During the first seven years of the program, however, the state legislature appropriated funds at a level of only 68% of the amount required by the voter initiative (64). Proposition 99 expenditures for tobacco education and prevention declined from $86 million during the first year of the program to $42 million during the seventh year, a drop of more than 50% (64, 65). Funds diverted from tobacco control programs between 1989 and 1996 exceeded $273 million (12).

The diversion of funds from tobacco prevention and cessation, largely to medical care services (12, 16, 58, 72), was supported by Governor Pete Wilson, legislative leaders, and even by the California Medical Association (12, 58). It was only after an aggressive paid advertising and media advocacy campaign in 1996, spearheaded by the American Nonsmokers' Rights Foundation and the American Heart Association and challenging Governor Wilson and the California Medical Association's support of Proposition 99 funding diversions, that tobacco prevention and cessation programs were fully funded (12, 71). Despite optimism that the election of Governor Gray Davis in November 1998 would reverse efforts to weaken the tobacco control program, the Davis administration has opposed substantial increases in funding for tobacco prevention programs (33b).

In addition to being undermined by the general diversion of funds from tobacco control programs, the implementation of Proposition 99 was also hampered by attempts by Governor Pete Wilson and his administration to suspend or weaken the anti-smoking media campaign specifically (11, 12, 16, 35, 37). Governor Wilson suspended the media campaign completely during the 1992 fiscal year, prompting a lawsuit by the American Lung Association and a court order reinstating the campaign (12, 16, 35, 37). During the period from 1995 to 1997, the Wilson administration was able to mute the media campaign without suspending it outright: little new advertising was produced and existing advertisements aggressively challenging the legitimacy of tobacco industry marketing tactics were pulled or had their air time decreased (11, 36, 37, 72). The media campaign budget itself was cut nearly in half, falling from $12.2 million in the 1994-1995 fiscal year to $6.6 million in the 1995–1996 fiscal year (64, 65). Although Governor Gray Davis reversed the Wilson-era policy of not allowing advertisements that challenged tobacco industry practices, he maintained a cumbersome approval process for advertisements that continued to undermine the effectiveness of the media campaign (33b).

TOBACCO INDUSTRY RESPONSE   In response to Proposition 99, the tobacco industry greatly increased its political activity in California (16, 33b), raising its total political expenditures from $790,050 in 1985–1986 (the election before Proposition 99 passed) to $7,615,091 in 1991–1992 (16). There is strong evidence that the tobacco industry played an influential role in promoting the diversion of Proposition 99 funding (12, 16, 65). A 1990 Tobacco Institute memorandum outlines a plan to undermine tobacco control in California by lobbying the legislature and governor to mute the program—in particular, to weaken the media campaign (81).

In response to a proliferation of local clean indoor air ordinances in California associated with the implementation of Proposition 99, tobacco industry spending at the local level also increased drastically (16), to over $2.4 million in 1991–1992, mostly directed to repeal clean indoor air ordinances (16). The industry also attempted to overturn existing local ordinances and prevent the adoption of new ones by promoting preemption legislation (3, 17, 53, 74). In 1994, the tobacco industry spent $18.9 million promoting Proposition 188, a state ballot initiative that would have repealed all local clean indoor air ordinances in California (3, 53).

After the passage of Proposition 99, the tobacco industry's promotional expenditures in California increased, as did the aggressiveness of its targeting of youth, women, and minorities in California (75). Despite the highest expenditures for tobacco control programs in the nation's history, the diversion of Proposition 99 funding and intense tobacco industry marketing allowed the tobacco industry to maintain a 10:1 ratio of its marketing expenditures to state tobacco control program expenditures during the period 1993 to 1996 (64, 65).

Massachusetts

PROGRAM FUNDING AND IMPLEMENTATION   In 1992, Massachusetts voters approved Question 1, a ballot initiative that raised the state cigarette tax by 25 cents per pack and placed the revenues into a Health Protection Fund, one purpose of which was to fund tobacco use prevention and cessation programs (42, 51). Since fiscal year 1994 (the first year of program implementation), the legislature has allocated only 30% of Question 1 funds for tobacco control programs (14). The budget for the Massachusetts tobacco control program declined from approximately $43 million in fiscal year 1994 to $37 million in 1999, a reduction of about 15% (1, 2). Between fiscal years 1995 and 2001 (projected budget), Question 1 spending for tobacco control programs decreased by 27% in inflation-adjusted dollars (14).

As in California, the diversion of Question 1 funds from tobacco control programs to non-initiative–specified programs has been spearheaded primarily by the governor (14, 15). In 1995, Governor William Weld proposed diverting $40 million in Question 1 funds to finance an income tax cut (15). This diversion would have completely eliminated the tobacco control program (15). Because of strong public opposition, Weld modified his proposal to eliminate just the media campaign (63), although the legislature did not accept his proposal. Weld's successor, Paul Cellucci, also cut funding for the tobacco control program. In fiscal year 2001, the Massachusetts legislature allocated $23.7 million from Master Settlement Agreement funds to supplement the statewide tobacco control program and to correct for prior budget cuts (14). However, Governor Cellucci vetoed $10.7 million of this funding (14).

TOBACCO INDUSTRY RESPONSE   Tobacco company lobbying expenditures in Massachusetts rose from approximately $900,000 in 1993–1994 to more than $1.3 million in 1994–1995, an increase of 48% (14). There is strong evidence that the diversion of Question 1 funds to non-tobacco-related purposes was part of a strategy by the tobacco industry to undermine the effects of Question 1 (14). A December 1992 Tobacco Institute memorandum outlines a strategy to analyze "the state budget to identify other sources to which the initiative money may be targeted—to keep disbursement of initiative funds to local health boards to a minimum" (5). The memorandum also outlined a plan to block local clean indoor air policies by promoting a statewide preemption bill and by setting up community front groups to oppose new ordinances and to challenge existing ones (5). In fact, preemption legislation has been introduced, unsuccessfully, in the legislature, and the tobacco industry has worked with the Massachusetts Restaurant Association to promote state preemption legislation and oppose local smoke-free restaurant ordinances (70).

Arizona

PROGRAM FUNDING AND IMPLEMENTATION   In 1994, Arizona voters passed Proposition 200, which increased the cigarette excise tax by 40 cents per pack and allocated 23% of the resulting revenues to tobacco prevention and education programs (19). Despite several attempts to divert money from tobacco-related programs, a strong and united response from health groups was successful in preserving their full funding (18, 19).

Nevertheless, there were still two severe problems in the implementation of Proposition 200. First, for the first two years of the program, the Arizona Department of Health Services limited its target audience to youth and pregnant women (18, 19). Thus, promoting smoking cessation among adults was not included in the scope of the program (18, 19). Second, the state health department severely limited the scope of the media campaign (18, 19). Advertisements that challenged the legitimacy of the tobacco industry's marketing and public relations tactics, that increased awareness of the risk of secondhand smoke, or that dealt with nicotine addiction were not to be a major component of the media campaign (18, 19), which instead focused almost exclusively on portraying smoking as a disgusting and dangerous habit (18, 19). In 1998, the health department expanded the program's scope by developing and encouraging programs to promote smoking cessation among adults and the adoption of policies to protect citizens from exposure to secondhand smoke (19). However, it is not clear whether the media campaign will expand to target tobacco industry marketing and public relations tactics.

TOBACCO INDUSTRY RESPONSE   In response to the passage of Proposition 200, political activity by the tobacco industry increased in Arizona (18, 19). The number of paid tobacco industry lobbyists at the state Capitol rose from 4 to 18 (18). It has been suggested that this increased tobacco industry presence, combined with strong tobacco industry connections with Governor Fife Symington, may have influenced the decision of the executive branch to limit the scope and aggressiveness of the tobacco control program (18). In addition, the tobacco industry attempted (unsuccessfully) to move preemption legislation through the Arizona legislature in 1995, 1996, and 1997 (18, 19), and through the National Smokers Alliance and the Mesa Freedom Committee, attempted unsuccessfully to defeat a smoke-free workplace ballot initiative in Mesa in 1996 (18).

Oregon

PROGRAM FUNDING AND IMPLEMENTATION   Oregon's Measure 44, passed by voters in 1996, increased the state cigarette excise tax by 30 cents per pack and allocated 10% of the revenues for tobacco use reduction programs (22, 39). Unlike in California and Massachusetts, public health advocates in Oregon successfully defended against diversion of Measure 44 funds from tobacco control programs to other purposes and unlike in Arizona, a truly comprehensive tobacco control program was implemented, without limitation of its scope (38, 39).

TOBACCO INDUSTRY RESPONSE   After passage of Measure 44, the tobacco industry lobbied the legislature to try to prevent the allocation of funds to a comprehensive tobacco control program and to prevent the media campaign from including advertisements that attacked the industry (38, 39). Through the National Smokers Alliance, the tobacco industry attempted to defeat a 1997 ordinance in Corvallis that eliminated smoking in all workplaces (38). There is some evidence that the tobacco industry had a role in the legislature's consideration of state preemption legislation in 1997 (38). During the 2001 legislative session, the Oregon Restaurant Association promoted statewide preemption legislation (9, 9a); ultimately, the legislature enacted a compromise measure that preempted future local efforts to ban smoking in bars (9a). Whether the tobacco companies played any role in these efforts has not been determined.

Florida

PROGRAM FUNDING AND IMPLEMENTATION   In August 1997, Florida reached a settlement with the tobacco industry in its state Medicaid fraud lawsuit in which the industry agreed to pay $11.3 billion; a portion of these funds could be used to run a youth smoking prevention campaign for two years that could include a media campaign, although advertisements attacking the tobacco industry would not be permitted (34). In September 1998, the agreement was modified to eliminate the two-year time limit as well as the limitation on the scope of the media campaign (34). In the 1998 fiscal year, an aggressive smoking prevention campaign was initiated, highlighted by the "truth" campaign, a media campaign urging Florida youths to choose the "truth" as a brand rather than the tobacco industry's product, lies (43, 85).

The Florida legislature cut the program's funding by 36%, from $70.5 million in the 1998 fiscal year to $45.2 million in the 1999 fiscal year (34). Part of this reduction was supported by Governor Jeb Bush, who proposed an $8.5 million cut in the program budget, but the bulk of the funding cut was promoted by the legislature (34). One House subcommittee had actually recommended eliminating the tobacco control program entirely (34). After two additional funding vetoes by Governor Bush, the final 1999–2000 tobacco control program budget was only $38.5 million, a reduction of 45.1% from the previous year (34). The media campaign itself was cut from $26 million to $12 million, a reduction of 53.8% (34). Public health groups in Florida, unlike groups in Arizona and Oregon, and more recently in California, were unwilling to speak out publicly and hold specific legislators accountable for slashing the funding to the program (34).

TOBACCO INDUSTRY RESPONSE   Tobacco companies continue to make substantial contributions to legislators and the political parties in Florida (a total of $398,194 in 1997–1998) and these contributions probably help explain the vigorous opposition to the youth-focused tobacco control program in the state legislature (34). The tobacco industry also continues to work to prevent the repeal of statewide preemption legislation that does not allow for the adoption of local clean indoor air ordinances (34).

OUTCOME EVALUATION

California

CIGARETTE CONSUMPTION   A number of econometric studies have demonstrated an association between the implementation of Proposition 99 and reductions in the level of per capita cigarette consumption in California (25, 31–33, 35, 45–48, 65).

The two most recent studies provide the strongest evidence of an effect of Proposition 99 on cigarette consumption, by comparing statistically trends in consumption in California with trends nationwide (32, 65). Pierce et al. (65) reported that during the early program period (1989 to 1993), cigarette consumption in California declined 52% faster than during the pre-Proposition 99 period (1983 to 1989). During a later program period (1994 to 1996), cigarette consumption in California declined only 28% faster than during the pre-program period. In contrast, the rate of decline in cigarette consumption showed no significant change in the rest of the United States during the period 1989 to 1993, and cigarette consumption in the rest of the United States showed no significant change during the period 1994 to 1996.

Fichtenberg & Glantz (32) corroborated these findings, estimating that during the early years of Proposition 99 (1989 to 1992), the program accelerated the annual rate of decline in per capita cigarette consumption in California, relative to the rest of the nation, by 2.7 packs per year. From 1992 to 1997, however, the impact of the program was reduced and per capita cigarette consumption was falling only 0.7 packs per year faster in California than in the rest of the nation.

Of note, Pierce et al. (65) reported that the declines in cigarette consumption in California are not explained wholly by changes in cigarette price. They conclude that other elements of the tobacco control program, in addition to the increased cigarette tax, must have contributed to the decline.

The magnitude of the observed decline in per capita cigarette consumption in California was substantial. Fichtenberg & Glantz (32) estimated that between 1989 and 1997, the California tobacco control program reduced cigarette consumption in California by 2.9 billion packs, resulting in a loss of $4 billion in pretax sales for the tobacco industry.

The effect of Proposition 99 on per capita cigarette consumption in California is readily visible; the tobacco control program resulted in a substantial widening of the gap in per capita cigarette consumption between California and the remainder of the nation (60) (Figure 1). Prior to the start of the program (1988), per capita cigarette consumption in California was 22.5 packs lower than the national average; within about one decade (1999), per capita cigarette consumption in California fell to 40.4 packs lower, representing a near-doubling of the gap between California and the rest of the nation (Figure 1).

ADULT SMOKING PREVALENCE   Two studies have demonstrated that the California tobacco control program resulted in a significant decline in the prevalence of smoking among adults (65, 75). Pierce et al. (65) reported that smoking prevalence in California and in the rest of the United States was declining at a similar rate of 0.8 percentage points per year prior to Proposition 99. While the rate of decline of adult smoking prevalence in California accelerated significantly to 1.1 percentage points per year during the early implementation period of the tobacco control program (1989–1993), the rate of decline in smoking prevalence in the rest of the United States remained stable at about 0.6 percentage points per year. However, during the later program implementation period (1997–1996), no significant decline in smoking prevalence was recorded in either California or the remainder of the United States.

Siegel et al. (75) confirmed this finding of a significant acceleration in the rate of decline in adult smoking prevalence in the early years of Proposition 99. These authors reported that smoking prevalence in both California and the rest of the United States was declining by 0.5 to 0.6 percentage points per year during the period

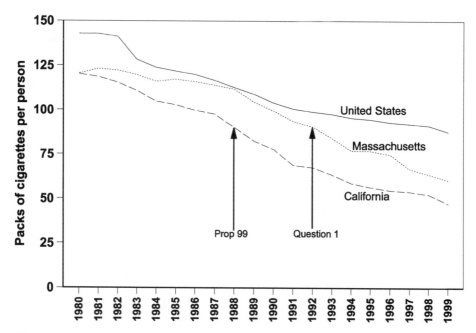

Figure 1   Trends in per capita cigarette consumption: California, Massachusetts, and the remainder of the United States (excluding California and Massachusetts), 1980–1999. Data, derived from Orzechowski & Walker (60), are for fiscal year ending June 30 of the year shown and are based on total population.

1978 to 1985, well prior to Proposition 99. From 1985 to 1990 (which includes the early years of the statewide tobacco control program), the rate of decline in smoking prevalence in California accelerated significantly to 1.2 percentage points per year; a smaller, but still significant, acceleration (to 0.9 percentage points per year) in the rate of decline in smoking prevalence also occurred in the rest of the United States during this period. From 1990 to 1994, smoking prevalence in California continued to decline significantly at a rate of 0.4 percentage points per year; in contrast, there was no significant change in smoking prevalence in the remainder of the United States.

YOUTH SMOKING PREVALENCE   The prevalence of current smoking (smoking in the past 30 days) among 12- to 17-year-olds in California remained stable at 9.2% from 1990 to 1993, but increased significantly to 12% in 1996 (64). Thus, Proposition 99 does not appear to have resulted in an early decline in youth smoking. However, to determine whether Proposition 99 had an effect on youth smoking in California, one would need to compare state with national trends. To date, no rigorous analysis comparing these trends has been published.

HEART DISEASE MORTALITY   Because the excess risk of heart disease among former smokers decreases rapidly after smoking cessation (52, 82), it is plausible that changes in heart disease mortality could be observed within one to two years after substantial reductions in cigarette consumption. Fichtenberg & Glantz (32) estimated that between 1989 and 1992, the California tobacco control program accelerated the annual rate of decline in heart disease mortality by 2.9 deaths per 100,000 population in California, relative to the rest of the United States. This difference in the annual rate of decline in heart disease mortality between California and the United States was reduced to 1.2 deaths per 100,000 population during the period 1993 to 1997. The authors estimate that during the entire study period, 1989 to 1997, the California tobacco control program resulted in 33,000 fewer deaths from heart disease in the state (compared with the total of 611,500 deaths from heart disease in California during this period). The validity of these findings is strengthened by the striking correlation between the trends in per capita cigarette consumption and in age-adjusted heart disease mortality in California. This study represents the strongest evidence to date that an aggressive, statewide tobacco control program can have a substantial impact on not only cigarette consumption, but on mortality rates as well, and that these effects can be observed within a relatively short time (one to three years) following implementation of such a program.

SPECIFIC EFFECTS OF ANTI-SMOKING MEDIA CAMPAIGN   Two studies have demonstrated a striking relationship between the presence of the anti-smoking media campaign in California and accelerated rates of decline in per capita cigarette consumption (35, 37). Glantz (35) estimated that prior to Proposition 99 (1981–1988), cigarette consumption in California was declining by 45.9 million packs per year, but that after implementation of the statewide tobacco control program (1989–1991), the rate of decline in cigarette consumption more than tripled to 164.3 million packs per year. However, the suspension of the media campaign in 1992 was associated with a dramatic slowing in the rate of decline in cigarette consumption to 19.4 packs per year. Subsequently, cigarette consumption began to decline more rapidly when the media campaign was reinstated (37).

In their econometric analyses of trends in cigarette consumption in California during the period 1980 to 1993, Hu et al. (46–48) estimated the independent effect of the media campaign on cigarette consumption by controlling for cigarette price and including a variable that reflected the cumulative expenditures for the state media campaign. The authors estimate that between 1990 and 1992, Proposition 99 was associated with a total reduction in cigarette consumption of 1.1 billion packs; they attribute a reduction of 819 million packs to the effects of the cigarette tax increase and a reduction of 232 million packs to the impact of the anti-smoking media campaign (47). Based on these estimates, approximately 21% of the overall reduction in cigarette consumption in California during the period from 1990 to 1992 was due to the anti-smoking media campaign.

Popham et al. (68), using data from a telephone survey of California smokers who quit during the initial media campaign in 1990–1991, estimated that the anti-smoking advertisements were an important stimulus in the quit decisions of

6.7% of California adults who quit smoking during this period. An additional 34.3% of former smokers in California reported that the anti-smoking advertisements played some role in their decision to quit. Thus, from 1990 to 1991 alone, the California anti-smoking media campaign is estimated to have played an important role in the quit decisions of 33,000 former smokers and at least some role in the quit decisions of an additional 173,000 former smokers.

SPECIFIC EFFECTS OF CLEAN INDOOR AIR ORDINANCE ACTIVITY   One of the most striking effects of Proposition 99 was its stimulation of local clean indoor air ordinance development, especially smoke-free bar and restaurant policies (4) (Figure 2). Prior to Proposition 99 (before 1989), no city or town in California had adopted a 100% smoke-free restaurant ordinance; during roughly the first decade of California's statewide tobacco control program (1989 to 2000), 139 such ordinances were adopted (4) (Figure 2). This compares with only 64 similar ordinances adopted in the remaining 48 states (excluding Massachusetts) (Figure 2).

The dramatic increase in local clean indoor air policy activity stimulated by Proposition 99 has been documented in the public health literature. Elder et al. (31) reported a dramatic increase, from 1% in 1990 to 53% in 1993, in the proportion

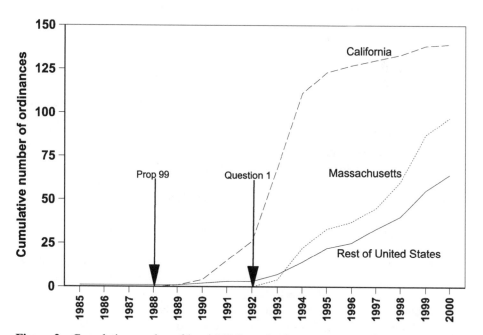

Figure 2   Cumulative number of local 100% smoke-free restaurant ordinances enacted in California, Massachusetts, and the remainder of the United States (excluding California and Massachusetts), 1985–2000. Data are from the American Nonsmokers' Rights Foundation Local Tobacco Control Ordinance Database© (4).

of local lead agencies in California that were involved in community-level policy interventions, the primary one being clean indoor air ordinances.

The literature also documents that the increase in local clean indoor air policy activity in California translated into both a higher proportion of smoke-free worksites and decreased exposure to secondhand smoke in the workplace (24, 56, 57, 64, 66). For example, Pierce et al. (64) reported that from 1990 to 1996, the proportion of California workers covered by a smoke-free worksite policy increased from 35% to more than 90%, and the proportion of indoor workers exposed to secondhand smoke at work decreased from 29% to 11.7%. By 1999, California ranked third in the nation in protection from secondhand smoke at work, with 76.9% of its private-sector indoor workers reporting a smoke-free workplace (71a).

SUMMARY   Proposition 99 resulted in a significant decline in per capita cigarette consumption and in the prevalence of smoking among adults in California. This decline was most dramatic during the early years of the program and waned considerably after 1992. It is not clear whether the program has had any significant effect on smoking behavior among youths. The media campaign specifically has been shown to have reduced cigarette consumption. Perhaps the most dramatic effect of the program was an increase in activity in local clean indoor air policies. These ordinances resulted in a substantial increase in protection of Californians from exposure to secondhand smoke. The program has been shown to have substantially reduced heart disease mortality within one to three years of its inception.

Massachusetts

CIGARETTE CONSUMPTION   Several studies suggest that Question 1 was associated with a significant decrease in per capita cigarette consumption in Massachusetts (2, 20, 21, 41). Biener et al. (21) reported that between 1988 and 1992, the annual rate of decline in cigarette consumption in Massachusetts and the United States (excluding Massachusetts and California) was similar (3.8% per year and 3.5% per year, respectively). In 1993, the rate of decline in cigarette consumption in Massachusetts jumped to 12%, while the rate of decline in the comparison states remained stable at 4%. From 1993 to 1999, cigarette consumption dropped annually by more than 4% in Massachusetts; in contrast, from 1993 to 1997, cigarette consumption declined annually by less than 1% in the comparison states. This finding of a significant effect of Question 1 on per capita cigarette consumption has been corroborated by the independent evaluation of the tobacco control program, which most recently reported a 32% decline in cigarette consumption in Massachusetts from 1992 to 1999, compared with an 8% decline in the rest of the country, excluding California, during the same period (2).

The effect of Question 1 on per capita cigarette consumption in Massachusetts is readily visible; the tobacco control program resulted in a substantial widening of the gap in per capita cigarette consumption between Massachusetts and the remainder of the nation (60) (Figure 1). Prior to the start of the program (in 1992), per capita cigarette consumption in Massachusetts was only 8.3 packs lower than in the United States; within seven years (by 1999), per capita cigarette consumption in Massachusetts was 27.2 packs lower than in the United States, representing more than a tripling of the gap between Massachusetts and the rest of the nation (Figure 1).

ADULT SMOKING PREVALENCE   Two studies have demonstrated a significant effect of Question 1 on the prevalence of smoking among adults in Massachusetts (21, 41). Most recently, Biener et al. (21) reported that adult smoking prevalence declined at a similar rate in Massachusetts and 41 comparison states (excluding California) prior to Question 1 (between 1989 and 1992). However, after Question 1 (from 1992 to 1999), smoking prevalence declined by 0.43 percentage points per year in Massachusetts while increasing by 0.03 percentage points per year in the comparison states.

YOUTH SMOKING PREVALENCE   Data from several surveys shows that the prevalence of smoking among youth in Massachusetts increased during the early years of Question 1 implementation and then began to decline in the late 1990s; thus, there was essentially no change in overall youth smoking prevalence associated with the implementation of Question 1 (26, 54, 55). Data from the Youth Risk Behavior Survey show an increase in 30-day smoking prevalence among ninth- to twelfth-grade students, from 30.2% in 1993 to 35.7% in 1995, with a decline to 30.3% in 1999 (54). In a survey conducted by Health and Addictions Research, Inc., 30-day smoking prevalence among sixth- to twelfth-grade students in Massachusetts increased from 23.1% in 1990 to 30.7% in 1996, but fell back down to 23% in 1999 (26, 55). It therefore appears that the observed reductions in cigarette consumption and smoking prevalence in Massachusetts in association with the early years of implementation of Question 1 were not attributable to any decrease in youth smoking. In the absence of any rigorous analysis of trends in youth smoking in Massachusetts compared with other states, however, it is impossible to evaluate whether the more recent declines in smoking among youth in Massachusetts are attributable to the tobacco control program.

SPECIFIC EFFECTS OF ANTI-SMOKING MEDIA CAMPAIGN   Siegel & Biener (73) provided evidence that the Massachusetts anti-smoking media campaign reduced the rate of smoking initiation among exposed youths in the state. They found that among youths aged 12 to 13 years at baseline in 1993, those who recalled having seen an anti-smoking television advertisement at baseline were half as likely to have progressed to established smoking (having smoked 100 or more cigarettes in their lifetime) over a four-year follow-up period than those who failed to recall seeing such an advertisement.

SPECIFIC EFFECTS OF CLEAN INDOOR AIR ORDINANCE ACTIVITY   One of the most striking effects of Question 1 was its stimulation of local clean indoor air ordinance policy development, especially smoke-free restaurant policies (4) (Figure 2). Prior to Question 1 (before 1993), no city or town in Massachusetts had adopted a 100% smoke-free restaurant ordinance; during the first eight years of the statewide tobacco control program (1993 to 2000), 97 such ordinances were adopted (4) (Figure 2). This compares with only 64 similar ordinances adopted in the remaining 48 states (excluding California) (Figure 2).

From 1992 to 1999, the proportion of Massachusetts residents covered by 100% smoke-free restaurant ordinances increased from 0.2% to 44% (2, 27). During the same period, the proportion of workers who had smoke-free worksites increased from 53% to 79%, and the average number of hours of exposure to secondhand smoke at work decreased from 4.5 to 2.1 per week (2). By 1999, Massachusetts ranked fourth in the nation in protection from secondhand smoke at work, with 76.8% of its private-sector indoor workers reporting a smoke-free workplace (71a).

SUMMARY   There is strong evidence that the Massachusetts tobacco control program has reduced per capita cigarette consumption and adult smoking prevalence. It is not clear whether the program has had any effect on youth smoking behavior, although recent declines in youth smoking prevalence warrant rigorous analysis with comparison to national data. Preliminary evidence suggests that exposure to the media campaign is reducing rates of progression to established smoking among youths. Perhaps the most dramatic effect of the Massachusetts tobacco control program is the proliferation of local clean indoor air ordinances and the striking increase in the protection of Massachusetts residents from exposure to secondhand smoke.

Arizona

CIGARETTE CONSUMPTION   Hogan (44) reported an 8.4% reduction in per capita cigarette consumption in Arizona during the first year following implementation of the increased cigarette tax imposed by Proposition 200. This observed reduction in cigarette consumption is in line with what would be expected from the price increase alone. Since the media campaign and other aspects of the tobacco control program were not implemented until 1996, it makes sense that the reduced per capita cigarette sales reflect the price increase alone. Analysis of more recent cigarette consumption data is needed to determine the effect of the Proposition 200 program elements on cigarette consumption and to assess the long-term repercussions of the cigarette tax increase.

ADULT SMOKING PREVALENCE   There has not been a published analysis comparing trends in adult smoking prevalence in Arizona with trends in other states to determine the effect of Proposition 200. Data from the Arizona Adult Tobacco Survey show a decline in adult smoking prevalence from 23.8% in 1996 to 18.8% in 1999 (8). Data from the Behavioral Risk Factor Surveillance System (BRFSS) show a similar decline in adult smoking prevalence in Arizona from 23.7% in

1996 (8) to 20% in 1999 (69). Viewed in light of national data showing that adult smoking prevalence in the United States was essentially stable during the same period (80), this change could reflect an effect of the tobacco control program. More rigorous analysis of trends in adult smoking in Arizona is needed before any definitive conclusions can be drawn.

YOUTH SMOKING PREVALENCE   Adequate data have not yet been presented to assess the impact of the Arizona tobacco control program on the prevalence of smoking among youth. Prevalence estimates from the 1997 Arizona Youth Tobacco Survey Baseline Report (7) and from the 2000 Arizona Youth Tobacco Survey (40) cannot be directly compared because the former was a telephone survey and the latter an in-school survey. The Arizona Criminal Justice Commission Substance Use Survey showed a decline in the 30-day prevalence of smoking among middle-school students from 18.7% in 1997 to 13% in 1999 and a decline among high school students from 31.3% in 1997 to 26.1% in 1999 (6). These trends need to be compared statistically to national trends to determine whether they reflect an outcome of the Arizona tobacco control program or whether they simply reflect secular trends in the nation.

CLEAN INDOOR AIR ORDINANCE ACTIVITY   Local efforts to protect citizens from secondhand smoke in public places, including workplaces and restaurants, were accelerated by the implementation of Proposition 200 (18). In particular, Project Rolling Thunder, whose goal was both to fight state preemption legislation and to assist communities in developing smoke-free ordinances, helped accelerate clean indoor air ordinance activity (18). Whereas Flagstaff and Tempe had enacted 100% smoke-free ordinances prior to Proposition 200, Mesa became the third city in Arizona to provide smoke-free restaurants in 1996, soon after the implementation of Proposition 200 (18).

SUMMARY   The price increase associated with Proposition 200 significantly reduced per capita cigarette consumption. Effects of the program elements of Arizona's tobacco control program on cigarette consumption and adult and youth smoking prevalence have not yet been conclusively established. Nevertheless, comparison of trends in adult and youth smoking prevalence in Arizona with national trends suggests a possible effect of Arizona's tobacco control program on both adult and youth smoking behavior. The passage of Proposition 200 does appear to have accelerated local efforts to develop clean indoor air policies.

Oregon

CIGARETTE CONSUMPTION   One study has reported a significant decline in per capita cigarette consumption in Oregon in association with the first two years of the statewide tobacco control program (67). Pizacani et al. (67) reported that during the pre-program period (1993 to 1996), per capita cigarette consumption increased

2.2% in Oregon and decreased 0.6% in the remainder of the United States (excluding California, Massachusetts, and Arizona). During the first two program years (1996 to 1998), cigarette consumption in Oregon declined by 11.3%; in contrast, cigarette consumption in the comparison states declined by only 1% during 1996 to 1997. The observed reduction in cigarette consumption exceeded that predicted by estimates of the price elasticity of demand for cigarettes, suggesting that the reduction in cigarette consumption was due not only to the price increase, but to other elements of the tobacco control program as well. A more recent report suggests that the observed effects of Measure 44 on cigarette consumption in Oregon continued through 1999 (59).

ADULT SMOKING PREVALENCE   No published analysis has compared trends in the prevalence of smoking among adults in Oregon with those in the nation to determine the impact of Measure 44 on adult smoking prevalence. Data from the BRFSS show a decline in adult smoking prevalence from 23.4% in 1996 to 21.4% in 1999 (59). In light of nearly stable adult smoking rates in the nation as a whole (80), this progress in Oregon could be related to Measure 44; however, statistical comparison of trends in Oregon with those in the nation is necessary to draw any conclusions about the effect of Oregon's tobacco control program.

YOUTH SMOKING PREVALENCE   Data from the Oregon Public School Drug Use Survey and Youth Risk Behavior Survey show that current smoking among Oregon eighth-grade students decreased from 22% in 1996 to 14.8% in 1999 (59). However, current smoking among eighth-grade students nationally decreased from 21% to 17.5% during the same period (59). Further analysis will be necessary to determine whether the decline in youth smoking in Oregon is statistically greater than the decline observed in the nation as a whole. A recent finding (70a) that the magnitude of decline in smoking prevalence between 1999 and 2000 among eighth-grade Oregon students varied with the level of implementation of school-based components of the statewide tobacco control initiative provides preliminary evidence that the observed declines may indeed be due to program activity.

CLEAN INDOOR AIR ORDINANCE ACTIVITY   The passage of Measure 44 stimulated local clean indoor air policy activity. The first two local 100% smoke-free restaurant ordinances in Oregon (Corvallis and Benton County) were enacted in 1997, the first year of the statewide tobacco control program (38).

SUMMARY   Oregon's tobacco control program has significantly reduced per capita cigarette consumption, and the observed effects are attributable both to the price increase and other elements of the tobacco control program. Effects of Measure 44 on the prevalence of smoking among adults and youths have not yet been conclusively established, but the observed declines in adult and youth smoking prevalence suggest possible effects on both adult and youth smoking behavior. Measure 44 stimulated local clean indoor air policy activity and resulted in the first local 100% smoke-free restaurant ordinances in Oregon's history.

Florida

Since Florida's tobacco control program is focused on smoking prevention among youth, potential effects on adult smoking behavior are not reviewed here.

YOUTH SMOKING PREVALENCE   Using data from the Florida Youth Tobacco Survey, Bauer et al. (13, 33a) reported significant declines in 30-day smoking prevalence among middle-school and high school students in Florida from 1998 (before implementation of the statewide tobacco program) to 2000 (second year of program implementation). Middle-school student smoking prevalence dropped from 18.5% to 11.1% and high school student smoking prevalence fell from 27.4% to 22.6%. Although there were also significant declines in 30-day youth smoking prevalence nationally, with rates among eighth-grade students dropping from 19.1% to 14.6% and rates among tenth-grade students falling from 27.6% to 23.9% during the same period (49), the observed declines in Florida were substantially greater.

A more rigorous analysis, with statistical comparison of youth smoking prevalence trends in Florida with national trends over the same time period, provides strong evidence that the sharp declines in youth smoking prevalence in Florida are attributable to the tobacco control program rather than to national secular trends (78). Using telephone surveys conducted in Florida and in the nation as a whole (excluding California, Massachusetts, Arizona, and Oregon), Sly et al. (78) found that while current smoking prevalence among youths in Florida decreased from 13.8% to 12.6% from 1998 to 1999, smoking prevalence among youths in the comparison states increased from 12.6% to 14.1%. Among youths ages 12 to 15, smoking prevalence in Florida fell significantly from 9.9% to 7.2%, whereas smoking prevalence in the comparison states increased significantly from 7% to 8.6%.

SPECIFIC EFFECTS OF ANTI-SMOKING MEDIA CAMPAIGN   One study has demonstrated a specific effect of exposure to the "truth" anti-smoking media campaign on smoking initiation among youths (79). Sly et al. (79) found that youths who reported high awareness of the media campaign at baseline were 2.4 times less likely to progress to established smoking over a ten-month follow-up period than those who did not report exposure to the media campaign. At lower levels of reported media awareness, youths were 1.8 times less likely to progress to established smoking. Sly et al. (77) confirmed these results over a longer follow-up period (up to two years) and demonstrated a dose-response relationship between confirmed awareness of television anti-smoking advertisements and risk of smoking initiation.

CLEAN INDOOR AIR ORDINANCE ACTIVITY   Because Florida has a state preemption law that prevents local communities from adopting smoke-free ordinances, there can be no local clean indoor air ordinance activity in the state. However, the implementation of the state tobacco control program appears to have stimulated efforts to overturn the state's preemption law, although without success to date (34).

SUMMARY   Within two years of implementation of Florida's tobacco control program, sharp declines in the prevalence of smoking among youth have been observed. These declines exceed those observed in the nation as a whole and appear to be a result of the aggressive and intensive Florida Tobacco Pilot Program. In addition, a specific effect of exposure to the "truth" media campaign on smoking initiation has been demonstrated.

DISCUSSION

When faithfully implemented, comprehensive statewide tobacco control programs are an effective public health intervention. These programs can produce dramatic declines in per capita cigarette consumption and in the prevalence of smoking among both adults and youths, and within a short time, these declines can produce a demonstrable reduction in mortality from heart disease. The magnitude of this reduction in morbidity and mortality can be substantial; during its first nine years, the tobacco control program in California is estimated to have saved 33,000 lives (from reduction in heart disease mortality alone) (32). There probably is no other public health intervention, even at a national level, that comes close to this degree of effect on the public's health. Tobacco use is the chief preventable cause of death in the United States; comprehensive statewide tobacco control programs should now be seen as the most critical public health intervention available.

Anti-smoking media campaigns, specifically, are the central and most critical component of a statewide tobacco control program. The suspension of these media campaigns and the limiting of their aggressiveness has resulted in demonstrable reversals of the effects of state tobacco control programs on cigarette consumption (35, 37). Exposure to aggressive anti-smoking television campaigns has been specifically shown to lower smoking prevalence (78) and to reduce progression to established smoking among youths (73, 79). Although statewide tobacco control interventions should not focus solely on a media campaign, the fact that the most successful programs have been those highlighted by an aggressive media campaign suggests that such a strategy may serve as a central core around which other essential units of tobacco control activity (29) can be molded. If properly coordinated with local programs, a statewide media campaign can help enable and support community-level initiatives.

Although a statewide media campaign appears to be a critical component of an effective state-level tobacco control program, intervention at the local level also appears to be essential. In fact, perhaps the most dramatic effect of statewide tobacco control programs has been the rapid proliferation of local clean indoor air ordinances. The number of local 100% smoke-free restaurant ordinances enacted in California and Massachusetts alone [236] after the passage of Proposition 99 and Question 1 exceeded by a factor of nearly four the number of similar ordinances [64] enacted in the remaining 48 states (4) (Figure 2). These interventions serve not only to protect citizens from the hazards of secondhand smoke but are also effective in reducing cigarette consumption and promoting smoking cessation (74). Along with anti-smoking media campaigns, the promotion of local clean indoor air policies should be viewed as a critical specific focus of statewide tobacco control programs. In order to allow such activity to take place, public health advocates must be prepared to fight vigorously against state preemption legislation. Such legislation has been promoted by the tobacco industry and other groups in almost every state where a comprehensive tobacco control program has been implemented. In states with preexisting preemption legislation (e.g., Florida), the repeal of preemption should be viewed as a critical focus of tobacco control program activity.

The approximate two-year lag between passage of both Proposition 99 and Question 1 and the actual proliferation of local clean indoor air ordinances (Figure 2) probably reflects the time needed to establish local clean indoor air coalitions, develop an infrastructure to support grassroots mobilization, conduct extensive public education campaigns about the health hazards of secondhand smoke, and mobilize public support for these ordinances. Public health practitioners who wish to repeat the successes of California's and Massachusetts' clean indoor air policy development in their own states must understand the importance of developing local infrastructure to support community education and mobilization efforts and of supporting this infrastructure for a sustained period of time. They should also recognize that the local level is where the most effective clean indoor air policies have been enacted and that attempts to enact statewide clean indoor air legislation are not only more difficult but risk having preemption language tacked onto a bill, a device that in many states has put a complete end to clean indoor air policy activity (74). Most recently, Oregon learned this difficult lesson when a 2001 state bill to eliminate smoking in all workplaces, restaurants, and bars was amended both to exclude bars and to preempt future local clean indoor air ordinances. It is much safer, as well as more effective, to concentrate on local clean indoor air ordinances, at least until these policies are so widespread that there is unshakable support for a comprehensive state law that provides 100% protection at all workplaces (as was the case in California, which provides 100% protection for workers at virtually all workplaces, including bars and restaurants).

Based on the experience of the five state programs reviewed here, although these programs can work, their effectiveness depends on the intensity and aggressiveness of program implementation. Proposition 99 in California had dramatic effects on both cigarette consumption and the prevalence of smoking among adults, although both results waned greatly after program funding was cut. Florida's "truth" media campaign had dramatic repercussions on the prevalence of smoking among youths, but it is difficult to see how these positive results can be maintained in light of a 54% cut in the media campaign budget.

Not only are overall funding levels critical to the success of statewide tobacco control programs, the scope of program activity is also critical. The most dramatic effects on smoking behavior have been observed in states where aggressive campaigns were waged. These campaigns directly confronted the legitimacy of marketing practices by the tobacco industry, widely publicized the health hazards of secondhand smoke, and supported local initiatives to promote policies to protect nonsmokers from secondhand smoke in public places, including bars and restaurants. The tobacco industry's attempts to prevent aggressive television advertising campaigns that directly confront the legitimacy of their marketing practices should confirm for public health practitioners the potential effectiveness of such campaigns. Similarly, the tobacco industry's efforts to preempt local clean indoor air ordinance activity corroborates the potential value of those policies.

Whereas the tobacco industry's drive to limit program funding, scope, and aggressiveness is understandable because of its interest in preserving corporate profits, concurrence by public health officials in some states in limiting program scope and aggressiveness make less sense. For example, it took two years before the Arizona tobacco control program expanded to include adult smoking cessation and protection of citizens from secondhand smoke (18, 19), and it is still not clear whether the program will address marketing tactics by the tobacco industry. In suggesting that they do not want to "attack" the tobacco industry in their ads, public health officials are implying a willingness to limit the effectiveness of their advertising campaign. The most dramatic success of any of the five tobacco control programs on youth smoking prevalence occurred in Florida, where the entire media campaign is focused on exposing the lies the tobacco industry has told and on creating a new brand to promote to kids, the truth. Advertisements that educate youths about the marketing tactics used by the tobacco companies to recruit and addict youth smokers should not be viewed as "attacks" on anyone. These advertisements are simply telling the truth—they are educational advertisements about corporate marketing practices—and based on observed effects in multiple states, they are likely to be effective in changing smoking behavior among youth.

Recent data from Florida suggest that youth attitudes toward tobacco industry marketing techniques are one of the strongest predictors of smoking initiation and that these attitudes can be changed by an aggressive media campaign (76, 77). The observed declines in cigarette smoking in Florida were closely tied to youths' attitudes about the extent of tobacco industry manipulation in advertising, the precise focus of the campaign (77). Youths with a high level of appreciation of the tobacco industry's manipulation of youths in its advertising were nearly 14 times less likely to start smoking over an 18-month follow-up period than youths with a low level of appreciation of these manipulative tactics (77).

Ensuring that anti-smoking media campaigns will be aggressive and will use the techniques found to be most effective in previous research presents a continuing challenge in the implementation of new programs. For example, Virginia recently announced the allocation of $28 million of tobacco settlement funds over three years to an anti-tobacco marketing and advertising campaign (23). The campaign developers were reportedly directed to design a campaign that respects the tobacco industry's historic and economic heritage in the state and that does not directly confront the industry's behavior (23). The chances of developing an effective campaign under the constraints imposed by that political directive seem minimal.

Equally unfortunate is the failure of public health organizations to aggressively fight against proposed reductions in budgets for tobacco control programs and to hold governors and legislators who promote such cuts publicly accountable. The experiences of the five state programs reviewed here demonstrate that in order to successfully protect program funding, public health groups must publicly hold officials accountable for their actions. Political factors have influenced and will continue to influence the initial funding, development, execution, and sustained funding of anti-smoking media campaigns and comprehensive statewide tobacco control programs. Public health practitioners must be prepared to stand up to political interference.

Statewide tobacco control programs are not implemented in a vacuum. The tobacco industry's reactions to these interventions are strong and predictable. The response includes more intensive and aggressive marketing; increased political activity at the state and local level; attempts to limit program funding, scope, and aggressiveness; promotion of state preemption legislation; and funding of local groups to fight against local clean indoor air ordinances. Counteracting the tobacco industry's response to statewide tobacco control programs should constitute an integral part of the program itself. Public health practitioners should expect, monitor, and plan for action from the tobacco industry.

As public health practitioners in other states look to replicate the successful tobacco control programs in California, Massachusetts, Arizona, Oregon, and Florida, many are looking to tobacco settlement funds to implement such programs. However, convincing state legislators to allocate tobacco settlement funds to tobacco control programs has had limited success. As of the end of 2000, only 15 states had allocated substantial settlement funds to tobacco prevention and cessation efforts and only 6 states were funding these programs at minimum levels recommended by the Centers for Disease Control and Prevention's best practices guidelines (28, 29). In fiscal year 2001, only 5 of the 46 states participating in the Master Settlement Agreement had committed the minimum recommended level to tobacco control programs (30). The U.S. General Accounting Office estimated that as of April 2001, the 46 signatories to the tobacco settlement had allocated only 7% of settlement funds for tobacco control, only slightly higher than the percentage of funds (6%) allocated for tobacco growers and economic development in tobacco-growing states (82a). Only four states had allocated more than 20% of their settlement funds for tobacco control (82a). The most recent report, issued by the National Conference of State Legislatures, found that from fiscal years 2000 to 2002, only 5% of tobacco settlement funds were allocated to tobacco prevention and cessation programs (57a).

There is nothing wrong with trying to convince legislators to allocate tobacco settlement funds for tobacco control programs, but there simply is no substitute for the model established by California in which the initiative process is used to establish a comprehensive statewide tobacco control program funded by dedicated revenues from an increased cigarette excise tax. Legislatures face too many fiscal pressures and demands from conflicting political constituencies, and tobacco control is not at the top of their agendas. The experience to date with convincing legislators to allocate substantial settlement funds for tobacco control has been dismal, and there is little hope for change. The time and resources of tobacco control organizations might better be spent in trying to educate the public on the primacy of tobacco control. The initiative process itself may be an effective tobacco control intervention. Evidence from California suggests that the initial acceleration in the decline in cigarette consumption preceded the implementation of Proposition 99, coinciding instead with the period during which this voter initiative was publicized and debated (75). Moreover, organization and planning required to mount an initiative campaign is probably a minimal prerequisite for developing a successful statewide tobacco control program. Allocating resources for tobacco control programs in the absence of an existing infrastructure and a comprehensive, unified strategic plan is unlikely to be as effective as spending several years in organizing, building infrastructure, and strategic planning prior to attempting to run a program. Finally, there is a strong disincentive for states to mount successful anti-smoking campaigns with their settlement funds, as the Master Settlement Agreement calls for substantial decreases in payments to states if tobacco consumption falls. This is not a structural arrangement under which tobacco control is likely to flourish in the long term, even if a state allocates settlement funds to tobacco control in a given year. In states where the initiative process is not available, public health practitioners might look to legislated increases in the cigarette excise tax as a source to fund comprehensive tobacco control programs, especially where legislatures have shown no interest in using settlement funds for this purpose.

Ultimately, if public health practitioners are interested in making a statewide tobacco control program a permanent part of the public health infrastructure, they should focus on promoting a voter initiative (or state law where the initiative process is not available) to develop a comprehensive statewide tobacco control program funded by cigarette excise tax revenues. Where possible, the specific proportion of revenues to be allocated to tobacco control programs should be specified in the initiative. Once such an initiative is passed, public health practitioners should direct their attention to preserving full funding for the program and to ensuring that the most aggressive and comprehensive program is implemented. Given the evidence of the weight these programs bring to bear on smoking behavior and on mortality, it is difficult to imagine any more worthwhile allocation of public health effort and resources.

ACKNOWLEDGMENTS

Local tobacco control ordinance data were provided by the American Nonsmokers' Rights Foundation Local Tobacco Control Ordinance Database©.

Visit the Annual Reviews home page at www.annualreviews.org

LITERATURE CITED

1. Abt Associates Inc. 1995. *Independent Evaluation of the Massachusetts Tobacco Control Program: First Annual Report.* Cambridge, MA: Abt Assoc. Inc.
2. Abt Associates Inc. 2000. *Independent Evaluation of the Massachusetts Tobacco Control Program: Sixth Annual Report.* Cambridge, MA: Abt Assoc. Inc.
3. Aguinaga S, Macdonald H, Traynor M, Begay ME, Glantz SA. 1995. *Undermining Popular Government: Tobacco Industry Political Expenditures in California, 1993–1994.* San Francisco: Inst. Health Policy Stud., Sch. Med., Univ. Calif., San Francisco
4. American Nonsmokers' Rights Foundation. 2001. *American Nonsmokers' Rights Foundation Local Tobacco Control Ordinance Database©.* Berkeley, CA: Am. Nonsmokers' Rights Found.
5. American Tobacco Company. 1992. *The Massachusetts Plan. Draft #4, 12/3/92, KLM Remarks for the 12/10 Exec. Comm. Meet.* http://www.bw.aalatg.com/public. asp. Document ID: 60207992
6. Arizona Criminal Justice Commission. 2000. *Substance Abuse in Arizona: 1999.* http://www.acjc.state.az.us/pdfs/Full Report2000.PDF
7. Arizona Dep. Health Services. 1998. *1997 Arizona Youth Tobacco Survey Baseline Report.* http://www.tepp.org/evalua tion/1997youthbaseline
8. Arizona Dep. Health Services. 2000. *1999 Arizona Adult Tobacco Survey Report.* http://www.tepp.org/evaluation/1999 adultsurvey
9. Associated Press. 2001. *Restaurants launch campaign to fight smoking ban.* Feb. 7. http://www.kgw.com/kgwnews/oregon wash_story.html?StoryID=13749
9a. Associated Press. 2001. *Senate panel approves bill to thwart future anti-smoking*

bans. July 3. http://www.katu.com/news/ story.asp?ID=26675
10. Bal DG, Kizer KW, Felten PG, Mozar HN, Niemeyer D. 1990. Reducing tobacco consumption in California: development of a statewide anti-tobacco use campaign. *JAMA* 264:1570–74
11. Balbach ED, Monardi FM, Fox BJ, Glantz SA. 1997. *Holding Government Accountable: Tobacco Policy Making in California, 1995–1997.* San Francisco: Inst. Health Policy Stud., Sch. Med., Univ. Calif., San Francisco
12. Balbach ED, Traynor MP, Glantz SA. 2000. The implementation of California's tobacco tax initiative: the critical role of outsider strategies in protecting Proposition 99. *J. Health Polit. Policy Law* 25 (4):689–715
13. Bauer UE, Johnson TM, Hopkins RS, Brooks RG. 2000. Changes in youth cigarette use and intentions following implementation of a tobacco control program: findings from the Florida Youth Tobacco Survey, 1998–2000. *JAMA* 284(6):723–28
14. Begay ME. 2000. *Undermining the Mandate: How Massachusetts Spent Tobacco Education and Prevention Funds, 1994–2001 Fiscal Years.* Amherst, MA: Dep. Commun. Health Stud., Sch. Public Health and Health Sci., Univ. Mass., Amherst
15. Begay ME, Glantz SA. 1997. Question 1 tobacco education expenditures in Massachusetts, USA. *Tob. Control* 6:213–18
16. Begay ME, Traynor M, Glantz SA. 1993. The tobacco industry, state politics, and tobacco education in California. *Am. J. Public Health* 83(9):1214–21
17. Begay ME, Traynor M, Glantz SA. 1994. *The Twilight of Proposition 99: Reauthorization of Tobacco Education Programs and Tobacco Industry Political Expenditures in 1993.* San Francisco: Inst. Health

Policy Stud., Sch. Med., Univ. Calif., San Francisco

18. Bialous SA, Glantz SA. 1997. *Tobacco Control in Arizona, 1973–1997*. San Francisco: Inst. Health Policy Stud., Sch. Med., Univ. Calif., San Francisco

19. Bialous SA, Glantz SA. 1999. Arizona's tobacco control initiative illustrates the need for continuing oversight by tobacco control advocates. *Tob. Control* 8:141–51

20. Biener L, Aseltine RH, Cohen B, Anderka M. 1998. Reactions of adult and teenaged smokers to the Massachusetts tobacco tax. *Am. J. Public Health* 88 (9):1389–91

21. Biener L, Harris JE, Hamilton W. 2000. Impact of the Massachusetts tobacco control programme: population based trend analysis. *Br. Med. J.* 321:351–54

22. Bjornson W, Sahr RC, Moore J, Balshem H, Fleming D, et al. 1997. Tobacco tax initiative—Oregon, 1996. *Morbid. Mortal. Wkly. Rep.* 46(11):246–48

23. Blackwell JR. 2001. Foundation to spend $28 million on youth no-smoking campaign. *The Richmond Times-Dispatch* (online version), March 12. Accessed March 31, 2001. http://www.timesdispatch.com/business/MGBFPCLF7KC.html

24. Borland R, Pierce JP, Burns DM, Gilpin E, Johnson M, Bal D. 1992. Protection from environmental tobacco smoke in California: the case for a smoke-free workplace. *JAMA* 268(6):749–52

25. Breslow L, Johnson M. 1993. California's Proposition 99 on tobacco, and its impact. *Annu. Rev. Public Health* 14:585–604

26. Briton NJ, Clark TW, Soldz S, Krakow M. 1997. *Adolescent Tobacco Use in Massachusetts: Trends Among Public School Students, 1984–1996*. Boston: Health Addict. Res., Inc.

27. Brooks DR, Mucci LA. 2001. Support for smoke-free restaurants among Massachusetts adults, 1992–1999. *Am. J. Public Health* 91(2):300–3

28. Campaign for Tobacco-Free Kids. 2001. *Show Us the Money: An Update on the States' Allocation of the Tobacco Settlement Dollars*. Washington, DC: Campaign for Tobacco-Free Kids, Am. Cancer Soc., Am. Heart Assoc., Am. Lung Assoc.

29. Cent. Dis. Control Prev. 1999. *Best Practices for Comprehensive Tobacco Control Programs—August 1999*. Atlanta: U.S. DHHS, CDC, Natl. Cent. Chronic Dis. Prev. Health Promot., Off. Smoking Health

30. Cent. Dis. Control Prev. 2001. *Investment in Tobacco Control: State Highlights—2001*. Atlanta: U.S. DHHS, CDC, Natl. Cent. Chronic Dis. Prev. Health Promot., Off. Smoking Health

31. Elder JP, Edwards CC, Conway TL, Kenney E, Johnson CA, Bennett ED. 1996. Independent evaluation of the California tobacco education program. *Public Health Rep.* 111:353–58

32. Fichtenberg CM, Glantz SA. 2000. Association of the California Tobacco Control Program with declines in cigarette consumption and mortality from heart disease. *N. Engl. J. Med.* 343(24):1772–77

33. Flewelling RL, Kenney K, Elder JP, Pierce J, Johnson M, Bal DG. 1992. First-year impact of the 1989 California cigarette tax increase on cigarette consumption. *Am. J. Public Health* 82(6): 867–69

33a. Florida Dep. Health. 2001. *Assessing the Impact of Florida's Pilot Program on Tobacco Control: 1998 to 2000. A Comprehensive Analysis of Data from the Florida Youth Tobacco Survey*. Tallahassee: Fla. Dep. Health, Bur. Epidemiol.

33b. Givel MS, Dearlove J, Glantz SA. 2001. *Tobacco Policy Making in California 1999–2001: Stalled and Adrift*. San Francisco: Inst. Health Policy Stud., Sch. Med., Univ. Calif., San Francisco

34. Givel MS, Glantz SA. 1999. *Tobacco Industry Political Power and Influence in Florida from 1979 to 1999*. San Francisco: Inst. Health Policy Stud., Sch. Med., Univ. Calif., San Francisco

35. Glantz SA. 1993. Changes in cigarette consumption, prices, and tobacco industry revenues associated with California's Proposition 99. *Tob. Control* 2:311–14

36. Glantz SA. 1996. Editorial: preventing tobacco use—the youth access trap. *Am. J. Public Health* 86(2):156–58

37. Goldman LK, Glantz SA. 1998. Evaluation of antismoking advertising campaigns. *JAMA* 279(10):772–77

38. Goldman LK, Glantz SA. 1998. *Tobacco Industry Political Expenditures and Tobacco Policy Making in Oregon: 1985–1997.* San Francisco: Inst. Health Policy Stud., Sch. Med., Univ. Calif., San Francisco

39. Goldman LK, Glantz SA. 1999. The passage and initial implementation of Oregon's Measure 44. *Tob. Control* 8:311–22

40. Gowda VR. 2001. *The 2000 Arizona Youth Tobacco Survey: Middle School, Grades 6–8.* Phoenix: AZ Dep. Health Serv. http://www.tepp.org/evaluation/2000youthsurvey

41. Harris JE, Connolly GN, Brooks D, Davis B. 1996. Cigarette smoking before and after an excise tax increase and an antismoking campaign—Massachusetts, 1990–1996. *Morbid. Mortal. Wkly. Rep.* 45(44):966–70

42. Heiser PF, Begay ME. 1997. The campaign to raise the tobacco tax in Massachusetts. *Am. J. Public Health* 87 (6):968–73

43. Hicks JJ. 2001. The strategy behind Florida's "truth" campaign. *Tob. Control* 10:3–5

44. Hogan TD. 1996. *The Impact of Proposition 200 on Cigarette Consumption in Arizona.* Tempe: AZ State Univ.

45. Hu T, Bai J, Keeler TE, Barnett PG, Sung H. 1994. The impact of California Proposition 99, a major anti-smoking law, on cigarette consumption. *J. Public Health Policy* 15:26–36

46. Hu T, Keeler TE, Sung H, Barnett PG. 1995. The impact of California antismoking legislation on cigarette sales, consumption, and prices. *Tob. Control* 4(Suppl. 1):S34–38

47. Hu T, Sung H, Keeler TE. 1995. Reducing cigarette consumption in California: tobacco taxes vs an anti-smoking media campaign. *Am. J. Public Health* 85(9):1218–22

48. Hu T, Sung H, Keeler TE. 1995. The state antismoking campaign and the industry response: the effects of advertising on cigarette consumption in California. *AEA Pap. Proc.* 85(2):85–90

49. Institute for Social Research. 2000. *Long-term Trends in Prevalence of Use of Cigarettes for Eighth, Tenth, and Twelfth Graders (Table 1).* Ann Arbor: Univ. Mich., Inst. Soc. Res., Surv. Res. Cent., Monitoring the Future Study. http://monitoringthefuture.org/data/00data/pr00cig1.pdf

50. Institute of Medicine. 2000. *State Programs Can Reduce Tobacco Use.* Washington, DC: Natl. Cancer Policy Board, Inst. Med., Natl. Res. Counc. Board Health Promot. Dis. Prev.

51. Koh HD. 1996. An analysis of the successful 1992 Massachusetts tobacco tax initiative. *Tob. Control* 5:220–25

52. Lightwood JM, Glantz SA. 1997. Short-term economic and health benefits of smoking cessation: myocardial infarction and stroke. *Circulation* 96:1089–96

53. Macdonald H, Aguinaga S, Glantz SA. 1997. The defeat of Philip Morris' 'California Uniform Tobacco Control Act.' *Am. J. Public Health* 87(12):1989–96

54. Mass. Dep. Educ. 2000. *1999 Massachusetts Youth Risk Behavior Survey Results: May 2000.* Malden, MA: Mass. Dep. Educ.

55. Mass. Dep. Public Health. 2000. *Adolescent Tobacco Use in Massachusetts: Trends Among Public School Students, 1996–1999.* Boston: Mass. Dep. Public Health

56. Moskowitz JM, Lin Z, Hudes ES. 1999. The impact of California's smoking ordinances on worksite smoking policy and

exposure to environmental tobacco smoke. *Am. J. Health Promot.* 13(5):278–81

57. Moskowitz JM, Lin Z, Hudes ES. 2000. The impact of workplace smoking ordinances in California on smoking cessation. *Am. J. Public Health* 90(5):757–61

57a. Natl. Conf. State Legislatures. 2001. *State Management and Allocation of Tobacco Settlement Revenue—1999 to 2001.* Washington, DC: Natl. Conf. State Legis.

57b. Novotny TE, Romano RA, Davis RM, Mills SL. 1992. The public health practice of tobacco control: lessons learned and directions for the states in the 1990s. *Annu. Rev. Public Health* 13:287–318

58. Novotny TE, Siegel MB. 1996. California's tobacco control saga. *Health Aff.* 15(1):58–72

59. Oregon Health Division. 2000. *Oregon Tobacco Facts.* Portland: OR. Health Div., Dep. Hum. Serv., Tobacco Prev. Educ. Progr. http://www.ohd.hr.state.or.us/tobacco

60. Orzechowski and Walker. 2000. *The Tax Burden on Tobacco: Historical Compilation, Vol. 34, 1999.* Arlington, VA: Orzechowski & Walker

61. Pechmann C. 1997. Does antismoking advertising combat underage smoking? A review of past practices and research. In *Social Marketing: Theoretical and Practical Perspectives*, ed. ME Goldberg, M Fishbein, SE Middlestadt, 12:189–216. Mahwah, NJ: Lawrence Erlbaum

62. Pechmann C, Reibling ET. 2000. Antismoking advertising campaigns targeting youth: case studies from USA and Canada. *Tob. Control* 9(Suppl. 2):ii18–ii31

63. Phillips F. 1995. Funds vs. smoking appear to be safe; Weld, eyeing poll, softens proposal. *The Boston Globe*, Dec. 8, p. 37

64. Pierce JP, Gilpin EA, Emery SL, Farkas AJ, Zhu SH, et al. 1998. *Tobacco Control in California: Who's Winning the War? An Evaluation of the Tobacco Control Pro-*

gram, 1989–1996. La Jolla, CA: Univ. Calif., San Diego

65. Pierce JP, Gilpin EA, Emery SL, White MM, Rosbrook B, Berry CC. 1998. Has the California Tobacco Control Program reduced smoking? *JAMA* 280(10):893–99

66. Pierce JP, Shanks TG, Pertschuk M, Gilpin E, Shopland D, et al. 1994. Do smoking ordinances protect non-smokers from environmental tobacco smoke at work? *Tob. Control* 3:15–20

67. Pizacani B, Mosbaek C, Hedberg K, Bley L, Stark M, et al. 1999. Decline in cigarette consumption following implementation of a comprehensive tobacco prevention and education program—Oregon, 1996–1998. *Morbid. Mortal. Wkly. Rep.* 48(7):140–43

68. Popham WJ, Potter LD, Bal DG, Johnson MD, Duerr MJ, Quinn V. 1993. Do antismoking media campaigns help smokers quit? *Public Health Rep.* 108(4):510–13

69. Reese S, Owen P, Bender B, Potts G, Davis B, et al. 2000. State-specific prevalence of current cigarette smoking among adults and the proportion of adults who work in a smoke-free environment—United States, 1999. *Morbid. Mortal. Wkly. Rep.* 49(43):978–82

70. Ritch WA, Begay ME. 1999. *Strange Bedfellows: The History of Collaboration Between the Tobacco Industry and the Massachusetts Restaurant Association.* Amherst, MA: Dep. Commun. Health Stud., Sch. Public Health and Health Sci., Univ. Mass.

70a. Rohde K, Pizacani B, Stark M, Pietrukowicz M, Mosbaek C, et al. 2001. Effectiveness of school-based programs as a component of a statewide tobacco control initiative—Oregon, 1999–2000. *Morbid. Mortal. Wkly. Rep.* 50(31):663-66

71. Sherman R. 1996. Shaming Big Tobacco's friends in California. *Tob. Control* 5:189–91

71a. Shopland DR, Gerlach KK, Burns DM, Hartman AM, Gibson JT. 2001. State-specific trends in smoke-free workplace policy coverage: the Current Population Survey Tobacco Use Supplement, 1993 to 1999. *J. Occup. Environ. Med.* 43(8):680–86

72. Siegel M, Biener L. 1997. Evaluating the impact of statewide anti-tobacco campaigns: the Massachusetts and California tobacco control programs. *J. Soc. Issues* 53(1):147–68

73. Siegel M, Biener L. 2000. The impact of an antismoking media campaign on progression to established smoking: results of a longitudinal youth study. *Am. J. Public Health* 90(3):380–86

74. Siegel M, Carol J, Jordan J, Hobart R, Schoenmarklin S, et al. 1997. Preemption in tobacco control: review of an emerging public health problem. *JAMA* 278(10):858–63

75. Siegel M, Mowery PD, Pechacek TP, Strauss WJ, Schooley MW, et al. 2000. Trends in adult cigarette smoking in California compared with the rest of the United States, 1978–1994. *Am. J. Public Health* 90(3):372–79

76. Sly DF, Heald G, Hopkins RS, Moore TW, McCloskey M, Ray S. 2000. The industry manipulation attitudes of smokers and nonsmokers. *J. Public Health Manag. Pract.* 6(3):49–56

77. Sly DF, Heald G, Ray S. 2000. *Preventing Youth Smoking Behaviors: How Florida's "Truth" Works: Final Report on the 2000 Follow-Up Survey of Florida Youth and Early Young Adults.* Tallahassee: FL State Univ.

78. Sly DF, Heald GR, Ray S. 2001. The Florida "truth" anti-tobacco media evaluation: design, first year results, and implications for planning future state media evaluations. *Tob. Control* 10:9–15

79. Sly DF, Hopkins RS, Trapido E, Ray S. 2001. Influence of a counteradvertising media campaign on initiation of smoking: the Florida "truth" campaign. *Am. J. Public Health* 91(2):233–38

80. Subst. Abuse and Mental Health Serv. Admin. 2000. *Summary of Findings from the 1999 National Household Survey on Drug Abuse.* Rockville, MD: U.S. DHHS. http://www.samhsa.gov/oas/NHSDA/1999/TitlePage.htm

81. The Tobacco Institute. 1990. *Memorandum to the Members of the Executive Committee* (April 18). Washington, DC. http://www.tobaccoinstitute.com. TIMN 298436–298440

82. U.S. Dep. Health and Hum. Serv. 1990. *The Health Benefits of Smoking Cessation.* Atlanta: CDC, Cent. Chronic Dis. Prev. Health Promot., Off. Smoking and Health. DHHS Publ. No. (CDC) 90–8416

82a. U.S. Gen. Account. Off. 2001. *Tobacco Settlement: States' Use of Master Settlement Agreement Payments. Report to the Honorable John McCain, Ranking Minority Member, Committee on Commerce, Science, and Transportation, U.S. Senate.* Washington, DC: U.S. Gen. Account. Off.

83. Wakefield M, Chaloupka F. 1999. *Effectiveness of Comprehensive Tobacco Control Programs in Reducing Teenage Smoking: A Review.* Chicago: Univ. Ill., Chicago

84. Wakefield M, Chaloupka F. 2000. Effectiveness of comprehensive tobacco control programmes in reducing teenage smoking in the USA. *Tob. Control.* 9:177–86

85. Zucker D, Hopkins RS, Sly DF, Urich J, Kershaw JM, Solari S. 2000. Florida's "truth" campaign: a counter-marketing, anti-tobacco media campaign. *J. Public Health Manag. Pract.* 6(3):1–6

Annu. Rev. Public Health 2002. 23:73–91

Direct Marketing of Pharmaceuticals to Consumers

Alan Lyles

*Health Systems Management, University of Baltimore, Baltimore, Maryland 21202;
e-mail: alyles@ubmail.ubalt.edu*

Key Words DTC advertising, prescription drugs, pharmaceutical marketing, drug information, direct-to-consumer advertising

■ **Abstract** Revised FDA regulations governing pharmaceutical companies' broadcast advertisements directed to consumers produced substantial increases in direct-to-consumer advertising (DTCA) expenditures. Proponents of DTCA claim it supports patient autonomy in the patient-physician relationship and has motivated some consumers to seek a physician's care for conditions they previously had not discussed with a doctor. However, DTCA's blend of promotion and information has produced more prescription drug awareness than knowledge—it has been largely ineffective in educating patients with medical conditions about the medications for those conditions. The evidence for DTCA's increase in pharmaceutical sales is as impressive as is the lack of evidence concerning its impact on the health of the public. Broadcast advertisements are too brief to include extensive technical information; consequently, the impact of FDA regulations to assure a fair balance of risk and benefit in DTCA is still being assessed.

INTRODUCTION

Changes in Food and Drug Administration (FDA) regulations governing pharmaceutical companies' broadcast advertisements directed to consumers produced substantial increases in direct-to-consumer advertising (DTCA) expenditures, yet there is little evidence of their effect on public health. This article examines the motivations for DTCA, its evolution, and the limited evidence of its results. Financial aspects are considered; however, the focus concerns health services and outcomes.

The lack of information on DTCA's health impact has not prevented key stakeholders from identifying strong and often opposing positions. DTCA supporters view it as an appropriate extension of patient empowerment, opponents reject it as inappropriate and misleading for its intended audience, whereas others see a role for DTCA under specific circumstances and with additional safeguards. Alan Holmer, president of the Pharmaceutical Research and Manufacturers of America, cites the extent of undiagnosed or undertreated chronic illnesses such as diabetes, hypercholesterolemia, hypertension, and depressive illness, for which DTCA may

0163-7525/02/0510-0073$14.00

motivate consumers to seek a physician's care. Mr. Holmer asserts both the "right and responsibility" of pharmaceutical companies to advertise their products, arguing that the drug companies do not determine the physician's prescribing decision (38). Noting that FDA relaxed standards for marketing prescription drugs directly to consumers in the absence of "rigorous, independent studies," Matthew Hollon emphasizes the mixed incentives influencing communications from the pharmaceutical industry. Industry's legitimate profit motive makes the quality of the information it provides "suspect" so Hollon proposes stronger regulation until "well designed, independent studies" demonstrate the public health value of the information provided (37).

The Academy of Managed Care Pharmacy discourages product-specific DTCA (2); however, many organizations share the perspective of the American Association of Retired Persons (AARP) that "FDA should regulate all direct-to-consumer (DTC) advertising and promotion of prescription drugs to ensure that it is balanced and accurate and includes information on any adverse effects" (3). Information provided through DTCA under these safeguards could complement the prescription drug initiatives of *Healthy People 2010*, a national initiative to identify and reduce the leading preventable threats to health. Under *Healthy People 2010*, FDA's objectives include increasing the proportion of patients (*a*) receiving drug information with their new prescriptions, and (*b*) receiving verbal counseling on appropriate medication use and risks (36).

The growth of managed care in the United States both expanded the number of people with prescription drug insurance but restricted their options for coverage of specific drugs: Greater choice among the marketed pharmaceuticals typically requires greater patient cost-sharing (47). Managed care controls that limit the physician's prescriptive authority also reduce the potential impact of promotional activities targeting physicians; consequently, pharmaceutical companies have responded by seeking alternative ways to influence physician prescribing (45). Managed care arrangements that produce time constraints on patient-physician interactions and financial incentives for physicians have contributed to erosion of the patient's trust (49). One fourth of respondents in a recent national poll trust their doctor less than in recent years, and over half believe their health plan is more worried about saving money than about providing the best treatment (61). DTCA reflects the consumer's growing role in prescription drug decisions in managed care, desire for information, and distrust in their providers.

BACKGROUND: REGULATORY

Self-medication and DTCA have a long history (see Table 1). Contrasting drug advertising expenditures circa 1930 with those of 1972, 90% of the former was in newspapers and popular magazines—with detailing, samples, and technical journal advertisements totaling 5%, whereas the latter categories represented 75% by 1972 (68). Testimony by the chief of the FDA and a subsequent U.S. House

TABLE 1   Chronology of selected issues relevant to DTCA

Year	Event/Issue	Relevance to drug marketing
1906	Federal Food and Drug Act	Prohibited interstate commerce of misbranded drugs
1938	Federal Food, Drug and Cosmetic Act	Required evidence of safety prior to marketing approval testimony that it would "make self-medication safer and more effective" (69)
	Wheeler-Lea Act	Federal Trade Commission (FTC) jurisdiction over all drug advertising
1951	Durham-Humphrey Amendment	Defined separate classes for prescription and over-the-counter drugs
1962	Kefauver-Harris Amendment	Required evidence of safety and efficacy prior to marketing Required risk and benefit information for advertisements in medical journals Gave FDA jurisdiction for prescription drug advertising
1968	Caution on isoproterenol inhalers	Instituted FDA's first labeling directed to patients
1970	Information for patients on oral contraceptive's risks and benefits	Instituted FDA's first required Patient Package Insert
1981–1982	Beginning of product-specific public promotions	
1982	Cancellation of Pilot Patient Package Insert program	FDA's reliance on voluntary initiatives for patient information
1983	FDA Commissioner requests moratorium on prescription drug DTCA	Time to assess evidence on risk and benefit communications in DTCA
1985	Withdrawal of moratorium on DTCA	Same marketing regulations for physician and for consumer audiences
1990s	Increase in managed care enrollments (47)	More restrictions and oversight of insurance benefit Marketing competition increased
1992	Prescription Drug User Fee Act (60)	Required manufacturer's fees to support hiring additional FDA reviewers, expedited pre-marketing product reviews, increased new product competition
1997	Draft Guidance for Industry on DTC Broadcast Advertisements	Allowed broadcast advertisements to contain limited risk and benefit information Required adequate provision for alternate sources of complete labeling information
1999	Final Guidance for Industry on DTC Broadcast Advertisements	Retained the main features of the Draft Guidance Made commitment to evaluation within two years
2001	ASPE conference on the effects of DTCA on health care use, costs and outcomes	Focused attention on research methodology and the need for empiric evidence of DTCA's effects

Sources: 24, 25, and as noted in individual references.

of Representatives Report on what would become the Food, Drug and Cosmetic Act of 1938 (FDCA) were clear that the FDCA was "not intended to restrict in any way the availability of drugs for self-medication. On the contrary, it is intended to make self-medication safer and more effective" (69). For the next 13 years, manufacturers determined what was, and was not, a prescription drug, although FDA could sue if it disagreed (1). The Durham-Humphrey Amendment of 1951 (21) finally clarified the distinction between over-the-counter (OTC) and prescription drugs, requiring prescription drugs to display the legend "CAUTION: Federal law prohibits dispensing without a prescription."

Until 1962, the Federal Trade Commission (FTC) regulated advertising both for OTC and for prescription drugs. During the thalidomide tragedy the Kefauver-Harris Amendment, passed to strengthen the drug approval process (42), placed prescription drug advertising under FDA's jurisdiction. Consequently, different criteria regulate the content of OTC vs prescription drugs advertised directly to consumers.

The FDCA does not define what constitutes a prescription medicine advertisement; consequently, the FDA has interpreted it to "include information (other than labeling) that is sponsored by a manufacturer and is intended to supplement or explain a product" (43). Under the FDCA, drug advertising must not be false, misleading or lacking in material facts, and its information must represent a *fair balance* of the drug risks and benefits. Specifically, it has to contain a *brief summary* from the approved product label (the package insert), consisting of "the product's adverse event profile, contraindications, warnings and precautions" (31). Clearly, the brief summary was likely to be anything but brief.

Consumers cannot directly purchase prescription medications in the United States, so DTCA was a minor aspect of prescription drug promotions from the 1950s through the 1970s. Changes began in the 1980s with the first product-specific DTCA, a price advertisement for Rufen®, a branded generic of ibuprofen (58). A 1981 advertisement in *Reader's Digest* for pneumococcal vaccine (Pneumovax®) and a 1982 *Washington Post* advertisement for acyclovir at People's Drug Store signaled a growing interest in DTCA, though the companies referred to these as public service campaigns (7). Pfizer's "Healthcare Series" in 1982 was an early example of *help-seeking* promotions: It described symptoms and diseases, but did not mention specific drug products (7). The 1982 campaign for Oraflex® (benoxaprofen) changed the direction of DTCA from price or general information to product-specific promotion by distributing press kits and videotapes for the broadcast media. However, the drug was soon associated with adverse events and deaths, leading the manufacturer to withdraw it from the market voluntarily (7). This experience illustrates a substantial concern for DTCA—that it promotes drugs recently approved for marketing at a time when their side effects are less understood, particularly if these side effects are less common, have a long induction period, or result from interaction with other agents or patient characteristics (62).

Based on many DTCA proposals, in 1983 the Commissioner of the FDA requested a moratorium on direct-to-consumer advertising of prescription drugs (43). During this moratorium, the FDA encouraged (*a*) a dialogue among consumers, health professionals and industry; and (*b*) research and interpretation of findings on DTCA. The moratorium ended in 1985 with the FDA concluding that the existing regulations, intended for physicians, provided adequate consumer protection and would be applied to all prescription drug advertisement audiences (16). FDA also requested pre-dissemination submission of DTCA; even though many companies voluntarily sought prior review of promotional materials, it has never been a requirement. The *brief summary* and *fair balance* requirements effectively eliminated broadcast advertisements from pharmaceutical companies' consideration and lessened print advertisements' promotional appeal since their effectiveness message might be negated in the viewer's mind by the contraindications and side-effect warnings that would follow.

FDA recognizes three categories of DTCA: (*a*) *Product-claims* promote a specific product and must present a *brief summary* with a *fair balance* of benefits and of risks; (*b*) *Help-seeking advertisements* provide information on diseases or conditions—they encourage consumers to consult their physician regarding treatment options; specific prescription drugs or treatments cannot be mentioned, nor can the advertisement contain linkages to materials identified with a specific product; and (*c*) *Reminder advertisements*: these materials cannot contain or suggest the clinical role of the product (17).

Although pharmaceutical companies have sponsored *reminder* and *help-seeking* advertisements, not having both the product name and the condition it treated in the same promotional communication meant that they provided little helpful information to consumers (58). However, the growing use of *reminder* and *help-seeking* advertisements coupled with their limited utility as a source of consumer information led to a reconsideration of the guidelines for broadcast advertisements. FDA Commissioner David Kessler was opposed to expanding broadcast DTCA; consequently, his departure in January 1997 removed one of the remaining barriers to change for DTCA (58).

Broadcast advertisements pose special challenges to communicating risk effectively: They are too brief to include information as extensive and as technical as a *brief summary*. Thus, the 1997 Draft Guidance on DTC Broadcast Advertisements permitted broadcast media (radio, television advertisements, or telephone communications) to address risk differently: A *major statement* containing the most important product risks had to be either in the audio or in the audio and visual segments of the advertisement, but *adequate provision* was required for consumers to access the full package labeling (31). *Adequate provision* required the advertisement to contain four additional sources from which the consumer could obtain the labeling information: (*a*) a toll-free telephone number, (*b*) a currently running print advertisement that contained the information, (*c*) referral to a health care provider, and (*d*) an Internet web page address. In this draft FDA committed to "evaluating the effects of the guidance [within two years of the publication of the final guidance], including effects on the public health of DTC promotion, and specifically of consumer-directed broadcast advertising" (20).

FDA "is unaware of any data supporting the assertion that the public health . . . is being harmed, or is likely to be harmed, by the Agency's actions in facilitating consumer-directed broadcast advertising" (29). Consequently, the final Guidance, issued August 1999, is essentially the same as the draft (28). Surveillance and enforcement of the Guidance covering DTCA is the responsibility of the Division of Drug Marketing, Advertising and Communications in the FDA (26). Advertisements that do not satisfy regulatory requirements may result in enforcement actions, ranging from an Untitled Letter to a Warning Letter, to "recalls, seizures, injunctions, administrative detention and criminal prosecution" (29).

Examples of print DTCA for tamoxifen (Figure 1, see color insert) and for simvastatin (Figure 2, see color insert) demonstrate the *major statement* and *adequate provision* requirements. In addition, these advertisements illustrate information on risk factors for the specific condition (Figure 1) and on nondrug alternatives (Figure 2).

In summary, current regulations have not eliminated the strong, divergent positions that stakeholders have regarding DTCA. Proponents assert that DTCA: (*a*) provides educational information, (*b*) enhances the physician-patient relationship, (*c*) improves adherence to prescription drug regimens, (*d*) stimulates competition, and (*e*) results in lower prices for pharmaceuticals. Opponents counter that: (*a*) consumers lack the expertise to assess the quality of the content of the advertisements, (*b*) the promotional aspect of advertising will not communicate risk information effectively, (*c*) it will harm the physician-patient relationship, (*d*) it will lead to increased drug prices, (*e*) it will lead to increased liability and litigation, and (*f*) it will encourage overuse of medications (17).

BACKGROUND: PATIENT AUTONOMY

Patient autonomy has become a primary feature of the patient-physician relationship, demonstrated through measures such as informed consent, advance directives, and shared decision-making among treatment options (64). Autonomy extends to health promotion, emphasizing the need for increased control over factors influencing one's health; for example, the Ottawa Charter for Health Promotion specifically included access to information as one of the factors (13).

Surprisingly, patients want more information on their medical conditions and treatment options than they express directly to their physician (22, 63). The gap between the information that consumers want and what is routinely provided is small for instructions on medication use (3%), but substantial for serious side effects (22%), for possible drug interactions (23%), for how the medication works (23%), and for how much it costs (19%) (61). National, cross-sectional surveys from 1982 to1994 indicate that physician counseling has increased, mostly on risk information, but only slightly (52).

By raising consumer awareness about prescription medications, DTCA increases the likelihood that patients may discuss these products with their physician. Supporting patient autonomy, however, will require physicians to employ a variety of communication skills to encourage patients to be active partners in their own care

(63). When patients evaluated the quality of communication with their physician as low, they have been less likely to accept their doctor's decision not to prescribe a requested advertised drug without considering other actions or ways to get the drug (9). Another consequence of effective communications is that adherence to medical recommendations is higher among satisfied patients (63) and when client preferences are included in the therapeutic selection (14). Twenty-five percent of a national survey's respondents reported trusting their doctor's advice less than in previous years, whereas 18% were dissatisfied with the information they received about their medical conditions and treatment options (61). Across many medical conditions and dosing regimens patient adherence too often ranges from suboptimal to subtherapeutic (35), emphasizing the importance of the patient-physician relationship for effective pharmacotherapy. Some physicians may require training to develop their communication skills; a study using objective evidence, including video analysis, demonstrated that physicians overestimated how much they communicated with patients regarding the patient's view of a treatment regimen and of medication risks (48).

Patient Package Inserts are another potential source of prescription drug information for patients. Patient Package Inserts, according to FDA, "provide patients with information that will promote safe and effective use and . . . provide patients with adequate and meaningful information sufficient for them to participate in evaluating the benefits, risks, and proper use of drug products" (32). In 1968, FDA's first labeling directed to patients was a brief caution on isoproterenol inhalers, not to exceed the recommended dose (overuse could produce a paradoxical, fatal response). However, even a diminished pilot program was cancelled in 1982 based on the anticipated program costs and the intervening growth of voluntary patient information initiatives. For example, the National Council on Patient Information and Education was formed in 1982 as a nonprofit coalition "to stimulate and improve communication of information on the appropriate use of medicines to consumers and health care professionals" (53).

CONCEPTUAL FRAMEWORK

DTCA is one component of a broader marketing and communication plan for businesses; as such, it represents an investment of resources that can be evaluated by its return-on-investment. Although purely financial models may measure the achievement of business goals, they are silent on health consequences. Useful research models must also provide insight into the behavioral components of health care, permit interactions among the participants, and accommodate levels of analysis ranging from the individual patient to the pharmaceutical industry. There is no single, comprehensive framework that organizes the diverse behavioral, economic, policy, and business models that may be applied to DTCA research. Consequently, alternate conceptual frameworks may be appropriate depending on the specific issues being examined and on the perspectives of the research.

The Office of the Assistant Secretary for Planning and Evaluation (ASPE) of the U.S. Department of Health Human Services convened a conference on May 30, 2001, to stimulate the examination of methodological issues concerning the effects of DTCA on health care use, costs, and outcomes (54). The ASPE-sponsored workshop highlights the importance of a broadly applicable model of DTCA and its effects: A common conceptual framework would encourage increased and consistent rigor in the analyses undertaken, and a cumulative body of results for research findings.

EVIDENCE AND PERSPECTIVES

Promotional expenditures for prescription drugs have experienced unprecedented growth during 1996–2000; over this four-year period total promotional spending increased 71%. Although DTCA increased 216% in absolute dollars, it was just 57% of the increase in product-sampling to office-based physicians and only 8.1% greater than the increase in office promotional expenditures (39). These collective expenditures represent an expanded marketing strategy to influence the prescription drug decisions of physicians and patients.

Although the dollar increase in DTCA is large, it is a selective strategy. DTCA tends to be concentrated in a small number of products; 24 brands represented 74% of 1999 spending. These same 24 brands had a 42% increase in 1999 sales compared with a 14.4% increase for all other drugs. Three antiallergy medications together accounted for 4.4% of the increase in all prescription drug expenditures in 1999, while the increase in sales of atorvastatin, a cholesterol-reducing agent, represented 5.5% of the total increase in 1999 prescription drug expenditures. Taken together, these 24 brands represented 34% of the increase in all prescription drug spending from 1998 to 1999 (23).

Both the magnitude of the increase in DTCA and the shift in media purchased for promotional activities are striking. Television consumed 27% of the DTCA spending in 1997, whereas magazines were 62% and newspapers 10% of the expenditures. This distribution is consistent with the guidance on broadcast advertisements not being released until August 1997. Preliminary data for 2000 report television expenditures at 64%, magazines at 30%, and newspapers at 5% (66) (Table 2).

FDA SURVEILLANCE

FDA's continuing surveillance and review of DTCA against regulatory requirements focus resources on priorities; the first in a class of advertisements may have a more vivid or durable impact, thus it will be reviewed in more detail than will subsequent submissions in the class. During July and August 2000, for example, there were four first-in-class submissions; by contrast, during May to August 2000 per-month DTC broadcast submissions ranged from 9 to 28. FDA's enforcement actions against pharmaceutical companies for broadcast DTCA were most

TABLE 2   U.S. pharmaceutical prescription market

	Promotional expenditures 1996–2000 (numbers in thousands)						
	1996	1997	1998	1999	2000 (*Est)	% Increase 1996–2000	$ Increase 1996–2000
Professional spending	8,372,925	9,921,825	11,157,102	12,020,012	13,200,876	58%	4,827,951
Office promotion	2,457,785	2,785,320	3,386,247	3,606,675	4,037,702	64%	1,579,917
Hospital promotion	552,206	579,232	670,681	712,989	765,261	39%	213,055
Journal advertising	458,627	510,268	497,782	470,435	484,430	6%	25,803
Retail value of samples	4,904,307	6,047,005	6,602,392	7,229,913	7,913,483	61%	3,009,176
Direct-to-consumer spending	791,402	1,068,773	1,316,701	1,847,593	2,500,000	216%	1,708,598
Total promotion	9,164,327	10,990,598	12,473,803	13,867,605	15,700,876	71%	6,536,549

Source: IMS HEALTH & Competitive Media Reporting. Integrated Promotional Services May 10, 2001. Plymouth Meeting, PA.

numerous (13) during the first year following the 1997 Draft Guidance. Product claim advertisements received the most enforcement actions, for reasons such as statements or suggestions that efficacy was greater than the labeling supported, that minimized risk, lacked fair balance, or contained implied, unsubstantiated claims (55).

The absolute number of enforcement actions is small; however, reviewing advertisements after they have been broadcast may not offer sufficient protection. The American Public Health Association resolution on DTCA calls for increased FDA funding and more assertive reviews (12), while the American College of Physicians-American Society of Internal Medicine's position supports mandatory pre-broadcast clearance (4). Regulatory oversight is critical since many consumers believe television advertising implies drug safety. Of people who had seen a doctor within the last three months, 29% believed "only the safest prescription drugs are allowed to be advertised to the public" (30). A separate study reported that 43% believed drugs could be advertised only if they were completely safe: People with these and similar misconceptions regarding regulatory oversight view DTCA more positively (8). These beliefs provide the context within which risk information and potential benefits of an advertised drug are considered, as such they suggest a positive bias for some consumers and a potential filter if corrections are required following FDA's review. Almost half of the people who see a DTCA do not pursue the sources required by *adequate provision* for additional information and, thus, miss the opportunity for a more balanced, comprehensive assessment of benefit and risk. Having the four specific alternate sources for additional information is intended to provide formats that address the diversity in consumers' information processing abilities and in their preferences for privacy. Those who do seek more information most often get it from a doctor (81%) or a pharmacist (52%), and, much less frequently, the advertisement's toll-free number (18%), the Internet (18%), a magazine (14%), or a newspaper (7%) (30).

FDA has planned to evaluate the effects of the Guidance within two years of its publication in final form. Pending authorization by the Office of Management and

Budget, FDA anticipated conducting two national telephone surveys on DTCA in 2001, one directed to physicians and one to patients who have seen a physician within the last three months.

PATIENT AWARENESS AND ACTIVATION

Unaided consumer awareness of prescription drug advertisements increased from 63% in 1997 to 81% in 1999, though it was flat for 2000 (80%) and higher for those taking medications. However, in response to questions concerning advertisements for ten named prescription medicines, 91% of consumers were aware of advertisements for at least one. Among respondents who had the medical condition for which the advertised medicine is indicated, only two of the ten medications had consumer awareness greater than 50%, suggesting a failure of DTCA to reach its intended audience. Awareness of DTCA varies by race or ethnicity, socioeconomic strata, and gender; it is lower among minorities, particularly Hispanics, and those with annual household incomes below $25,000. Women are, in general, more likely to be aware of prescription drug advertisements than are men (61).

From a public health perspective, inappropriate patient demand for advertised prescription drugs wastes resources at best and, at worst, may lead to the use of unnecessary or inappropriate medications. Appropriately targeted messages might lead consumers who are not currently in treatment but might benefit from it to seek care for their condition(s). However, the failure of a large portion of DTCA to reach its target audience, at a time when it might influence decisions and in a form that the audience can comprehend, means that alternative approaches, tailored to specific groups, are required. The information needs of patients with chronic conditions are particularly important, because patients are assuming a larger role in managing their chronic conditions (34). Since pharmaceutical companies not only continue but increase their spending on DTCA despite this failure suggests that they are (a) basing their decisions on early financial results and (b) learning how to use these new broadcast marketing options most effectively.

The impact of different advertising media (TV vs magazine advertisements) and the format of the benefit and risk information were studied long before FDA's 1997 Guidance on DTCA. Research comparing fictitious prescription drug advertisements on television and in magazines concluded that patients had a greater sense of empowerment in prescription drug decisions after reading magazine advertisements, which contained comparatively more information. Television advertisements, by contrast, led consumers to seek more specific drug information and to be more likely to consult a physician. To provide effective guidance and oversight of DTCA, regulations governing risk communication must be adaptable to diverse media, formats, and consumer information processing styles (50).

The percent of patients being advised of side effects and precautions for their medications, though improving during 1992 to 1998, is below 40% for physician offices and 25% for pharmacies. In the past, few patients requested information

(<10%), and, perhaps, patient questions were pre-empted by distributing printed instruction sheets and brochures (27). Although consumers reported that they were more likely to take their medication if they believed they had received adequate risk information, few (40%) report reading at least half of the information in small print, although more (93%) felt they would if they were especially interested in the drug (30). Broadcast advertisements are only required to include the most important product risks, making this, alone, an incomplete source of information for viewers.

Beyond raising basic awareness regarding prescription drugs, the educational potential of DTCA appears to be failing. Of ten heavily promoted products, only one had consumer awareness both of the product and of its indication above 70% (Claritin®), one at 40% (Lipitor®), and the remainder at 32% or less. These statistics, calculated on the basis of those who were aware of the advertisement for any of the ten medications, may overstate the effectiveness of DTCA messages since products are also mentioned in news reports, press releases, and in other forms that may elevate awareness for specific agents (61).

From 1997 to 2000, about 30% of consumers who saw a DTCA spoke with their physician about it. Women more often than men spoke with their doctor, and people currently taking a prescription drug did so more often than those not taking one. Conversely, 78% of consumers who felt that DTCA provided inadequate risk information, and 82% who felt the benefit information was inadequate, did not discuss the drug with a doctor (61). Advertising aims to increase not only awareness but also sales; therefore, a central question is whether DTCA viewers request those specific, advertised medications when they do speak with their doctor. Of the 32% of consumers who spoke with their doctor about an advertised prescription drug, 26% requested that drug, with higher percentages for the younger and lower percentages for the older age groups (61).

Improved adherence to pharmacotherapy is another potential benefit of DTCA. Some consumers who are taking a prescription medicine and see an advertisement for it report feeling better about the product's safety (36%) and that they are more likely to take their medicine (22%). The reported likelihood of taking their medication increases if the consumers' doctor provides information on serious side effects or if the drug's mechanism of action is explained (61).

DTCA has the potential to support the belief in patient autonomy in clinical decisions. Forty-seven percent of persons who had seen or heard a prescription drug advertisement agreed that "Advertisements for prescription drugs help me make better decisions about my health," and 62% of those who had seen a physician within the last three months believed that "Advertisements for prescription drugs help me have better discussions with my doctor about my health" (30). Based on their self-report, the prescription drug advertisement motivated 27% of survey respondents to discuss a medical condition or illness that they had not previously discussed with a physician (30). These responses, however, reflect beliefs and not necessarily that patient autonomy is actually increasing. DTCA still does not provide enough risk (30%) or benefit (25%) information for many consumers to speak with their physician about the advertised drug. For those 55 plus years of age, a population at high risk for medical conditions and for prescription drug use, DTCA is least adequate in providing the necessary information on risks or benefits to lead them to discuss it with their doctor (61).

Experiments that assessed factors conducive to risk communication in television prescription drug promotions demonstrate its complexity. Risk information was conveyed more effectively when both audio and visual information were presented, rather than video alone; when the risk information was dispersed throughout the commercial rather than in a single warning at the end; and when specific rather than general disclosures were used. Formats with more opportunities for consumers to process information increased awareness and knowledge of risks. However, consumers appear to trade-off risk and benefit information; recalled benefits declined as the number of risks included in the commercial increased (51).

An advertisement for a prescription drug had led 51% of respondents in an FDA survey to seek more information, most often from their doctors and/or a pharmacist. However, some consumers may get a different message. Twenty-four percent of those who had seen or heard a DTCA agreed that "Prescription drug advertisements make it seem like a doctor is not needed to decide whether a drug is right for me" (30). A better understanding of risk communication is essential to avoid consumer overconfidence.

PHYSICIAN REACTION AND RESPONSE

DTCA effectiveness in promoting communication between a patient and his or her physician depends, in part, on the physician's support of the patient's participation. Physicians' participatory decision-making styles vary with their patients' characteristics; it is generally lower with patients who are 75 plus years of age, less educated, a minority or male, but it increases with the continuity of the physician-patient relationship (40).

Communication and intuition of both the physician's and the patient's prior expectations also influence subsequent drug-prescribing decisions. When a patient expects to receive a medication, the odds of it occurring increase; however, when the physician believes the patient expects a medication, the odds increase even more (15).

National data from 1992 through 1997, the years preceding the 1997 Guidance on broadcast advertisements, established a relationship between the modest DTCA occurring then and the physician diagnosing and prescribing an advertised product (70). More recently, 71% of consumers who requested an advertised medicine from their physician received a prescription for that product, whereas 10% received a prescription for a different product; only 19% did not receive a prescription (61). An earlier study, predating the FDA's guidance for broadcast DTCA, reported that the most frequent reason physicians gave for suboptimal prescribing was patient demand (65). There are no data on the appropriateness of the

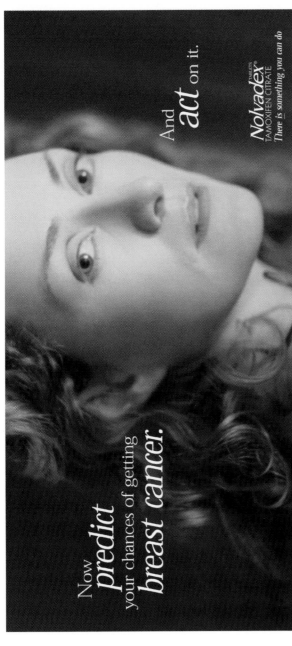

Figure 1 Direct-to-consumer advertisement for Tamoxifen Citrate. Source: AstraZeneca

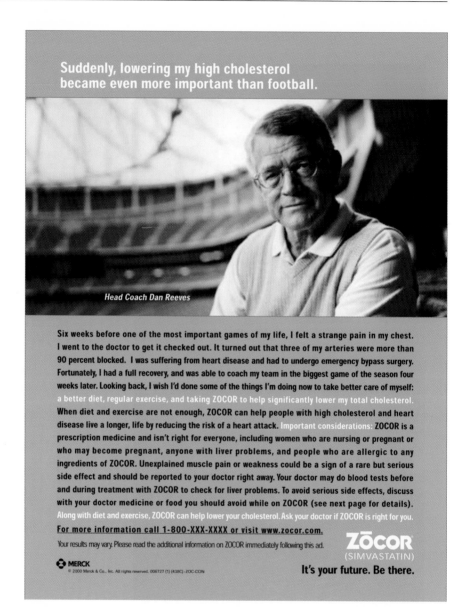

Figure 2 Direct-to-consumer advertisement for Simvastatin. Source: Merck & Co., Inc.

prescribing for those who request and receive the advertised drug; nor a contrast with those who request prescription drugs for reasons other than DTCA. An alternative approach to understanding the impact of DTCA is to test consumers directly for the appropriateness of their medication. When patients receiving one of three nonsedating antihistamines, nasal steroids, or both received specific IgE testing, 65% were determined not to have allergies, suggesting that the nonsedating antihistamines might be eliminated appropriately in these patients (67). Does DTCA cause patients and physicians to overlook nondrug options? Physicians provided information on nondrug therapies to 53% of consumers who asked about an advertised medication, but this was higher for certain conditions: diabetes (77%), high cholesterol (92%), or being overweight (84%). When these nondrug therapies are discussed, patients report greater trust in their doctor's advice and are less worried that the health plan is more concerned about money than about what is their best treatment (61).

In FDA's survey, 13% of persons who had seen a physician within the last three months mentioned an advertisement or brought something about the drug to the visit with the physician. Eighty-one percent of these people reported that the physician seemed to welcome the questions, but 4% said the doctor seemed to get angry or upset; overall, 85% were satisfied with the doctor's reactions to questions about the advertised drug. Although 50% of the patients received the prescription drug requested, 29% were counseled to make behavioral or lifestyle changes (30).

The physician's perspective of this interaction may be less positive than the consumer's. In a systematic sample of active members of the American Academy of Family Physicians, 84% held negative views of television and radio advertisements, many seeing them as biased and misleading. Overall, 80% felt DTCA was not a good idea, though 56% felt DTCA informed consumers who might seek care for conditions that otherwise may have been neglected (46). These paradoxical findings reflect the multiple realities concerning DTCA. An American Medical Association Member Pulse poll reported similar reservations; most respondents (72%) believed that DTCA's impact on their practice was negative (5).

MEDIA

The values the marketing industry brings to DTCA are demonstrated in the criteria weights for the second annual *DTC Excellence Awards*: 60% for "creativity and breakthrough execution of the marketing strategy" and 40% for "bottom-line results in achieving marketing objectives and growing sales" (44).

Content analysis of advertisements from popular magazines from 1989 to 1998 reported the drug information quality to be inconsistent, with information on alternative treatments mentioned in only 29% of the advertisements, lifestyle changes in 24%, and the success rate for the advertised drug in just 9% (10).

The imminent transition of leading branded products from brand only to brand plus generic options has intensified consumer marketing for these agents. As some brand name–only prescription drugs reach the end of their patent life, manufacturers are introducing versions of their products that may require fewer doses, thus potentially improving compliance but also securing a patent extension for these versions. DTCA for some products extends to inducements such as coupons for discounts or a free period of supply, such as a month. Others are raising the level of competition by assuring the achievement of targeted therapeutic endpoints or the price of the medication will be refunded (43). Consequently, complete information with a fair balance of drug risks and benefits is more necessary than ever.

Direct marketing to consumers also includes the Internet. Most people over 50 do not use the Internet (57), yet most who do have used it to obtain health-related information (56). Online prescription drug information was more likely to be sought by women, current prescription drug users, and people who reported less trust in their doctor's advice. Minorities and people living in households with annual incomes below $25,000 have lower rates of Internet use (61). Internet sites sponsored by pharmaceutical companies must also conform to the Guidance for DTCA and are monitored by FDA's Division of Drug Marketing, Advertising and Communications. Consequently, a product-specific website will typically use its home page to direct consumers and health care professionals to separate areas for information. However, health information on the Internet may require that consumers have advanced reading levels to comprehend it, reinforcing the need for health care professionals to "individualize" the information for patients (11).

UNINTENDED CONSEQUENCES

DTCA may alter existing standards and perceptions of liability. Courts have held that physicians are the "learned intermediary" between pharmaceutical companies and patients, and that they are responsible for judging a prescription drug's benefit and risk for their patients. Consequently, the "learned intermediary" doctrine has protected pharmaceutical companies from having to provide patients with product warnings directly. Litigation against pharmaceutical companies challenge this doctrine when the companies communicate directly with patients (33). With DTCA the manufacturer's liability may increase, particularly if FDA requires corrective actions subsequent to a pharmaceutical company's consumer-directed broadcast advertisement.

By communicating directly with consumers and bypassing health plans, pharmaceutical companies may have provoked health plans to bypass pharmaceutical companies and initiate actions with the FDA directly. DTCA of prescription nonsedating antihistamines has been substantial, as have the sales for these products. Wellpoint Health Networks filed a citizens' petition to have these drugs switched from prescription to OTC status, claiming that they are safer than the current OTC antihistamines. FDA's Advisory Committees agreed that these drugs are safe for OTC use (6), though FDA may lack authority to require a pharmaceutical company to market its approved prescription product as an OTC instead.

Another potential consequence of DTCA is civil litigation against pharmaceutical companies based on advertised claims for their products. In August 2001, a consumer coalition of more than 50 groups, the Prescription Access Litigation project (59), initiated a class action lawsuit against Schering-Plough Corporation based on the content of its DTCA for Claritin® (18). The coalition alleges that research reports Claritin's success to be 50%, but the lawsuit alleges that the advertisements contain "numerous statements of unqualified and absolute effectiveness and no mention of the limited usefulness of Claritin® products" (19). At the time of the news reports, Schering-Plough had not seen the charges and so did not comment on the contents of the lawsuit (18).

DISCUSSION

Direct marketing of pharmaceuticals to consumers follows social and economic trends that recognize patient autonomy in medical care and increasingly require consumers to consider costs in their prescription drug decisions. DTCA is also a reaction of the pharmaceutical industry to more restrictive prescription drug benefits and to the uncertain effectiveness of relying only on traditional marketing activities such as medical journal advertisements and detailing individual physicians.

The evidence for DTCA's impact on pharmaceutical sales is as impressive as is the lack of evidence concerning its impact on the health of the public. The limited research on DTCA suggests that there has been some improvement in communicating risk and benefit information since August 1997, but it is modest and insufficient. The values for excellence in marketing, increasing brand awareness and sales, are not those of public health. The postmarketing period for a new drug requires what has been termed pharmacovigilence, i.e., active identification and follow-up of unexpected consequences as experience is gained with the new prescription drug product. Experimental research, employing sound methodologies and examining actual consumer decisions and their health consequences, is needed to guide effective communications on drug risk and benefit in different media. Although the available evidence suggests that advertisements containing adequate risk information are more likely to motivate consumers to speak with their doctor, a substantial portion of consumers still believe the risk information in DTCA is inadequate. It may indicate the limits of traditional marketing approaches that most people having the conditions treated by the most heavily promoted DTCA cannot associate the product with the condition it treats.

Recognizing the blend of promotion and information contained in DTCA, physicians and the American Pharmaceutical Association are ambivalent about product-specific advertisements directed to consumers because many consumers may be unable to separate the two. Yet one appeal of these advertisements for consumers arises from the failure of physicians and pharmacists to provide drug information to them. Empirical evidence of DTCA's impact on physicians' and pharmacists' practices and on patient health outcomes is needed; does DTCA lead to meaningful dialogue and empowered patients or merely to motivated but ill-informed purchasers? When used alone, patient leaflets are an inadequate and ineffective response to the consumer's need for information. As the preferred information source, health care professionals should communicate directly with their patients and employ the leaflet as a reminder rather than as the main message. However, changing clinical practice to accommodate more time for patient communications will be exceedingly difficult if it must occur as an uncompensated, additional task in an already compressed schedule.

Much of the drug information on the Internet is not provided through the support, sponsorship, or promotion of a pharmaceutical company and, therefore, is beyond FDA's jurisdiction. As a practical matter, rescinding the DTCA guidance would not remove the consumer's exposure to drug information. The unregulated information would continue to exist (and likely increase), but it would no longer be balanced by communications that must meet a standard of fair balance in representing a pharmaceutical's effectiveness, side effects, and contraindications. If anything, it is FDA's mandatory review of advertisements after broadcast that should be reconsidered. What is the evidence that corrective advertisements actually change the consumer's initial perception?

The practice and regulation of DTCA must move beyond the positions and interests of stakeholders to an evidence-based examination of impacts. DTCA is unlikely to disappear; consequently, the central issues are how to create and how to regulate the communications most effectively. The resurgence of health care costs may result in more people receiving health insurance benefits as defined contributions by their employer rather than as defined benefits. Under that arrangement more choices and trade-offs will be made by the individual consumer, raising the significance and potential impact of DTCA that address prescription drug concerns from the patient's perspective.

Visit the Annual Reviews home page at www.annualreviews.org

LITERATURE CITED

1. Abood RR, Brushwood DB. 2001. *Pharmacy Practice and the Law*, p. 104. Gaithersburg, MD: Aspen Publ. 3rd ed.
2. Acad. Managed Care Pharm. 2001. *AMCP Position Statement on Direct-to-Consumer Advertising*. http://www.amcp.org/public/legislative/position/014.html. Accessed June 26
3. Am. Assoc. Retired Persons (AARP). 2001. Health care. In *The Policy Book: AARP's Public Policies 2001*, pp. 6–129. http://www.aarp.org/ppa/chapter6.pdf
4. Am. Coll. Physicians—Am. Soc. Intern.

Med. (ACP-ASIM). 1998. 9 Oct. *Direct to Consumer Advertising of Prescription Drugs, Executive Summary*. http://www.acponline.org/hpp/pospaper/dtcads.htm
5. Am. Med. Assoc. (AMA). 2001. *Direct-to-Consumer Advertising Gets Physicians Attention*. AMA Member Pulse poll. http://www.ama-asn.org/ama/pub/article/1615-3027.html. Accessed June 11
6. Am. Pharmaceut. Assoc. (APhA). 2001. *FDA Advisory Panels State Antihistamines Safe for OTC Use*. http://www.aphanet.org/lead/safeOTCuse.html. Accessed May 27

7. Basara LR. 1992. Direct-to-consumer advertising: today's issues and tomorrow's outlook. *J. Drug Issues* 22(2):317–30

8. Bell RA, Kravitz RL, Wilkes MS. 1999. Direct-to-consumer prescription drug advertising and the public. *J. Gen. Intern. Med.* 14(11):651–57

9. Bell RA, Wilkes MS, Kravitz RL. 1999. Advertising induced prescription drug requests: patients' anticipated reactions to a physician who refuses. *J. Fam. Pract.* 48(6):446–52

10. Bell RA, Wilkes MS, Kravitz RL. 2000. The educational value of consumer-targeted prescription drug print advertising. *J. Fam. Pract.* 49(12):1092–98

11. Berland GK, Elliott MN, Morales LS, Algazy JI, Kravitz RL, et al. 2001. Health information on the Internet: accessibility, quality, and readability in English and Spanish. *JAMA* 285(20):2612–21

12. Bradley LR, Zito JM. 1997. Direct-to-consumer drug advertising. *Med. Care* 35(1):86–92

13. Can. Public Health Assoc. (CPHA). 1986. 17-21 Nov. *Ottawa Charter for Health Promotion.* Ottawa: Can. Public Health Assoc. First Int. Conf. Health Promot., Ottawa, Canada

14. Chewning B, Sleath B. 1996. Medication decision-making and management: a client-centered model. *Soc. Sci. Med.* 42(3):389–98

15. Cockburn J, Pit S. 1997. Prescribing behavior in clinical practice: patients' expectations and doctors' perceptions of patients' expectations—a questionnaire study. *Br. Med. J.* 315:520–23

16. Direct-to-consumer advertising of prescription drugs; withdrawal of moratorium. 1985. 9 Sept. 50 *Fed. Regist.* 174:36677–78

17. Direct-to-consumer promotion; public hearing. 1995. 16 Aug. 60 *Fed. Regist.* 158:42581–84

18. Dooren JC. 2001. Consumer groups sue Schering-Plough to stop Claritin ads. *Wall Street J.*, Aug. 9. http://interactive. wsj.com/archive/retrieve.cgi?id=DI-CO-20010809-006125.djm. Accessed Aug. 10

19. Dow Jones Newswires. 2001. Schering-Plough accused of making false ads for Claritin. *Wall Street J.*, Aug. 9. http:// interactive.wsj.com/archive/retrieve.cgi?id =DI-CO-20010809-005998.djm. Accessed Aug. 10

20. Draft Guidance for Industry. 1997. 12 Aug. Consumer-directed broadcast advertisements: availability. 62 *Fed. Regist.* 155:43171–73

21. Durham-Humphrey Prescription Drug Amendment of 1951. 1997. 21 U.S.C. §§ 353, 355

22. Elwyn G, Edwards A, Kinnersley P. 1999. Shared decision-making in primary care: the neglected second half of the consultation. *Br. J. Gen. Pract.* 49:477–82

23. Findlay SD. 2001. Direct-to-consumer promotion of prescription drugs: economic implications for patients, payers and providers. *Pharmacoeconomics* 19(2):109–19

24. Food and Drug Admin. Consumer. 2001. The story of the laws behind the labels. June 1981. http://vm.cfsan.fda.gov/~lrd/histor1b.html. Accessed July 27

25. Food and Drug Admin. Cent. Drug Eval. Res. 2001. Timeline: chronology of drug regulation in the United States. http:// www.fda.gov/cder/about/history/time1htm. Accessed July 27

26. Food and Drug Admin. Div. Drug Mark., Advert. Commun. (DDMAC). 2001. http:// www.fda.gov/cder/handbook/ddmacrev. htm. Accessed May 26

27. Food and Drug Admin. Div. Drug Mark., Advert. Commun. 2001. National surveys of prescription medicine information received by consumers. http://www.fda.gov/ cder/ddmac/y2ktable.htm. Accessed May 28

28. Food and Drug Admin. 1999. Aug. Guidance for industry: consumer-directed broadcast advertisements. http://www.fda. gov/cder/guidance/index/htm

29. Food and Drug Admin. 2001. Guidance for industry: consumer-directed broadcast advertisements, questions and answers. http://www.fda.gov/cder/guidance/1804q &a.htm. Accessed May 28

30. Food and Drug Admin. Off. Med. Policy Div. Drug Mark. Advert. Commun. 1999. Attitudes and behaviors associated with direct-to-consumer (DTC) promotion of prescription drugs, preliminary survey results. http://www.fda.gov/cder/ddmac/DTC title.htm. Accessed May 28, 2001

31. Food and Drug Admin. 1999. *Prescription Drug Advertising*. 21 Code of Federal Regulations Pt. 202.1(e)

32. Food and Drug Admin. 1980. 12 Sept. Prescription drug products: patient package insert requirements. 45 *Fed. Regist.* 179:60759

33. Gemperli MP. 2000. Rethinking the role of the learned intermediary: the effect of direct-to-consumer advertising on litigation. *JAMA* 284(17):2241

34. Green LW, Mullen PD, Friedman RB. 1986. An epidemiological approach to targeting drug information. *Patient Educ. Couns.* 8:255–68

35. Haynes RB, McKibbon KA, Kanari R. 1996. Systematic review of randomized trials of interventions to assist patients to follow prescriptions for medications. *Lancet* 348:383–86

36. Healthy People 2010. Nov. 2000. Leading health indicators. http://www.health.gov/ healthypeople/document/HTML/Volume 2/17 Medical.htm. Accessed June 21, 2001

37. Hollon MF. 1999. Direct-to-consumer marketing of prescription drugs: creating consumer demand. *JAMA* 281(4):382–84

38. Holmer AF. 1999. Direct-to-consumer prescription drug advertising builds bridges between patients and physicians. *JAMA* 281(4):380–82

39. *Houston Chronicle*. 2001. Drug firms use coupons in marketing blitz. 4 June, Bus. Sect., p. 5

40. IMS HEALTH/Competitive Media Reporting. 2001. 10 May. *Integrated promotional services, U.S. pharmaceutical prescription market 1996–2000*. Plymouth Meet., PA

41. Kaplan SH, Gandek B, Greenfield S, Rogers W, Ware JE. 1995. Patient and visit characteristics related to physicians' participatory decision-making style. *Med. Care.* 12:1176–87

42. Kefauver-Harris Amendment: Drug Amendments of 1962. 2000. 21 U.S.C §§ 321, 355

43. Kessler DA, Pines WL. 1990. The federal regulation of prescription drug advertising and promotion. *JAMA* 264(18):2409–15

44. Koberstein W. 2000. TC excellence awards. *Pharm. Exec.* 20(6):156–59

45. Kravitz RL. 2000. Direct-to-consumer advertising of prescription drugs: implications for the patient-physician relationship. *JAMA* 284(17):2244

46. Lipsky MS, Taylor CA. 1997. The opinions and experiences of family physicians regarding direct-to-consumer advertising. *J. Fam. Pract.* 45(6):495–99

47. Lyles A, Palumbo FB. 1999. The effect of managed care on prescription drug costs and benefits. *Pharmacoeconomics* 15(2):129–40

48. Makoul G, Arntson P, Sekofield T. 1995. Health promotion in primary care: physician-patient communication and decision making about prescription medications. *Soc. Sci. Med.* 4(9):1241–54

49. Mechanic D. 2001. The managed care backlash: perceptions and rhetoric in health care policy and the potential for health care reform. *Milbank Q.* 79(1):35–54

50. Morris LA, Brinberg D, Kleinberg R, Rivera C, Millstein LG. 1986. The attitudes of consumers toward direct advertising of prescription drugs. *Public Health Rep.* 101(1):82–89

51. Morris LA, Magis MB, Brinberg D. 1989. Risk disclosures in televised prescription drug advertising to consumers. *J. Public Policy Mark.* 8:64–80

52. Morris LA, Tabak ER, Gondek K. 1997.

Counseling patients about prescribed medication: 12 year trends. *Med. Care* 35(10): 996–1007

53. Natl. Counc. Patient Inform. Educ. 2001. http://www.talkaboutrx.org/about.html. Accessed Sept. 1

54. Off. Assist. Sec. Plan. Eval., Dep. Health Hum. Serv. (ASPE). 2001. *Assessing the Impact of Direct-to-Consumer Advertising on Health Care Use, Costs and Outcomes.* 30 May. Washington, DC: GPO

55. Ostrove NM. 2000. Update on DTC promotion. 11 Sept. http://www.fda.gov/cder/ddmac/ostrFDLI900/index.htm. Accessed May 28, 2001

56. Pew Internet/Am. Life Proj. 2000. The online health care revolution: How the web helps Americans take better care of themselves. http://www.pewinternet.org/. Accessed June 21, 2001

57. Pew Internet/Am. Life Proj. 2000. Who's not online: 57% of those without Internet access say they do not plan to log on. http://www.pewinternet.org/. Accessed June 21, 2001

58. Pines WL. 1999. A history and perspective on direct-to-consumer promotion. *Food Drug Law J.* 54:489–518

59. Prescription Access Litigation. 2001. http://www.prescriptionaccesslitigation.org. Accessed: Sept. 1

60. Prescription Drug User Fee Act of 1992. PL 102–571. *Congr. Rec.* H9099–100. Sept. 22

61. Prevention Magazine. 2001. *International Survey on Wellness and Consumer Reactions to DTC Advertising of Rx Drugs: 2000–2001.* Emmaus, PA: Rodale Press

62. Rogers AS. 1991. Unintended drug effects: identification and attribution. In *Pharmacoepidemiology: An Introduction,* pp. 64–74. Ohio: Harvey Whitney Books. 2nd ed.

63. Roter DL, Hall JA. 1992. *Doctors Talking to Patients/Patients Talking to Doctors: Improving Communication in Medical Visits.* Westport, CT: Auburn House

64. Schneider CE. 1998. *The Practice of Autonomy.* New York: Oxford Univ. Press

65. Schwartz RK, Soumerai SB, Avorn J. 1989. Physician motivations for nonscientific drug prescribing. *Soc. Sci. Med.* 28(6):577–82

66. Scott-Levin. 2001. DTC advertising audit. *Pharm. Exec.* 21(2):110–16

67. Szeinbach SL, Boye M, Muntendarn P, O'Connor R. 2001. 28 March. *Diagnostic assessment and resource utilization in patients prescribed non-sedating antihistamines.* Presented at Am. Coll. Osteopath. Fam. Physicians (ACFP), Philadelphia

68. Temin P. 1980. *Taking Your Medicine: Drug Regulation in the United States.* Cambridge, MA: Harvard Univ. Press

69. US Congress. 1938. *Food, Drug, and Cosmetic Act.* HR 2139, 75th Congr., 3rd sess., 1938, p. 8; quoted in Ref. 68, p. 45

70. Zachry W III. 2000. *A study of the relationship of direct-to-consumer advertising to epidemiologic indices.* PhD thesis. Univ. Texas at Austin

Annu. Rev. Public Health 2002. 23:93–113

CHALLENGES IN MOTOR VEHICLE SAFETY

Patricia F. Waller

Transportation Research Institute, University of Michigan, 1779 Crawford Dairy Road, Chapel Hill, North Carolina 17516; e-mail: pwaller@umich.edu

Key Words   motor vehicle injury, federal motor vehicle safety standards, drunk driving, occupant restraints, motorcycle safety

■ **Abstract**   Reductions in motor vehicle injury and death represent a major public health success. Since the advent of the federal program in highway safety in 1966, motor vehicle deaths have dropped dramatically, not only in rates per miles driven but also in absolute numbers. Key to this success has been the broad-based comprehensive approach promoted by the program's first administrator, a public health physician. The federal program provided leadership and coordination that leveraged national, state, and local programs to bring about safer vehicles, improved traffic records, more effective enforcement, enormously improved emergency medical services, more responsible judicial systems, and many other accomplishments. Although progress has been made on many fronts, major areas addressed here include federal motor vehicle safety standards, alcohol safety programs, occupant restraint laws and usage, and speed limits. The achievements in motor vehicle safety provide a model for other injury control efforts.

MAGNITUDE OF MOTOR VEHICLE INJURY PROBLEM

Injury, both intentional and unintentional, is the leading cause of death from ages 1 to 45; because it so disproportionately strikes the young, it also accounts for more years of potential life lost before age 75 than either cancer or heart disease. Motor vehicle injury is the largest single component of these losses (6). The National Highway Traffic Safety Administration (NHTSA) estimates that in the year 2000, 41,800 people died in traffic crashes in the United States, and an additional 3,219,000 were injured (29). The International Federation of Red Cross and Red Crescent Societies identifies traffic accidents as "a worsening global disaster destroying lives and livelihoods, hampering development and leaving millions in greater vulnerability" (19, p. 20). Traffic crashes are identified as the ninth leading cause of death worldwide, and it is estimated that by the year 2020 traffic crashes will be the third largest cause of death and disability in the world, "far ahead of war, HIV and other infectious disease. Most of this increase will take place in the cities of developing nations" (19, p. 8).

0163-7525/02/0510-0093$14.00

BACKGROUND

The record of motor vehicle injury prevention nevertheless represents a major success in public health in the United States. Historically, motor vehicle deaths in the United States climbed as the number of motor vehicles and the miles driven increased. Except for decreases in the early years of the Great Depression and during World War II, the annual death toll rose steadily until in 1966 it was over 53,000.

The U.S. Congress responded with the National Highway Traffic and Motor Vehicle Safety Act and the Highway Safety Act of 1966, creating a new federal program to address motor vehicle safety. Under this legislation, the federal government has the power to establish safety standards for new motor vehicles and to create standards for a variety of highway safety programs implemented at the state level.

Traffic deaths continued to rise until they reached a high of 56,278 in 1972, declined somewhat in response to the energy crisis in the mid-1970s, then rebounded and fell until dropping below 40,000 in 1992, for the first time since 1961. Since then the numbers have fluctuated between 40,000 and 42,000. Exposure to risk, as measured by vehicle miles traveled, has increased more or less steadily, so that the fatality rate per hundred million vehicle miles has declined dramatically. In 1966 it was 5.5, and 3 was viewed as a barrier that could probably never be broken. In 1999 it dropped to 1.5 but increased to 1.6 in 2000. If the 1966 rate had continued, in 1999 there would have been over 147,000 motor vehicle fatalities in the U.S. This remarkable achievement is attributable to many factors, but very significant among these is the leadership at the inception of the federal program.

A PUBLIC HEALTH APPROACH

The first head of the National Highway Safety Bureau, subsequently the National Highway Traffic Safety Administration (NHTSA), was a public health physician, William Haddon. In addition to establishing motor vehicle safety standards, he developed standards for a wide range of state-administered programs to promote traffic safety, such as driver licensing, alcohol-impaired driving, motorcycle safety, and traffic records. States were required to show satisfactory progress toward meeting these standards, with potential loss of funding for failure to do so. Two other important components of the program were funding provided to every state to create a highway safety program, headed by a Governor's Highway Safety Representative, and a research program to develop much-needed information to improve highway safety practices.

Historically, motor vehicle crashes have been attributed primarily to human error. Even today it is often stated that "Research indicates that approximately 85 percent of the causation factors associated with crashes are attributed to the driver" (1). However, the way many studies are conducted largely determines the outcome. Primary focus is on driver behavior, and in-depth investigation of the vehicle and roadway is rarely conducted. State crash reporting forms include few options for recording vehicle or highway factors that may contribute to the crash. In contrast, there are many options for deciding whether a driver factor was involved. Whenever "driver error" is given as an explanation, it should be asked, "What modifications in the vehicle design, the highway design, or the overall circumstances may have reduced the likelihood that the driver would behave in such a way that a crash occurred?" It is this approach that the federal program brought to motor vehicle safety.

Initially, much of the focus was on environmental changes, particularly the motor vehicle itself. Because crashes could not be totally prevented, structural changes to make vehicles more "crashworthy" were implemented. Steering columns were made to be energy absorbent, so that they collapsed upon impact, rather than penetrating the driver's chest. Windshields were modified so that on impact from an unrestrained occupant, the windshield deformed but did not break apart; the energy was absorbed but the occupant was not subjected to jagged glass that could sever carotid arteries. Vehicle doors and latches were strengthened so that doors did not fly open in a collision but rather retained occupants within the vehicle. Safety belts became standard equipment in all new passenger vehicles, and programs were implemented to promote their use.

One of the most important contributions Haddon made to highway safety, and indeed to injury control in general, was his conceptual approach to the problem, illustrated by the Haddon Matrix. This matrix is based on the epidemiological model that includes host, agent, vector, and environment. Gordon (11) had previously described such an approach to injury prevention, and subsequently Gibson (10) identified uncontrolled exchange of energy as the causal factor in injury. However, Haddon (12) organized the potential points of intervention in a way that facilitates the identification of countermeasures. Rather than focusing primarily on the driver in the precrash phase, countermeasures may occur within any of the cells (see Figure 1). This was the first comprehensive public health approach to a major injury problem.

DATA SYSTEMS

There has been a serious lack of adequate data for sound evaluation of countermeasures. Even figures for traffic fatalities varied from one source to another, in part because different criteria were used, e.g., death at the scene of the crash, within 24 hours, 30 days, 120 days, or 365 days. Definitions of injury and injury severity vary from one jurisdiction to another, and the threshold for a reportable property-damage-only crash still varies. Some states do not require a police report unless there is an injury, precluding meaningful comparisons across states.

In 1975, NHTSA initiated a national database of all crashes involving at least one motor vehicle, occurring on roadways open to the public, and resulting in at least one fatality (e.g., vehicle occupant, pedestrian, cyclist). Originally labeled the Fatal Accident Reporting System (FARS), and currently known as the Fatality Analysis Reporting System, it is compiled from existing state documents, with most information coming from police reports. Other sources include vehicle

Factors

Phases		Human	Vehicle	Physical Environ-ment	Socio-economic Environ-ment
	Pre-Crash	Alcohol Use Fatigue	Brakes Tires Mainten-ance	Sight Distance Rumble Strips	Speed Limits DWI Laws
	Crash	Belt Use Age/ Fragility	Vehicle Size Air Bags	Guardrails Breakaway Signs	
	Post-Crash	Alcohol Use Physical Condition	Fuel System Integrity	EMS Response Rehab Care	EMS Training Trauma Care Systems

Figure 1   Haddon matrix. (Adapted from Reference 12)

registration files, driver license files, highway department data, vital statistics, death certificates, medical examiner or coroner reports, hospital records, and emergency medical data. This database is a census and in 1999 included 127 data elements covering the crash itself (e.g., time of day, day of week, weather, light condition, number of vehicles, roadway features, traffic controls); the vehicle (e.g., body type, make and model, vehicle weight, impact point, extent of deformation, registered owner); driver (e.g., height and weight, license status, drinking, violations charged); and persons (e.g., age and sex, seating position, restraint system use, injury severity).

Although FARS data from the early years are not as complete or reliable as in subsequent years, especially for variables such as alcohol, this database has been invaluable for monitoring problems and progress in highway safety. It is used by NHTSA for its own purposes and is available to researchers for independent analyses. The progress that has been made is in large part attributable to our ability to identify and describe problems and evaluate effectiveness of solutions based on careful analyses of FARS and related data systems. Opinion is replaced with factual evidence—the data make the case for where we should put our resources, as well as the outcome of such investments.

Because of important differences between fatal and nonfatal crashes, NHTSA developed the General Estimate System, or GES, based on a nationally representative sample of crashes involving at least one motor vehicle traveling on a traffic way and resulting in property damage, injury, or death. All information in the GES is based on police crash reports; no other sources are accessed. In 1999 it included 91 data elements. These data are used in conjunction with FARS to get a more comprehensive picture of traffic crashes in the United States. NHTSA and other federal agencies compile other databases that are also relevant to motor vehicle injury prevention.

Both FARS and GES build on programs in place at the state level, but the federal program uses a single format that is comparable across jurisdictions. Local data are often insufficient for in-depth analyses of causes and effectiveness of interventions, but analyses of national data provide information that can be applied at a local level. These data systems are an excellent illustration of federal leadership and coordination to create resources useful to the entire field and jurisdictions at every level. The cost of the national databases is relatively low because they build on existing state databases. The importance of good data cannot be overemphasized. They are essential for a science of injury control.

Four major motor vehicle safety issues are described that illustrate the importance of the multifaceted approach espoused by Haddon: the Federal Motor Vehicle Safety Standards (FMVSS), drunken driving, occupant restraints, and speed limits. In each area we have witnessed remarkable progress, although in the latter case much of the success was short-lived. Factors contributing to the success, as well as the failure, of countermeasures are described.

FEDERAL MOTOR VEHICLE SAFETY STANDARDS

Legislation enacted in 1966 requires the federal government to establish safety standards for new motor vehicles sold in the United States, whether of domestic or foreign manufacture (24). These FMVSS apply only to new vehicles, so that their full effect is not realized immediately but rather extends over eight or more years. The standards usually apply initially only to passenger cars; when light trucks and utility vehicles became popular, they often did not have to comply.

Early FMVSS, including softer instrument panels, head restraints, energy-absorbing steering columns, and high penetration-resistant windshields, have saved thousands of lives and prevented tens of thousands of injuries. Some, such as improved braking systems and improved side lighting, have also prevented hundreds of thousands of crashes. Table 1 shows estimates of lives saved annually from selected FMVSS, once all vehicles on the road meet the standard (C. Kahane, personal communication). Note that most estimates shown include lives saved for passenger cars only, although some standards now include light trucks as well.

Other FMVSS apply to occupant restraints and motorcycles helmets. FMVSS stipulate that safety belts meeting certain standards be available for use, and that child safety seats and motorcycle helmets meet certain requirements. Based on 1998 usage rates, Table 2 shows estimated annual savings attributable to these FMVSS.

TABLE 1   Estimated lives saved and injuries prevented annually by selected FMVSS, assuming all vehicles are equipped[a]

Standard	Safety device		Estimates for	
			Lives saved	Injuries prevented
105	Dual master cylinder/front disc brakes	pc*	320	24,000
108	Side marker lamps	pc + lt	—	93,000
108	Center high mounted stop lamps	pc + lt	—	55,000 hospitalizations
201	Softer/wider instrument panels	pc[b]	550	8000
202	Head restraints	pc[b]	—	85,000 whiplash injuries
203/4	Energy-absorbing steering columns	pc[b]	1300	24,000 hospitalizations
205	High-penetration resistant windshields	pc[b]	—	47,000 AIS[c] 2–4, 189,000 total
208	Air bags	pc + lt	3066	?
214	Side door beams	pc[b]	480	9500 hospital, 24,500 total

[a]C. Kahane, personal communication; reference 24.
[b]NHTSA has so far estimated benefits for passenger cars only, even though the standard now also applies to light trucks.
[c]Abbreviated Injury Scale (2).

FMVSS shown in Table 1 are effective even if human error occurs. Improvements in steering columns, windshields, and side door beams are operative even if the driver is drunk, inexperienced, medically disabled, or otherwise functioning at less than optimal performance. In contrast, for FMVSS in Table 2, additional measures are needed to ensure that the devices are used appropriately. Obviously,

TABLE 2   Estimated lives saved annually by FMVSS for occupant protection, based on 1998 usage rates[a]

Standard	Safety device		Estimates for	
			Lives saved	Injuries prevented
208	Safety belts—front seat	pc + lt	11,088	?
208	3 pt. belts—back seat	pc[b]	277	?
212	Child safety seats	pc + lt	299	?
218	Motorcycle helmets	mc	500	?

[a]C. Kahane, personal communication; reference 24.
[b]NHTSA has so far estimated benefits for passenger cars only, even though the standard now also applies to light trucks.

one cannot wear a safety belt if none is available, but simply providing a belt is not sufficient for protection. Education, legislation, and enforcement must be added to these FMVSS for maximum benefits.

DRUNKEN DRIVING

History

In 1904, not long after the first motor vehicle fatality in the United States, the *Journal of Inebriety* reported:

> We have received a communication containing the history of twenty-five fatal accidents occurring to automobile wagons. Fifteen persons occupying these wagons were killed outright, five more died two days later, and three persons died later.... A careful inquiry showed that in nineteen of these accidents the drivers had used spirits within an hour or more of the disaster.... [T]he ... management of automobile wagons is far more dangerous for men who drink than for driving of locomotives on steel rails.... The precaution of railroad companies to have only total abstainers guide their engines will soon extend to the owners and drivers of these new motor wagons (50).

The United States was one of the first nations to identify drunken driving as a criminal offense. Before World War I, both California and New York enacted laws prohibiting impaired driving (51). As other states followed suit, it became apparent that there were major difficulties in defining "impairment" or "drunk driving." The advent of chemical tests enabled objective measure of blood alcohol concentration (BAC), but initially such testing required a blood sample. Drunken driving occurs primarily at night and on weekends, and blood tests required that a police surgeon be available to draw the sample. Not until the development of an inexpensive breath test, which did not require a health professional to administer, was it possible to obtain BAC information routinely. Even with objective BAC data, there was argument as to whether everyone was impaired at a given level. There was little evidence relating BAC to crash risk per se.

Establishing Crash Risk

The first study that compared alcohol use in crash-involved injured drivers with alcohol use by drivers not involved in crashes but using the same roads was reported in 1938 (14). Based on BACs of both driver groups, Holcomb found that injured drivers were 12-1/2 times more likely to have been using alcohol. Although subsequent studies strongly suggested that alcohol increased crash risk, it was the Grand Rapids Study that clearly established increasing risk of crash as BAC increases (3). Comparison drivers, using the same roads at a time and day corresponding to those at which the crash occurred, were tested. The full range of crashes was included, and driver interviews provided additional background information. Almost 6000 crash-involved drivers and over 7500 comparison drivers were included. Data analyses clearly demonstrated elevated crash risk as BAC rises. At BAC 0.08% crash risk is about fourfold the risk at zero BAC; at BAC 0.10%, tenfold; and at 0.15%, 25-fold. A subsequent major study in Vermont confirmed these figures, although the study population was statewide and primarily rural (33).

Alcohol Safety Action Programs

Early on, the federal program placed major emphasis on combating drunken driving. In 1969, Alcohol Safety Action Programs (ASAPs) were established throughout the nation, addressing drinking and driving from a systems approach, taking into account many factors that contribute to the problem. Eventually there were ASAPs in 35 communities. They included programs in five categories of countermeasures: enforcement, judicial and legislative, presentence investigation and probation, rehabilitation, and public information and education.

Unfortunately, there was uneven implementation of program components, and so many interventions were occurring at once that it was almost impossible to determine what made how much difference. Although enormous effort was devoted to analyzing the data and heroic attempts were made to show beneficial effects, the evidence is weak, at best (20). Nevertheless, the ASAPs provided the foundation on which to build broad-based comprehensive programs to combat drunken driving.

Other Countermeasures

In the 1970s, drunken behavior was still generally acceptable, a natural part of growing up, and was even portrayed as humorous in movies and other entertainment venues. Efforts to curb drunken driving were tolerated but not widely taken seriously. Although the ASAPs did not achieve their intended goal, they were instrumental in raising public awareness of a drunk-driving problem and the need to address it. The federal program provided support for exploring the dimensions of the drunk-driving problem, and information was accumulating. In 1978, a summary of what was known about alcohol and highway safety was published (20), documenting the magnitude of the problem, as well as what was then known about countermeasures.

The *Zeitgeist* was changing, for both alcohol use and drinking and driving. The per capita consumption of pure alcohol, whether consumed as beer, wine, or spirits, peaked in 1980 but began a decline in 1982 that continued until about 1990, after which it appears to have stabilized, at least through 1995 (32, 44). Abstention rates increased for whites, African Americans, and Latinos, and for both women and men. Frequent heavy drinking also decreased or remained the same, except for Latinos, who showed some increase. During this same period, the proportion of fatal crashes involving alcohol also decreased. (Prior to 1982, national data on alcohol involvement in fatal crashes are not reliable.)

Citizen Action Groups

In 1978, Remove Intoxicated Drivers (RID) was organized in New York State, and in 1980, another group began in California, Mothers Against Drunk Drivers (MADD, later becoming Mothers Against Drunk Driving). By the time these organizations were created, a wealth of information already linked alcohol to highway injury and death, but there was still not general acceptance of existing countermeasures. Mandatory sanctions for conviction of drunken driving were rarely imposed because convictions were likely to be reversed on appeal by juries who considered the sanctions too draconian. Judges accepted plea bargaining to reduced offenses to ensure that some sanction would be imposed. The advent of the citizen action groups appears to be a critical factor in changing societal attitude toward drunken driving.

These groups were created by persons who had experienced the loss of a family member or friend as a result of a drunk driver. They spoke with undeniable credibility and pursued activities that neither researchers nor state agencies could have explored. Members of RID and MADD monitored courtrooms and compiled records on conviction rates of individual judges. Tragic stories of injury and death at the hands of drunken drivers, as well as lenient consequences imposed by judges, were widely disseminated. These groups took their message to state and national legislators, making sure the media were involved. They also provided counseling to new victims and helped them channel their grief into action. When then President Reagan declared that the minimum drinking age was a state, not a federal, concern, these groups generated enormous publicity and were represented at the signing of federal legislation creating a national minimum drinking age. Although still relatively small in number, RID and MADD have had an enormous influence in translating research findings into public policy.

It is instructive to note the opposition to these efforts. In December 14–16, 1988, the U.S. Surgeon General convened a national workshop on drunk driving, assembling a wide array of experts. In contrast to most such meetings, this workshop addressed more than simply enforcement, traditional education, and treatment, and included such topics as pricing and availability of alcohol, advertising and marketing, and citizen advocacy. The National Association of Broadcasters, the American Association of Advertising Agencies, and the Association of National Advertisers were all invited to participate, but all refused, suggesting that the workshop lacked "good balance." All three suggested that the workshop be cancelled, and one claimed that "At best, this workshop is designed to politicize the emotional tragedy of drunk driving. At worst, it is a total abuse of the policy-setting process" (49, p. 96).

The National Commission Against Drunk Driving was to speak at the opening plenary session, but it, too, refused at the last minute. On the day the workshop began, the National Beer Wholesalers Association filed in the U.S. District Court to cancel the meetings. The workshop was allowed to continue, but with the provision that other interested parties could contribute comments until January 31, 1989;

final workshop recommendations would not be made before February 28, 1989, and comments received subsequent to the workshop would be considered in the final recommendations (49). There was a virtual blackout of news coverage of the workshop. This experience clearly highlights the influence and strength of vested interests opposed to major public health efforts.

Initially, MADD focused completely on the drunk driver and punitive measures. From the outset, RID took a broader approach, addressing factors that may encourage drunk driving, such as alcohol advertising. This more comprehensive approach alienated the media, which were dependent on alcohol advertising money. Consequently, RID was slower to grow and gain recognition. MADD, focusing only on the offender and ignoring issues such as advertising and underage drinking, garnered much broader support, including from the alcohol industry. However, over time MADD extended its agenda to include factors that contribute to the problem. Perhaps it was necessary initially to emphasize only the offender and punitive measures in order to achieve an effective public image.

In 1982, 57% of traffic fatalities were alcohol related, whereas in 1999, only 38% were alcohol related. The proportion of drivers in fatal crashes who have been drinking has decreased for all age groups and both sexes (25, Table 15, 18; Figure 10).

OCCUPANT RESTRAINTS

Safety Belts

Safety belts were first made available to the public in the late 1950s, but to acquire them required enormous effort on the part of the consumer. Not surprisingly, they were rarely installed, although usage rates were high for those who had them. In 1966, the federal government required new passenger cars sold in the United States to be equipped with lap belts for the driver and outboard passenger in the front seat. Shoulder belts were required beginning in 1969. However, there was no concerted effort nationwide to promote belt usage. In 1970, Victoria, Australia, implemented safety belt usage legislation, and showed an increase in use from 30% to 80%. Other nations gradually followed suit, but in the United States there was strong feeling that a person has the right to decide for himself or herself whether to use such protection, and legislators were sympathetic to this position.

Robert Sanders, a county health department pediatrician in Tennessee, set out to address a problem that affected his patients but over which he had little control. He recognized that infants and small children were at risk in moving vehicles, but there was no requirement that they be transported safely. Working with other pediatricians in the state, in 1978 he succeeded in obtaining the very first legislation requiring that infants and small children be transported in approved child safety seats. No one could reasonably argue that infants and small children should decide for themselves whether to be transported safely.

Interestingly, once the legislation was enacted, the police made no effort to enforce it. When pediatricians met with the police, they were told that police saw their role as fighting crime, not ticketing mothers with young children. Together pediatricians and police developed a program whereby police carried in their patrol cars an approved child safety seat. When a driver was ticketed, the police offered to install the seat and show the driver how to use it properly. When the driver appeared in court and returned the seat, if proof of purchase of an approved seat could be shown, the ticket was dropped. This stratagem may be the best example of a carrot-and-stick approach to promote a highway safety measure.

The Tennessee example was replicated elsewhere. Since 1985 child restraint use laws have been in effect all 50 states. However, as parents and others learned of the importance of occupant restraints, their concern extended to other children and to their own welfare. The initial measures to protect small children, never a large part of the occupant safety problem, became the basis for occupant protection for the rest of the population. As of May 2001, 49 states and the District of Columbia had laws requiring the use of seat belts for at least some vehicle occupants (17).

Because of FMVSS and improvements in highway design, motor vehicles are much safer today than they were 30 or 40 years ago. Even so, safety belt use enormously improves the probability of surviving a crash. For front seat occupants in passenger cars the risk of fatal injury is reduced about 45%, and the risk of moderate to critical injury is reduced about 50%. For light trucks, the corresponding figures are 60% and 65%, respectively (26).

Occupant restraint laws vary in who is covered (17). Most belt use laws apply only to front seat occupants. Laws applying to children vary in both age at which law is applicable and location in the vehicle (18). Fines for offenses also vary, from $10 to $500. Only three states assess driver record points for violations.

Most seat belt laws entail secondary enforcement, that is, an officer may not apprehend a person for a seat belt violation unless the stop is made initially for some other reason. With primary, or standard, enforcement, the person may be apprehended for the seat belt violation alone. It is more difficult for police to enforce secondary laws, not only because the driver must have committed some other violation, but also because the other violation usually takes precedence, and the seat belt violation is dropped. As of May 2001, only 17 states, the District of Columbia, and Puerto Rico had enacted primary enforcement laws. There is good evidence that, for the same level of ticketing, primary enforcement results in significantly higher rates of belt use (about 15 percentage points) and thus lower injury rates (5, 26).

Based on a nationwide survey conducted routinely by NHTSA, belt use as of the fall of 2000 was 71% (30). However, the survey included only passenger vehicles (passenger cars, vans and sports utility vehicles, and pickups), driver, and outboard passenger in the front seat, during daylight hours. Belt use varies among these vehicle types and across regions of the country. There is also strong reason to believe that belt use rates are lower at night and in other seating positions. Nevertheless, belt use rates have soared above early estimates of what could be achieved in the U.S. Increasing these rates further offers one of the most promising means of reducing motor vehicle injury and death.

Air Bags

Perhaps no other highway safety measure has been as controversial as air bags. First proposed in the 1960s, their implementation became embroiled in bitter political battles that included industry, government, and the research community. Some early supporters touted them to the exclusion of seat belts, focusing on the desirable public health goal of making protection passive so as not to require active participation of those being protected. The argument often became one of either belts or bags. Because the U.S. standard required air bags to provide adequate protection for an unbelted male driver of 170 pounds, the driver air bag had to be much larger and more forceful than that required in Europe, where it was considered a supplemental protective device.

The more powerful air bag used in the U.S. had unfortunate consequences. Small drivers, especially older women, seated close to the steering wheel, and infants and children in the front seat became victims of the air bag. By April 2001, there had been 175 confirmed air bag-related fatalities, 104 of whom were children. At least 71 of the child fatalities were unrestrained or improperly restrained. Of the 71 adult fatalities, most were not using seat belts, and at least 27 were females with a height of 62 inches or less (31). Although on balance the air bags are saving lives (see Table 1), the resulting fatalities are totally unacceptable. A federally mandated protective device simply may not result in so many fatal injuries, especially to children.

Air bags are now generally recognized as supplemental devices that are most effective when the occupant is properly restrained in a seat belt. It is recommended that infants and small children be in the back seat, or, if the vehicle has no back seat, that there be a device to deactivate the air bag. Drivers are advised to sit at least 10 inches back from the steering wheel. Efforts are being made to devise "smart" air bags that will respond in a way appropriate to occupant characteristics, including position and weight, and crash characteristics, including point of contact and level of impact.

Initially, air bags were designed for protection in frontal crashes, but side air bags are now available on some vehicle models to provide protection in side impacts. Eventually, there may be inflatable devices distributed widely throughout the vehicle, including air bag protection from the front, the side, the roof, and the foot well of the vehicle, as well as inflatable seat backs and/or head restraints (35). Safety belts are becoming more "intelligent," so as to provide several levels of restraint depending on how the occupant loads the belt in a given crash. Belts are also becoming easier to use, especially for older occupants and others who may have difficulty reaching and fastening belts.

Motorcycle Helmets

In 2000, there were 2680 fatalities to motorcycle riders, an increase from 2472 in 1999. Injuries also increased, from 50,000 to 58,000 (29). There may be no other highway safety measure that has been so thoroughly demonstrated to be effective in reducing serious injury and death as motorcycle helmets. Under the best of circumstances, motorcycles are inherently more dangerous to operate than four-wheeled vehicles. Their death rate per mile driven is about 16 times that of passenger cars (27). When the federal standards were established, few states required use of motorcycle helmets. Helmet laws were included in the motorcycle safety standard, and guidance and assistance were provided to states to move toward compliance. Although there was no time frame for implementation, the federal government monitored progress and brought pressure to bear in the absence of reasonable movement toward compliance. Ultimately, NHTSA could invoke sanctions against a state, in the form of loss of funds for highway safety and highway construction.

By 1975 all but two states required helmet use by motorcyclists.[1] Injuries and deaths plummeted. California had no law, and a strong organized opposition emerged. The author was told by the California Office of Traffic Safety that state legislators had received threats to their homes and families should they support such a law. NHTSA moved to invoke sanctions, whereupon Congress was inundated with letters of protest from across the country. In response, in 1976 Congress removed NHTSA's authority to invoke sanctions in the absence of permission from Congress and expressly removed motorcycle helmet laws from any such consideration. Seventeen states revoked their laws, and another 19 states seriously weakened theirs by limiting required use to younger ages, usually below age 18 (15). Predictably, helmet use went down, and motorcyclist deaths increased.

After witnessing increases in casualties, some states reinstated their motorcycle helmet laws (23), and in 1991 Congress created incentives for states to implement helmet laws. These incentives were discontinued in 1996, and again state laws were weakened or rescinded. Again, motorcycle fatalities increased. Arkansas and Texas seriously weakened their laws in 1997. Previously, all motorcyclists were required to use helmets, but in August and September 1997, Arkansas and Texas, respectively, limited the requirement to riders under 21 and/or riders who had not had rider education or did not carry ample medical insurance. Helmet use in Texas decreased from over 97% to 66%, and in Arkansas usage fell from 97% to 51% (36).

A comprehensive analysis of the impact of helmet laws in the United States, covering a 22-year period and taking into account other factors such as speed limits, alcohol control policies, seat belt laws, level of enforcement, climate, age distribution of the population, and hospital density per square mile, found that helmet laws are associated with a 29% to 33% decrease in annual per capita motorcyclist fatalities (39). The authors conclude that the value of the law is

---

[1]California and Illinois had no law. Utah required helmet use only where the speed limit was 35 mph or higher.

considerable. In 1997, when half the states had helmet laws for at least part of the year, there were 2102 motorcyclist fatalities, but there would have been at least 763 more had there been no laws. The authors applied a value of $3 million per life, for a savings of $2.29 billion.

In 1999, only 21 states, the District of Columbia, and Puerto Rico required helmet use by all motorcycle operators and passengers (27). Interestingly, California is one of them. Three states have no laws, and another 26 states require helmet use only for persons under a specified age, usually 18 (16). Age-limited laws result in usage rates similar to those in states with no laws requiring helmet use. The age of a rider cannot be ascertained without stopping the vehicle, so that these laws are essentially unenforceable. The only effective helmet use law is one that requires all riders to wear helmets.

Motorcycle helmet laws illustrate an important point in highway safety, as well as other public health measures. When the effectiveness of a countermeasure requires active participation of the individual, there must be broad public support for laws and enforcement to be effective. NHTSA estimates that helmets are 67% effective in preventing brain injuries (27), and in the event of injury, the bulk of costs are borne by the larger society (37). A federal court has upheld the legality of helmet laws, saying:

> The public has an interest in minimizing the resources directly involved. From the moment of the injury, society picks the person up off the highway; delivers him to a municipal hospital and municipal doctors; provides him with unemployment compensation, if after recovery, he cannot replace his lost job; and, if the injury causes permanent disability, may assume the responsibility for his and his family's continued subsistence. We do not understand the state of mind that permits the plaintiff to think that only he himself is concerned.

This decision was subsequently affirmed by the U.S. Supreme Court (41).

Today few would argue that helmets are not effective. The reasons for rescinding laws or failing to enact them have more to do with individual rights and the freedom to choose. Historically, this balance between society's legitimate health interests and personal freedom has wavered as public policy was formulated on issues such as child labor, sanitation measures, and fluoridation of water. With fewer than half the states requiring helmet use for all motorcycle riders, motorcycle helmet laws are a current illustration of such disagreement on a major public health measure of demonstrated effectiveness.

SPEED LIMITS

In roadway travel, speed in and of itself does not kill; only when a collision occurs does speed become a factor, with higher speeds increasing impact exponentially. The difference between 55 mph and 60 mph is much greater than the difference between 40 mph and 45 mph.

Based on early research, it was generally accepted that speed variation rather than speed per se contributes to increased probability of crash, and that speeds below the average speed of traffic are as likely to cause crashes as those above (43). Subsequent work has seriously challenged this assumption, and more recent research (40) concludes that the evidence is equivocal so far as lower speeds are concerned. It is clear, however, that crash risk increases with increasing speed, other things being equal. Drivers in the top 15th percentile of speed pose a much greater risk than those traveling in the bottom 15th percentile (22). On all road types, risk of injury or fatality increases with increasing speed. Shinar (40) concludes that the costs of speed-related crashes are much higher than the relationship between speed and crash probability would indicate, because high-speed crashes are associated with more serious, and hence more costly, injury.

In 1974 a National Maximum Speed Limit (NMSL) of 55 mph was implemented, primarily to conserve fuel. Highway fatalities dropped dramatically, but the reasons were unclear. At the request of Congress, a review of the evidence was conducted by the Transportation Research Board (7). Their report made the following points.

Fuel Economy   The 55 NMSL was enacted for purposes of fuel economy. Even though additional reserves have since been discovered, the total amount of fossil fuel on the planet is finite. Fuel consumption rises disproportionately as speed increases.

Safety   Although there was a dramatic decrease in motor vehicle deaths, much of the decrease was attributable to factors other than the speed limit, e.g., reduced exposure, elimination of much discretionary driving. Nevertheless, the report estimated that lower speeds continued to save lives, with between 2000 and 4000 lives saved in 1983. In addition, 2500 to 4500 fewer serious, severe, and critical injuries, as well as 34,000 to 61,000 fewer minor and moderate injuries in same year could be attributed to the lower speed limit.

Motor Vehicle Injury Costs   The costs associated with motor vehicle injuries constitute a significant proportion of the nation's health care expenditure. These costs cross state lines. A driver licensed in one state may drive in other states, and if an injury occurs elsewhere, the emergency care and medical attention must be provided there. Even if one is not injured, costs incurred through taxes and health and auto insurance premiums reflect increases in injury-associated costs. The cost of motor vehicle injuries is a national problem, not a state or local one. Currently, the U.S. Department of Transportation estimates the average societal costs of a motor vehicle fatality to be about $2.7 million, so that the 41,800 deaths in 2000 represent societal costs of almost $113 billion.

Time Savings   The greatest controversy surrounding the 55 mph NMSL concerns the increase in travel time. It was found that, "On the basis of average trip lengths and average speeds, most personal vehicle travel slowed down by the 55 mph speed limit involved time losses of less than 3 minutes" (7, p. 115). Over a year's time, on a per-licensed-driver basis, the lower speed limit added about 7 hours of driving. One committee member observed, "Over a year's time the 55 NMSL would cost me perhaps a day and a half. However, if my day were broken up into two and three minute pieces, I could not get anything done." In other words, time savings in small pieces do not translate into time units that are realistically useable.

It was further found that it cost "roughly 40 years of driving per life saved and serious injury averted." However, "the average life expectancy of motor vehicle accident victims in 1982 was about 41 years" (6, p. 120). This comparison does not consider the enormous time costs incurred by family and friends of the killed and injured, or the time costs associated with the more numerous injuries that are less serious or crashes involving property damage only. Crashes are also the primary cause of traffic delays, creating enormous time costs to travelers. Thus, when all time costs are considered, the total societal time costs are less at 55 mph than they are at higher speeds.

Equity   There is an issue of equity in relation to distribution of time costs. With the lower speed limit, whatever time costs are incurred are distributed more evenly across the entire traveling public, usually in small segments of time for any one traveler. In contrast, at higher speed limits, time costs are borne disproportionately by those involved in crashes, especially those who are injured and killed, and those who are delayed in traffic by the incidents. The trade-off between arriving at a destination a few minutes later versus sacrificing a young life should not be difficult to choose.

Other issues not addressed in the report but relevant to the speed limit debate include the presence of large trucks on the highway, size variation in the vehicle fleet, consumer costs, national security, balance of payments, environmental impact, and the changing demographics of our population, especially our driving population. Each of these is discussed briefly below.

Trucking

In 2000, of 5307 people killed in large truck crashes, only 747 were in the large truck (29). When the 55 mph NMSL was enacted, the trucking industry requested, and obtained, authority for longer, wider, heavier trucks, arguing for additional cargo to offset the lower speeds. However, lower speeds were associated with more than commensurate savings in fuel consumption, maintenance, and safety. Most of the trucking industry (but not independent operators) still supports the 55 NMSL. As speed limits have subsequently increased, there has been no corresponding decrease in truck size and weight.

Vehicle Fleet

It is sometimes argued that our interstate highways were designed for speeds higher than 55 mph, but they were designed for a vehicle fleet different from the current one. The design standards were for passenger cars averaging around 4000 pounds and smaller, lighter trucks. Today, passenger cars average closer to 2000 to 3000 pounds, although the use of light trucks and SUVs has increased enormously. Trucks are larger and heavier than they were in 1974. Although passenger vehicles today are safer than 20 years ago, as speed increases, safety features become increasingly less effective. Increasing speeds compromise safety gains achieved through other measures.

Consumer Expenditures

Lower speeds translate into greater fuel economy, reducing vehicle operating costs. Both fuel and maintenance costs are lower with lower speeds.

National Security

Reduced fuel consumption reduces dependence on foreign oil supplies. In 1973, U.S. net imports of petroleum made up 35% of domestic consumption. In 2000, this figure had risen to over 50% and is estimated to reach 64% by 2020 (46). In 1999, 46% of our imported oil was from OPEC nations (47). The costs of the Persian Gulf War were directly related to our dependence on petroleum imports from that part of the world, and the United States still maintains a costly military presence in the Middle East, including heavy subsidies to allies in the vicinity.

Balance of Payments

In 1974, U.S. import of petroleum exceeded export by almost $24 billion. In 2000, our petroleum imports were almost $109 billion more than our exports, accounting for 28% of our balance-of-payments deficit (48, 45). Reductions in oil consumption would help reduce our balance-of-payments deficit.

Environmental Impacts

Motor vehicle fuel consumption contributes to greenhouse gases and global warming. Realistic efforts to reduce global warming will require reduced fuel consumption. Although remarkable progress has been made in reducing motor vehicle emissions, the increase in vehicle mileage has offset much of the gain (4). Other environmental pollution results from oil spills and underground leakage from pipelines and tanks. Noise pollution from motor vehicle transportation is an increasing problem in urban areas.

Changing Demographics

Perhaps the most significant, as well as the most ignored, factor in considering speed limits is the aging of our population. Prior to the Industrial Revolution, those age 65 and older comprised no more than 2% to 3% of the world's population. Today, in the developed world, their proportion is 14% and it is estimated to rise to as much as 25% by 2030 (34). The proportion of older drivers in the driving population is increasing even faster. In the United States, older people, especially older women, are obtaining and retaining driver licensure at ever higher rates, and older drivers are increasing both their trips and their mileage (38).

In 1999, 7088 persons age 65 and older were killed in motor vehicle crashes in the United States. Most were drivers (60%), with 24% passengers, 15% pedestrians, and 1% pedal cyclists (25). Given the increases in the older population, these numbers will certainly grow. There is undeniable loss of driving proficiency with advancing age. Whereas some of this loss may be attributable to the more frequent medical conditions associated with increasing age, "normal" aging also brings performance reductions. Loss of visual functioning occurs as early as in the 40s, and divided attention becomes more difficult with age. Increased crash risk based on mileage driven does not appear until the late 50s or early 60s, but by then older drivers are self-restricting. One of the earliest and widespread self-restrictions is nighttime driving (42). In spite of self-restriction, the crash risk increases at an accelerating rate until in the 80s it may equal or exceed that of teenage drivers (8, 28). At the same time, older persons are more vulnerable to serious or fatal injury in a crash of specified dimensions (8, 13). Thus both crash risk and risk of resulting injury increase for older people.

As drivers age and lose driving proficiency, they respond as other drivers do when the task becomes complex—they reduce speed. Older drivers are increasing their presence on the road, and many drivers cannot function at higher speeds. Prohibiting older drivers on the interstate system means removing them from the safest highway system ever developed. Finally, everyone will eventually join the ranks of elderly drivers. What policies do we really want to establish?

On the basis of virtually any dimension considered, the 55 mph NMSL should have been retained. Fuel economy, safety, consumer costs, time costs, environmental impacts, and national security issues all argue in support of the lower speed limit. Yet in 1995, Congress saw fit to remove the federal requirement that states retain the 55 mph. In those states that raised their speed limits, traffic fatalities increased 17% (9).

The public is clearly ambivalent about speed and speed limits on the highway. There have been important and effective measures to enhance safety, but the primary purpose of our highway system is mobility. If safety were truly our overriding concern, we could limit speed to 20 mph, with governors on vehicles to prevent higher speeds, and traffic injury would decrease dramatically. Clearly, we are not interested in safety at such a cost. What, then, is an acceptable trade-off between mobility and safety? There is far from unanimous agreement.

IMPORTANCE OF THE FEDERAL PROGRAM

There are other success stories that, because of space limitations, are not addressed here, including young drivers, pedestrians, bicyclists, and large trucks, as well as data capabilities. Of broader interest is the overall success in reducing motor vehicle injury and death. NHTSA, the federal program with jurisdiction in this area, is relatively modest as federal programs go. At its inception, training in traffic safety programs was limited and uncoordinated; there was essentially no training in traffic safety research. Crashes and injuries were generally viewed as accidents about which little could be done.

Two major factors were critical to the success of NHTSA. The first is leadership that, for the most part, worked collaboratively with state and local programs. With little expertise and limited funding, the federal program provided overall leadership and coordination that organized and guided state and local programs, providing them with some funding, but, more importantly, generating new knowledge that made demonstrable differences. The second critical factor is the creation of national databases that are publicly available and are used extensively by researchers worldwide to generate new and useful information.

There remain serious limitations. There is little support for investigator-initiated research; there is only limited input from independent researchers to the federal research program; there is no support for students interested in training in this field; and there is no support to sustain research careers (6). The federal program did not always run smoothly, but overall NHTSA has succeeded far beyond what could be envisioned at its outset. This success is the result of federal leadership and enormous effort on the part of organizations and agencies at every level of government and in the private sector. The highway safety program in the United States provides a model that those concerned with other injury issues would do well to consider.

Visit the Annual Reviews home page at www.annualreviews.org

LITERATURE CITED

1. Am. Assoc. State Highw. Transp. Off. 2001. Accessed June 20. http://safetyplan. tamu.edu/plan/goal.asp?GID = 7

2. Assoc. Adv. Automot. Med. 1990. *The Abbreviated Injury Scale (AIS) 1990 Revision.* Des Plaines, IL: Assoc. Adv. Automot. Med.

3. Borkenstein RF, Crowther RF, Shumate RP, Ziel WB, Zylman R. 1964. *The Role of the Drinking Driver in Traffic Accidents.* Bloomington, IN: Ind. Univ., Dep. Police Admin. (Subsequently publ. in 1975 Blutalkohol. 11[Suppl. 1]). 263 pp.

4. Bur. Transp. Stat. 2001. *National Transportation Statistics 2000.* Washington, DC: US Dep. Transp., Tables 4-38, 4-49, 4-50-40-53

5. Campbell BJ. 1988. The association between enforcement and seat belt use. *J. Saf. Res.* 19:159–63

6. Comm. Injury Prev. Control. 1999. *Reducing the Burden of Injury.* Washington, DC: Natl. Acad. Press

7. Comm. Study Benefits Costs 55 MPH Natl. Maximum Speed Limit. 1984. *55: a decade of experience.* Transp. Res. Board Spec. Rep. 204. Washington, DC: Natl. Res. Counc.

8. Evans L. 1991. *Traffic Safety and the Driver.* New York: Van Nostrand Reinhold. 417 pp.

9. Farmer CM, Retting RA, Lund AK. 1999. Changes in motor vehicle occupant fatalities after repeal of the national maximum speed limit. *Accid. Anal. Prev.* 31:537–43

10. Gibson JJ. 1961. The contribution of

experimental psychology to the formulation of the problem of safety: a brief for basic research. In *Association for the Aid of Crippled Children. Behavioral Approaches to Accident Research*, pp. 77–89. New York: Assoc. Aid Crippled Children

11. Gordon JE. 1949. The epidemiology of accidents. *Am. J. Public Health* 39:504–15

12. Haddon W Jr. 1980. Options for the prevention of motor vehicle crash injury. *Isr. J. Med.* 16:45–68

13. Hakamies-Blomqvist L. 2002. Safety of older persons in traffic. In *Transportation in an Aging Society: A Decade of Experience*, ed. SB Herbel. Washington, DC: Transp. Res. Board. In press

14. Holcomb RL. 1938. Alcohol in relation to traffic accidents. *JAMA* 111:1076–85

15. Insur. Inst. Highw. Saf. 2000. Accessed June 9, 2001. http://www.highwaysafety. org/safety_facts/qanda/helmet_use.htm#8

16. Insur. Inst. Highw. Saf. 2000. Accessed June 9, 2001. http://www.highwaysafety. org/safety_facts/state_laws/helmet_use.htm

17. Insur. Inst. Highw. Saf. 2001. Accessed May 22. http://www.highwaysafety.org/ safety_facts/state_laws/restrain3.htm

18. Insur. Inst. Highw. Saf. 2001. Accessed May 22. http://www.highwaysafety.org/ safety_facts/state_laws/restrain2.htm

19. Int. Fed. Red Cross Red Crescent Soc. 1998. *World Disasters Report 1998*, ed. N Cater, P Walker. Langport, Somerset, UK: Oxford Univ. Press. 198 pp.

20. Jones RK, Joscelyn KB. 1978. *Alcohol and Highway Safety 1978: A Review of the State of Knowledge*. Washington, DC: Natl. Highw. Traffic Saf. Admin. DOT HS-803 714

21. Deleted in proof

22. McCarthy P. 1998. Effect of speed limits on speed distributions and highway safety: a survey of the literature. In *Managing Speed. Review of Current Practice for Setting and Enforcing Speed Limits*, ed. NA Ackerman, pp. 277–358. Washington, DC: Natl. Acad. Press

23. McSwain NE, Willey AB. 1984. *Impact of the Re-Enactment of the Motorcycle Helmet Law in Louisiana*. Washington, DC: Natl. Highw. Traffic Saf. Admin. DOT HS 806 760

24. Natl. Highw. Traffic Saf. Admin. 2000. Accessed Aug. 25. http://www.nhtsa.dot. gov/cars/rules/regrev/evaluate

25. Natl. Highw. Traffic Saf. Admin. 2000. *Traffic Safety Facts 1999*. Washington, DC: Natl. Highw. Traffic Saf. Admin. DOT HS 809 100

26. Natl. Highw. Traffic Saf. Admin. 2000. *Traffic Safety Facts 1999: Occupant Protection*. Washington, DC: Natl. Highw. Traffic Saf. Admin. DOT HS 809 090

27. Natl. Highw. Traffic Saf. Admin. 2000. *Traffic Safety Facts 1999: Motorcycles*. Washington, DC: Natl. Highw. Traffic Saf. Admin. DOT HS 809 089

28. Natl. Highw. Traffic Saf. Admin. 2000. *Traffic Safety Facts 1999: Older Population*. Washington, DC: Natl. Highw. Traffic Saf. Admin. DOT HS 809 091

29. Natl. Highw. Traffic Saf. Admin. 2001. Accessed June 10. http://www.nhtsa.dot. gov/people/ncsa/pdf/2Kassess_rev4.pdf

30. Natl. Highw. Traffic Saf. Admin. 2001. *Observed Belt Use Fall 2000 National Occupant Protection Use Survey*. Res. Note. Feb. Washington, DC: Natl. Highw. Traffic Saf. Admin.

31. Natl. Highw. Traffic Saf. Admin. 2001. Accessed June 9. http://www.nhtsa.dot. gov/people/ncsa/SCIFiles/04_01rpt.html

32. Natl. Inst. Alcohol Abuse Alcoholism. 1997. *Alcohol and Health, 9th Spec. Rep. US Congr.* NIH Publ. 97 4017

33. Perrine MW, Waller JA, Harris LS. 1971. *Alcohol and Highway Safety: Behavioral and Medical Aspects*. Washington, DC: Fed. Highw. Admin. DOT HS 800 599

34. Peterson PG. 1999. Gray dawn: the global aging crisis. *For. Aff.* Jan./Feb., pp. 42–55

35. Pike JA. 2002. Protecting the older driver—vehicle concepts. In *Transportation in an Aging Society: A Decade of Experience*, ed. SB Herbel. Washington, DC: Natl. Acad. Sci. In press

36. Preusser DF, Hedlund JH, Ulmer RG. 2000. *Evaluation of Motorcycle Helmet Law Repeal in Arkansas and Texas.* Washington, DC: Natl. Highw. Traffic Saf. Admin. DOT HS 809 131

37. Rivara FP, Dicker BG, Bergman AB, Dacey R, Herman C. 1988. The public costs of motorcycle trauma. *JAMA* 260: 221–23

38. Rosenbloom S. 2002. The mobility of the elderly: There's good news and bad news. In *Transportation in an Aging Society: A Decade of Experience,* ed. SB Herbel. Washington, DC: Transp. Res. Board. In press

39. Sass TR, Zimmerman PR. 2000. Motorcycle helmet laws and motorcyclist fatalities. *J. Regul. Econ.* 18:195–215

40. Shinar D. 1998. Speed and crashes: a controversial topic and an elusive relationship. In *Managing Speed. Review of Current Practice for Setting and Enforcing Speed Limits,* ed. NA Ackerman, pp. 221–76. Washington, DC: Natl. Acad. Press

41. Simon v Sargent, 346 F. Supp. 277, 279 (D. Mass. 1972), affirmed 409 U.S. 1020, 1972

42. Smiley A. 2002. Adaptive strategies of older drivers. In *Transportation in an Aging Society: A Decade of Experience,* ed. SB Herbel. Washington, DC: Transp. Res. Board. In press

43. Solomon D. 1964. *Accidents on Main Rural Highways Related to Speed, Driver, and Vehicle.* Washington, DC: Bur. Public Roads, US Dep. Comm.

44. Trauma Found. 2000. Accessed July 25. http://www.tf.org/tf/alcohol/ariv/facts/consum3.html

45. US Dep. Comm., Bur. Econ. Anal. 2001. Accessed June 22. http://www.bea.doc.gov/bea/newsrel/trans101.htm

46. US Dep. Energy, Energy Inf. Admin. 2001. *Energy Price Impacts on the US Economy.* Accessed June 22. http://www.eia.doe.gov/oiaf/economy/energy_price.html

47. US Dep. Energy, Energy Inf. Admin. 2001. *Petroleum Imports by Country of Origin, 1960–1999.* Accessed June 12. http://www.eia.doe.gov/pub/energy.overview/aer1999/txt/aer0504.txt

48. US Dep. Energy, Energy Inf. Admin. 2001. *Merchandise Trade Value.* Accessed June 19. http://www.eia.doe.gov/pub/energy.overview/monthly.energy/txt/mer1-6

49. US Dep. Health Hum. Serv. 1989. *Surgeon General's Workshop on Drunk Driving Proceedings.* Washington, DC

50. US Dep. Transportation: *Alcohol and Highway Safety. Report to the US Congress.* 1968. Washington, DC: US GPO. Quoted in Jones RD, Joscelyn KD. *Alcohol and Highway Safety, 1978: Review of the State of Knowledge,* DOT HS 803-714; Washington, DC: Nat. Highw. Traffic Saf. Admin., pp. 1–2

51. Voas RB, Lacey JH. 1989. Issues in the enforcement of impaired driving laws in the United States. In *Surgeon General's Workshop on Drunk Driving. Background Papers,* pp. 136–56. Rockville, MD: US Dep. Health Hum. Serv.

Annu. Rev. Public Health 2002. 23:115–34

HALYS AND QALYS AND DALYS, OH MY:
Similarities and Differences in Summary Measures of Population Health

Marthe R. Gold[1], David Stevenson[2], and Dennis G. Fryback[3]

[1]Department of Community Health and Social Medicine, City University of New York Medical School, 138th Street and Convent Avenue, New York, New York 10031; e-mail: Goldmr@med.cuny.edu

[2]Program in Health Policy, Harvard University, Cambridge, Massachusetts 02138; e-mail: Stevens@fas.harvard.edu

[3]Department of Population Health Sciences, University of Wisconsin-Madison, Madison, Wisconsin 53705-2397; e-mail: Dfryback@facstaff.wisc.edu

Key Words burden of disease, cost-effectiveness analysis, health-related quality of life

■ **Abstract** Health-adjusted life years (HALYs) are population health measures permitting morbidity and mortality to be simultaneously described within a single number. They are useful for overall estimates of burden of disease, comparisons of the relative impact of specific illnesses and conditions on communities, and in economic analyses. Quality-adjusted life years (QALYs) and disability-adjusted life years (DALYs) are types of HALYs whose original purposes were at variance. Their growing importance and the varied uptake of the methodology by different U.S. and international entities makes it useful to understand their differences as well as their similarities. A brief history of both measures is presented and methods for calculating them are reviewed. Methodological and ethical issues that have been raised in association with HALYs more generally are presented. Finally, we raise concerns about the practice of using different types of HALYs within different decision-making contexts and urge action that builds and clarifies this useful measurement field.

INTRODUCTION

Health has long been evaluated by mortality-based indicators, both in the United States and internationally. Life expectancy, all-cause and disease-specific mortality, and infant mortality are compared by region, by nation, and across nations. Death rates and life expectancies are disaggregated and presented by sociodemographic and ethnic descriptors in efforts to evaluate population health and, at times, to monitor the impact of health interventions. Although mortality-based rates are useful in a cursory way, they provide insufficient information with which

0163-7525/02/0510-0115$14.00

to make any but the most basic judgments about the health of a population or the comparative impact of an intervention. The contribution of chronic disease, injury, and disability to population health goes unrecorded.

As commitment to monitoring health and rational allocation of health resources has grown in the United States and internationally, so too have the methods that researchers and policymakers use to evaluate health and medical outcomes in individuals and in populations. Health-adjusted life years (HALYs) are summary measures of population health that allow the combined impact of death and morbidity to be considered simultaneously. This feature makes HALYS useful for comparisons across a range of illnesses, interventions, and populations. A 1998 Institute of Medicine report (15) found these measures to be "increasingly relevant to both public health and medical decision makers" and of late, HALYs have gained higher visibility in policy circles, both domestically and internationally.

An umbrella term for a family of measures, HALYs includes disability-adjusted life years (DALYs) and quality-adjusted life years (QALYs). The morbidity or quality of life component of HALYs is referred to as health-related quality of life (HRQL) (22), and is captured on a scale of 0 to 1.0, representing the extremes of death and full health. The HRQL associated with different conditions of health and disease is multiplied by life expectancy, and then, depending on the underlying methodology, produces an estimate of DALYs or QALYs associated with different levels of health. Health-adjusted life expectancy (HALE), a related type of summary measure of population health, estimates the average time in years that a person at a given age can expect to live in the equivalent of full health. Life tables, such as those created by the US census, are combined with cross-sectional age-specific HRQL data. Note that in HALE the contribution of any specific disease or condition to decrements in health is not presented. Rather, HALE seeks to provide an overarching view of the morbidity and mortality burden of a population.

Although both QALYs and DALYs interweave estimates of morbidity and mortality, their original purposes are somewhat at variance and their methods of calculation differ. This paper provides an overview of their origins and their key features. Our intention is to better familiarize public health professionals with the differences and, importantly, the similarities between these tools. In addition, we flag methodological and ethical issues that have been raised in association with HALYs generally so that readers may more critically examine study and report findings. We conclude with a discussion of the implications of the use of the different types of HALYs within decision-making settings and explore approaches that could help build the field.

HEALTH-ADJUSTING LIFE YEARS: A BRIEF HISTORY OF QALYs AND DALYs

QALYs

Following on early work to develop a descriptive measure combining time lived with functional capacity (34, 52, 54), QALYs were developed in the late 1960s by economists, operations researchers, and psychologists, primarily for use in cost-effectiveness analysis (CEA) (13, 29, 43). In this setting, they represented an important breakthrough in conceptualizing the health outcome (denominator) in a cost-effectiveness (CE) ratio. A CE ratio describes the incremental price of obtaining a unit of health effect from a health intervention—be it preventive or curative, population-based, or clinical—when compared with an alternative intervention. When the denominator of the CE ratio is computed using QALYs, the cost-effectiveness analysis is referred to as cost-utility analyses (CUA).

Cost-utility analysis is appropriate in situations where quality of life is "the" or "an" important outcome of health care, and when it is necessary to have a common unit of measurement to compare between types of interventions and programs (55). Cost-utility analyses of medical interventions have been conducted for over 30 years; Klarman and coauthors published a CUA of chronic renal disease in 1968 (29). Quality-adjusted life years are routinely used in assessments of medical care, technology, and public health interventions; these studies have proliferated over the past two decades (9).

Given a specific budget constraint, QALYs are maximized by increasing the "utility" of individuals and aggregates of individuals. Utility can be understood as the value, or preference, that people have for health outcomes along a continuum anchored with death (0) and perfect health (1.0) (for a fuller discussion, see Reference 55). The original formulation of QALYs was drawn from the theoretical underpinnings of welfare economics and expected utility theory (46). In welfare economics, a social utility function is the aggregate of individuals' utilities, and economists hold that maximizing the social utility function is the primary goal for resource allocation. Quality-adjusted life years are often seen as inexorably linked with utilitarianism, a social theory that dictates that policies designed to improve social welfare should do the greatest good for the greatest number of people. We return to this when we explore ethical concerns that have been raised more generally about HALYs.

DALYs

In 1993, a World Bank and World Health Organization collaboration resulted in the publication of a volume that sought to quantify the global burden of premature death, disease, and injury and to make recommendations that would improve health, particularly in developing nations (66). The Global Burden of Disease (GBD) study, an ongoing effort that has continued to evolve from the initial World Bank effort, had three major objectives, "to facilitate the inclusion of nonfatal health outcomes in debates on international health policy, to decouple epidemiological assessment from advocacy so that estimates of the mortality or disability from a condition are developed as objectively as possible, and . . . to quantify the burden of disease using a measure that could be used for cost-effectiveness analysis" (35).

Disability-adjusted life years (DALYs) were developed to quantify the burden of disease and disability in populations, as well as to set priorities for resource allocation. Disability-adjusted life years measure the gap between a population's health and a hypothetical ideal for health achievement. Internationally, a number of countries have either completed or are conducting national burden of disease studies that use DALYs as their metric (36). A recent U.S. study has used DALYs to look at the burden of disease in Los Angeles County, demonstrating significant differences in rankings by ethnicity, gender, and area of residence (6).

As we discuss in greater detail below, the aspects of health that are valued as well as the populations from whom values are gathered differ between QALYs and DALYs. Life expectancy is also handled in divergent ways within the two frameworks. Finally, DALYs, in their original formulation, place different value weights on populations based on their age structure so that DALYs in the very young and the very old are discounted compared to other age groups.

CALCULATING QALYs AND DALYs: METHODS AND IMPLICATIONS

There are three general steps in calculating a HALY: (a) describing health, i.e., as a health state or as a disease/condition; (b) developing values or weights for the health state or condition, which are called HRQL weights here; and (c) combining values for different health states or conditions with estimates of life expectancy. Each of these steps includes methodological choices that affect the estimates that are obtained.

Describing Health: QALYs

Traditional QALYs are built using HRQL weights that are attached to individual experiences of health. These HRQL weights are not linked to any particular disease, condition, or disability. Rather, HRQL weights are based on the values of individuals for either their own health state (patient weights) or the health states of others that are described to them (community weights). The health states that are valued are comprised of component "attributes," "dimensions," or "domains" for which there exists general consensus on their centrality to health.[1] To create QALYs, health states—which are often, but not necessarily associated with a particular disease or condition—are first described along their component domains.

Measuring health status in a standardized way requires a conceptualization of the thorny issue of what exactly constitutes "health." The universe of health states that individuals experience is immense, and the challenge of any health status measure is to capture the complexity of these states in a manageable way that is resonant with shared views of health across ages, cultures, and gender. A number of descriptive systems that include all or some of key domains such as physical, psychological, and social/role function, health perceptions, and symptoms, have

---

[1]These terms are used in describing generic elements of health status and largely represent differences in vocabulary rather than in concept.

been developed over the past 30 years with the intention of filling this requirement. Descriptive health status measures that have been used to create QALYs include the Health Utilities Index (HUI) (8, 56), the Quality of Well-Being Scale (QWB) (28), the EQ-5D (EuroQoL) (12), and the Health and Activity Limitation Index (HALex) (11).

Because the domains or health attributes described are particular to each instrument, not surprisingly, each portrays a different picture of health status. Much controversy has swirled around the validity of these measures; investigators are appropriately concerned with the question of whether these systems are measuring what they intend to measure. Given an absence of a benchmark of health, determining criterion validity—comparing the results achieved to an accepted gold standard—is impossible. Researchers therefore rely on other forms of validity, such as convergent validity—an indication that results achieved using the same method for similar individuals are compatible—and content validity—an indication of the extent to which a measure is consistent with an intended domain of content.

Although different conceptualizations of health, together with differing techniques for valuing the states (described briefly in the next section) result in variations in HRQL scores when they are attached to specific disease entities (27, 37, 39), overall correlations among the instruments have been shown to be quite reasonable (18, 20). A number of reviews of these instruments are available to the interested reader who wishes to gain a fuller understanding of the structure of each of the systems (22, 32, 38, 44).

Describing Health: DALYs

In contrast to QALY methods, DALY architects chose to attach estimates of HRQL to specific diseases, rather than to health states. In part this was done for pragmatic reasons, given the difficulties of collecting comparable primary data from the vast numbers of countries for which a global burden of disease is calculated. In addition, DALY developers have voiced concerns about self-assessments of health, viewing them as potentially misleading, especially for purposes of cross-cultural comparisons. World Health Organization researchers give as an example the aboriginal population in Australia, whose mortality experience is greater than the rest of Australians, but who are less likely to rate their health as either "poor" or "fair" (35). When objective tests of health are viewed as a type of criterion validity, use of self-assessment data across-countries is found wanting by the WHO.[2]

Given these concerns, Murray and colleagues have relied on secondary data and expert opinion to identify and describe disease, placing different conditions along a continuum of disability (35, 36). Rather than creating a classification scheme of generic health states as is done with all other HRQL measures, DALYs use the

---

[2]Self-assessment is distinguished here from "self-report." In point of fact, disease prevalence rates, which are used to build DALYs estimates, in many countries are based on self-report.

conceptualization of nonfatal health outcomes drawn from the International Classification of Impairments, Disabilities, and Handicaps (ICIDH) (35, 67), focusing on disability, or the impact of a disease or condition on the performance of an individual. Descriptions of the specific ICIDH disabilities are generated by health professionals; values for the undesirability of specific diseases and conditions are based on their descriptions, as we describe later.

Disability states in DALYs do not take account of comorbid conditions. For aging populations in industrialized nations, comorbidities are the norm rather than the exception, and someone with angina is quite likely to have coincident illnesses such as diabetes and hypertension. There is no provision in DALY weights to simultaneously consider all of these illnesses within the same individual (or population). A corollary to this occurs at the level of intervention evaluation. A therapy that creates unwanted side effects cannot be captured within the DALY framework. For example, if treatment of arthritis with nonsteroidal antiinflammatory medications resulted in peptic ulcers, there is no method within the DALY lexicon to describe the accompanying alteration in HRQL that accompanies abatement of arthritic symptoms and simultaneous onset of the symptoms that accompany peptic ulcer disease. Because the QALY family of measures is grounded in domains of health, rather than descriptions of specific diseases and disability, it is at least theoretically possible to describe, and therefore value, combinations of illness.

Generating Values for Health and Disease

Once an illness, condition, or disability is described, its desirability (or lack of such) must be valued in a manner that allows it to be combined with units of life expectancy. Although this process differs somewhat for valuation of HRQL in QALY as compared to DALY calculations, generation of the values share certain common requirements.

First, by convention, each measure is anchored on a 0 to 1.0 scale of health. Quality-adjusted life years are a measure of health expectancy (a "good" to be maximized); DALYs are a measure of a health gap (a "bad" to be minimized). Consequently, the scale for each measure is reversed from the other—a valuation of 1 represents full health on the QALY scale and full disability (death) on the DALY scale; 0 represents the lowest possible health state (death) on the QALY scale and no disability or full health on the DALY scale.

Second, the health scales in each system are created so that they have interval scale properties, i.e., changes of equal amount anywhere on a scale of 0 to 1.0 can be interpreted as equivalent to one another. This means that an improvement in health (using the QALY orientation) from 0.4 to 0.6 would be numerically equivalent to an improvement from 0.7 to 0.9. This requirement occurs because years of life and HRQL must be combined into a single metric such that more QALYs (or fewer DALYs) can be influenced equivalently by changes in life expectancy and health status.

Third, HRQL weights must reflect preferences that people have for different states of health or disease. Dimensions of health that can be affected at different levels must ultimately be summarized into scores representing the relative trade-offs in desirability between these different components of health, or impacts of disease. Health-related quality of life weights used in QALYs are assigned to health states based on how people make trade-offs between different dimensions of health. Disability-adjusted life years do this by assigning a disability weight (which can be seen as a preference) to a specific disease or health condition.

Generating Values: QALYs

Preferences, or values for HRQL for use in QALYs, are generated by a number of techniques. The most commonly used methods include standard gamble, time trade-off, and rating or visual analogue scales. Standard gamble and time trade-off methods ask respondents to value health states by making explicit what they would be willing to sacrifice (in terms of time or risk of death) in order to return from the health state being described (or experienced) to perfect health. These techniques are preferred by many economists, who hold that eliciting preferences in this manner is consistent with utility theory, a model for how people make decisions under conditions of uncertainty (60). The theoretical foundations of CUA lie, at least in part, in expected utility theory (19). The Health Utility Index (HUI), developed in Canada and applied both in clinical (14) and population health settings (63), was scaled using the time trade-off method to assess preferences.

In rating scales or visual analogue scales, respondents must designate a point on a scale, or "feeling thermometer," that corresponds to the strength of their preference for a given health state. Many investigators believe that the cognitive burden to respondents is less with these scales, since they are familiar to most people from a variety of everyday experiences where they are asked to fill out questionnaires or respond to queries regarding their strength of preference. Both the Quality of Well-Being (QWB) scale and the EuroQol EQ-5D (in part) use rating scales in assessment of values. Fuller descriptions of these methods together with discussions of their advantages and limitations are covered elsewhere (22, 38, 44, 55).

The different methods employed by the varied valuation techniques give rise to inconsistencies in values for like health states or illnesses (27, 42, 48, 59). These variations arise for a number of reasons, including the differential sensitivity of the measures to particular domains of health that are affected by illness, the differences in how individuals comprehend and implement the weighting tasks, and scaling properties particular to the technique that is used.

Another potential source of variation in HRQL scores for health states and illnesses arises from the elicitation of values from different groups of people. Values can be elicited from people with experience of the illness/condition (patient preferences), a representative population sample who would be affected by resource allocation decisions (community preferences), study investigators, and experts—generally health professionals who have good understanding of the symptoms associated with the disease entities under investigation. Although some evidence suggests that values for health states are fairly consistent across groups in general (3, 4, 12, 31), health professional experts have been found to provide lower values than others in ranking illnesses (35). In addition, the literature suggests that patients often adapt to their illness and value their health states higher than those who do not have experience with the disease (10, 51, 53).

The Panel on Cost Effectiveness in Health and Medicine (PCEHM), an expert group appointed by the Department of Health and Human Services to improve standardization of cost-effectiveness methodology in the health care arena, recommended that any CEA designed to inform resource allocation decisions use a societal perspective that incorporates the costs and the effects of the intervention to all members of society. As an extension of that recommendation, the Panel found that "the best articulation of society's preferences . . . would be gathered from a representative sample of informed members of the community"[3] (23).

Generating Values: DALYs

In DALYs, values for diseases and other nonfatal health outcomes were obtained through an iterative, deliberative process that attempted to reconcile differences in the preferences of health professional expert groups with respect to the desirability of different conditions and injuries. Framers of the DALY argue for using experts for valuation on the grounds of feasibility and efficiency (convenience samples of WHO and affiliated health workers were used rather than gathering community data in multiple locations), as well as on a methodologic basis. Concerns that potential variation of community health perceptions across cultures could inhibit cross-national comparisons, uncertainty of how to handle adaptation by people with disabilities,[4] and the cognitive burden of preference weighting techniques on respondents, all influenced DALY developers who utilize a single technique for value elicitation (35).

The DALY valuation exercise was built upon a person trade-off (PTO) method (40, 45) that explicitly addresses trade-offs between life and HRQL for people with different diseases. Champions of the PTO method have argued that this technique

---

[3]Relying on a community perspective is not without controversy. Advocates for people with disabilities posit that individuals with specific conditions should be the ones to value that particular health state, since health professionals and community members both tend to rate disability states more negatively than individuals who have actually experienced them. Depending on the intervention in question (e.g., prevention or treatment of disability versus treatment of someone who is disabled for a condition unrelated to their disability), this difference could make an intervention look better or worse as a societal investment.

[4]WHO researchers refer to this as the "happy slave" phenomenon, implying that some people with disabilities become more satisfied with their quality of life over time simply because of the way in which they have coped, despite the underlying functional disability remaining unchanged.

is better than standardly applied QALY techniques to embed the notion of resource allocation within the measurement of population health.

DALY architects used the person trade-off method on a series of 22 "indicator" health conditions selected to represent different dimensions of disability and non-fatal health outcomes. Some of the indicator conditions create limitations that are predominantly physical (e.g., blindness and deafness); others have more significant cognitive and psychological impact (e.g., Down syndrome, unipolar major depression.) Pain, along a continuum ranging from sore throat to severe migraine, is a feature of some of the illnesses. Conditions affecting sexual and reproductive function were also evaluated (35).

Health experts were first asked to establish "equality" in life extension between healthy people and people with the indicator conditions. For example, informants were asked whether they would prefer to purchase an intervention that provided one year of health for 1000 fully healthy people, or 2000 people with angina. Next, they were asked to consider what trade-off they would make between raising the quality of life for people with angina to a state of full health versus extending by one year the life of individuals who were already healthy. Although both of these PTO exercises yield weights, they typically differed from one another and needed to be made internally consistent to arrive at a final score.

Deliberation is integral to the DALY weighting process. It is promulgated on the basis that individuals should be faced with the policy implications of their choices. In valuing nonfatal outcomes, it has been used to reconcile individual discrepancies regarding weights, as well as to align a larger group in generating a consensus set of values. For the Global Burden of Disease project, nine expert groups participated in the weighting process. Good correlations between the ordinal rankings as well as the cardinal values of the indicator conditions are reported by WHO[5] (35). Based on these results, DALY investigators created seven disability classes that lie along the spectrum from full health to death. Included within disability class 5, for example, are conditions such as unipolar major depression, blindness, and paraplegia, which ranged in severity from 0.619 to 0.671. Once preference scores for a set of index conditions were established, weights for hundreds of other conditions were mapped by extrapolation (35).

Combining Values for Health with Life Expectancy

In a general sense, HALYs are created by multiplying values for health states or conditions by life expectancy. Because QALYs emerge from a clinical tradition, life expectancy is handled in a more heterogenous fashion than in DALYs, which are expressly designed to look at disease burden from a population perspective with an average life expectancy. The clinical tradition is accustomed to measuring the effectiveness (in life extension and symptom relief) of specific

---

[5]Some participants have, however, described difficulties with creating consistency across the two exercises and felt "led" in order to harmonize the results of the PTO exercises (2).

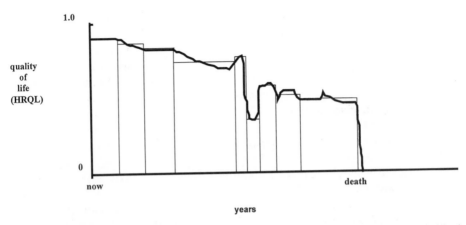

Figure 1   The life path of changing health-related quality of life (HRQL) for an individual from "now" to that person's death is shown by the irregular line. After a steady decline for some years followed by a brief improvement, the person suffers a major event from which he or she briefly recovers some HRQL, but this recovery is followed by fluctuating HRQL until a precipitous decline and death. The area under this curve is the QALYs accumulated by the person over this portion of his or her lifetime. The area is approximated by summing the areas of the rectangles as described in the text.

interventions on groups of individuals. Much of the life-expectancy information drawn on for QALY calculations relies on data from observational studies and clinical trials, as well as standard population life tables.

Combining—QALYs

The calculation of QALYs is explained with reference to Figure 1. The irregular line graphs the HRQL life path of a hypothetical individual over time from "now" forward. Ideally, we compute QALYs attained between "now" and the individual's death by determining the area under this shaded line—i.e., the product of instantaneous HRQL times a small time increment summed over the individual's remaining lifetime. Of course, we have no way of knowing the individual's HRQL at each possible point in time. Alternatively, we suppose that this individual's HRQL has been measured at various times (centered in each vertical rectangle but not marked on the graph, to preserve clarity), using a standardized instrument [such as the Health Utilities Index or the EuroQol (57)]. The standardized HRQL instrument is used to classify the individual's health state at each point in time on a system of health attributes (e.g., degree of mobility, mental status, social functioning, sensory capabilities, etc.), and the scoring function associated with the instrument is used to assign an HRQL to each state. We approximate the area under the curve by computing areas of the rectangles, which are drawn assuming the measured HRQL is constant between measurement intervals. The area of each rectangle is the product of an HRQL weight and the time for which the individual is assumed to experience that HRQL level. The result of summing the areas of the rectangles is an approximation of the QALYs attained by the individual from "now" onward. The more points at which HRQL is measured, the better the approximation.

For example, consider the "normal" life path of health for a white non-Hispanic American woman, with a life expectancy of 79 years. She might spend the first 40 years of her life in excellent health, with HRQL valued at 0.95,[6] experience a little nonspecific wear and tear that decreases her HRQL to 0.9 from age 40 to age 60, have the onset of other constellations of symptoms decreasing her HRQL to 0.8 from age 60 to age 70, and then at age 70, experience further declines that decrease her HRQL to 0.70 for a final 12 years of her life. That path would provide her with 72.4 QALYs $\{[40] (0.95) + [20] (0.9) + [10] (0.8) + [12] (0.7)\}$. Although she actually lived 82 life years, 3 years more than her life expectancy at birth, she accumulates 72.4 QALYs. Note that decrements in her HRQL could be associated with onset of specific illnesses (for example, hypertension or allergies) or might simply be associated with loss of vigor, onset of ill-defined symptoms, less ability to function in her role. No specific "diagnosis" is required in order for her HRQL to decrease. If at age 60, the drop from 0.9 to 0.8 was averted through successful replacement of an arthritic hip, maintaining her HRQL at 0.9 until age 70, when she developed symptoms associated with diabetes and dropped to 0.7, she would have a life path that yielded an additional 1.0 QALYs, for a total of 73.4. Alternatively, if she had a bad outcome from her hip replacement, her HRQL might have dropped to 0.7 at age 60 and persisted there until age 82, losing a total of 1.0 QALYs. Had she died at 60 as a result of her surgery, her life path sum of QALYs would have been 56.[7]

Although our example has computed QALYs retrospectively, looking back over the life path of the described individual, individual decision problems are usually projected forward in time using a mathematical model of the anticipated life path based on observations from clinical trials, observational cohorts, and population epidemiology. In a population, cross-sectional surveys using HRQL instruments can be used along with stationary population actuarial techniques to compute the average QALYs expected to be attained by an individual (49, 64).

Note that QALYs might also be calculated to look at specific segments of life, for example, the QALYs gained or lost following successful (or unsuccessful)

---

[6]Many investigators believe that it is inappropriate to assume that people have "perfect" health, so that even at younger ages when people are presumably at their healthiest, a score of 1.0 is viewed as inaccurate (see 18a).

[7]For simplicity, QALY modelers frequently omit adjusting for gradations of HRQL during different segments of a life path—once a diminution in health has occurred it is frequently handled as persisting throughout the remaining years of life.

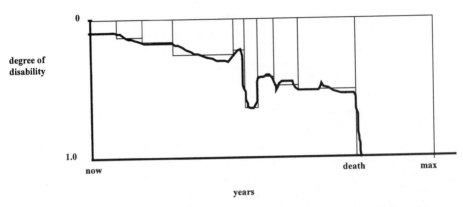

Figure 2   The same life path as in Figure 1 is shown by the irregular line. Added to the graph is a point, "max," which is the ideal sex-specific life expectancy for humans as determined by the WHO researchers. To compute DALYs, the area lost from the ideal lifetime, living to the maximum life expectancy in full health, is computed approximately by summing the areas of the rectangles.

chemotherapy for cancer. And they might be calculated to look more closely at subpopulations. For example, low-income women have lower life expectancy and poorer HRQL, in general, than do more affluent women.

Combining—DALYs

The computation of DALYs, in principle, proceeds in the same fashion as QALYs, but as shown in Figure 2, the area being computed is that above the life path and extending out to the ideal life expectancy, to approximate the total area lost from the "ideal" life path of living in perfect health for the entire ideal life expectancy. As DALYs measure health gaps, specific ideal life expectancies are used for males and females from which to calculate the gaps. DALYs take as their standard a life-expectancy at birth of 82.5 years for women, and 80 years for men; these numbers are chosen to represent the average life expectancy of the Japanese, who at present have the longest overall life expectancy in the world. Note that these imply age-specific life expectancies that are greater than average life expectancies when considering individuals who have lived to a given age (e.g., a male at age 50 is assumed to have a life expectancy of 30.99 years, since he has avoided mortality hazards affecting men in their first 50 years). World Health Organization investigators have selected these life expectancies for universal application (i.e., regardless of sociodemographic characteristics) on equity grounds, arguing that all nations should be able to obtain the survival results of the most successful. In Figure 2, this point is denoted "max."

In practice, the DALY weighting system for disability adjustments is tied to diseases and not to generic, descriptive dimensions of health. Disability weights have been assigned to typical time courses of health in cohorts of persons after onset of a particular disease. Population burden due to a particular disease is computed using these weights, data about the incidence of the disease in the particular population, and average age of onset. Total population disease burden is computed by summing attributable DALYs across diseases.

If DALYs were used to describe the life course of the woman above, the first decrement that would be recorded would be for osteoarthritis, at age 60. Until that time she would be considered to be "fully" healthy, with disability weighted at 0. With the onset of osteoarthritis, a disability decrement of 0.158 (untreated), or 0.108 (treated), would be tallied. This level of decrement would be counted as if it lasted for her life expectancy (ideally 24.83 years in a woman who has attained an age of 60 years), resulting in a loss of (24.83) (0.158) DALYs (treated) or (24.83) (0.108) DALYs (untreated). The added decrement in her health resulting from the onset of diabetes would be incorporated by adding the full weight of the decrement coming from the diabetes scores (ranging from .012 to 0.078) and decreases in actual life expectancy (i.e., the loss of life years relative to the ideal) due to diabetes and its complications, to the decrement already extant for osteoarthritis. If she suffered death as a complication of hip replacement surgery at age 60, she would be denoted as losing 22.5 DALYs.

In our example as presented, we do not make two added adjustments to DALY computation that are made by WHO researchers. The first of these is an age-weighting that is applied similarly to an HRQL weighting. Building this weighting into the DALY formula gives greater value to years lived in young adulthood and less to years lived at the beginning and end of the life span. The WHO researchers present age weights as consistent with community values and reflective of the reliance of the old and the young on support by the middle-age groups (35). In response to some astringent critiques that hold age-weighting to be unethical and discriminatory (1, 5), DALY researchers have countered that age-weighting does not discriminate between individuals but simply differentiates between differently productive periods of life for a cohort. DALY researchers also report that sensitivity analyses have shown that age-weighting makes little difference in ranking conditions by burden of disease (35). The final adjustment to the DALY formula is to discount time in the future at a discount rate of 3%. To simplify our comparisons here we have omitted this further adjustment.

Although QALY measures in principle could incorporate weighting schemes that value time lived at different ages differently, this approach has not been adopted in QALY-based CEAs (62); instead, life years are valued equally across individuals. When age-weighting is used (as with DALYs), it appears that age is essentially counted "against" older people twice—once because of the greater incidence of functional impairment among older people (making saving their life years less "valuable" overall) and again because of embedded judgments about the intrinsic worth of a year of life at older ages. When QALYs are used in cost-effectiveness analyses, they are regularly discounted to present value in a similar manner to DALYs.

ETHICAL CHALLENGES TO HALYs

Both QALYs and DALYs are designed to support a resource allocation frame-work that is largely utilitarian in its orientation. In that capacity, the goal of each of the measures is to accurately represent outcomes that can be generated most efficiently per dollar spent so that the total "good" for a population is maximized. Although an efficiency-oriented approach maximizes overall health, however it is defined, the practical and distributional implications of such an approach can be problematic to individuals and to particular subgroups who fare less well in the HALY calculus.

Several critiques of QALYs and DALYs highlight the ways in which these measures can be used counter to "societal values" (1, 2, 25, 33, 58). Methodological problems that bear on ethical issues remain contentious. We have previously flagged concerns about the sources of values (patients versus health experts versus community members) and, in the case of DALYs, the use of differential age-based weights. Additional objections that are primarily ethical in nature can be grouped into three broad categories (the first two of which are distributional concerns): QALYs and DALYs fail to give priority to those who are worst off (e.g., on the basis of ill health or low social class); they discriminate against people with limited treatment potential (e.g., those with preexisting disability or illness); and they fail to account for qualitative differences in outcomes (e.g., life saving versus health improving) because of the way in which morbid and mortal outcomes are aggregated.

In the first instance, critics argue that HALYs, as currently calculated, discriminate against those members of society who are already at health or social disadvantage. These potential consequences strike many as unfair (25, 26, 30, 47); indeed, this orientation does not adequately reflect the concern that people often have for those who are least well off (5, 7). Detractors from the HALY approach suggest that absent incorporating a socially sanctioned and empirically valid "equity weight," distributional effects of resource allocation based solely on HALYs will always be unjust and those most in need by reason of health or social disadvantage will remain most in need (1, 33).

Related to this concern is the problem that certain groups of individuals—older persons and people with extensive disabling conditions refractory to significant amelioration—are comparatively bad investments. This is the case because older people have a finite number of years that can be gained, and because some illnesses can only improve a small amount. Limitations on either type of improvement yield fewer HALYs. With respect to age in particular, there is considerable debate about its pertinence as a criterion for priority setting (1, 25), although some have argued that social values and empirical findings support giving priority to younger persons who have not had the opportunity to achieve their "fair innings" (61). Countering concerns of systematic bias against those with lessened capacity to benefit is the argument put forward by the PCEHM that cost-effectiveness studies primarily evaluate the comparative economic efficiency of interventions and do not disaggregate people into subgroups based on age or comorbid status (23, 50). However, others have pointed out that some interventions are targeted to diseases that are heavily concentrated in the elderly or in subpopulations whose life expectancy is markedly decreased (e.g., persons with cystic fibrosis), and when compared with interventions that are beneficial to a younger population, the aged or chronically ill will always come up short (33).

A third major concern is one of "aggregation"; i.e., how values for health states and diseases are combined across individuals, as well as along the spectrum of alive to dead. Critics of HALYs say that failure to treat life-saving interventions as conceptually distinct from health-improving interventions is at odds with how society views life and death medical decisions (24, 33). Similarly, some question whether minor benefits accruing to many should be viewed as equivalent to more significant benefits accruing to few (7).

In response to the dilemmas detailed above, two general approaches have been suggested. The first argues for changes in how measures are constructed. The desire to "build a better machine" for CEA stems from the view that policymakers often take economic pronouncements at face value, and it is therefore incumbent upon researchers to incorporate societal values into the ratio. This would be possible because although welfare economics seeks to maximize a social utility function (an aggregate of individual utilities), it does not prescribe how individual utilities should be aggregated. Different types of people could therefore receive different weights in counting HALYs (for a fuller discussion see References 23, p. 32; 62). Techniques attempting to better reflect social judgments about equity have been proposed (41, 58). These techniques are in early stages of development, and they have not yet been fully justified on a theoretical basis, nor implemented in real-world situations. Concerns about how to factor in the complexity of many social judgments into a single moral calculus have been raised (7).

The second approach, favored by the PCEHM, is that cost-effectiveness studies be seen as only one of multiple inputs to decision making (23). Consideration of distributional issues for those with greater needs, of allocation priorities for illnesses that are rare or expensive, and of the balance between health status improvement and life saving, need to remain part of the political and clinical decision-making process in which HALYs may be one factor, instead of entering as distortions in the HALY calculations. Economic efficiency, the PCEHM argues, should never be the sole criterion for resource allocation. If QALYs or DALYs were to lead policymakers to make decisions based solely on economics, they would be being used inappropriately.

CONCLUSIONS

As initially conceived, DALYs were primarily intended to document information about the comparative health of populations. Accuracy and responsiveness to more nuanced changes in health status at the individual level were less important than accumulating a database that could provide reliable data with respect to the descriptive epidemiology of fatal and nonfatal health outcomes. At their start, QALYs focused on the evaluation of medical interventions. Developers of HRQL measures placed a greater emphasis on issues such as measure responsiveness, sensitivity and reliability (16, 17, 44), paying less attention to generating overall models of disease distribution, severity, and mortality.

Although not without detractors, DALYs and QALYs have proved serviceable for their initially intended uses. As each measure extends across the chasm that separates population health and medical care, however, inevitable differences will be seen in the outputs of their estimates of disease burden. And different outputs may imply different priorities. One study that compared HALYs for five common medical conditions, using DALY- and QALY-associated HRQL weights, but keeping life-expectancy calculations identical, found differences in disease-burden estimates as well as changes in rank order of the illnesses (21).[8] As Murray points out, once a measure is used it influences policy, permeates the thinking of decision makers, and becomes normative (35). More than one normative measure at play in the same fields may contribute to significant confusion.

Important objectives for any health care system are to maximize the aggregate health of its populace and to minimize disparities within subgroups. Although social factors and social policies have a dominant influence on the overall health of populations, public health and clinical interventions are the tools that are available to health professionals. Understanding gaps in health achievement and maximizing effectiveness in intervention implementation require measures that can reliably capture the duration of life and its quality. Summary measures of population health such as HALYs offer the possibility of more rational allocation of health-related interventions at both clinical and population levels.

In a perfect measurement world, HALYs would be used at the macro level to track population health and monitor population-based interventions (e.g., health education, environmental protection, health-related legislative actions) and at the micro (clinical) level to assess the effectiveness of preventive, palliative, and curative therapies. Statistics Canada has taken an approach to monitoring and policy development that relies on use of the Health Utility Index (57) in both clinical and population settings. They have reasoned that a common metric, employed in clinical trials and in population health monitoring, will build a rich and coherent evidence base. Reliable information about the effectiveness and efficiency of different interventions will be available to inform clinical as well as population health-based decision making (65).

The United States has taken a more laissez-faire attitude toward its summary measures. Many investigators believe that the science of these measures, particularly in the area of describing and valuing health, is not fully developed and selection of one particular system now would result in premature closure of an

---

[8]For example, in the case of asthma, the DALY system records a decrement of 0.06 for asthma, whereas the QALY-linked Quality of Well-Being Scale measures a 0.32 loss from full health. Similar inconsistencies can be seen in QALY-associated HRQL measures, but in the DALY/QALY comparison they are compounded by the different methods used in calculating life expectancy within the two systems.

important area of research. Others believe that failure to select a standard measure hinders rational policy development; they argue that the perfect measure will be hard to find. In the meantime, federal funding supports some studies that use DALYs and others that use QALYs. No investigations are currently under way to systematically compare outcomes/burden of disease inferred using the DALY approach to inferences based on QALYs computed with any of the many available HRQL measurement instruments. A careful consideration of the outputs of the two methods simultaneously could provide a better understanding of convergence or divergence in estimates. Convergence would bolster confidence in their validity; divergence would point the way to a better understanding of the performance characteristics of each of the methods and encourage more focused research. Either outcome would advance us toward resolution in this key measurement arena.

Visit the Annual Reviews home page at www.annualreviews.org

LITERATURE CITED

1. Anand S, Hanson K. 1997. Disability-adjusted life years: a critical review. *J. Health Econ.* 16(6):685–702
2. Arnesen T, Nord E. 1999. The value of DALY life: problems with ethics and validity of disability adjusted life years. *BMJ* 319(7222):1423–25. Erratum. 2000. *BMJ* 320(7246):1398
3. Balaban DJ, Sagi PC, Goldfarb NI, Nettler S. 1986. Weights for scoring the quality of well-being instrument among rheumatoid arthritics: a comparison to the general population weights. *Med. Care* 24:973–80
4. Boyle MH, Torrance GW. 1984. Developing multiattribute health indexes. *Med. Care* 22:1045–57
5. Brock D. 1998. Ethical issues in the development of summary measures of population health status. See Ref. 15, pp. 73–91
6. The burden of disease in Los Angeles County. A study of the patterns of morbidity and mortality in the county population. (http:/www.hsph.Harvard.edu/org anizations/bdu/papers/usbodi/index.html) The link on this is "US Patterns of Mortality by County and Race: 1965–1994" by CJL Murray, CM Michaud, M McKenna, J Marks

7. Daniels N. 1998. Distributive justice and the use of summary measures of population health status. See Ref. 15, pp. 58–71
8. Drummond MF, Stoddart GL, Torrance GW. 1987. *Methods for the Economic Evaluation of Health Care Programmes.* New York: Oxford Univ. Press
9. Elixhauser A, Halpern M, Schmier J, Luce BR. 1998. Health care CBA and CEA from 1991 to 1996: an updated bibliography. *Med. Care* 36(5 Suppl.):MS1–9, MS18–147
10. Epstein AM, Hall JA, Tognetti J, Son LH, Conant L. 1989. Using proxies to evaluate quality of life. *Med. Care* 27:S91–98
11. Erickson P, Wilson RW, Shannon I. 1995. *Years of Healthy Life.* Stat. Note No. 7. Hyattsville, MD: Natl. Cent. Health Stat.
12. EuroQol Group. 1990. EuroQol: a new facility for the measurement of health-related quality of life. *Health Policy* 16:199
13. Fanshel S, Bush JW. 1970. A health status index and its application to health-services outcomes. *Oper. Res.* 18:1021–66
14. Feeny DH, Furlong W, Barr RD, et al. 1992. A comprehensive multi-attribute

system for classifying the health status of survivors of childhood cancer. *J. Clin. Oncol.* 10:923–26

15. Field JM, Gold MR, eds. 1998. *Summarizing Population Health: Directions for the Development and Application of Population Metrics.* Inst. Med., Washington, DC: Natl. Acad. Press

16. Froberg DG, Kane RL. 1989. Methodology for measuring health-state preferences I. Measurement strategies. *J. Clin. Epidemiol.* 42:345–54

17. Froberg DG, Kane RL. 1989. Methodology for measuring health-state preferences II. Scaling Methods. *J. Clin. Epidemiol.* 42:459–71

18. Fryback DG, Dasbach EJ, Klein R, Klein BEK, Dorn N, et al. 1993. The Beaver Dam Health Outcomes Study: initial catalog of health-state quality factors. *Med. Decis. Mak.* 13:89–102

18a. Fryback DG, Lawrence WF. 1997. Dollars may not buy as many QALYs as we think: a problem with defining quality-of-life adjustments. *Med. Decis. Mak.* 17:276–84

19. Garber AM, Weinstein MC, Torrance GW, Kamlet MS. 1996. Theoretical foundations of cost-effectiveness analysis. See Ref. 23, pp. 25–53

20. Gold MR, Franks P, McCoy KI, Fryback DG. 1998. Toward consistency in cost-utility analyses. Using national measures to create condition-specific values. *Med. Care* 36(6):778–92

21. Gold MR, Muennig P. 2002. Measure-dependent variation in burden of disease estimates: implications for policy. *Med. Care.* 40:In press

22. Gold MR, Patrick DL, Torrance GW. 1996. Identifying and valuing outcomes. See Ref. 23, pp. 82–134

23. Gold MR, Siegel JE, Russell LB, Weinstein MC. 1996. *Cost-effectiveness in Health and Medicine.* New York: Oxford Univ. Press. 425 pp.

24. Hadorn DC. 1991. Setting health care priorities in Oregon. Cost-effectiveness meets the rule of rescue. *JAMA* 265:2218–25

25. Harris J. 1987. QALYfying the value of life. *J. Med. Ethics* 13(3):117–23

26. Harris J. 1988. Life: quality, value and justice. *Health Policy* 10(3):259–66

27. Hornberger JC, Redelmeier DA, Peterson J. 1992. Variability among methods to assess patients' well-being and consequent effect on a cost-effectiveness analysis. *J. Clin. Epidemiol.* 5:505–12

28. Kaplan RM, Anderson JP. 1988. A general health policy model: update and applications. *Health Serv. Res.* 23:203–35

29. Klarman HE, Francis JO, Rosenthal GD. 1968. Cost-effectiveness analysis applied to the treatment of chronic renal disease. *Med. Care* 6:48–54

30. Koch T. 2000. Life quality vs the 'quality of life': assumptions underlying prospective quality of life instruments in health care planning. *Soc. Sci. Med.* 51(3):419–27

31. Llewellyn-Thomas HA, Sutherland JH, Tibshirani R, Ciampi A, Till JE, Boyd NF. 1984. Describing health states: methodologic issues in obtaining values for health states. *Med. Care* 22:543–52

32. McDowell I, Newell P. 1996. *Measuring Health: A Guide to Rating Scales and Questionnaires.* New York: Oxford Univ. Press

33. Menzel P, Gold MR, Nord E, Pinto-Prades JL, Richardson J, Ubel P. 1999. Toward a broader view of values in cost-effectiveness analysis of health. *Hastings Cent. Rep.* 29(3):7–15

34. Moriyama I. 1968. Problems in the measurement of health status. In *Indicators of Social Change*, ed. E Sheldon, WE Moore, pp. 573–600. New York: Russell Sage Found.

35. Murray CJL, Lopez AD. 1996. *The Global Burden of Disease: A Comprehensive Assessment of Mortality and Disability from Diseases, Injuries, and Risk Factors in 1990 and Projected to 2020.* Global Burden of Disease and Injury Series, Vol.

1. Cambridge, MA: Harvard Sch. Public Health/WHO/World Bank. 990 pp.

36. Murray CJ, Lopez AD. 2000. Progress and directions in refining the global burden of disease approach: a response to Williams. *Health Econ.* 9(1):69–82

37. Nease RF, Kneeland GT, O'Connor W, Sumner W, Lumpkins C, et al. 1995. Variation in patient utilities for outcomes of the management of chronic stable angina: implications for clinical practice guidelines. *JAMA* 273:1185–90

38. Neumann PJ, Goldie SJ, Weinstein MC. 2000. Preference-based measures in economic evaluation in health care. *Annu. Rev. Public Health* 21:587–611

39. Nord E. 1992. Methods for quality adjustment of life years. *Soc. Sci. Med.* 34(5):559–69

40. Nord E. 1995. The person trade-off approach to valuing health care programs. *Med. Decis. Mak.* 15(3):201–8

41. Nord E, Pinto JL, Richardson J, Menzel P, Ubel P. 1999. Incorporating societal concerns for fairness in numerical valuations of health programmes. *Health Econ.* 8:25–39

42. O'Leary JF, Faircloth DL, Jankowski MK, Weeks JC. 1995. Comparison of time trade-off utilities and rating scale values of cancer patients and their relatives: evidence for a possible plateau relationship. *Med. Decis. Mak.* 15:132–37

43. Packer A. 1968. Applying cost-effectiveness concepts to the community health system. *Oper. Res.* 16:227–53

44. Patrick DL, Erickson P. 1993. *Health Status and Health Policy: Allocating Resources to Health Care.* New York: Oxford Univ. Press

45. Patrick DL, Bush JW, Chen MM. 1973. Methods for measuring levels of wellbeing for a health-status index. *Health Serv. Res.* 8(3):228–45

46. Pliskin JS, Shepard DS, Weinstein MC. 1980. Utility functions for life years and health status. *Oper. Res.* 28:206–24

47. Rawles J. 1989. Castigating QALYs. *J. Med. Ethics* 15(3):143–47

48. Read JL, Quinn RG, Berwick DM, Fineberg HV, Weinstein MC. 1984. Preferences for health outcomes: comparisons of assessment methods. *Med. Decis. Mak.* 4:315–29

49. Rosenberg MA, Fryback DG, Lawrence WF. 1999. Computing population-based estimates of health-adjusted life expectancy. *Med. Decis. Mak.* 19:90–97

50. Russell LB, Gold MR, Siegel JE, Daniels N, Weinstein MC. 1996. The role of cost-effectiveness analysis in health and medicine. *JAMA* 276:1172–77

51. Sackett DL, Torrance GW. 1978. The utility of different health states as perceived by the general public. *J. Chronic Dis.* 31:697–70

52. Sanders B. 1964. Measuring community health levels. *Am. J. Public Health* 54(7):1063–70

53. Slevin ML, Stubbs L, Plant HJ, Wilson P, Gregory WM, et al. 1990. Attitude to chemotherapy: comparing views of patients with cancer with those of doctors, nurses, and general public. *BMJ* 300:1458–60

54. Sullivan D. 1966. *Conceptual Problems in Developing an Index of Health.* Washington, DC: U.S. Dep. HEW

55. Torrance GW. 1986. Measurement of health state utilities for economic appraisal. A review. *J. Health Econ.* 5:1–30

56. Torrance GW, Boyle MH, Horwood SP. 1982. Application of multi-attribute utility theory to measure social preferences of health states. *Oper. Res.* 30:1043–69

57. Torrance GW, Furlong W, Feeny D, Boyle M. 1995. Multi-attribute preference functions. Health Utilities Index. *Pharmacoeconomics* 7:503–20

58. Ubel PA, Nord E, Gold MR, Menzel P, Pinto-Prades JL, Richardson J. 2000. Improving value measurement in cost-effectiveness analysis. *Med. Care* 38(9):892–901

59. Van Wijck EE, Bosch JL, Hunink JM.

1998. Time-trade-off values and standard gamble utilities assessed during telephone interviews versus face-to-face interviews. *Med. Decis. Mak.* 18:400–5

60. Von-Neumann J, Morgenstern O. 1944. *Theory of Games and Economic Behavior.* Princeton, NJ: Princeton Univ. Press

61. Williams A. 1996. QALYS and ethics: a health economist's perspective. *Soc. Sci. Med.* 43(12):1795–804

62. Williams A. 1999. Calculating the global burden of disease: time for a strategic reappraisal? *Health Econ.* 8:1–8

63. Wolfson M. 1994. POHEM—a frame-work for understanding and modeling the health of human populations. *World Health Stat. Q.* 47(3):157–76

64. Wolfson MC. 1996. Health-adjusted life expectancy. *Health Rep.* 8:41–46

65. Wolfson MC. 1999. Measuring health—visions and practicalities. *Stat. J. U. N. ECE* 16:1–17

66. World Bank. World Dev. Rep. 1993. *Investing in Health.* New York: Oxford Univ. Press/World Bank

67. World Health Organ. 1980. International Classification of Impairments, Disability and Handicap. Geneva: WHO

Annu. Rev. Public Health 2002. 23:135–50

MORBIDITY AND MORTALITY FROM MEDICAL ERRORS: An Increasingly Serious Public Health Problem

David P. Phillips and Charlene C. Bredder

Department of Sociology, University of California at San Diego, La Jolla,
California 92093; e-mail: dphillip@weber.ucsd.edu, cbredder@weber.ucsd.edu

Key Words   prescription medications, death, trends

■ **Abstract**   From 1983 to 1998, U.S. fatalities from acknowledged prescription errors increased by 243%, from 2,876 to 9,856. This percentage increase was greater than for almost any other cause of death, and far outpaced the increase in the number of prescriptions. Many nonfatal prescription errors also occur, but estimates of the frequency of these errors vary widely, because various definitions, geographic settings, and institutions have been used. Efforts to reduce fatal and nonfatal prescription errors have encountered perceptual, legal, medical, and cultural barriers. It may be possible to reduce prescription errors by instituting a central agency responsible for collecting, analyzing, and reporting harmful or potentially harmful drug events, and for issuing recommendations and directives.

INTRODUCTION

With the introduction of Medicare's prospective pricing system in 1983, governmental and nongovernmental organizations have increasingly pressured hospitals to control the costs of patient care (1). Partly in response to these financial pressures hospitals have decreased the average length of stay for patients and have increasingly substituted outpatient for inpatient services. From 1979–1998 the number of outpatient visits increased by 125% (1) while the number of inpatient days decreased by 45% (1) and the average hospital stay decreased by 21% (1). Have these large-scale efforts to reduce medical costs also reduced the quality of medical care?

One way to examine this question is to estimate the number of fatal and nonfatal medical errors, including errors in diagnoses, surgery, and prescriptions. Studies (14, 15, 27, 33, 37, 39, 46, 60) indicate that prescription errors outnumber other types and appear in a wide range of medical settings. In this review we focus mainly on prescription errors. There is considerable potential for such errors: 2.9 billion retail U.S. prescriptions were filled in 2000, up 62% from a decade earlier (50).

0163-7525/02/0510-0135$14.00

According to the ninth revision of the *International Classification of Diseases (Clinical Modification)*, fatal and nonfatal errors from prescription medicines fall into three general categories. These (with their ICD-9 codes) are listed below:

1. **Acknowledged prescription errors** (E850–E858)   These are accidental errors from prescription medicines, in which errors by the patient or by medical staff have been officially acknowledged. Errors in this category resulted from an "accidental overdose of drug, wrong drug given or taken in error, and drug taken inadvertently" (61).

2. **Unacknowledged prescription errors** (E930–E949)   These are accidental errors from prescription medicines, in which there is no obvious mistake by patient or by medical staff. Errors in this category resulted from an unexpected reaction to the "correct drug properly administered in therapeutic or prophylactic dosage" (61).

3. **Undetermined prescription errors** (E980.0–E980.5)   These are errors from prescription medicines in which it is unclear whether the death resulted from homicide, suicide, or accident, and (if accidental) whether the death resulted from correct or incorrect medical procedures (61).

The E-code section of the International Classification of Diseases is used to classify external causes of death. Thus, the E-codes are used whenever a medical official records a death from non-natural causes, such as gunshot, automobile accident, drowning, suicide, or prescription medicine. Medical officials may sometimes have difficulty distinguishing between the three types of prescription errors listed above. However, given that acknowledged prescription errors are legally the most problematic of the three types, it seems likely that a physician would assign a death to this category only if the evidence pointed clearly in this direction.

When examining medical errors, researchers have generally adopted either of two major strategies. They have sought errors in nationwide mortality data or in a relatively small number of local institutional settings. Because each research strategy has different strengths and weaknesses, the two approaches are complementary and together provide a fuller and richer picture of the scope of the problem. Nationwide studies can provide an overview and can indicate whether there is a long-term increase in medical errors. Studies of this type examine a very large number of cases, in a wide geographic area, over a long time period. However, nationwide studies are also limited, because they focus exclusively on fatal errors. In contrast to national studies, local studies typically examine both fatal and nonfatal errors and provide richer descriptions of the processes leading to errors. In addition, local studies can identify with greater precision the medical settings and occupations most prone to error. Alternatively, local studies are limited because they examine relatively few cases in limited geographic and temporal settings. Each type of study is discussed below.

NATIONWIDE STUDIES OF FATAL PRESCRIPTION ERRORS

Only two investigations have used nationwide U.S. mortality data to examine fatal prescription errors. The first of these (18) compared fatal prescription errors as reported to the FDA with those recorded on death certificates. Chyka (18) found 206 U.S. death certificates that recorded prescription errors as the primary cause of death. However, although nominally interested in all fatal prescription errors, Chyka (18) chose to examine only the smallest subcategory: unacknowledged prescription errors (E930–E949). He did not examine acknowledged prescription errors (E850–E858), which accounted for many more deaths in the year of his study (8021 versus 206 in 1995).

In contrast to Chyka, Phillips et al. (55) examined all three types of prescription errors listed above. Their study spanned 11 years (1983–1993) and showed that U.S. deaths from prescription errors increased markedly over this period. Of the three categories of prescription errors, acknowledged prescription errors (APE) increased most, by 157% (7391 in 1993/2876 in 1983). The increase in mortality from prescription errors far exceeds the increase in the number of prescriptions during the study period. Overall, mortality from APE increased more than mortality from any other leading cause of death, except for AIDS. The largest increase in APE occurred in outpatient settings: a 748% rise in deaths, versus a 137% rise for inpatients. In 1993 the proportion of deaths from APE was 6.5 times greater for outpatients than for inpatients, a risk-ratio that rose steadily during the study period.

Since this study appeared, more recent mortality data have become available, which indicate a continued, upward trend in deaths from prescription medicines. From 1983 to 1998 all mortality from APE increased by 243% (9856/2876), (62) while outpatient mortality from APE increased by 907% (1733/172) (62). This 907% increase is much greater than would be expected from the overall increase in outpatient visits (1) and from the increase in outpatient deaths from other causes (62).

Figure 1 indicates that APE deaths increased more steeply than did other deaths resulting from the misuse of solid and liquid substances. At the beginning of the study period the number of APE deaths was about the same as the number of deaths from suicides using prescriptions. However, at the end of the study period, fatal accidents from APEs far outnumbered suicides from prescriptions. In fact, APE deaths outnumbered all other plotted deaths from solid and liquid poisoning combined (9856 versus 8924 in 1998). Aside from APE deaths, only one other category markedly increased: deaths from prescription medicines for which it is undetermined whether the misuse is purposeful (in the form of suicide or homicide) or accidental. These undetermined prescription deaths increased by 207%.

The statistics plotted in Figure 1 indicate an increasingly serious, nationwide public health problem resulting from prescription errors. Local institutional studies

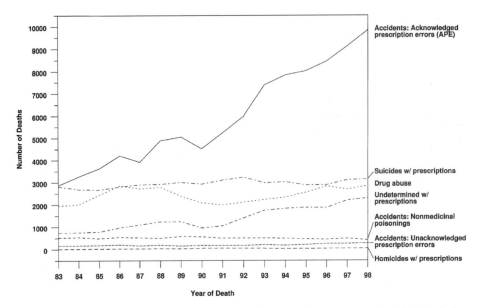

Figure 1   Trends in U.S. deaths from prescriptions and related causes, 1983–1998. This figure is a modified and updated version of one originally presented by Phillips et al. (55), which covered 1983–1993. Mortality data come from computerized death certificates provided by the National Center for Health Statistics (62). Currently these data are not available beyond 1998. The causes plotted (with their *International Classification of Disease* codes) are accidents from prescriptions for which error is acknowledged (E850–E858); suicides with prescription medicines (E950.0–E950.5); dependent and nondependent drug abuse (304–305); prescription medicines, for which it is undetermined whether death resulted from purposeful or accidental acts (E980.0–E980.5); accidental poisonings by nonmedicinal solid and liquid substances (E860–E866); accidents from prescriptions for which error is not acknowledged (E930–E949); and homicides with prescription medicines (E962.0).

provide a more detailed picture of the circumstances, personnel, and medical procedures contributing to this problem.

LOCAL INSTITUTIONAL STUDIES OF FATAL AND NONFATAL MEDICAL ERRORS

The literature on this topic is in an early, exploratory phase, partly because the complexity of the U.S. health-care system makes it difficult to study and partly because researchers have chosen to focus on many different aspects of this system (27, 36, 44, 66). In addition, when studying errors, researchers have often applied different methods and definitions to a wide variety of types and sizes of institutions in many parts of the United States. Because of these considerations, it may be premature to provide a definitive, systematic, and generalizable overview of errors in U.S. health care. Despite these difficulties, certain themes recur in the literature, and these will be examined in turn.

DIFFERENT METHODS FOR IDENTIFYING MEDICAL ERRORS

In document-based studies researchers have identified diagnostic, surgical, and prescription errors by intensively reviewing hospital records (15, 19, 38–40, 46, 60). In more focused studies of this sort investigators have identified errors by reviewing prescriptions before they were filled (43). In interview-based studies researchers have asked medical staff to report on their own errors and also on errors they observed (3). Studies of this sort have tried to identify errors that actually occurred and errors that would have occurred in the absence of intervention. In observational studies researchers have followed medical staff during their daily rounds and have noted both actual and potential errors (2, 21). In quasi-experimental studies researchers have installed computerized systems for checking and suggesting prescriptions and have then compared error rates in the postcomputer and precomputer phases (4, 13, 19, 23–25, 67).

FREQUENCY AND COSTS OF MEDICAL ERRORS FOUND

It is difficult to create an overview of error rates and costs because research designs have employed a wide variety of definitions, institutions, locations, time periods, and sample sizes. Three of the most comprehensive, multi-hospital studies (14, 15, 46, 60) found overall hospital error rates of 2.9% (Utah and Colorado in 1992), 3.7% (New York in 1984), and 4.6% (California in 1977). These studies found that prescription errors accounted for between 18.8% and 19.3% of all hospital errors. Smaller studies of prescriptions measured error rates in different ways: Leape et al. (37) found 6.1 adverse drug events and 4.8 potential adverse drug events per 100 admissions; Lesar et al. (38) found 3.99 prescription errors per 1000 medication orders. Bates et al. (3) found 6.5 adverse drug events (ADE) per 100 patient admissions (where an ADE is defined as an injury resulting from administering a drug). Bowman (11) found 29.7 ADEs per 100 patient admissions (where an ADE is defined as any adverse experience associated with the use of a drug, including experiences rated "possible" on the Naranjo scale). A General Accounting Office report (27) cites a 6-month hospital study that found an ADE rate of 1 per 10,000 drug administrations. Another study found that 15% of prescriptions filled at retail pharmacies contained medication errors (63).

In a study of a single teaching hospital in Utah (19), researchers found that 2.4% of admissions experienced an adverse medical event, resulting in excess hospitalization costs of nearly $4.5 million over a 4-year period. Other studies (5, 23, 27) found extra costs ranging from $1939 to $2595 for each patient who experienced an ADE. According to the Harvard Medical Study (14, 15), preventable ADEs generated 4.6 extra days of hospital stay and $4685 of additional costs for each patient.

RISK FACTORS FOR PRESCRIPTION ERRORS

Many studies have found that prescription errors are more frequent for certain types of settings, patients, staff, and procedures. Risk factors for error can be usefully classified under four general headings, each of which is discussed in turn.

Risk Factors Associated with Characteristics of Medical Setting and Staff

As noted above, hospitals have decreased the average length of stay for patients and have increasingly substituted outpatient for inpatient services. Studies indicate that these changes can sometimes result in medical errors. A 9-year hospital investigation found that as the length of stay decreased, the number of medications ordered per patient-day increased twofold and, at the same time, the number of prescription errors increased (39). Mills et al. found that a higher rate of drug-related errors involved nonhospital settings (46). Phillips et al. found that the risk of fatal prescription errors was 6.5 times greater for outpatients than for inpatients (55).

Other types of errors may result because patients have begun to use a combination of local, mail-order, and web-based pharmacies (34, 51, 58, 63). Pharmacists in one of these three categories may not know about prescriptions filled by pharmacists in the other categories, and hence there is increased potential for overprescribing and for adverse drug interactions (32, 59). Additional errors are possible because web-based pharmacies cannot positively identify the person ordering medications (26) and because some U.S. residents have used the web to order medications not currently approved by the FDA (26).

These problems result from factors outside the hospital; other problems arise from factors inside the hospital. For example, medication errors seem to be more likely in certain departments (pediatric, emergency, and ICU) (39, 60), and within each hospital department, error rates are also influenced by characteristics of the staff. Safety is reduced during staff shortages (54) and when continuity of care is disrupted, either in the case of nurses (52) or physicians (42, 54). Other risk factors include poor interstaff communication (13), inexperienced staff (54), new residents (68), and introduction of new medical techniques (3, 38, 69).

Throughout the hospital, cost controls are increasingly emphasized and physicians are spending less time per patient. Consequently doctors may sometimes have inadequate knowledge of their patients and may prescribe inappropriately. Several studies (37, 38, 60) found that this lack of knowledge was the most important predictor of prescription error.

Risk Factors Associated with Characteristics of the Patient

Errors are generated not only by medical staff, but also by patients. One study (20) found that 11% of all elderly patients were admitted to a hospital because of their noncompliance with medication regimes. Medical errors are linked not only to patients' behavior, but also to their medical condition. For example, prescription errors frequently result from failure to adjust dosages for the patient's age, allergies, body mass, and for decreased renal, cardiac, or liver function (19, 27, 37, 38). In addition, seriously ill patients may require more medicines and nonstandard treatments; the risk of prescription error is greater under these circumstances (2, 13–15, 17, 37).

Risk Factors Associated with Drugs

Leape et al. (37) found that 29% of prescription errors were caused by mistakes in the dissemination of drug information, whereas 12% were caused by mistakes in the checking of identity and dosage. According to a report by the General Accounting Office, errors also occur because of confusion resulting from similarly named drugs (27). Other errors occur when drugs are inappropriately prescribed to treat conditions for which they were ineffective (38). Lesar et al. (38) noted that the risk of error is increased because the rapid development of pharmaceuticals makes it difficult for physicians to keep up with new drugs, dosages, effects, and interactions.

Some of the above errors arise from lack of information. However, even when medical staff are fully informed about a drug, errors may occur. Drugs frequently associated with medication errors include narcotic analgesics, sedatives, psychotropics, antibiotics, and cardiovascular and chemotherapeutic agents (3, 4, 27, 28, 39). The inclusion of a drug on this list need not necessarily imply that the drug is inherently dangerous: The number of errors associated with a drug may be high merely because the drug is frequently used, rather than because it has a high error rate. However, some drugs are associated with medical errors even when they are used relatively seldom, because their pharmacological properties make them "difficult to use, even when administered in generally recommended doses" (27). Examples include the anticoagulant warfarin and the cardiac stimulant digoxin.

Risk Factors Associated with Determining, Ordering, Administering, and Checking a Prescription Drug

Studies have found various impediments to correct determination and administration of drug dosages. Dosage errors can arise because of deficiencies in some nurses' mathematical and conceptual skills (52). Even when dosages have been correctly calculated, medical staff may still administer an incorrect dose because they have misread a confusing, incomplete, or handwritten prescription (52). In addition, a prescription that may have been written and read correctly at one stage of the ordering process may have been transcribed incorrectly at another (37, 52). Even when a prescription has been correctly written, transcribed, and read, errors may still occur when the drug is administered (3, 4). For example, correct procedure might require that the patient receive the drug with food, but the drug is administered without food (3, 4). This type of error is a subset of a larger category, in which medical staff fail to follow general hospital procedures (52). Several studies (4, 13, 23, 38, 53) have found that many of these errors can be reduced when data on drugs, prescriptions, and patients have been computerized.

The studies reviewed suggest that medical errors are increasingly significant and occur in a wide range of settings. We now consider some ways in which these errors can be reduced.

A COMPARISON OF EFFORTS TO REDUCE ERRORS IN MEDICINE AND TRANSPORTATION

Although the destruction of the World Trade Center indicates that airplanes can be used purposefully to cause many deaths, nonpurposeful deaths are rare in the aviation industry. Because of the rarity of aviation accidents, some have suggested that medical errors could be reduced if they were treated in a manner similar to that prevailing in aviation (16) or other industries (6, 8, 56). We summarize levels and trends for fatal errors in medicine and transportation. Then we briefly describe techniques used by the National Transportation Safety Board (NTSB) to investigate and reduce transportation errors. Finally, we note that efforts to study and regulate medical errors are less thorough than parallel efforts in transportation.

Figure 2 compares 20-year trends in accidental deaths from prescription medicines with trends in accidental deaths from aircraft, watercraft, trains, and motor vehicles. To facilitate comparison, all data are plotted on the same ratio scale, with 1979 = 1. In 1998, the latest data-year available, the number of accidental deaths from prescriptions was five times the number of accidental deaths from aircraft, watercraft, and trains combined (10,133/1,887 = 5.37). Fatal transport accidents in each sector have either decreased or remained approximately level; in contrast, fatal prescription accidents have increased markedly.

This marked difference in trends may arise partly because transport accidents are studied and regulated far more thoroughly than prescription accidents. For more than 33 years, the NTSB has investigated transport accidents, both fatal and nonfatal, commercial and noncommercial (48). It has issued 11,000 safety recommendations to 1,300 recipients in federal, state, and local governments, industry, associations, media, and law, as well as to consultants and private individuals (47, 49). Although the NTSB, an independent accident investigation agency, has no regulatory powers, 82% of its recommendations have been implemented (47).

The primary purpose of the NTSB is to identify facts, conditions, circumstances, and probable cause of individual accidents and to issue directives and recommendations that will reduce the recurrence of any errors uncovered in NTSB investigations (48). In addition, the NTSB produces an Annual Review of aircraft

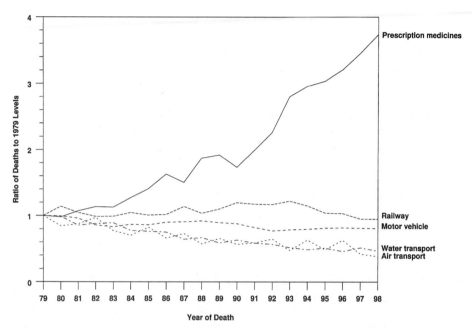

Figure 2   Trends in U.S. deaths from prescriptions and from different types of transportation accidents, 1979–1998 (1979 = 1). To facilitate comparison of trends, mortality levels have been expressed in terms of a ratio: deaths in a given year/deaths in 1979. Thus, for example, the number of accidental deaths from prescription medicines in 1998 is nearly four times the number in 1979. Mortality data come from computerized death certificates provided by the National Center for Health Statistics (62). The period covered begins in 1979, with the introduction of the ninth revision of the *International Classification of Diseases*, and ends with 1998, the latest data year available. The causes plotted (with their *International Classification of Disease* codes) comprise prescription and transportation accidents: prescriptions with acknowledged and unacknowledged error (E850–E858, E930–E949); railway (E800–E807); motor vehicle traffic (E810–E819); water transport (E830–E838); and powered aircraft (E840–E841).

accident data, public records, pamphlets, and press releases (48). Staff members also communicate their findings in an Annual Report to Congress and in speeches and testimony (48). The agency maintains a publicly available aviation accident database, consisting of 46,000 cases, each of which is typically described in terms of 600 data elements (48, 49). The NTSB conducts safety studies to determine whether government regulations have indeed reduced error and whether additional regulations are advisable (48).

In addition to providing information to the public and appropriate organizations, the NTSB also promotes a flow of information in the opposite direction: The agency has established a 24-hour communications center (49) and a "Most Wanted List" of transportation improvements recommended by the public (49).

It is noteworthy that the NTSB commits enormous resources to investigating, reporting, analyzing, summarizing, and reducing fatal and nonfatal air, water, and train accidents, even though the number of deaths caused by these accidents is small and diminishing. In marked contrast, there is a much larger and increasing number of deaths from prescription accidents, and these are not investigated or reported with the same thoroughness. Several federal agencies, e.g., the FDA, help reduce certain types of medical errors. However, for the detection, investigation, and control of medical errors, there is no federal agency whose scope, function, and powers are equivalent to the NTSB.

SOME BARRIERS TO REDUCING MEDICAL ERRORS

Why has the medical industry not developed as much as transportation industries with respect to the detection, investigation, analysis, reporting, and control of fatal errors? This relative lack of development has occurred partly because prior to the current report (Figure 2) there was no published comparison of levels and trends in deaths from prescription accidents versus levels and trends in deaths from air, water, and rail accidents. Consequently policy makers have not been fully aware of the paradox we have noted—few resources devoted to solving a larger problem and many resources devoted to solving a smaller one. Some additional barriers to reducing medical errors are discussed below.

Perceptual Barriers: Perceived Risk versus Actual Risk of Death

The NTSB investigates every commercial and noncommercial plane crash, even those involving only one fatality. Each crash is investigated partly because death is viewed as a startling and avoidable outcome of travel. Fatal plane crashes are typically publicized; the cause of death is clear and frequently elicits outrage. In contrast, deaths from prescription error are not typically publicized; the cause of death may not be clear and rarely elicits public outrage. Unlike airplane accidents, hospital deaths are not startling: They are common (963,320 people died as U.S. inpatients in 1998) (62) and sometimes unavoidable. In short, plane crash fatalities are highly visible (though infrequent), whereas prescription deaths are less visible (though more frequent). Because of these considerations, policymakers and the public have a distorted perception of the relative risk of death from air travel versus prescriptions. This difference in perceived risks may help to explain why more national resources are invested in the reduction of accidents caused by airplanes rather than prescriptions. Aside from these perceptual factors, there are also legal and medical barriers to the reduction of medical errors.

Legal Barriers

Tort law is structured to assign fault to individuals rather than to systemic problems, (10, 12, 15, 29, 64), and medical staff frequently share this attitude. These legal and medical views hinder the free, open, and voluntary reporting of prescription errors (35). Different conditions hold for the reporting and analysis of aviation errors. The aviation industry has learned that pilots are more willing to report incidents and near-misses if the threat of punishment is eliminated (37), and fault is frequently assigned to systemic factors rather than to individuals. In addition, the NTSB is a fact-finding rather than a punitive agency: The errors it uncovers are used to improve safety, and the NTSB's "analysis of factual information and its determination of probable cause cannot be entered as evidence in a court of law" (48, p. 1).

Medical Barriers

The delivery of medical care is not as systematically integrated as the delivery of aviation services. Even now (45), computers are not used everywhere to track patients, medications, illnesses, and dosages. In addition, doctors' computer systems may not be integrated with those used by pharmacists (32, 45, 63), and computer systems used by one pharmacy network may not be linked to systems used by other pharmacy networks (32, 63). Unlike airports, which are in frequent, routine contact, hospitals do not communicate problems and solutions daily in a nationwide system. This nonsystematic communication between hospitals has hindered the standardized development of error checks and redundant controls (31). These are present in many medical settings, but are not as pervasive as in aviation.

The free flow of information is not only restricted between hospitals but also within them. For example, because of the hierarchical nature of medicine, some nurses may be unwilling to report errors to physicians and some physicians may be unwilling to hear them (52, 64, 65). As Wears et al. noted, "Strong professional values (such as autonomy) and the lack of organizational structures in health care systems prevent awareness of errors and near misses, even without any intent to conceal" (64, p. 58). Despite these perceptual, legal, and medical barriers it should be possible to reduce the risk of medical error. Some recommendations are listed below.

RECOMMENDATIONS TO REDUCE MEDICAL ERRORS

Congress should create a federal agency that deals with medical errors in the same way the NTSB deals with transportation errors. This medical agency should have the same scope and powers as the NTSB and should perform the following functions:

Centralized collection of information of medical errors   This information should be solicited and recorded in standardized form and should include variables that describe the time, place, and circumstances in which the error occurred. The reporting of fatal medical errors should be mandatory, whereas voluntary, anonymous reporting of nonfatal errors should be encouraged (33, 41, 64).

Centralized archiving of information on medical errors   These archives should be in at least two forms: (*a*) narrative reports on each individual, fatal medical error and (*b*) an internet-accessible database consisting of all fatal medical errors, described in a systematic, standardized format. This database should not include information that identifies staff members.

Analysis of medical errors   The information produced by the agency should be analyzed, not only by the agency but also by researchers, educators, administrators, and practitioners. Currently most analysis of medical errors is restricted to a small number of hospitals and data years. Future analyses should have a broader scope: They should (*a*) not be confined primarily to hospitals but should also cover outpatient settings, including the home; (*b*) examine multiyear, nationwide trends; and (*c*) systematically compare trends in medical errors with trends in other types of errors monitored by the federal government.

Dissemination of information on medical errors   The agency should produce an annual report to Congress, an annual review of medical errors, pamphlets, and press releases. In addition, members of the agency should give speeches and testimony on medical safety and errors. Information should not flow in one direction only: The agency should create a 24-hour hotline and should solicit safety suggestions from medical staff and the public (a "most wanted list"). In addition, the agency should encourage medical institutions to share information on medical errors, not only with the agency but also with each other (30).

Discussion of medical errors and ways to reduce them   The agency should sponsor symposia and conferences (33) for practitioners, administrators, educators, researchers, and manufacturers of medical equipment and drugs.

Recommendation of procedures for the control and reduction of medical errors   The agency (like the NTSB) should not be a punitive body, but instead should focus on identifying causes of error and on ways to reduce them (65). To facilitate this reduction, the agency should issue recommendations to hospitals, nursing homes, clinics, professional associations, universities, and manufacturers of medical devices and drugs. Some of these recommendations should include ways of increasing the number of standardized procedures, error-checks and redundant controls (22, 65).

Evaluation of effectiveness of safety recommendations   The agency should conduct safety studies to evaluate the effectiveness of its recommendations and of medical procedures in general.

CONCLUSION

Reduction of medical errors cannot be achieved by government fiat alone, but will also require changes in the medical culture, both in training centers and in the field. Currently medical courses devote time and resources to the detection, prevention, and control of specific diseases, e.g., viral hepatitis. However, little teaching time is devoted to the recognition, avoidance, and reduction of medical errors. However, in 1998 there were many more U.S. deaths from acknowledged prescription errors (9856) than from viral hepatitis (4821) (62). In the future, medical, nursing, and pharmacy courses should devote increased time to the discussion of medical errors (33).

Practitioners as well as students would benefit from a change in attitude toward medical errors. Errors would probably be reduced if medical staff came to realize that some errors originate in systemic problems or in poor design of equipment and procedures, rather than in individual malfeasance (7, 16, 65). Safe medical practices can be more easily achieved if medical staff recognize the benefits of reporting, discussing, and learning from errors (8, 9, 22, 57).

Educational efforts should be directed not only to medical students and practitioners, but also to the public. When contemplating risks generated by an industry, the public is sometimes more apprehensive than the experts and more concerned than is warranted by the data. In the medical industry, however, the situation is reversed: At present, the public is not strongly preoccupied with the risk of death from medical errors, even though this risk is significant and increasing. It is desirable to increase public awareness of the problem, and this can best be done through education and publicity. Ultimately the responsibility for avoiding errors rests not only on government agencies and medical staff, but on the public as well.

ACKNOWLEDGMENTS

This paper was partially funded by the Marian E. Smith Foundation.

Visit the Annual Reviews home page at www.annualreviews.org

LITERATURE CITED

1. American Hospital Association. 1979–98. *Hospital Statistics: The AHA Profile of the United States Hospitals.* Chicago: Am. Hosp. Assoc., yearly volumes
2. Andrews LB, Stocking C, Krizek T, Gottlieb L, Krizek C, et al. 1997. An alternative strategy for studying adverse events in medical care. *Lancet* 349:309–13
3. Bates DW, Cullen DJ, Laird N, Petersen LA, Small SD, et al. 1995. Incidence of adverse drug events and potential adverse drug events: implications for prevention. *JAMA* 274:29–34
4. Bates DW, Leape LL, Cullen DJ, Laird N, Peterson LA, et al. 1998. Effect of computerized physician order entry and a team intervention on prevention of serious medication errors. *JAMA* 80:1311–16
5. Bates DW, Spell N, Cullen DV, Durdick E, Laird N, et al. 1997. The costs of adverse drug events in hospitalized patients. *JAMA* 277:307–11
6. Berwick DM. 1989. Continuous improvement as an ideal in health care. *N. Engl. J. Med.* 320:53–56
7. Berwick DM. 1994. Eleven worthy aims for clinical leadership of health system reform. *JAMA* 272:797–802

8. Blumenthal D. 1994. Making medical errors into "medical treasures." *JAMA* 272:1867–68

9. Blumenthal D, Kilo CM. 1998. A report card on continuous quality improvement. *Milbank Q.* 76(4):625–48

10. Bogner MS, ed. 1994. *Human Error in Medicine.* Hillsdale, NJ: Erlbaum

11. Bowman L. 1994. Incidence of adverse drug reactions in adult medical inpatients. *Can. J. Hosp. Pharm.* 47:209–16

12. Brennan TA. 2000. The Institute of Medicine report on medical errors: Could it do harm? *N. Engl. J. Med.* 342:1123–25

13. Brennan TA, Hebert LE, Laird NM, Lawthers A, Thorpe KE, et al. 1991. Hospital characteristics associated with adverse events and substandard care. *JAMA* 264:3265–69

14. Leape LL, Brennan TA, Laird NM, Lawthers AG, Localio AR, et al. 1991. The nature of adverse events in hospitalized patients: results of the Harvard medical practice study II. *N. Engl. J. Med.* 324:377–84

15. Brennan TA, Leape LL, Laird NM, Hebert L, Localio AR, et al. 1991. Incidence of adverse events and negligence in hospitalized patients. Results of the Harvard medical practice study I. *N. Engl. J. Med.* 324:370–76

16. Chassin MR. 1998. Is health care ready for six sigma quality? *Milbank Q.* 76(4):565–91

17. Chassin MR, Galvin RW. National Roundtable on Health Care Quality. 1998. The urgent need to improve health care quality. *JAMA* 280:1000–5

18. Chyka PA. 2000. How many deaths occur annually from adverse drug reactions in the United States? *Am. J. Med.* 109:122–30

19. Classen DC, Pestonik SL, Evans SR, Lloyd JF, Burke JP. 1997. Adverse drug events in hospitalized patients. *JAMA* 277:301–6

20. Col N. 1990. The role of medication non-compliance and adverse drug reactions in hospitalizations of the elderly. *Arch. Int. Med.* 150:841–45

21. Donchen Y, Gopher D, Olin M, Badihi Y, Biesky M, et al. 1995. A look into the nature and causes of human errors in the intensive care unit. *Crit. Care Med.* 23:294–300

22. Editorial. 1997. Zeroing in on medication errors. *Lancet* 349:369

23. Evans RS, Pestotnik SL, Classen DC, Bass SB, Burke JP. 1993. *Prevention of Adverse Drug Events Through Computerized Surveillance. 16th Annual Symposium on Computer Applications in Medical Care.* New York: McGraw-Hill

24. Evans RS, Classen DC, Stevens LE, Pestotnik SL, Gardner RM, et al. 1994. *Using a Hospital Information System to Assess the Effects of Adverse Drug Events. 17th Annual Symposium on Computer Applications in Medical Care.* New York: McGraw-Hill

25. Evans RS, Pestotnik SL, Classen DC, Clemmer TP, Weaver LK, et al. 1998. A computer-assisted management program for antibiotics and other infective agents. *N. Engl. J. Med.* 338:232–38

26. Freeman M. 2000. Customers outpacing pharmacy ID developments. *Chem. Druggist.* http://www.pharmacy.uk.co/itm00037.htm

27. GAO Report. 2000. *Adverse drug events: the magnitude of health risk is uncertain because of limited incidence data.* GAO/HEHS-00-21. Washington, DC: GAO

28. GAO Testimony. 2000. *Adverse events: surveillance systems for adverse events and medical errors.* GAO/T-HEHS-00-61. Washington, DC: GAO

29. Glasson J, Orentlicher D. 1993. Caring for the poor and professional liability: Is there a need for tort reform? *JAMA* 270:1740–41

30. Grumbach K, Anderson GM, Luft HS, Roos LL, Brook R. 1995. Regionalization of cardiac surgery in the United States and Canada. *JAMA* 274:1282–88

31. Kahn K. 1995. Above all "do no harm":

How shall we avoid errors in medicine? *JAMA* 274:75–76

32. Kirking DM, Ascione FJ, Richards JW. 1990. Choices in prescription-drug benefit programs: mail order versus community pharmacy services. *Milbank Q.* 68(1):29–47

33. Kohn LT, Corrigan JM, Donaldson MS, eds. 1999. *To Err is Human: Building a Safer Health System.* Washington, DC: Natl. Acad. Press

34. Laver R. 1997. Drugs and dirty tricks. *Macleans* 110:66

35. Leape LL. 1994. Error in medicine. *JAMA* 272:1851–57

36. Leape LL. 2000. Institute of Medicine medical error figures are not exaggerated. *JAMA* 284:95–96

37. Leape LL, Bates DW, Cullen DJ. 1995. Systems analysis of adverse drug events: ADE prevention study group. *JAMA* 274:35–43

38. Lesar TS, Briceland L, Stein DS. 1997. Factors related to errors in medication prescribing. *JAMA* 277:312–17

39. Lesar TS, Lomaestro BM, Pohl H. 1997. Medication prescribing errors in a teaching hospital: a nine year experience. *Arch. Intern. Med.* 157:1569–76

40. Localio AR, Lawthers A, Brennan TA. 1996. Identifying adverse events caused by medical care: degree of physician agreement in retrospective chart review. *Ann. Intern. Med.* 125:457–64

41. Macklis RM, Meier T, Weinhous MS. 1998. Error rates in clinical radiotherapy. *J. Clin. Oncol.* 16:551–56

42. Markson LE, Nash DB, eds. 1995. *Accountability and Quality in Health Care: The New Responsibility.* Oakbrook Terrace, IL: Joint Commission on Accreditation of Health Care Organizations

43. McDonald CJ. 1976. Protocol-based computer reminders, the quality of care and the non-perfectability of man. *N. Engl. J. Med.* 295:1351–55

44. McDonald CJ, Weiner M, Hui SL. 2000. Deaths due to medical errors are exaggerated in Institute of Medicine report. *JAMA* 284:93–95

45. Menduno M. 1999. Apothecary now. *Hosp. Health Networks* 73(7):34–38

46. Mills DH, Boyden JS, Rubsamen DS. 1977. *Report on the Medical Insurance Feasibility Study.* San Francisco: Sutter

47. National Transportation Safety Board. 1998. *We Are All Safer.* Washington, DC: NTSB

48. National Transportation Safety Board. 2001. About the NTSB. http://www.ntsb. gov/abt_ntsb/invest.htm

49. National Transportation Safety Board. 2001. Recommendations and accomplishments. http://www.ntsb.gov/recs

50. NDC Health. 1991–1998. National prescription audit. Yardley, Pa: NDC. http://www.ndchealth.com

51. Nordenberg T. 2000. Make no mistake: Medical errors can be deadly serious. http://www.fda.gov/fdac/features/2000/500_err.html

52. O'Shea E. 1999. Factors contributing to medication errors: a literature review. *J. Clin. Nurs.* 8:496–504

53. Pestonik SL, Classen DC, Evans RS, Burke JP. 1996. Implementing antibiotic practice guidelines through computer-assisted decision support: clinical and financial outcomes. *Ann. Intern. Med.* 124:884–90

54. Petersen LA, Brennan TA, O'Neil AC, Cook EF, Lee TH. 1994. Does housestaff discontinuity of care increase the risk for preventable adverse events? *Ann. Intern. Med.* 121:866–72

55. Phillips DP, Christenfeld N, Glynn LM. 1998. Increase in US medication-error deaths between 1983 and 1993. *Lancet* 351:1656–57

56. Reason J. 1990. *Human Error.* New York: Cambridge Univ. Press

57. Risser DT, Rice MM, Salisbury ML, Simon R, Jay GD, Berns SD. 1999. The potential for improved teamwork to reduce errors in the emergency department. *Ann. Emerg. Med.* 34:373–83

58. Sanborn G. 2000. Internet industry challenged to provide physicians with valuable online applications. http://www.cyberdia logue.com/news/releases/2000/12-05-cch-pulse.html

59. Spurgeon D. 1995. Advent of mail-order pharmacy causes concern among some pharmacists. *Can. Med. Assoc. J.* 152(9): 1485–86

60. Thomas EJ, Studdert DM, Burstin HR, Orav EJ, Zeena T, et al. 2000. Incidence and types of adverse events and negligent care in Utah and Colorado. *Med. Care* 38:261–71

61. U.S. Dep. Health and Human Services. 1994. *Public Health Service. International Classification of Diseases, 9th Revision, Clinical Modification.* Vols. 1, 2

62. U.S. Dep. Health and Human Services. National Center for Health Statistics. *Vital Statistics of the United States, Annual,* Vol. 2. *Mortality. Part A,* Table I-24. Washington, DC: GPO

63. Walsh PJ. 2000. E-pharmacy systems: prescription and medication fulfillment come of age. *MD Comput.* 17(3):45–48

64. Wears RL, Janiak B, Moorhead JC, Kellermann AL, Yeh CS, et al. 2000. Human error in medicine: promise and pitfalls, part I. *Ann. Emerg. Med.* 36(1):58–60

65. Wears RL, Janiak B, Moorhead JC, Kellermann AL, Yeh CS, et al. 2000. Human error in medicine: promise and pitfalls, part II. *Ann. Emerg. Med.* 36(2):142–44

66. Weingart SN, Wilson RM, Gibberd RW, Harrison B. 2000. Epidemiology of medical error. *Br. Med. J.* 320:774–77

67. Whiting-O'Keefe QE, Simborg DW, Epstein WV, Warger A. 1985. A computerized summary medical record system can provide more information than the standard medical report. *JAMA* 254:1185–92

68. Wilson JG, McArtney RG, Newcomb RG, McArtney RJ, Gracie J, et al. 1998. Medication errors in paediatric practice: insights from a continuous quality improvement approach. *Eur. J. Pediatr.* 157: 769–74

69. Wu AW, Folkman S, McPhee SJ, Lo B. 1991. Do house officers learn from their mistakes? *JAMA* 265:2089–94

Annu. Rev. Public Health 2002. 23:151–69

THE IMPORTANCE OF THE NORMALITY ASSUMPTION IN LARGE PUBLIC HEALTH DATA SETS

Thomas Lumley, Paula Diehr, Scott Emerson, and Lu Chen

Department of Biostatistics, University of Washington, Box 357232, Seattle, Washington 98195; e-mail: tlumley@u.washington.edu

Key Words parametric, nonparametric, Wilcoxon test, rank test, heteroscedasticity

■ **Abstract** It is widely but incorrectly believed that the t-test and linear regression are valid only for Normally distributed outcomes. The t-test and linear regression compare the mean of an outcome variable for different subjects. While these are valid even in very small samples if the outcome variable is Normally distributed, their major usefulness comes from the fact that in large samples they are valid for any distribution. We demonstrate this validity by simulation in extremely non-Normal data. We discuss situations in which in other methods such as the Wilcoxon rank sum test and ordinal logistic regression (proportional odds model) have been recommended, and conclude that the t-test and linear regression often provide a convenient and practical alternative. The major limitation on the t-test and linear regression for inference about associations is not a distributional one, but whether detecting and estimating a difference in the mean of the outcome answers the scientific question at hand.

INTRODUCTION

It is widely but incorrectly believed that the t-test and linear regression are valid only for Normally distributed outcomes. This belief leads to the use of rank tests for which confidence intervals are very hard to obtain and interpret and to cumbersome data-dependent procedures where different transformations are examined until a distributional test fails to reject Normality. In this paper we re-emphasize the uncontroversial statistical facts that the validity of the t-test and linear regression in sufficiently large samples depends only on assumptions about the variance of the response and that violations of those assumptions can be handled easily for the t-test (and with slightly more difficulty for linear regression). In addition to reviewing the literature on the assumptions of the t-test, we demonstrate that the necessary sample size is relatively modest by the standards of today's public health research. This is true even in one of the most extreme kinds of data we have encountered, annualized medical costs. We should note that our discussion is entirely restricted

0163-7525/02/0510-0151$14.00

to inference about associations between variables. When linear regression is used to predict outcomes for individuals, knowing the distribution of the outcome variable is critical to computing valid prediction intervals.

The reason for the widespread belief in a Normality assumption is easy to see. If outcomes are indeed Normally distributed then several different mathematical criteria identify the t-test and ordinary least squares regression as optimal analyses. This relatively unusual convergence of criteria makes the Normal theory an excellent example in mathematical statistics, and leads to its popularity in both theoretical and applied textbooks. The fact that the Normality assumption is sufficient but not necessary for the validity of the t-test and least squares regression is often ignored. This is relatively unimportant in theoretical texts, but seriously misleading in applied books.

In small samples most statistical methods do require distributional assumptions, and the case for distribution-free rank-based tests is relatively strong. However, in the large data sets typical in public health research, most statistical methods rely on the Central Limit Theorem, which states that the average of a large number of independent random variables is approximately Normally distributed around the true population mean. It is this Normal distribution of an average that underlies the validity of the t-test and linear regression, but also of logistic regression and of most software for the Wilcoxon and other rank tests.

In situations where estimation and comparison of means with the t-test and linear regression is difficult because of extreme data distributions, it is important to consider whether the mean is the primary target of estimation or whether some other summary measure would be just as appropriate. Other tests and estimation methods may give narrower confidence intervals and more powerful tests when data are very non-Normal but at the expense of using some other summary measure than the mean.

In this review we begin by giving the statistical background for the t-test and linear regression and then review what the research literature and textbooks say about these methods. We then present simulations based on sampling from a large data set of medical cost data. These simulations show that linear regression and the t-test can perform well in moderately large samples even from very non-Normal data. Finally, we discuss some alternatives to the t-test and least squares regression and present criteria for deciding which summary measure to estimate and what statistical technique to use.

DEFINITIONS AND THEORETICAL ISSUES

Least-Squares Techniques

We will discuss first the two-sample t-test, and then linear regression. While the t-test can be seen as merely a special case of linear regression, it is useful to consider it separately. Some more details of the calculations and a review of the Central Limit Theorem can be found in Appendix 1.

The t-Test

Two different versions of the two-sample t-test are usually taught and are available in most statistical packages. The differences are that one assumes the two groups have the same variance, whereas the other does not. The t-statistic, which does not assume equal variances, is the statistic in Equation 1. In Appendix 1 we show that, because of the Central Limit Theorem, this is normally distributed with unit variance when the sample size is large, no matter what distribution Y has. Thus, this version of the t-test will always be appropriate for large enough samples. Its distribution in small samples is not exactly a t distribution even if the outcomes are Normal. Approximate degrees of freedom for which the statistic has nearly a t distribution in small samples are computed by many statistical packages.

$$t = \frac{\overline{Y}_1 - \overline{Y}_2}{\sqrt{\frac{s_1^2}{n_1} + \frac{s_2^2}{n_2}}}. \qquad 1.$$

We next mention the version of the t-statistic that assumes the variances in the two groups are equal. This, the original version of the test, is often used in introductory statistics because when the data do have a Normal distribution, the statistic in Equation 2 has exactly a t distribution with a known number of degrees of freedom. One would rarely prefer this statistic in large samples, since Equation 1 is more general and most statistical programs compute both versions. However, Equation 2 is useful in illustrating the problem of *heteroscedasticity*.

$$t = \frac{\overline{Y}_1 - \overline{Y}_2}{\sqrt{\frac{(n_1 - 1)s_1^2 + (n_2 - 1)s_2^2}{n_1 + n_2 - 2}} \sqrt{\frac{1}{n_1} + \frac{1}{n_2}}}. \qquad 2.$$

Equation 2 differs from Equation 1 in combining the two group variances to estimate a pooled standard deviation. It is identical to that in Equation 1 if either $n_1 = n_2$ or $s_1^2 = s_2^2$. The two forms will be similar if n_1 and n_2 or σ_1^2 and σ_2^2 are similar, as is often the case. However, it is possible for them to differ in extreme situations. Suppose n_1 is much larger than n_2. In that case, the denominator of the t-statistic in Equation 1 can be seen to be primarily a function of s_2^2, while the denominator of the t-statistic in Equation 2 is primarily a function of s_1^2. If the variances in the two groups are different, this can result in the two t-statistics having different denominators. For example, if n_1 is ten times as big as n_2, and the two variances also differ by a factor of 10, then Equation 1 will still be appropriate but Equation 2 will be too small or too large by a factor of about 2, depending on which group has the larger variance. In such an extreme case, it would be possible to make an incorrect inference based on Equation 2. That is, the Central Limit Theorem guarantees that the t-statistic in Equation 2 will be normally distributed, but it may not have variance equal to 1. This is not a problem in practice because we can always use Equation 1, but severe heteroscedasticity will cause problems for linear regression, as is discussed below.

Linear Regression

As with the t-test, least-squares linear regression is usually introduced by assuming that Y is Normally distributed, conditional on X. This is not quite the same as saying that Y must be Normal; for example, Y for men and women could each have a different Normal distribution that might appear bimodal when men and women are considered together. That they were Normally distributed when controlling for sex would satisfy the usual Normality assumption. Normality is not required to fit a linear regression; but Normality of the coefficient estimates $\hat{\beta}$ is needed to compute confidence intervals and perform tests. As $\hat{\beta}$ is a weighted sum of Y (see Appendix 1), the Central Limit Theorem guarantees that it will be normally distributed if the sample size is large enough, and so tests and confidence intervals can be based on the associated t-statistic.

A more important assumption is that the variance of Y is constant. As with the t-test, differences in the variance of Y for different values of X (heteroscedasticity) result in coefficient estimates $\hat{\beta}$ that still have a Normal distribution; as with Equation 2 above, the variance estimates may be incorrect. Specifically, if the predictor X has a skewed distribution and Y has different variance for large and small values of X, the variance of $\hat{\beta}$ can be estimated incorrectly. This can be related to the conditions for t-test (2) to be incorrect by writing the t-test as a linear regression with a single binary predictor variable. A binary predictor X is skewed when the proportions p with $X = 0$ and the proportion $q = 1 - p$ with $X = 1$ are different [the skewness is equal to $(q - p)pq$]. Thus the condition that X is skewed and Y is heteroscedastic in this linear regression is the same as the condition that n and σ^2 both differ between groups for the t-test. Modifications analogous to t-test{1} to provide reliable inference in the presence of substantial heteroscedasticity exist but are not widely implemented in statistical software. In the case of the t-test, we saw that heteroscedasticity must be extreme to cause large biases; in our simulations below we examine this question further for linear regression.

LITERATURE REVIEW

An unwritten assumption of much of the literature on the t-test is that all two-sample tests are effectively testing the same null hypothesis, so that it is meaningful to compare the Type I and Type II error rates of different tests. This assumption is frequently untrue, and testing for a difference in means between two samples may have different implications than testing for a difference in medians or in the proportion above a threshold. We defer until later a discussion of these other important criteria for selecting an estimator or test. Most of the literature on the assumptions of the t-test is concerned with the behavior of the t-test in relatively small samples, where it is not clear if the Central Limit Theorem applies.

For linear regression, the statistical literature largely recognizes that heteroscedasticity may affect the validity of the method and non-Normality does not. The literature has thus largely been concerned with how to model heteroscedasticity and with methods that may be more powerful than linear regression for non-Normal data. These issues are outside the scope of our review.

A number of authors have examined the level and power of the t-test in fairly small samples, without comparisons to alternative tests. Barrett & Goldsmith (4) examined the coverage of the t-test in three small data sets, and found good coverage for sample sizes of 40 or more. Ratcliffe (22) looked at the effect on the t distribution of non-Normality, and provided an estimate of how large n must be for the t-test to be appropriate. He examined sample sizes of up to 80 and concluded that "extreme non-Normality can as much as double the value of t at the 2.5% (one tail) probability level for small samples, but increasing the sample sizes to 80, 50, 30, and 15 will for practical purposes remove the effect of extreme skewness, moderate skewness, extreme flatness, and moderate flatness, respectively." We note that the one-tailed tests he studied are more sensitive to skewness than two-tailed tests, where errors in the two tails tend to compensate. Sullivan & d'Agostino (32) found that t-tests produced appropriate significance levels even in the presence of small samples (50 or less) and distributions in which as many as 50% of the subjects attained scores of zero.

Sawilowsky & Blair (23) examined the robustness of the t-test to departures from Normality using Monte Carlo methods in 8 data sets with sample sizes up to 120. They found the t-test was robust to Type II error. Sawilowsky & Hillman (24) showed that power calculations based on the t-test were appropriate, even when the data were decidedly non-Normal. They examined sample sizes up to 80.

The bootstrap (12) provides another method of computing confidence intervals and significance levels using the t-statistic. The bootstrap is a general-purpose method for estimating the sampling distribution of any statistic computed from independent observations. The sampling distribution is, by definition, the distribution of the statistic across repeated samples from the same population. The bootstrap approximates this by assuming that the observed sample is representative of the population and by taking repeated samples (with replacement) from the observed sample. The bootstrap approach usually requires some programming even in statistical packages with built-in bootstrap facilities [e.g., Stata (29) and S-PLUS (17)]. There is a wide theoretical and applied literature discussing and extending the bootstrap, much of which is summarized in books by Efron & Tibshirani (12) and Davison & Hinkley (9).

Bootstrapping for comparing means of non-Normal data has been evaluated in the context of cost and cost-effectiveness studies. Barber & Thompson (3) recommended a bootstrap approach for testing for differences in mean costs. They presented two examples, with sample sizes of 184 and 32 patients, respectively. In both cases, the p-values and the confidence intervals were very similar using the t-test and using the bootstrap procedure. Rascati et al. (21) concluded that the bootstrap was more appropriate, but they only examined the distribution of the cost data, not the more relevant sampling distribution of the mean.

In a practical setting, the t-test should be discarded only if a replacement can perform better, so comparisons with other tests are particularly important. Cohen &

Arthur (8) looked at samples of 25 per group and found that t-tests on raw, log, and square transformed data; the Wilcoxon test; and a randomization test all exhibited satisfactory levels of alpha error, with the randomization test and the t-test having the greatest power. Stonehouse & Forrester (30) found that the unequal-variance form of the t-test performed well in samples drawn from non-Normal distributions but with different variances and sample sizes. The Wilcoxon test did not perform as well. Zimmerman (34) compared the t-test to the Wilcoxon test when data were non-Normal and heteroscedastic and found that the t-test performed better than the Wilcoxon. Zimmerman & Zumbo (35) found that rank methods are as influenced by unequal variances as are parametric tests, and recommended the t-test. Skovlund & Fenstad (27) also found that the t-test was superior to the Wilcoxon when variances were different.

Theoretical results on the properties of the t-test are mostly over 30 years old. These papers mostly examine how the skewness and kurtosis of the outcome distribution affects the t-statistic in fairly small samples. In principle, they could be used to create a modified t-statistic that incorporated estimates of skewness and kurtosis. At least one such test (7) has achieved some limited applied use. The original references appear to be to Gayen (14) and Geary (15), who approximated the distribution of the t-statistic in non-Normal distributions. They were followed by other authors in producing better approximations for very small samples or extreme non-Normality.

In contrast to the t-test, there has been little empirical research into the behavior of linear regression for non-Normal data. Such research typically focuses on the effects of extreme outliers, under the assumption that such outliers are caused by errors or at least may be excluded from the analysis. When residuals are not Normally distributed, these robust regression methods may be useful for finding the line that best fits the majority of the data, ignoring some points that do not fit well. Robust regression methods do not model the mean of Y but some other summary of Y that varies from method to method. There is little literature on robust regression at an elementary level, but chapters by Berk (5) and Goodall (16) are at least addressed to the practising statistician rather than the theoretician.

Textbooks of biostatistics frequently describe linear regression solely in the context of Normally distributed residuals [e.g., Altman (2), Fisher & van Belle (13), Kleinbaum et al. (18)] where it is the optimal method for finding the best-fitting line; however, the least-squares method was invented as a nonparametric approach. One of the inventors, Legendre [quoted by Smith (28)], wrote,

> Of all the principles which can be proposed for that purpose, I think there is none more general, more exact, and more easy of application, that of which we made use in the preceding researches, and which consists of rendering the sum of squares of the errors a minimum.

Discussions of linear regression that do not suppose Normality are relatively rare. One from an impeccable statistical authority is that of Stuart et al. (31). More commonly, a Normality assumption is presented but is described as less important than other assumptions of the model. For example, Kleinbaum et al. (18, p. 117) wrote,

> [Normality] is not necessary for the least-squares fitting of the regression model but it is required in general for inference making ... only extreme departures of the distribution of Y from normality yield spurious results.

This is consistent with the fact that the Central Limit Theorem is more sensitive to extreme distributions in small samples, as most textbook analyses are of relatively small sets of data.

SIMULATIONS

The simulations in much of the statistical literature we reviewed refer to sample sizes far smaller than those commonly encountered in public health research. In an effort to fill part of this gap, this section describes some simulations that we performed with larger samples. We used data from the evaluation of Washington State's Basic Health Plan, which provided subsidized health insurance for low-income residents, starting in 1989 (10, 19). The 6918 subjects in the study were enrolled in four health plans, 26% in a health maintenance organization (HMO) and 74% in one of three independent practice associations (IPA). Subjects were aged 0 to 65 (mean 23 years) and were followed for an average of 22 months (range 1 to 44 months). Length of follow-up depended on when the person joined the program relative to the end of the evaluation period, and is probably not related to the person's health. During the study period 79% used some services. As examples we use the variables "cost of outpatient care," age, sex, and self-rated general health. The last variable is abbreviated EVGFP, for "excellent/very good/good/ fair/poor."

Example of Central Limit Theorem

The Central Limit Theorem depends on the sample size being "large enough," but provides little guidance on how large a sample might be necessary. We explored this question using the cost variable in the Washington Basic Health Plan data. Annualized outpatient cost has a very long right tail, as shown in Figure 1. We truncated the histogram at $3000 so that the distribution for lower values could be seen, but use the full distribution in the following analysis. The actual costs ranged from $0 to $22, 452, with a mean of $389. The standard deviation is $895, standardized skewness is 8.8, and standardized kurtosis is 131.

Figure 2 shows the sampling distribution of 1000 means of random samples of size 65, 129, 324, and 487 from this very non-Normal distribution (approximately 1%, 2%, 5%, and 7.5% of the population). The graph shows a histogram and a smooth estimate of the distribution for each sample size. It is clear that the means are close to Normally distributed even with these very extreme data and with sample sizes as low as 65.

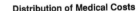

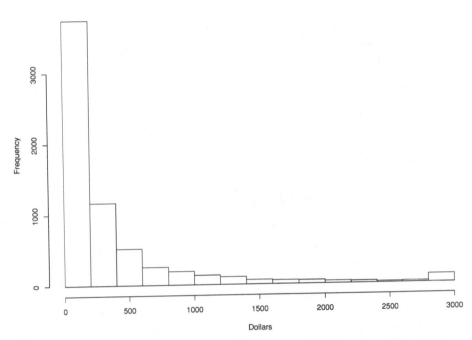

Figure 1   Distribution of annualized medical costs in the Washington Basic Health Plan.

Example for Linear Regression

Medical costs usually have the very non-Normal distribution we see here, but transformations are undesirable as our interest is in total (or mean) dollar costs rather than, say, log dollars (11). We considered the 6918 subjects to be the population of interest and drew samples of various sizes to determine whether the test statistics of interest had the distribution that was expected.

In addition, there is substantial heteroscedasticity and a somewhat linear relation between the mean and variance. In Figure 3 we divided subjects into groups by age and sex and calculated the mean and standard deviation of cost for each group. It is clear that the standard deviation increases strongly as the mean increases. The data are as far from being Normal and homoscedastic as can be found in any real examples.

We used these data to determine how large a sample would be needed for the Central Limit Theorem to provide reliable results. For example, as illustrated on the first line of Table 1, we drew 1000 1% samples, of average size 65, from the population. For each sample we calculated the regression of cost on age, sex, self-rated health, and HMO (IPA = 0) versus Fee for Service (IPA = 1). For each parameter in the regression model we calculated a 95% confidence interval and then checked

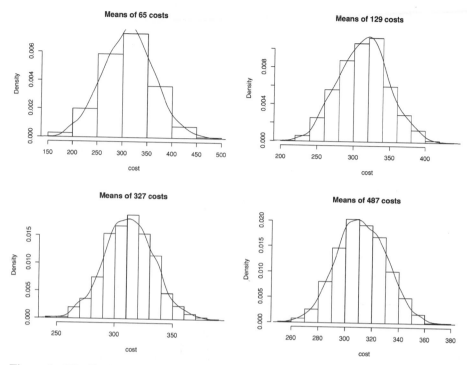

Figure 2   Distribution of means of samples of annualized costs.

to see whether the confidence interval contained the true value. The percent of times that the confidence interval included the value computed from the entire population of 6918 is an estimate of the true amount of confidence (coverage) and would be 95% if the data had been Normal to start with. For samples of size 65 and 129, some of the confidence interval coverages are below 90%. That means that the true alpha level would be 10% or more, when the investigator believed it to be 5%, yielding too many significant regression coefficients. Note that for sample sizes of about 500 or more, the coverage for all regression coefficients is quite close to 95%. Thus, even with these very extreme data, least-squares regression performed well with 500 or more observations.

These results suggest that cost data can be analyzed using least-squares approaches with samples of 500 or more. Fortunately, such large samples are usually the case in cost studies. With smaller samples, results for variables that are highly significant (p < .001, for example) are probably reliable. Regression coefficients with p-values between .001 and .10, say, might require additional analysis if they are important.

For data without such long tails much smaller sample sizes suffice, as the examples in the literature review indicate. For example, at one time a popular method of generating Normally distributed data on a computer was to use the sum

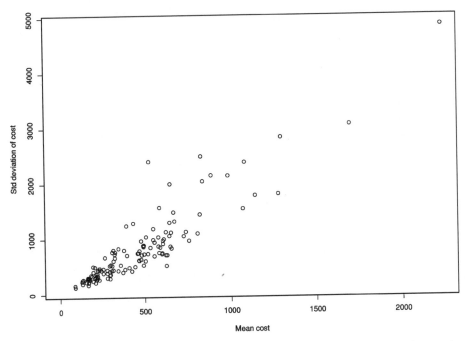

Figure 3   The relationship between mean and standard deviation of annualized costs, in age-sex subgroups.

of a sample of 12 uniformly distributed random numbers. The resulting distribution was not just close enough to Normal for statistical purposes, it was effectively indistinguishable from a Normal distribution. Similarly, the familiar rule that 2×2 tables should have expected counts of at least 5 for a χ^2 test comes from applying the Central Limit Theorem to binary variables.

ALTERNATIVES TO LEAST-SQUARES APPROACHES

The literature summarized above and our simulations illustrate that linear regression and the t-test can perform well with data that are far from Normal, at least in the large samples usual in public health research. In this section we examine alternatives to linear regression. In some disciplines these methods are needed to handle small samples of non-Normal data, but in reviewing their appropriateness for public health research we focus on other criteria. These methods usually come with their own sets of assumptions and they are "alternatives" to least-squares methods only when no specific summary statistic of interest can be identified, as we discuss in the next section.

We examine the Wilcoxon rank-sum test as an alternative to the t-test and the logistic and proportional odds models as alternatives to linear regression.

TABLE 1   Coverage[a] results for the mean and coefficients from multivariable regression. (Based on 1000 replicates)

% of population	N in sample	Mean	b-age	b-sex	b-EVGFP	b-IPA
1	65	88.5	89.7	96.4	88.8	93.1
2	129	90.5	89.9	96.3	88.4	91.5
5	324	92.4	89.9	97.5	91.3	93.8
7.5	487[b]	94.0	90.3	97.3	92.3	94.0
10	649[c]	94.9	91.2	97.7	92.5	94.7
15	973	95.8	92.9	98.3	94.3	96.0
20	1297	96.2	92.6	98.4	95.0	97.1

[a]Coverage is the % of time that the (nominal) 95% confidence included the true mean, out of 1000 replicates.
[b]Not always the same because some of the data are missing—468 to 500.
[c]Range from 629–669 because of missing data.

Wilcoxon and Other Nonparametric Tests

The Wilcoxon two-sample test is said to be nonparametric because no particular distribution is assumed for the data. The test simply ranks all of the data and calculates the sum of the ranks for one of the groups. It is possible to test how likely that sum would be under the null hypothesis that the two distributions were identical. The Wilcoxon test can thus be performed without distributional assumptions even in very small samples. It is sometimes described as a test for the median, but this is not correct unless the distribution in the two groups is known *a priori* to have the same shape. It is possible to construct distributions with arbitrarily different medians for which the Wilcoxon test will not detect a difference.

The Wilcoxon test is widely known to be more powerful than the t-test when the distribution of data in the two groups has long tails and has the same shape in each group but has been shifted in location. Conversely, it is less powerful than the t-test when the groups differ in the number and magnitude of extreme outlying distributions, as recognized in EPA guidelines for testing for environmental contamination in soil (33). Although its power relative to other tests depends on the details of the null and alternative hypotheses, the Wilcoxon test always has the disadvantage that it does not test for equality in any easily described summary of the data. This is illustrated by the analysis of Rascati et al. (21) in comparing overall medical costs for asthmatics prescribed steroids compared with other treatments. Although the mean cost was lower in the steroid group, a Wilcoxon test reported significantly higher costs for that group. A related disadvantage is that it is not easy to construct confidence intervals that correspond to the Wilcoxon test.

EXAMPLE   As an example, we compared the outpatient cost for people who rated themselves in poor health to those in fair health (n = 103 and 340, respectively). The t-test showed that the mean costs in the poor and fair groups were $960 and

$727, respectively; the mean difference is $234; the 95% confidence interval for the difference ($-$72$ to $+ 540); $t = 1.51$; $p = 0.133$. The Wilcoxon test provides the information that the mean rank of costs in the poor and fair groups were 245.51 and 214.88; that the sum of ranks was 25288 versus 73058; the Wilcoxon statistic was 73058 and the p-value 0.033. The Wilcoxon test thus yielded a more significant result than the t-test, but did not provide any useful descriptive statistics. The data for the two groups did not seem to have the same shape, based on a histogram.

Logistic Regression

When the dependent variable is binary, the most common analytic method is logistic regression. In this approach the assumptions fit the data. Further, the (exponentials of the) regression parameters can be interpreted as odds ratios, which are nearly identical to relative risks when the event under study is rare.

Another possible approach is least-squares linear regression, letting Y be the 0/1 binary variable. Such an approach is not usually considered appropriate because Y is not Normally distributed; however, the Central Limit Theorem ensures that the regression coefficients will be Normally distributed for large enough samples. Regression estimates would be a weighted sum of the $Y's$, which are 0' and 1's. The usual rule for the binomial distribution is that proportions are approximately Normal if $np > 5$ and $n(1 - p) > 5$, which should hold for the large data sets we are considering. Another objection to the linear regression approach is that estimated proportions can be below 0 or greater than 1. This is a problem if the goal is to predict a probability for an individual, and the sample is small. It will rarely be a problem when the goal is to assess the effects of independent variables on the outcome. A final objection is that the homoscedasticity assumption is violated, since the variance is a function of the mean. The usual rule of thumb is that if proportions are between, say, 0.2 and 0.8, the variance is approximately constant and heteroscedasticity is not a serious problem.

Linear regression might actually be preferred in some situations. Logistic regression assumes a multiplicative model, whereas linear regression provides an additive model which is sometimes more biologically plausible. The public health significance of estimates of risk and risk difference provided by a linear model is often clearer than that of odds ratios. Odds ratios can be hard to interpret when the event is not rare. This was dramatically demonstrated by a recent study of racial bias in referrals for cardiac catheterization (25), when an odds ratio of 0.6 was widely quoted in the mass media as showing a 40% percent lower chance of referral for blacks. The relative risk was actually 0.87 (26). Although logistic regression is the standard of practice for binary dependent variables, the investigator may sometimes find linear regression useful and should not be deterred by perceived problems with non-Normality.

EXAMPLE   As an example, we calculated a regression to predict use of any outpatient services as a function of gender, using both logistic and OLS regression.

The linear regression of use (0/1) from sex (0/1) yielded a coefficient of 0.0663 ($t = 6.78$); the interpretation is that the use of services was 6.63 percentage points higher for women than for men. The same analysis run as a logistic regression yielded a slope of 0.402, and an estimated odds ratio of 1.495, Wald statistic $= 45.4$. The square root of the Wald statistic is 6.74, about the same as the t-statistic from linear regression.

Linear and logistic regression both give valid results in this example, but the information that the utilization among women is about 7% higher than among men may be more interpretable than the 50% relative increase in odds of utilization. It is of interest that although the odds ratio is 1.5, the relative risk is about 1.1.

Proportional Odds Model

Ordered categorical data commonly arise from assigning values to a scale that cannot be readily quantified. In our example data, participants are asked if their health is "excellent, very good, good, fair, or poor," producing a variable with five ordered categories. As there is no unique objective way to assign numerical values to these categories, it is often argued that the analysis should not depend on any particular assignment of scores.

In estimation and particularly in regression modeling, however, we would often like a single summary that describes how the outcome varies with the predictors. The behavior of a five-level category cannot be reduced to a single summary statistic without imposing some restrictions.

One popular model for analyzing ordered data is the ordinal logistic regression or proportional odds model. An ordered categorical response can be collapsed into a binary (proportional odds) model (1, 20). This model is based on the binary variables created by dichotomizing the ordinal response at any threshold C, giving the model

$$\text{logit } P[Y > C] = \alpha_C + \beta_1 X_1 + \beta_2 X_2 + \cdots + \beta_p X_p.$$

Dichotomizing at a different level C necessarily changes α_C as this is related to the proportion of outcomes above C. The proportional odds model assumes that this is the only change and that $\beta_1, \beta_2, \ldots, \beta_p$ remain the same. Although it does not make distributional assumptions, it does makes strong assumptions about the relationships between categories.

An alternative approach is to assign numerical scores to the categories, either using a default 1, 2, 3, 4, 5 or basing the scores on scientific knowledge about the underlying scale. It is then possible to analyze ordered categorical data by ordinary least squares regression. If two groups have the same probability distribution, the mean measurement will be the same, no matter how numbers are assigned to each possible level of outcome. Furthermore, if there is in fact a tendency for higher measurements to predominate in one group more than the other, the mean will tend to be shifted in that direction. In this setting, however, there is no clear scientific interpretation of the size of a nonzero difference in the means, leading to the difficulties in interpretation similar to those with the Wilcoxon and other nonparametric tests. There is also a potential problem with heteroscedasticity in assigning scores, but as with binary data, this is only likely to be important if a large majority of the observations are in the highest or lowest categories.

EXAMPLE   We predicted whether an adult's health would be excellent, very good, good, fair, or poor based on whether or not he or she had less than a high school education. We examined the assumption that dichotomization at any level of EVGFP gave the same level. If we compared excellent to the other four categories, the odds ratio (OR) was 0.50; breaking at very good, the OR was 0.45; at good, the OR was 0.42; and the OR from dichotomizing below Fair was 0.70. The last odds ratio was not significantly different from the others (95% confidence interval of 0.38 to 1.30). The ordered logistic regression gave a common odds ratio of 0.46. The interpretation is that wherever one cuts the health variable, the odds of being in the healthy group are about half as high for persons with only a high school education. As above, the odds ratio is not the same as the relative risk, since being in the "high" health category is not a rare outcome.

A linear regression where Y takes on the values from 1 (poor) to 5 (excellent) achieves a coefficient of -0.42 and a t-statistic of -7.55. The interpretation is that adults with low education are about a half-category lower in health than those with more education. The t-statistics for the linear and the ordered logistic regressions are nearly identical. While neither model is ideal in terms of scientific interpretation, it is easier to give a precise description of the results for the linear model than for the proportional odds model. In the absence of any strong reason to trust the proportional odds assumption the linear model would be a sensible default analysis.

REASONS FOR CHOOSING AN ESTIMATOR OR TEST

It is rarely necessary to worry about non-Normality of outcome variables. It is necessary to worry about heteroscedasticity in linear regression, though, as the example shows, even with significant heteroscedasticity the performance of linear regression is often good.

The fact that these methods are often valid does not mean that they are ideal in all cases, merely that the reasons for choosing other analyses are different from those often given. The t-test and linear regression both estimate differences in the mean of the outcome. In some cases, this is precisely what is of interest: Health care suppliers, for example, care about the mean cost of care. In other cases, some other summary is appropriate: Median income or percentage living in poverty may be more relevant in considering access to health care. Although costs and income are both measured in dollars, and both have strongly skewed distributions, different questions lead to different choices of summary statistic.

In other examples, the choice between mean, median, and percentage below some threshold may be less obvious. The decision of whether to base a data analysis on a particular summary measure, if any, should be based on the following criteria (in order of importance): clinical or scientific relevance of the summary measure, scientific plausibility that the groups would differ with respect to the summary measure, and statistical precision with which the groups can be compared using the summary measure.

If the question under investigation identifies the preferred analysis, as with comparing total medical care costs, other criteria are irrelevant. It may be easier to estimate differences in, say, the median, but differences in the median need not be a good guide to differences in the mean and so are of little interest. This is what happened in the analysis of Rascati et al. (21) discussed above, where a Wilcoxon test indicated significant cost differences in the opposite direction to the difference in mean costs.

On the other hand, we may not know which summary measure is most important, but have some idea which summary measure is most likely to be affected. Consider a cholesterol-lowering drug, where it might be the case that the treatment is thought to work only in individuals whose initial cholesterol measurement is extremely high. In this setting, there may be no difference between treated and untreated populations with respect to the median cholesterol level, though the mean cholesterol level in the treated group would be lower, as would the proportion of individuals exceeding some high threshold. However, if in that same example the drug is thought not to have effect in individuals with the most severe disease, then neither the median cholesterol level nor the proportion of individuals having cholesterol higher than, say, 350 mg/dl might differ between the control and treatment groups. The mean cholesterol level might still differ between the groups owing to the segment of the population with moderately high cholesterol for whom the treatment was effective. A t-test would then detect this difference, but a comparison of medians might not.

Finally, we may have no real knowledge of which summary statistic is most likely to differ between different groups of people. In this case, we may still have a preference based on statistical sensitivity or on convenience or other factors. For example, if a measurement (such as serum cholesterol) has a very long right tail, the mean is hard to estimate reliably. This would be a valid argument against using a t-test if we had no particular interest in the mean as a summary and no particular knowledge of how cholesterol varies between groups of people. The median or the geometric mean might be better summaries, leading to a different test or to a t-test based on transformed data.

This discussion has been phrased in terms of the t-test, but the same criteria apply in considering alternatives to linear regression. There are many alternative regression methods, like the proportional odds model for categorical data or more robust median regressions for long-tailed data. These quantify the effects of a predictor variable in different ways. Sometimes it will be possible to identify the desired method based on the scientific question to be answered. On other occasions we may know whether the effect is likely to be a small increase in most values (perhaps favoring a robust regression) or a large increase in a few outliers (which would be ignored by a robust regression).

SUMMARY AND CONCLUSIONS

The t-test and least-squares linear regression do not require any assumption of Normal distribution in sufficiently large samples. Previous simulations studies show that "sufficiently large" is often under 100, and even for our extremely non-Normal medical cost data it is less than 500. This means that in public health research, where samples are often substantially larger than this, the t-test and the linear model are useful default tools for analyzing differences and trends in many types of data, not just those with Normal distributions. Formal statistical tests for Normality are especially undesirable as they will have low power in the small samples where the distribution matters and high power only in large samples where the distribution is unimportant.

While the large-sample properties of linear regression are well understood, there has been little research into the sample sizes needed for the Normality assumption to be unimportant. In particular, it is not clear how the necessary sample size depends on the number of predictors in the model.

The focus on Normal distributions can distract from the real assumptions of these methods. Linear regression does assume that the variance of the outcome variable is approximately constant, but the primary restriction on both methods is that they assume that it is sufficient to examine changes in the mean of the outcome variable. If some other summary of the distribution is of greater interest, then the t-test and linear regression may not be appropriate.

APPENDIX 1

The Central Limit Theorem

The classical version of the Central Limit Theorem taught in introductory statistics courses deals with averages of identically distributed data. This suffices for the t-test but not for linear regression, where the regression coefficients are computed from averages of the outcome multiplied by the covariates. To cover both cases we use the Lindeberg-Feller Central Limit Theorem (6). An approximate translation of this result is that if $Y_1, Y_2, \ldots Y_n$ are a large collection of independent random variables with variances $s_1^2, s_2^2, \ldots, s_n^2$ the average

$$\overline{Y} = \frac{1}{n} \sum_{i=1}^{n} Y_i$$

is approximately Normally distributed, with mean equal to the average of the means of the Ys and variance equal to the average of their variances, under two conditions:

1. The variance of any single observation is small compared to the sum of the variances.
2. The number of outcomes that are extreme outliers, more than $\sqrt{n}$ standard deviations away from their mean, is small.

These conditions both restrict the impact any single observation can have on the average. Extreme outliers and very unequal variances (such as might be caused by outlying covariate values in linear regression) are allowed, but imply that larger sample sizes are needed.

This result does not answer the perennial question "How large is large?," and theoretical results are not particularly helpful. In order to understand how the required sample size varies for different sorts of data, we need to rely on simulations that reflect the sort of data we typically use. We do know that the important features of such a simulation are how the sample size relates to the differences in variance and the prevalence of extreme outliers; this information will help us generalize from the simulations to other sorts of data.

The t-Statistic

Let $\overline{Y}_1$ and $\overline{Y}_2$ be the mean of Y in groups 1 and 2 respectively. By the Central Limit Theorem, if n_1 and n_2 are large enough $\overline{Y}_1 \sim N(\mu_1, \sigma_1^2)$ and $\overline{Y}_2 \sim N(\mu_2, \sigma_2^2/n_2)$, so

$$\overline{Y}_1 - \overline{Y}_2 \sim N\left(\mu_1 - \mu_2, \frac{\sigma_1^2}{n_1} + \frac{\sigma_2^2}{n_2}\right)$$

and thus

$$\frac{\overline{Y}_1 - \overline{Y}_2}{\sqrt{\frac{\sigma_1^2}{n_1} + \frac{\sigma_2^2}{n_2}}} \sim N(\mu_1 - \mu_2, 1).$$

Now in a large sample, s_1^2 and s_2^2 are close to σ_1^2 and σ_2^2, so we may replace the population variance by the sample variance to arrive at the unequal-variance form of the t-statistic.

Linear Regression

The parameter estimates in least-squares linear regression are given by the matrix formula

$$\hat{\beta} = (X^T X)^{-1} X^T Y$$

This formula shows that each coefficient is a weighted average of the Y values with weights that depend in a complicated way on the covariates X. That is, we can write each coefficient as

$$\hat{\beta}_j = \frac{1}{n} \sum_{i=1}^{n} w_i Y_i.$$

This is an average of variables $w_i Y_i$ that have different distributions depending on X, but the Central Limit Theorem still applies. In this case extreme values of Y or of X will increase the required sample size.

Visit the Annual Reviews home page at www.annualreviews.org

LITERATURE CITED

1. Agresti A. 1990. *Categorical Data Analysis*. New York: Wiley
2. Altman DG. 1991. *Practical Statistics for Medical Research*. London: Chapman & Hall
3. Barber JA, Thompson SG. 2000. Analysis of cost data in randomized trials: an application of the non-parametric bootstrap. *Statist. Med.* 19:3219–36
4. Barrett JP, Goldsmith L. 1976. When is n sufficiently large? *Am. Stat.* 30:67–70
5. Berk RA. 1990. A primer on robust regression. In *Modern Methods of Data Analysis*, ed. J Fox, JS Long, pp. 292–324. Newbury Park, CA: Sage
6. Billingsley P. 1995. *Probability and Measure*. New York: Wiley. 3rd. ed.
7. Chen L. 1995. Testing the mean of skewed distributions. *J. Am. Stat. Assoc.* 90:767–72
8. Cohen ME, Arthur JS. 1991. Randomization analysis of dental data characterized by skew and variance heterogeneity. *Comm. Dent. Oral.* 19:185–89
9. Davison AC, Hinkley DV. 1997. *Bootstrap Methods and their Application*. Cambridge: Cambridge Univ. Press
10. Diehr P, Madden C, Martin DP, Patrick DL, Mayers M. 1993. Who enrolled in a state program for the uninsured: Was there adverse selection? *Med. Care* 31:1093–105
11. Diehr P, Yanez D, Ash A, Hornbrook M, Lin DY. 1999. Methods for analyzing health care utilization and costs. *Annu. Rev. Public Health* 20:125–44
12. Efron B, Tibshirani R. 1993. *An Introduction to the Bootstrap*. New York: Chapman & Hall
13. Fisher LD, van Belle G. 1993. *Biostatistics: A Methodology for the Health Sciences*. New York: Wiley
14. Gayen AK. 1949. The distribution of Student's t in random samples of any size drawn from non-normal universes. *Biometrika* 36:353–69
15. Geary RC. 1936. The distribution of Student's ratio for non-normal samples. *J. R. Stat. Soc.* 3 (Suppl.):178–84
16. Goodall C. 1983. M-estimators of location: an outline of the theory. In *Understanding Robust and Exploratory Data Analysis*, ed. DC Hoaglin, F Mosteller, JW Tukey, pp. 339–41. New York: Wiley
17. Insightful. 2000. *S-PLUS 2000*. Seattle, WA: Insightful Corp.
18. Kleinbaum DG, Kupper LL, Muller KE, Nizam A. 1998. *Applied Regression Analysis and Multivariable Methods*. Pacific Grove, CA: Duxbury. 3rd ed.
19. Martin D, Diehr P, Cheadle A, Madden C, Patrick D, Skillman S. 1997. Health care utilization for the "newly insured": results from the Washington Basic Health Plan. *Inquiry* 34:129–42
20. McCullagh P. 1980. Regression models for ordinal data. *J. R. Stat. Soc. B* 42:109–42
21. Rascati KL, Smith MJ, Neilands T. 2001. Dealing with skewed data: an example using asthma-related costs of Medicaid clients. *Clin. Ther.* 23:481–98
22. Ratcliffe JF. 1968. The effect on the t distribution of non-normality in the sampled population. *Appl. Stat.* 17:42–48
23. Sawilowsky SS, Blair RC. 1992. A more realistic look at the robustness and type II error properties of the t test to departures from population normality. *Psychol. Bull.* 111:352–60
24. Sawilowsky SS, Hillman SB. 1993. Power of the independent samples t test under a prevalent psychometric measure distribution. *J. Consult. Clin. Psychol.* 60:240–43
25. Schulman KA, Berlin JA, Harless W, Kerner JF, Sistrunk S, et al. 1999. The effect of race and sex on physicians' recommendations for cardiac catheterization. *New Engl. J. Med.* 340:618–26
26. Schwartz LM, Woloshin S, Welch HG.

1999. Misunderstandings about the effect of race and sex on physicians' referrals for cardiac catheterization. *New Engl. J. Med* 341:289–93

27. Skovlund D, Fenstad GU. 2001. Should we always choose a nonparametric test when comparing two apparently nonnormal distributions? *J. Clin. Epidemiol.* 54:86–92

28. Smith DE. 1959. *A Source Book in Mathematics*. Dover

29. StataCorp. 2001. *Stata Statistical Software: Release 7.0.* College Station, TX: Stata Corp.

30. Stonehouse JM, Forrester GJ. 1998. Robustness of the t and U tests under combined assumption violations. *J. Appl. Stat.* 25:63–74

31. Stuart A, Ord K, Arnold S. 1999. *Kendall's Advanced Theory of Statistics: 2A Classical Inference and the Linear Model.* London: Arnold. 6th ed.

32. Sullivan LM, D'Agostino RB. 1992. Robustness of the t test applied to data distorted from normality by floor effects. *J. Dent. Res.* 71:1938–43

33. US EPA. 1994. *Statistical Methods for Evaluating the Attainment of Cleanup Standards, Vol. 3: Reference-based Standards for Soils and Solid Media.* EPA/230-R-94-004. Off. Policy Plan. Eval. US EPA, Washington, DC

34. Zimmerman DW. 1998. Invalidation of parametric and nonparametric statistical tests by concurrent violation of two assumptions. *J. Exp. Educ.* 67:55–68

35. Zimmerman DW, Zumbo DW. 1992. Parametric alternatives to the student t test under violation of normality and homogeneity of variance. *Percept. Motor. Skill.* 74:835–44

Annu. Rev. Public Health 2002. 23:171–212

GAMBLING AND RELATED MENTAL DISORDERS:
A Public Health Analysis

Howard J. Shaffer

*Division on Addictions, Harvard Medical School, 350 Longwood Avenue, Suite 200,
Boston, Massachusetts 02115; e-mail: howard_shaffer@hms.harvard.edu*

David A. Korn

*Department of Public Health Sciences, University of Toronto Faculty of Medicine,
Toronto, Ontario, Canada, M4S 2S7; e-mail: david.korn@utoronto.ca*

Key Words epidemiology, comorbidity, prevalence, pathological gambling, construct validity, syndrome

■ **Abstract** This article reviews the prevalence of gambling and related mental disorders from a public health perspective. It traces the expansion of gambling in North America and the psychological, economic, and social consequences for the public's health, and then considers both the costs and benefits of gambling and the history of gambling prevalence research. A public health approach is applied to understanding the epidemiology of gambling-related problems. International prevalence rates are provided and the prevalence of mental disorders that often are comorbid with gambling problems is reviewed. Analysis includes an examination of groups vulnerable to gambling-related disorders and the methodological and conceptual matters that might influence epidemiological research and prevalence rates related to gambling. The major public health problems associated with gambling are considered and recommendations made for public health policy, practice, and research.

> *The enduring value of a public health perspective is that it applies different
> 'lenses' for understanding gambling behaviour, analysing its benefits and
> costs, as well as identifying strategies for action.*
>
> *Harvey A. Skinner (160, p. 286)*

BACKGROUND

Throughout recorded history, gambling has been viewed through multiple prisms—moral, mathematical, economic, social, psychological, cultural and, more recently, biological (8, 26, 40, 132, 137, 138, 156, 159, 171). The last decade of the twentieth century witnessed a remarkable growth of gambling accompanied by health and social science research into gambling-related disorders (e.g., 43).

This article aims to stimulate and promote public health attention toward gambling issues by reviewing the literature on the prevalence of gambling and its related mental disorders. This discussion covers the public health issues in the gambling field and concludes with implications for public health policy, practice, and research. Focus on the prevalence of mental disorders should not suggest that gambling is unrelated to other disorders of consequence, such as repetitive movement disorders, orthopedic distress, sexual dysfunction, gastrointestinal problems, and cardiovascular or other physical ailments (e.g., 39, 68, 74, 126, 127). However, discussion is limited to the distribution and determinants of disordered gambling and associated mental disorders.

In the United States, there are questions as to whether this rapid expansion of gambling might be accompanied by extraordinary social costs. Consequently, former President Clinton was prompted to establish the National Gambling Impact Study Commission (1). This Commission, in turn, requested that the National Research Council (NRC) conduct a scientific review of pathological gambling and that the National Opinion Research Center (NORC) provide new data on the extent of gambling-related problems in America. The NRC published its findings (123) and NORC released its findings twice (56, 57), reflecting the politically charged circumstances surrounding this research. Finally, a Republican congressman, Representative Frank Wolf, called upon the General Accounting Office (GAO) to independently review the findings proffered by both of these bodies and the National Gambling Impact Study Commission (55). Findings from these reports are included in this article.

Although public health perspectives were gaining strength with respect to other addictive behaviors (e.g., 37, 65, 110, 158, 174, 197–199), this viewpoint remained peculiarly absent (87–89, 131) from the contemporary dialogue on gambling and its fallout. Until the monograph by Korn & Shaffer on gambling and the health of the public (87), public health strategies and perspectives had not been applied to gambling-related problems. For example, in 1998, a comprehensive search of MEDLINE, HealthSTAR, Current Contents, and Web of Science databases identified fewer than 20 gambling-related articles in public health or related peer-reviewed journals (87).

Contemporary public health perspectives are not limited to the biological and behavioral dimensions related to gambling and health, but also can address socioeconomic determinants such as income, employment, and poverty. A public health viewpoint can lead to the design of more comprehensive and effective strategies for preventing, minimizing, and treating gambling-related pathologies and encourages public policy makers to distinguish acceptable from unacceptable risks. It promotes an epidemiological examination of gambling and gambling-related disorders to better understand the distribution and determinants of gambling as well as the factors that influence a transition to disordered states.

Korn & Shaffer suggested that by understanding gambling and its potential effects on the public's health, policy makers and practitioners could minimize the negative results and appreciate its potential benefits. A multidimensional public health framework, they suggest, could stimulate a better understanding of gambling, elucidate the determinants of disordered gambling, and point to a range

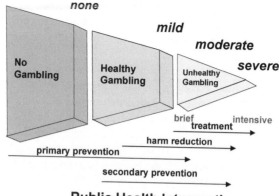

Public Health Interventions

Figure 1 Public health perspective on gambling and gambling-related problems (87).

of interventions. The classic public health model for communicable disease, which examines the interaction among host, agent, environment, and vector, also could be instructive for gambling.

For gambling, the host is the individual who chooses to gamble and who might be at risk for developing problems, depending upon his or her neurobiology, psychology, and behavior patterns. The agent represents the specific gambling activities in which players engage (e.g., lotteries, slot machines, casino table games, bingo, horse or dog race betting). The vector can be thought of as money, credit, or something else of value. The environment is both the microenvironment of the gambling venue, family, and local community and the socioeconomic, cultural, social policy, and political context within which gambling occurs (e.g., whether it is legal, how available it is, and whether it is socially sanctioned or promoted). Like most public health matters, there is a complex relationship among multiple determinants. This confluence can produce a variety of possible outcomes ranging from desirable to undesirable. Applied to gambling, this public health paradigm invites consideration of a broad array of prevention, harm reduction, and treatment strategies directed toward various elements of the model. Figure 1 summarizes a public health perspective on gambling, its potential consequences, and opportunities for multilevel interventions.

GAMBLING

Gambling activities risk something of value on the outcome of an event when the probability of winning or losing is less than certain (87). Gamblers have variable awareness that they are putting something of value at risk, that the bet is irreversible, and that the outcome of the gambling is determined by chance (e.g., 92). As a human endeavor, gambling has been well described since ancient times (51). During various periods in history, problems associated with this activity have been recognized and characterized in personal, social, and economic terms (e.g., greed, crime, and social costs).

Gambling resides on a behavioral continuum that can range from none to a great deal. This quantitative continuum has been transformed into discrete categories, with labels such as at-risk, problem, subclinical, pathological, probable patholog-ical, extremely pathological, in-transition, compulsive. Recent evidence suggests that subclinical or problem gambling is a milder form of pathological gambling (161). Similar to alcohol, most population-based harms are associated, by virtue of their greater numbers, with the group of subclinical gamblers and not the most severe cases (20).

Public Policy and the Growth of Gambling During the Modern Era

Korn & Shaffer noted three primary forces have encouraged the growth of gam-bling throughout North America: the desire of governments to identify new sources of revenue without invoking new or higher taxes; development by tourism en-trepreneurs of new destinations for entertainment and leisure; and the rise of new technologies and forms of gambling [e.g., video lottery terminals (VLTs), Powerball™ mega-lotteries, and Internet offshore gambling] (87).

The growth of gambling activities has occurred within the context of a new and expanded public policy framework. The United States has promoted the leisure and recreational aspects of gambling, whereas Canada has emphasized the social benefit to charities, nonprofit, and community service agencies (21). Since New Hampshire reintroduced a legalized state-sponsored lottery more than 30 years ago, North Americans have embraced legalized gambling in unprecedented numbers and new ways. For example, while the United States permits both government and privately sponsored gambling, in Canada only governments can manage and con-duct gaming ventures or authorize charitable gaming under license (i.e., regulated under the 1892 Criminal Code of Canada). Private sector ownership is prohibited. Over the years, periodic amendments to the sections on gambling have permitted its growth, but only since the 1970s have lotteries and casinos operated legally. In 1985, computers, video, and slot devices were legalized and the provinces were given exclusive control of gambling (21).

During the 1990s, the fiscal and economic needs of states, provinces, and local governments provided the primary driving force behind the expansion of gambling in North America. The strategy has been to stimulate local economic development through gambling-related jobs, thereby creating new government revenues without increasing taxes. Associated with this strategic shift was a dramatic increase in the types of gambling available (e.g., casino, lottery, charity bingo) and the locations where gambling is accessible (e.g., expansion to Native American reservations, riverboats, and border communities). In the United States, the proliferation of cruise ship and riverboat gaming has been a mechanism to circumvent or comply with gambling restrictions imposed by existing state laws. To attract customers, the casino industry has expanded the packages offered at tourist destinations such as Las Vegas, Nevada; Atlantic City, New Jersey; and Niagara Falls, Ontario, to include nongaming entertainment.

Gambling Participation, Psychoeconomics, and Health Policy

In the United States, between 1975 and 1999, adult gambling increased from 67% to 85%, gambling expenditures increased from 0.3% to 0.74% of personal income, and gambling patterns among women grew to resemble those of men. The most dramatic increase in lifetime gambling occurred in the 65+ age group, from 35% of older adults to 80% (56). Corporate profits in the gaming entertainment and related hospitality industries have soared. Gambling revenues in the United States leisure economy in 1996 grossed over $47 billion, which was greater then the combined revenues of almost $41 billion from film box office, recorded music, cruise ships, spectator sports, and live entertainment (24). During 1996, 82% of Canadian households spent money on government and nongovernment lotteries, raffles, casinos, slot machines, or bingo. In 1997, Canadians wagered $6.8 billion (Can) on some form of government-run gambling activity, 2.5 times the amount wagered in 1992, with casinos and VLTs accounting for almost 60% of all government gambling revenue. Profits for provincial governments have also risen dramatically. By 1997, all provinces were receiving at least 3% of total government revenue from gambling (111).

There has been considerable interest in the relation between gambling and socioeconomic status. For example, Canada's Family Expenditure Survey (111) reports that gambling participation rates in general increase with household income, a trend that holds for the purchase of government and nongovernment lottery tickets, spending at casinos, and use of slot machines.[1] High-income households spent more than low-income households on gaming activities (i.e., lotteries, casinos, slot machines, VLTs, and bingo); however, lower-income households spend proportionately more of their money on gambling than higher-income households. Given that some gambling revenue goes to the government (e.g., lotteries), these data encourage the view that gambling expenditures represent a regressive tax (25, 111).

Poverty often is associated with increased financial risk-taking, perhaps because of the psychoeconomics of gambling (108)—a primary driving force behind the epidemiology of gambling. People living in poverty perceive greater potential to change their lives from a gambling win than people living in wealth. For example, people of lesser means played the lottery more than people of greater means (e.g., 25). The opposite also is true: People with wealth perceive little opportunity

---

[1]Bingo was the only gambling activity for which there was an inverse correlation with income.

to change their lives from a gambling win—unless the magnitude of the potential win is particularly meaningful. This psychoeconomic driving force is powerful: It can subdue public health and other social forces that encourage abstinence or moderation. Consequently, in addition to increased rates of many other health risks, the poor also are at increased risk for intemperate gambling and its potential consequences (25, 108). The psychoeconomics of gambling is a complex determinant for gambling frequency and intensity; it also has multiple correlations with many other determinants of health status such as smoking and drinking. Consequently, it provides the landscape against which pro- and antigambling forces interact to shape gambling patterns among various segments of the population.

ASSESSING THE IMPACT OF GAMBLING ON THE PUBLIC HEALTH

General Considerations

A public health approach to gambling offers a broad viewpoint on gambling and is not restricted to a narrow focus on gambling addiction. This position is similar to public health approaches toward alcohol, tobacco, and other drugs. The public policy arena only recently has provided the setting to examine and debate the long-term social, economic, and health ramifications of the dramatic expansion of gambling (e.g., 122). Controversy consistently surrounds the shifting social and political environment that has permitted the growth of gambling. For governments, there is considerable ambivalence as to the appropriate balance between permitting new gambling programs and regulating policies. For example, the government of Ontario, Canada, one of the largest owners of gambling operations in North America, reversed its policy to expand charity casinos throughout the province following widespread local controversy. Some religious groups oppose the expansion of gambling on moral and ethical grounds. In the United States, the casino industry strenuously lobbies states and municipalities for opportunities to offer its gaming entertainment. Local communities vigorously debate the effect of gambling on the community [e.g., safety and quality of life for their neighborhoods and families (63)]. State and provincial councils on compulsive or pathological gambling provide public education, help lines and referral services, as well as advocacy for individuals and their families affected by gambling-related problems that require treatment services and insurance reimbursement for such care.

Considering Costs and Benefits

A public health position recognizes that gambling yields both potential costs and benefits that affect all aspects of the community, including health and socioeconomic dimensions. A cost-benefit analysis that incorporates the distribution of costs and benefits among a range of subgroups and vulnerable populations is essential to any evaluation of community impact. Only after such analysis can a public health strategy be developed that resolves important apprehensions and supports worthwhile initiatives.

The Costs: The Potential Adverse Consequences of Gambling

The scientific literature and the popular media have attributed a range of difficulties for individuals, families, and communities either indirectly or directly to gambling (e.g., 90, 99). These unintended negative consequences can include gambling disorders, a term used to encompass a spectrum of problems experienced along the continuum that incorporates the constructs of problem and pathological gambling (e.g., 151); family dysfunction and domestic violence including spousal and child abuse (12, 61, 67, 106, 109, 119, 191); youth and underage gambling (e.g., 42, 148, 151, 153); alcohol and other drug problems (29, 35, 104, 157, 162, 168, 169); psychiatric conditions including major depression, bipolar disorder, antisocial personality, anxiety, and attention deficit disorder (e.g., 14, 29, 35, 64, 86, 114, 141, 157); suicide, suicidal ideation, and suicide attempts (12, 29, 35, 113, 128); significant financial troubles including bankruptcy, loss of employment, and poverty as a direct result of wagering (15, 49, 56, 57, 90, 99, 111); and criminal behavior ranging from prostitution and theft to drug trafficking and homicide (19, 56, 97, 123, 164).

Determining the causal role of gambling, if any, in these adversities is highly controversial. Research suggests that gambling can have a negative impact on health because of associated crime, substance abuse, poverty, and domestic violence (e.g., 123). However, it is difficult to separate cause from effect. Do criminals gamble, or do gamblers become criminals? Do people with psychological disturbance gamble to treat their emotional circumstance (e.g., 66, 81), or does gambling stimulate these emotional disturbances (e.g., 176)? Like the use of psychoactive substances, these relationships likely are "dose"-related (i.e., the amount of money gambled, frequency of gambling, and the duration of engagement or exposure to gambling). As with the positive consequences of gambling, more research is necessary to resolve these important questions.

The relationship between accessibility to gambling settings and gambling problems is controversial. Investigators for the National Gambling Impact Study Commission (NGISC) reported in a combined patron and telephone survey that the availability of a casino within 50 miles is associated with double the prevalence rates of problem and pathological gamblers (56). However, it is not possible to determine if (*a*) the availability of gambling caused this inflated prevalence rate, (*b*) more people with gambling problems settled in areas closer to major opportunities to gambling, (*c*) casinos locate in areas that already have a high rate of disordered gambling, or (*d*) casinos locate in areas with a disproportionately vulnerable population. To understand fully the overall repercussions of gambling on society, a significant research effort is necessary to document the complex interaction among these health and socioeconomic variables, as well as their short- and long-term costs.

The NRC and the NGISC concluded that it was not yet possible to determine if gambling causes crime, bankruptcy, domestic violence, and other perceived social consequences (122, 123). Some observers anticipated another set of findings. Therefore, to assure the integrity and validity of these conclusions, the GAO conducted an independent review of the evidence and conclusions of the NGISC (55) and added their own research on the Atlantic City area. The GAO concluded, "Neither NGISC nor our Atlantic City case study was able to clearly identify the social effects of gambling for a variety of reasons. The amount of high quality and relevant research on social effects is extremely limited. While data on family problems, crime, and suicide are available, tracking systems generally do not collect data on the causes of these incidents, so they cannot be linked to gambling. Sometimes data were available only at the county level, not for Atlantic City. Further, while studies have shown increases in social costs of pathological gamblers, it is difficult to isolate whether gambling is the only factor causing these problems because pathological gamblers often have other behavior disorders. While NGISC and our case study in Atlantic City found some testimonial evidence that gambling, particularly pathological gambling, has resulted in increased family problems (such as domestic violence, child abuse, and divorce), crime, and suicides, NGISC reached no conclusions on whether gambling increased family problems, crime, or suicide for the general population. Similarly, we found no conclusive evidence on whether or not gambling caused increased social problems in Atlantic City" (55, p. 3).

The GAO also failed to find a relationship between gambling and bankruptcies. It can appear that gambling causes social problems, and it even might be that gambling is a cause of these social problems. However, the current state of scientific research simply does not permit this conclusion (55, 123).

The Benefits: The Potential Positive Health Impact of Gambling

Most gambling research has focused on its adverse mental health and social consequences. Until Korn & Shaffer formally introduced the idea of healthy gambling, health care, addictions, and public health professionals had not considered the possibility of positive health benefits (87). To date, with one notable exception (139), the study of gambling behavior has ignored the possibility of health gains associated with gambling.

Gambling holds potential direct and oblique benefits for both the individual and the community. For example, population health research has examined the relationship between health status and socioeconomic variables including income and employment (46, 73, 192). A particular focus of this work is the variance and inequities in health status indicators among subgroups within the general population. Population health studies demonstrate that economic well-being in general and income in particular are key determinants of health and the quality of life of individuals, families, and communities. Wealth and its generation or loss is correlated with the health status of various demographic segments. In the future, analyses of the linkage between economic and social policy to health can provide a vehicle to analyze and understand the questions and controversies central to the study of gambling and health.

Gambling affects the emotional, intellectual, physical, and social dimensions of an individual's health. The concept of mental health promotion provides a promising new frame of reference and vocabulary for examining the potential health benefits involved. This approach examines the population segments affected by gambling, their mental health promotion goals, and the settings within which these are realized. For example, gambling can provide a sense of connectedness and socialization through discretionary leisure time entertainment. Like going to a movie, sitting in a pub, or participating in physical activity, going to a casino or horse race may provide a healthy change and respite from everyday demands or social isolation. This may be particularly important for older adults.

Gambling is a form of adult play (163). While the importance of play has been long recognized for the healthy development of children (189), play also is important for adults (2, 41, 75). For example, whereas children play card, board, and video games, adults play blackjack, bingo, and video slot machines. In addition to providing fun and excitement, some forms of gambling can enhance coping strategies by building skills and competencies such as memory enhancement, problem solving through game tactics, mathematical proficiency, concentration, and hand-to-eye physical coordination.

The mental health literature demonstrates that physical activity such as cycling, jogging, yoga, fencing, or weight lifting can reduce stress, anxiety, and depression (7, 60, 112, 134). Some individuals derive similar compensations from certain forms of gambling. Like exercise, certain gambling activities might be associated with the ability to manage stress,[2] which can in turn affect a person's vulnerability to disease.

Health benefits can accrue to communities through gambling-related economic development. Gambling enterprises can provide significant economic stimulus to local communities, particularly those in economically deprived areas (123). Casinos, for example, can act as a community catalyst for economic development. Job creation in the gaming industry in turn stimulates other sectors such as tourism and hospitality. However, projected community health status improvements associated with gambling expansion and local economic development should be interpreted with caution because these economic gains must be sustainable for any positive health benefit to accrue. As yet, other than for originally impoverished areas, the long-term economic gains predicted for communities have not been substantiated and currently rest on a complex analysis of projected economic benefit and wealth generation (120, 122, 123).

---

[2]Gambling might act as a buffer against the development or progression of mental health problems. Extrapolating from Rado's consideration of heroin addiction, gambling involvement can "catch" people and keep them from progressing to a more disordered state of mental illness by occupying their attention and shifting their subjective focus (133).

Estimating the Cost and Benefits

For communities, groups, and individuals, the central question in public health is whether gambling adds to or detracts from the quality of life. Estimates of the health and socioeconomic costs of problem and pathological gambling have been proposed but the methodologies require further refinement (123). An example of an unsupported but commonly cited estimate (e.g., 59) for the annual cost to society of each pathological gambler is $13,200 (U.S.) or $20,000 (Can). The NGISC estimated that the annual cost for problem and pathological gamblers is $5 billion (U.S.) per year and an additional $40 billion (U.S.) in lifetime costs for productivity reductions, social service, and creditor losses. Where casinos have been introduced into a community, unemployment rates, unemployment insurance, and welfare payments decline by one seventh and earnings rise in construction, hospitality, transportation, recreation, and amusements sectors (56). Politzer et al. suggest that problem gamblers each negatively affect 10 to 17 people around them including family, employer, and government (129). A recent report by the Canadian Tax Foundation on the benefits and costs of gambling in 1995 estimates the net benefits to society at $3044 million and the net benefits to government of $2330 million (175). However, taken together, research on the current state of gambling costs and benefits rarely highlights the distribution of costs and benefits and fails to provide certainty about the nature of this relationship at either the community or the individual level of analysis.

THE EPIDEMIOLOGY OF GAMBLING AND GAMBLING DISORDERS

An epidemiological review of gambling and gambling-related disorders revolves around the distribution and determinants of gambling and the factors that can influence its transition to disordered states. The distribution and onset of gambling and its associated disorders across population segments comprises the study of prevalence and incidence. Prevalence represents the number of people with a specific disorder at a point or period in time. Incidence represents the number of people who acquire the disorder during a point or period in time. As of fall 2001, there were more than 200 existing studies of prevalence related to gambling and its consequences but no true incidence studies (123, 149). Further, there are few studies of the contextual determinants of gambling and disordered gambling. Most of the research on the causes of disordered gambling has focused on psychological factors at the expense of the social environment (43).

The Origins of Disordered Gambling Prevalence Studies

During the mid-1970s, a research team (71) undertook to describe the nature and scope of gambling activities in the United States on behalf of the U.S. Commission on a National Policy Toward Gambling. One objective was to determine the extent of compulsive gambling. While this national survey was being conducted, Robert

Custer was offering the American Psychiatric Association Task Force a description of compulsive gambling for use in the Diagnostic and Statistical Manual (DSM) (71, p. 73).

Lacking an instrument with which to measure compulsive gambling, Kallick and her colleagues created an 18-item scale, based upon concepts from the extant literature that seemed related to compulsive gambling. This first research instrument became known as the ISR (Institute for Social Research) scale. Only one other researcher subsequently used Kallick et al.'s gambling scale (i.e., 33). Nevertheless, the process of attempting to accurately measure the construct of disordered gambling had commenced and the era of gambling-related epidemiological research was under way.

The results of advice and guidance to the American Psychiatric Association by Custer and others on the subject of gambling first surfaced in the third edition of the *Diagnostic and Statistical Manual* (DSM-III) (4). In 1980, the diagnosis of pathological gambling joined pyromania, kleptomania, and intermittent and isolated explosive disorders as an impulse disorder in the DSM-III (4). Since 1980, many researchers and instrument developers have used the DSM-III or subsequent DSM-based instruments (e.g., DSM-III-R, DSM-IV) to assess and measure the prevalence of pathological gambling. For example, in 1987, to develop a "consistent, quantifiable, structured instrument that could be administered easily by nonprofessional as well as professional interviewers" (101, p. 1184), Lesieur & Blume developed *The South Oaks Gambling Screen* (SOGS). These investigators used the DSM-III-R criteria to guide both the development and validation of the SOGS, which rapidly became the instrument of choice among researchers estimating disordered gambling prevalence. Now, there are over 27 instruments for identifying gambling disorders, with many more in development.

Observers of the disordered gambling prevalence field have described the evolution of prevalence instruments and methodological issues in gambling research (e.g., 32, 98, 105, 151, 178, 184). For example, Culleton questioned the appropriateness of applying a clinical screening test (e.g., the SOGS) to a population-based sample to establish a prevalence rate (32) because screening for a low base rate disorder within the general population has low predictive value. That is, the SOGS fails to account for the increase in false positives when used within a population with low base rates of gambling pathology. New evidence suggests that Culleton might be correct (e.g., 6, 91, 151) and the SOGS might inflate the rate of gambling problems.

Culleton's concern with estimating the prevalence of low base rate behaviors represents a fundamental dilemma for the study of prevalence. By introducing positive predictive value to the gambling literature, Culleton reminded us that screening instruments are most capable of identifying a problem of interest (i.e., high positive predictive value) when measuring a phenomenon that is common among the sample population. The accuracy of any screening instrument diminishes, however, when investigators apply it to a sample where the base rate of the disorder is low. Even when an instrument has excellent criterion validity, "... the actual predictive value of the instrument could be much more limited, depending on the prevalence of the disorder of interest" (58, p. 236).

Alternatively, Lesieur (98) noted that most epidemiological surveys underestimate the extent of disordered gambling as a result of methodological flaws such as not including the homeless or hospitalized populations and not reaching gamblers at home in a telephone survey. Lesieur is correct on methodological grounds; however, investigators have failed to recognize that over- or underestimates of prevalence screening instruments can be identified only when a gold standard also exists to identify the attribute of interest.

The central question, then, is not whether the SOGS provides an overestimate or an underestimate, or whether the methodological weaknesses of research protocols offset the unique measurement characteristics of a screening instrument. It similarly would be incorrect to conclude that the SOGS yields a higher estimate of disordered gambling until scientists assure that comparison instruments do not over- or underestimate the prevalence of disordered gambling (151). Rather, the principal question is, with what independent standard can we compare the SOGS or any other estimate of prevalence? Only by evaluating a screening instrument against an independent and valid standard can we decide about the precision of its measurements. Unfortunately, most screening devices are incestuous, having been derived from each other and then used to test the development of their progeny. The result is a psychometric tautology. Because DSM was used as the standard for the development of the SOGS, the confusion around this issue—and the completion of the tautology—was evident when Volberg suggested, "In the case of the DSM-IV Screen we must use the SOGS as the 'gold standard' since this is the primary method that has been used to identify problem and pathological gamblers since the late 1980s . . ." (180, p. 34). Like many other psychiatric disorders, there is no epidemiological gold standard in the area of disordered gambling prevalence (6).

The history of the disordered gambling research field reflects the developmental process of shifting attempts to measure a singular phenomenon. Although various instruments are available to assess the prevalence of disordered gambling, each instrument is best understood by viewing it through an evaluative lens, which can focus on the context of its origin, driving motivation, relationship to funding, and its inherent strengths and weaknesses.

Prevalence Estimates of Gambling and Disordered Gambling

Since the prevalence of gambling in the United States was first examined, increasing numbers of people have tried gambling, both licit and illicit, fueling interest in excessive gambling from clinical, public policy, and scientific perspectives. During the past 25 years, the public has sensed that gambling problems have been increasing. Public policy makers have pushed repeatedly for review of gambling and its adverse consequences. In response, studies on the prevalence of gambling-related disorders have burgeoned (e.g., 43).

Shaffer et al. demonstrated that an assortment of different algorithms used to calculate the rate of disordered gambling in North America provide stable and similar estimates (149, 151, 152). A variety of international studies are consistent with this observation, although differences in reporting standards have made comparisons

TABLE 1 Mean gambling prevalence estimates and 95% confidence intervals for four study populations[a]

	Adult	Adolescent[b]	College	Treatment or prison
Level 3 lifetime	1.92 (1.52–2.33)	3.38 (1.79–4.98)	5.56 (3.54–7.59)	15.44 (11.58–19.31)
Level 2 lifetime	4.15 (3.11–5.18)	8.40 (5.61–11.18)	10.88 (4.86–16.89)	17.29 (11.05–23.53)
Level 1 lifetime	93.92 (92.79–95.06)	90.38 (86.49–94.29)	83.13 (74.71–91.55)	67.61 (58.10–77.11)
Level 3 past year	1.46 (0.92–2.01)	4.80 (3.21–6.40)	—	—
Level 2 past year	2.54 (1.72–3.37)	14.60 (8.32–20.89)	—	—
Level 1 past year	96.04 (94.82–97.25)	82.68 (76.12–89.17)		

[a]See Reference 149.

[b]Although mean past-year estimates are higher than mean lifetime estimates for adolescents, there is considerable overlap between the confidence intervals of these measures; adolescents' past-year gambling experiences are likely to be comparable to their lifetime gambling experiences. Differences between instruments that provide past-year estimates among adolescents and instruments that provide lifetime estimates among adolescents most likely account for these discrepancies.

difficult. Consequently, Shaffer & Hall proposed a universal system for reporting prevalence rates (148) that avoids pejorative and misleading language and reflects the underlying continuum of gambling; this system also is consistent with a public health perspective on populations. Level 0 represents the prevalence of nongamblers; level 1 represents respondents who do not report any gambling-related symptoms (i.e., not experiencing any gambling problems); level 2 represents respondents who are experiencing subclinical levels of gambling problems; and level 3 represents respondents who meet diagnostic criteria for having a gambling disorder. Note that level 2 gamblers can move in two directions: to a more disordered state (i.e., level 3), or to a less disordered state (i.e., level 1). New research suggests that these gamblers progress to level 3 less frequently than expected and move toward level 1 more frequently than the conventional wisdom would have predicted (150).

Table 1 summarizes the prevalence rates for lifetime and past-year gambling among adults from the general population in the United States and Canada. Table 2 revises these estimates using three methods (i.e., median, 5% outliers, and Andrews Wave M-estimator) to trim outliers and provide a more precise estimate of disordered gambling (149). Table 3 compares national estimates worldwide.[3]

Approximately half of the prevalence estimates reside in unpublished reports that have not been subjected to critical peer review. Nonetheless, prevalence estimates from published and unpublished reports do not differ significantly

---

[3]While these tables refer to "level 1 gamblers," it should be noted that, in these tables, this group includes non-gamblers as well as gamblers without any gambling-related symptoms.

TABLE 2 Trimmed gambling prevalence estimates[a]

Estimate	Time frame and statistic	Adult	Adolescent	College	Treatment or prison
Level 3 lifetime	Mean	1.92	3.38	5.56	15.44
	Median	1.80	3.00	5.00	14.29
	5% trimmed mean	1.78	3.33	5.14	15.07
	Andrews' wave M-estimator	1.73	2.74	4.64	13.49
Level 2 lifetime	Mean	4.15	8.40	10.88	17.29
	Median	3.50	8.45	6.50	15.64
	5% trimmed mean	3.76	8.35	9.83	17.01
	Andrews' wave M-estimator	3.31	8.22	6.51	16.59
Level 3 past year	Mean	1.46	4.80	—	—
	Median	1.20	4.37	—	—
	5% trimmed mean	1.27	4.77	—	—
	Andrews' wave M-estimator	1.10	4.65	—	—
Level 2 past year	Mean	2.54	14.60	—	—
	Median	2.20	11.21	—	—
	5% trimmed mean	2.25	13.83	—	—
	Andrews' wave M-estimator	2.15	11.26	—	—

[a]See Reference 149.

(149, 151). Further, the inconsistent quality of the various studies that generate prevalence rates seems not to influence the magnitude of these estimates (151).

Perhaps most notable about this evidence is the relative consistency of the prevalence rates observed in different venues, using different measures and methods. This observation indicates that disordered gambling is a relatively stable phenomenon. However, we should not mistake reliability of measurement for validity.

TABLE 3 International past-year prevalence rates[a]

	United States 1979	United States 2001	Sweden 2001	Switzerland 2000	New Zealand 2001	United Kingdom 2000
Level 1	97.05	96.75	98.00	97.00	98.7	99.3
Level 2	2.22	2.15	1.4	2.2	0.8	—
Level 3	0.73	1.10	0.6	0.8	0.5	0.7

[a]Sources available from the author(s) upon request.

It is not clear that gambling disorders such as pathological gambling are unidimensional and unique. Gambling problems often co-occur with other disorders (see below).

TRENDS IN POPULATION SEGMENTS

Some critics of gambling have likened it to both an environmental contaminant and an infectious agent. This view suggests that the presence of gambling opportunities causes adverse social and personal fallout (e.g., 28). This perspective reflects an exposure model of gambling and its effect on community health. During the 1990s, the increasing number of gambling-related problems attracted considerable attention and debate. As gambling opportunities expanded worldwide, some observers expressed alarm that the rate of gambling-related disorders also was increasing because of this exposure. The idea of social environmental exposure has its roots in McGuire's model of "resistance to persuasion" and "social inoculation" (115), which suggests that exposure to certain social events (e.g., gambling, advertising) correspond to the equivalent of exposure to germs. More specifically, exposure to gambling or activities and materials that promote it reflects a sequence of social contacts that conceptually act like germs or toxins that can lead to adverse health consequences. However, few studies provided empirical evidence about the nature of gambling exposure or its association with the prevalence of gambling disorders. Next, we consider the nature of gambling exposure and review the evidence associated with population segment prevalence rates, beginning with the trends among youth and adults.

Adolescents and Adults

In a rare longitudinal study of gambling-related behaviors, Winters et al. observed that the prevalence of adolescents with gambling disorders in Minnesota did not increase despite a shift away from informal games toward more legalized games (194). Similarly, Wallisch observed that the rate of gambling remained steady and the prevalence of gambling disorders actually diminished among adolescents in Texas between 1992 and 1995 (185, 186). Meta-analytic research showed that the rate of disordered gambling had increased during the last three decades of the twentieth century, but only among adults from the general population (149, 151, 152). Consistent with the few local studies that had monitored young people's gambling behavior, the rate of disorder was not increasing among youth or patients with psychiatric or substance use disorders (149, 151, 152).

Estimates of gambling disorders among young people suggest that they experience this problem at approximately 2.5 to 3.0 times the rate of their adult counterparts. Despite this observation, the NRC concluded that variation in methods, instrumentation, and conceptualization might influence these findings and therefore it is not yet possible to draw confident conclusions about the rate of gambling disorders among youth (123). This problem is evident in Table 1 where the evidence reveals that mean past-year rates are higher than lifetime rates. The considerable variation among estimates suggests a possible cohort effect, memory distortion, or other methodological difficulties associated with screening young people. New research suggests that SOGS-based youthful prevalence rates might simply be inflated (91), though this explanation still does not adequately address how past-year rates can exceed lifetime rates.

Shaffer et al. noted that although more people started to gamble as legalized gambling proliferated, the rate of gambling disorders increased only among adults from the general population (151, 152). For adults, they argued, legalized gambling provided an increasingly acceptable opportunity to try a new activity, whereas for young people, gambling remained illicit. For psychiatric patients, the social sanctions and proscriptions were less influential than for adults from the general population. As gambling became legalized, therefore, adults from the general populace were the population segment most responsive to these changes. Consequently, the finding that only these adults are reflecting an increasing rate of disorder should not be very surprising.

Regional state replications are emerging (e.g., 177, 182). The evidence regarding trends is mixed: Some reports show an increase in gambling disorders and others a decrease. Observed increases in past-year level 3 gambling might reflect a cohort-related artifact. For example, regions implementing replication studies initially might have had either higher or lower rates of level 3 gambling than the regions that do not conduct replication projects. Shaffer & Hall tested this hypothesis for a possible confounding effect (149). They compared the prevalence estimates obtained from the first available statewide adult population studies from states that later conducted replication studies with estimates derived from states without replication studies. Although initial prevalence estimates were consistently lower from the replication states, the paucity of these studies yielded insufficient statistical power to identify significant differences between replication and non-replication states (149). Further, despite Volberg's (178) earlier observation that Central and Midwestern states tend to have lower prevalence rates of problem and probable pathological gambling than states in the Northeast and West, Shaffer et al. did not detect any regional differences (151).

The magnitude of contemporary gambling suggests to some observers that North America is experiencing an "epidemic" of gambling (e.g., 3). Indeed, evidence suggests that adults from the general population are evidencing a low but gradually increasing rate of gambling disorders. If this trend continues unabated, it might become appropriate to characterize disordered gambling in the general adult population as pandemic. For now, however, to clarify this kind of characterization, prospective epidemiological studies are needed.

To date, the many and consistent findings derived from studies of adults from the general population suggest that—except for tracking the effect of public policy modifications—the era of general population prevalence research might be ending and the next phase of epidemiological research beginning. Young people, psychiatric patients, and prisoners reflect a stable but meaningfully higher rate of gambling-related problems that can be described as hyperendemic (151). Consequently, the next phase of epidemiological investigation needs to focus on more vulnerable and special needs segments of the population, for example, women, older adults, Aboriginals, and selected ethnocultural and lower socioeconomic groups. Nascent research has been completed on special population segments and the following section will review some of these studies.

Vulnerable and Special Needs Population Segments

As we described earlier, the social gradient (e.g., poverty and the psychoeconomics of gambling) disproportionately influences disordered gambling patterns across population segments (108). People with lower socioeconomic status experience gambling-related and other socioeconomically related problems at rates higher than those associated with high socioeconomic standing (95, 142, 147). This factor pervades considerations of gambling among vulnerable population segments. Given the early phase and preliminary nature of research on population segments, ironically, the current value of segment-specific research is generic. However, future research directed toward specific population segments holds important potential for future epidemiological gambling research. For example, Fisher reminds us that studies of population segments net significantly more problem gamblers from smaller samples. This strategy also has the potential to identify the proportion of problem gamblers attributable to each sector (50) and the nature of gambling within various population segments. For example, the first studies of homeless treatment seekers indicate that, like other psychiatric population segments, community service recipients (95) in general and the homeless in particular evidence elevated rates of gambling disorders (147). Past-year level 2 and 3 gambling disorders (i.e., 12.8 and 5.4 prevalence rates, respectively) among homeless treatment seekers at intake are significantly higher among this population than among the general adult population.

In the following discussion, we will examine in brief some other vulnerable and special needs populations. We illustrate the potential of sector-specific prevalence research by reviewing a selection of population segments. As research on the distribution and determinants of gambling matures, scientists likely will identify other population segments as vulnerable.

Women

Epidemiological research suggests that disordered gambling is more prevalent among men than among women (123, 151); adolescent boys are about four times more likely to be pathological gamblers than female adolescents. Some have speculated that women gamble to escape more often than men, who gamble for the action (e.g., 38), although there is little supporting experimental evidence. More likely, gender differences reflect complex attitudes and opportunities about recreational activities and the social milieus within which these occur (e.g., 10, 82).

Casino Employees

Casino employees represent a unique and conceptually important segment of the population, with full access and exposure to gambling compared to the general public. If gambling is the cause of adverse health and disordered gambling, then occupational experience is central to determining its effects. In the early days of epidemiology, John Snow argued that if a trade truly causes adverse health consequences, it should "... be extremely so to the workmen engaged in those trades ..." (107, p. 5). If gambling is the cause of adverse health, then those with the greatest gambling exposure should experience more health problems than those with less exposure. Alternatively, workers might seek employment in the gaming industry to satisfy their gambling interests. Studying gambling industry employees might serve as an important harbinger of gambling patterns that others will experience if gambling becomes even more widely available than now—a concern for public policy makers and opponents of gambling alike.

Casino employees have higher levels of gambling, smoking, drinking, and mood disorder compared to the general population (157). In addition, gambling problems, like the abuses of alcohol, tobacco, opiates, and cocaine, are more dynamic than the conventional wisdom suggests (148, 151). Shaffer & Hall propose transitional stages (155) from which people move toward more healthy or more disordered states during their involvement with gambling (e.g., 150, 151). Further, concurrent psychiatric and alcohol or other substance use problems are likely to influence transitions to more disordered states and impede changes to less disordered states (e.g., 18, 29, 54, 78, 102, 103, 152). For example, the first multiyear prospective study of casino employees (150) indicated that people troubled with gambling, drinking, or both shifted these behavior patterns regularly; in addition, these changes tended toward reduced levels of disorder rather than the increasingly serious problems often suggested by a traditional view of addictive behavior patterns (150). However, this study did not examine the pathways to recovery for casino employees. If gambling disorders are similar to other addictions, there is a vital gap in the literature since most people with gambling-related problems probably escape this circumstance without treatment (34, 154, 165, 183, 193). Prospective research designs are necessary to establish the extent of natural recovery and the determinants that influence the transition from problem to nonproblem gambling or abstinence.

Younger and Older Adults

While younger people have evidenced higher rates of gambling-related problems compared with their adult counterparts (e.g., 130), attention has recently shifted toward older adults and their increased risk. As gambling expanded and older adults sought more varied recreational activities, gambling junkets became more common. Investigators reported that older adults gambled to relax, pass time, get away for the day, avoid boredom, and take advantage of inexpensive meals (116). The prevalence of disordered gambling among this population segment is not yet determined. The reasons for gambling among the elderly are likely very similar to the reasons for gambling among adolescents.

Selected Ethnocultural Populations

Although there has been no systematic evaluation of the effects of culture on gambling and problem gambling, there is evidence in the literature of cultural variation in prevalence rates. Higher than average rates of gambling and gambling problems are found among African American, Aboriginal, and Latin American adolescents (170). Other studies point to group differences in gambling, which likely have ethnocultural roots. In Florida, for example, problem gamblers are disproportionately Latin American (31). Likewise, Asian groups in America show higher rates of gambling disorders compared with other groups (196). Gambling, including illegal gambling, continues to be popular in America's Chinese communities, with many working extra shifts to support this recreational activity (84). There is also evidence of gambling's popularity in Asia, for example, in Singapore where gambling is associated with substance abuse and other detrimental behaviors (173).

Evolving public policy on gambling has resulted in revenue creation and employment opportunities for Aboriginal communities. This potential benefit might, however, be offset by increased vulnerability to the negative consequences of gambling. In general, Aboriginal people evidence higher rates of problem and pathological gambling, poorer mental health status, as well as higher rates of substance-related problems compared with the general population (e.g., 44, 124, 125, 181, 187).

COMORBIDITY

Versions of the DSM that have included pathological gambling as a distinct disorder also have observed that other disorders may coexist with pathological gambling. For example, DSM-IV notes that pathological gamblers "may be prone to developing general medical conditions that are associated with stress. . . . Increased rates of Mood Disorders, Attention-Deficit Hyperactivity Disorder, Substance Abuse or Dependence, and Antisocial, Narcissistic, and Borderline Personality Disorders have been reported in individuals with Pathological Gambling" (5, p. 616).

Like casino employees with gambling problems, clinicians often report that patients who seek treatment for pathological gambling have a variety of social problems caused by gambling. However, treatment seekers are very different from people who have gambling problems but do not seek treatment. Treatment seekers typically have a greater variety and intensity of psychological problems compared with their counterparts who do not seek treatment (e.g., 29, 77, 135, 157). Among the group of gamblers who seek treatment, are the comorbid problems the cause or consequence of pathological gambling?

Comorbidity reflects the coexistence of gambling with other disorders—here, we are focusing on psychiatric disorders. This confluence makes it difficult to determine whether (a) gambling behavior causes a "gambling disorder" or (b) other disorders cause intemperate gambling and the problems that often accompany excessive gambling, or (c) both sets of problems reflect another underlying disorder. To illustrate, where X represents a comorbid condition, and PG represents level 3 gambling disorders, seven primary relationships can describe the association between disordered gambling and psychiatric comorbidity.

1. X contributes to, is a risk factor for, or causes PG;
2. X protects against or "treats" the occurrence of or progression to PG;
3. PG contributes to, is a risk factor for, or causes X;
4. PG protects against or "treats"[4] the occurrence of or progression to X;
5. X and PG co-occur/co-exist but are coincidental and completely independent;
6. X and PG share common determinants (i.e., biological, psychological, behavioral, or social);
7. X and PG combined are actually components of some larger entity, disorder, or syndrome.

Despite this organizing map of the complex relationships that can exist between gambling and comorbid disorders, ". . . [r]esearch on psychiatric comorbidity in pathological gambling is still very much in its infancy. While an overlap of symptoms belonging to a variety of diagnostic disorders is common, a more systematic analysis . . . reveals a much more tentative picture" (29, p. 48). To consider these complicating factors in more depth, the following section examines the comorbidity of gambling.

THE PREVALENCE OF RELATED MENTAL DISORDERS

Despite the disproportionately high levels of various mental disorders among disordered gamblers, empirical research about the comorbidity of gambling and other psychological disorders is scant. Research is currently under way into the relationship between gambling and other psychiatric disorders, e.g., the new, ongoing national comorbidity study (NCS) includes a gambling module (R.C. Kessler, personal communication).

Crockford & el-Guebaly published a seminal review on comorbid conditions and gambling (29), and Black & Moyer described the clinical features (11). In an important study from the St. Louis 1981 Epidemiological Catchment Area Study, the authors reported, "Recreational gamblers and problem gamblers had higher rates of most psychiatric disorders than nongamblers after adjustment for race, sex, and age effects. The association between gambling and antisocial personality

---

[4]When pathological gambling "treats" the occurrence of a coexisting disorder or the progression of these problems, gambling serves as a self-medication (80).

disorder was strongest—recreational gamblers and problem gamblers were at increased odds of meeting the diagnostic criteria for this disorder (ORs = 2.3 and 6.1, respectively). Using age-of-onset information, we found that problems with depression and phobias usually preceded gambling among problem gamblers with comorbid depression and phobias" (35, p. 1094). Cunningham-Williams et al. observed that 0.9% of their 1981 DIS/DSM-III screened sample evidenced a lifetime rate of pathological gambling and another 9.2% reported at least one gambling-related symptom. Like the seminal prevalence research conducted by Kallick et al. over 25 years ago (71), these 20-year-old data yielded an estimate of the most serious level of disordered gambling that is very similar to contemporary rates generated from international studies.

Substance Use Disorders

Most gambling studies on the relationship between gambling and other psychiatric conditions have focused on substance use and mood disorders (e.g., 48). Crockford & el-Guebaly report, ". . . between 25% and 63% of pathological gamblers meet criteria for a substance use disorder in their lifetime . . . . Correspondingly, 9% to 16% of patients with a substance use disorder are also found to be probable pathological gamblers" (29, p. 44). Alcohol is the most commonly abused substance; a high rate of nicotine use is also very common among pathological gamblers. When more than one substance is abused, the prevalence and severity of pathological gambling is increased as compared to individuals who abuse only one drug. Like the findings of Shaffer et al., Crockford & el-Guebaly note that there is considerable variation among study estimates of the comorbidity of substance abuse and gambling as well as the quality of these study methods (151).

Not only can alcohol intoxication reduce the perception of negative consequences of risk-taking (52), it also can encourage the perception of potential benefits so these reliably outweigh the negative consequences (53). Emerging evidence suggests common genetic risk factors for alcohol dependence and pathological gambling; however, the risk for alcohol dependence accounts for a significant but only modest proportion of the genetic and environmental risk for subclinical and DSM-III-R pathological gambling disorders (161).

Research from the Epidemiological Catchment Area (ECA) study found no difference in the rate of lifetime prevalence of pathological gambling among drug users from the community and those in drug treatment settings (36). The rate of level 2 and level 3 gambling among these groups is 22% and 11%, respectively (36). This study also reported that whereas most psychiatric disorders were not associated with gambling disorders, antisocial personality disorder was more prevalent among disordered gamblers than among recreational gamblers (36). Finally, another study of eight drug treatment settings in five Northeastern states found a similar rate of pathological gambling (13%); impulsivity and antisocial characteristics were also identified as important determinants associated with pathological gambling (94).

Mood Disorders

As we discussed earlier, evidence suggests that the prevalence of dysthymia, depression (uni-polar and bipolar), suicidal ideation, and suicide attempts is inflated among disordered gamblers. However, Lesieur & Blume did not identify an elevated prevalence of pathological gambling among patients treated for mood disorders (100). This observation runs counter to the often-observed relationship between these disorders. Consequently, an accurate rate of comorbidity might best be provided by a follow-up study (172) observing that about 18% of disordered gamblers experienced continued depression "... despite abstinence from gambling and improvement in their work and family lives—a percentage of depressive disorders similar to that seen in patients with substance use disorders" (29, p. 46).

Gambling, Suicide and Mortality

Clinical observations have associated gambling problems with suicidal thoughts and attempts. However, between 1980 and 1997, since pathological gambling entered the psychiatric nosology, no death certificate in the United States has listed gambling as the underlying cause of death (i.e., 0 deaths for 312.3, the ICD-9 code for impulse-control disorder, which includes pathological gambling (312.31) (23).[5] Nevertheless, there have been many attempts in the scientific literature and popular media to establish gambling as an indirect cause of death. The idea that gambling is a cause of suicide emerges primarily from (*a*) anecdotes about successful suicides that are preceded by episodes of losing at gambling (e.g., 93), (*b*) higher rates of reported depression among disordered gamblers, and (*c*) case studies (e.g., 13, 69). A definitive answer about the relationship between gambling and suicide will only emerge by conducting large-scale epidemiological research. Even with such research, the results can be confusing and difficult to interpret.

Two research teams have investigated this problem using epidemiological strategies. Both studies employ very different methodologies and report very different findings: Phillips et al. (128) imply that there is a link by virtue of elevated suicides proximate to gambling; McCleary et al. (113) argue against such a link. However, each research team employed differing methods to calculate suicide parameters. The Proportionate Mortality Rate (PMR) used by Phillips et al. represents the percentage of all "gambling destination" visitor-deaths attributable to suicide. By contrast, McCleary et al. use the suicide-specific mortality rate (SSMR), calculated by dividing the number of destination visitor suicides by the number of visitors. Depending on the statistical representation, very different conclusions can be drawn about the same data. Unfortunately, both studies use gambling settings

---

[5]The absence of pathological gambling as the underlying cause of death on the death certificate does not mean that no one has died of factors associated with pathological gambling. Medical examiners, who must identify the immediate cause and contributing causes of death on the death certificate, for any number of reasons, might be unaware of pathological gambling or unwilling to list it as a cause of death.

(i.e., destinations) rather than actual gamblers as their unit of analysis. It would have been interesting to know whether the visitors who committed suicide were in fact gamblers. This is not a small concern and, therefore, we cannot draw a meaningful conclusion about the relationship between gambling behavior and suicide.

A study of casino-related deaths in Atlantic City between 1982–86 showed that 83% of the total number of fatalities were cardiac sudden deaths. Although the stress of gambling activities could arguably induce sudden cardiac death (69), it has not yet been established that problem or pathological gamblers die at different rates compared with their nonproblem gambling counterparts.

There are many difficulties associated with determining gambling as a necessary and sufficient cause for adverse social consequences. Equally complex difficulties associated with identifying gambling as a partial cause continue to plague this area of investigation. In particular, psychiatric comorbidity is often evident among pathological gamblers; this influence significantly confuses the assessment of causality since mood disorders may antedate disordered gambling. Further, if we consider gambling as a source of behavioral "toxicity," then research also must establish a "dose-response" relationship between gambling and death, i.e., that more time spent gambling or higher stakes gambling cause an increased frequency of deaths. To date, no such relationship has been demonstrated. Absent this evidence, a relationship between gambling and mortality cannot be concluded. In their review of the NRC and the NGISC findings, the GAO arrived at the same conclusion (55).

Anxiety Disorders

Anxiety often appears as a hallmark of gamblers who seek treatment; however, this anxiety typically is more representative of anxious depression than anxiety disorders. Clinicians have described the signs and symptoms of anxiety (i.e., fear and stress) as common prior to becoming a gambler, whereas gambling as escape from these unpleasant emotions meets a DSM-IV diagnostic criterion for pathological gambling. However, clinical anxiety disorders are a complex grouping of specific mental disorders ranging from general anxiety disorder, panic attacks, obsessive-compulsive disorder to posttraumatic stress disorder. For these clinical conditions, "little is known about the association of anxiety disorders and problem gambling" (123, p. 138). After a careful review of the literature, Crockford & el-Guebaly concluded, ". . . despite an increased prevalence being reported in 3 studies, there would appear to be insufficient data to support the theory that anxiety disorders are comorbid with pathological gambling. In particular, there is little support for the comorbidity with obsessive-compulsive disorder (OCD)" (29, p. 47).

Personality Disorders

In spite of little empirical evidence to estimate the comorbidity of personality and gambling disorders, clinicians regularly describe a high level of narcissistic personality disorder among pathological gamblers. Two important general population studies found that problem gambling was associated with antisocial personality disorder and that pathological gambling always was secondary to this disorder (35, 36). Blaszczynski & Steel concluded, ". . . [M]ultiple overlapping personality disorders per subject [were] more the rule than the exception". . . . "On average, subjects met criteria for 4.6 DSM-III personality disorders" (14, pp. 60, 65). In addition, the number of personality disorders was significantly related to SOGS scores in a positive direction. "The results of this study indicate that pathological gamblers as a group exhibit rates of personality disorders that are comparable to those found in general psychiatric patient populations" (14, p. 65). Recent findings add support for the relationship between antisocial personality and pathological gambling among treatment-seeking cohorts (94).

Impulse and Other Disorders

Currently, DSM-IV (TR) places pathological gambling within the impulse disorders category, which also includes kleptomania, pyromania, and trichotillomania. It is reasonable to expect that pathological gambling would covary with these disorders of similar origin. However, despite the occasional appraisal of impulsiveness, gambling and the other diagnoses from the DSM impulse disorders category have not been investigated comparatively. Instead, gambling has been compared and contrasted with substance use disorders. Consequently, there is a paucity of evidence to inform us about the comorbidity of pathological gambling and the other impulse disorders.

Similarly, Crockford & el-Guebaly concluded that there is little evidence to suggest a comorbid relationship between gambling disorders and eating or sexual addictions (29). They also noted that despite clinical descriptions of dissociative-like symptoms among pathological gamblers, "[I]t would seem highly unlikely that this would be probable. . ." (29, p. 48). Compulsive shopping or oniomania has been identified as having similar etiology and comorbidity patterns to pathological gambling, with a very similar prevalence rate (i.e., 1.1%) (96). Blum et al. have suggested that pathological gambling and other excessive behavior patterns have a common etiology that is characterized by a reward deficiency syndrome (16). These investigators propose that addiction is ". . .a biogenetic disease" and that ". . .vulnerability to addiction (as well as impulsive and compulsive behaviors) is genetically transmitted. It is not necessary to establish that all addiction is caused by genetic vulnerability. Heavy exposure to alcohol and other drugs may set in motion perturbators of neurochemistry and receptors which may have similar end results" (16, p. 2). This common neurobiological vulnerability has linked the prevalence of pathological gambling to increased rates of Tourette's syndrome (26).

Neurobiological, neuropsychological, and clinical studies (e.g., 141) provide growing evidence of an increase in attention-deficit hyperactivity disorder among pathological compared with nonpathological gamblers (27, 62, 123, 167, 195). Preliminary evidence indicates that noradrenaline is associated with attention problems (e.g., attention-deficit hyperactivity disorder) and that dopamine level shifts might be associated with pathological gambling (8).

The Games People Play

Although we do not believe that using a specific object of addiction (e.g., heroin, cocaine, keno, lottery, or shopping) represents the necessary and sufficient cause to produce addictive behavior,[6] there is reason to examine the epidemiological relationship between gambling disorders and the specific games on which people wager. Understanding the biopsychosocial influences of specific games should provide insight into determinants that facilitate or inhibit the development of gambling disorders. A research synthesis examined the extent of participation in seven different common gambling activities among general population adults, adolescents, adults in treatment and prison populations, and college students (151). As expected, adolescents were found to participate significantly more than adults in gambling activities that are most socially accessible and do not require authorization, i.e., games of skill, non-casino card games, and sports betting. Adolescents can participate in these three activities within a group of school friends, with their families, or with their friends' families. Similarly, college students are betting more than adults in the general population on non-casino card games and games of skill, activities that are popular within a college setting. Not surprisingly, adults in the general population are gambling more than adolescents on casino games, the lottery, and pari-mutuel wagering. Generally, the vendor of these adult activities requires authorization from a licensing bureau or certification board. Although adolescents engage in these three activities despite their illegal status, the vast majority of participants in these legal forms of gambling are adults.

Deciphering relationships among specific gaming activities and disordered gambling requires sophisticated research that focuses on the nature of the relationships between an individual and the object of their addiction, i.e., their gambling activity of choice. Gambling researchers would do well to emulate lines of inquiry by substance abuse researchers, who have discovered many important and illuminating differences among various substances and their substance-specific physiological, psychological, and socioeconomic influences on users. For example, alcohol has "releasing" properties that tend to disinhibit users. Cocaine has antidepressant stimulating properties. Khantzian suggested that certain personality types are more attracted to each of these drug classes to produce a self-medicating effect (79–81). Similarly, Jacobs suggested that certain gambling activities (e.g., video poker machines) could produce dissociative effects that might differentially attract individuals with certain personality attributes (66). Much remains to be learned about the relationship between people and the games they choose to play (Table 4).

---

[6]We encourage interested readers to review other relevant works (144–146) for a more complete discussion.

TABLE 4   Prevalence of gambling activity by population segment[a]

	Adults (%)	Adolescents (%)	College (%)
Lifetime prevalence of gambling	81.19	77.55	85.04
Casino games—lifetime	32.32	7.74	40.59
Casino games—past year	14.95	12.56	60.83
Lottery—lifetime	61.25	34.89	50.29
Lottery—past year	49.05	30.16	60.18
Sports gambling—lifetime	26.83	38.17	28.45
Sports gambling—past year	14.76	30.69	30.5
Pari-mutuel—lifetime	25.11	10.88	27.17
Pari-mutuel—past year	7.13	11.24	8.9
Financial markets—lifetime	13.11	—	16.65
Financial markets—past year	5.81	—	4.2
Non-casino card games—lifetime	28.16	53.46	47.37
Non-casino card games—past year	15.89	39.61	36.1
Games of skill—lifetime	18.57	40.43	39.93
Games of skill—past year	10.25	31.61	23.93

[a]See Reference 151.

CONCEPTUAL AND METHODOLOGICAL ISSUES

Is Pathological Gambling a Primary and Unique Disorder?

The research methods associated with promulgating basic estimates of gambling prevalence have changed little during the past 20 years (149, 151). With some exceptions, the NRC noted the overall weakness of research methods in the area of gambling studies (123). Shaffer et al. noted that regardless of the quality of these studies, weak and strong methods seem to produce comparable estimates of disordered gambling prevalence (151). Nevertheless, two critically important conceptual and methodological questions face the study of gambling and related psychiatric disorders. First, is pathological gambling a primary and unique disorder or a multidimensional syndrome? Second, are existing estimates of disordered gambling prevalence accurate in the absence of a gold standard? These unresolved questions commingle and their confluence affects how we understand gambling disorders. For example, although clinicians might heed exclusion criteria in planning treatment, for the most part, the implications of exclusion criteria have been ignored (17) during the conduct of prevalence research. One research consequence of ignoring exclusion recommendations might be overestimation of the prevalence of pathological gambling. That is, if other primary disorders such as manic episodes are not identified by survey instruments and then excluded by the investigator, the evidence will yield inflated prevalence estimates of gambling disorders. In addition, between DSM-III and DSM-IV, the American Psychiatric Association shifted the exclusion criteria from antisocial personality disorder to mania. This change reflects an ongoing struggle to develop a clear definition of pathological gambling in the absence of a gold standard. The nature of the overlap and interaction among antisocial personality, manic episodes, and pathological gambling is poorly understood. Measuring the prevalence of related psychiatric disorders along with pathological gambling should provide important insight into these questions. Ultimately, the field of gambling studies is in need of research that can provide additional construct validity.

If pathological gambling represents a primary disorder, then it can emerge in the absence of other comorbidity and cause sequelae independent of any other condition(s). However, if it is a secondary disorder, subordinate to other dysfunctional behavior, then pathological gambling will only exist as a consequent of another condition [e.g., manic episode, antisocial personality, alcohol abuse, obsessive-compulsive disorder, or adolescence (70)]. In this case, pathological gambling is not a unique disorder but rather a cluster of symptoms associated with another disorder. Although worldwide prevalence estimates of disordered gambling have identified a relatively stable and robust phenomenon, investigators have not established with ample certainty that this phenomenon represents a unique construct. The implications of this failure are potentially significant for the development and planning of both treatment strategies and social policy initiatives designed to ameliorate or regulate gambling-related problems.

Symptoms or Syndrome

The symptoms associated with pathological gambling reflect a complex syndrome rather than a single disorder. The comorbidity and co-occurrence of pathological gambling with other diagnostic entities probably is an artifact of DSM-IV, misdirecting observers away from the likelihood that it is a syndrome. Overlapping symptoms can represent a common underlying factor. However, when a variety of symptoms are associated with a disorder but not all the symptoms are always present, a syndrome is in evidence.

Constructing pathological gambling as a syndrome suggests both common and unique components. A syndrome's common component (e.g., depression) is shared with other disorders (e.g., substance use disorders), whereas its unique component (e.g., betting increasing amounts of money) is specific to pathological gambling. The shared component, which accounts for the comorbidity evidence, reflects broad individual differences that can vary along multiple dimensions (e.g., intensity and duration); the unique component distinguishes pathological gambling from other disorders and is specific only to it (e.g., 190).

Although it has unique elements, pathological gambling has many signs and symptoms shared with other disorders (e.g., anxiety, depression, impulsivity); consequently, disordered gambling is best thought of as a syndrome. From this perspective, the most effective treatments for gambling problems will reflect a multimodal "cocktail" approach combined with patient-treatment matching. These multidimensional treatments will include combinations of psychopharmacology, psychotherapy, and financial, educational, and self-help interventions; such treatment elements are both additive and interactive to deal with the multidimensional nature of gambling disorders.

Because syndromes are multidimensional, these disorders typically do not respond favorably to a single treatment modality. Whether we view disordered gambling as primary or secondary, unique or syndromal, intemperate gambling inflicts human suffering. If pathological gambling is a primary disorder, it often will require professional assistance; if it is a disorder secondary to another problem, it still requires specialized modalities focusing on the gambling problems in addition to those related to the primary disorder. These theoretical, research, and clinical distinctions need to be clarified in future research.

Reconsidering Clinical Diagnoses as the Gold Standard

In the absence of a gold standard, some investigators have assumed that clinicians provide the proxy gold standard against which the accuracy of screening instruments can be measured (e.g., 101, 177, 188). For example, investigators often use the term probable pathological gambling rather than pathological gambling. "The term *probable* distinguishes the results of prevalence surveys, where classification is based on responses to questions in a telephone interview, from a clinical diagnosis" (177, p. 3). Similarly, others have concluded, "Because only a clinical evaluation using DSM-IV can diagnose pathological gambling, we have used the term 'probable' pathological gambling . . . . Since the survey is not a clinical diagnosis, we cannot say that respondents can be 'diagnosed' as pathological gamblers, rather we use the term 'probable' pathological gamblers" (188, pp. 5-2–5-5).

However, clinicians who perform diagnostic evaluations are not as reliable as often assumed (e.g., 117, 118, 140, 200). Clinicians are extremely vulnerable to biases in clinical judgment. Faraone & Tsuang emphasize that psychiatric diagnoses should not be considered a gold standard and that it is important to assess their adequacy (47). Therefore, the assumption that gamblers should be grouped into a tentative class, for example, probable pathological gamblers, is faulty. We suggest that all diagnostic classification—whether clinician- or instrument-based—be held as tentative and not final (e.g., 85, 143).

Considering False Positives and False Negatives: The Need for Theory

The often-repeated debate about false positives and false negatives contributes little to our understanding of gambling disorders. An instrument can yield useful prevalence indices even if it has only moderate sensitivity and specificity. So long as false positives are "balanced" by false negatives, an instrument will perform very well as a general population screen.[7] Only when these faulty classification assignments fail to balance does a screening instrument begin to deteriorate as an index of population prevalence. Debates surrounding faulty classification are subject to the same constraints as those about validity: To determine a false assignment, there must be a standard against which to judge the classification system. Without a gold standard, there is the risk of "infinite frustration"—always trying to refer to a higher standard for construct validity (30). Consequently, the only way out of this conceptual chaos is to develop what Cronbach & Meehl called a nomological network: an interlocking system of laws that constitutes a theory (30).

With few exceptions, the prevalence estimates reviewed here seem to have been promulgated, at best, by the question of "let's find out," and, at worst, in a conceptual vacuum. The goals and objectives of disordered gambling prevalence estimation have not been made sufficiently clear by those generating them. Without knowing whether the estimates of disordered gambling prevalence are designed to guide the development of public policy, allocate limited public health resources, expand scientific knowledge, identify economic needs, or inform some other activity, observers are left to project their own needs onto prevalence estimates. Absent a driving set of objectives, gambling epidemiologists have not provided policy makers with the basic information essential to building an effective system of treatment (e.g., estimates of the obstacles to treatment entry and how often people encounter these difficulties). Similarly, because prevalence research has not been driven by explicit theory, investigators have not identified the extent and direction of movement between level 2 gamblers either toward or away from more disordered states. Without such information, social cost estimates are less than precise, and the challenges to conceptual validity will continue.

Other Methodological Concerns

Although a full consideration of methodological problems is beyond the scope of this review, we offer a brief comment. Various methodological shortcomings can influence prevalence estimates and potentially diminish their accuracy (e.g., 98, 151). For example, failing to randomly select a sample of respondents can bias prevalence estimates. There also are problems with survey instruments, nonresponse rates, and refusal bias (98). Low response rates are common, and some investigators have defended these rates simply because they are consistent with other contemporary survey results (e.g., 179). Low response rates might provide biased estimates because a sample is not representative—however, low response rates also might reflect a representative sample that provides an accurate estimate. The burden of proof resides with the investigator to demonstrate that a low response rate is representative.

---

[7]In clinical practice, however, quality patient care requires a very different standard of accuracy; when only one case is under consideration, there is no one to "balance" a misdiagnosis. Therefore, the consequences of clinical errors can be severe.

Most investigators conducting prevalence research use telephone surveys as the primary sampling strategy. This methodology might present important problems. People with gambling disorders may have less access to telephones because of financial problems or may not be available to answer the phones because they are out gambling. Alternatively, disordered gamblers may be stuck at home feeling depressed and answer the phone at higher rates than their nongambling counterparts, thereby inflating the rate of gambling disorders. These uncertainties deserve empirical attention since each circumstance can bias prevalence estimates.

Finally, a considerable body of prevalence estimation research has emerged from in-treatment or treatment-seeking respondents. Since Berkson (9) first demonstrated that reliance on treatment seekers might be misleading (i.e., Berkson's bias), we must remember to interpret prevalence estimates from this population segment cautiously (123). Similarly, the methods employed to generate prevalence estimates have been relatively few, and investigators have tended to ignore the social desirability pressures that can influence respondents. Taken together, these forces might bias prevalence estimates; without additional research, however, it is not possible to determine in which direction.

AN OVERVIEW OF THE MAJOR PUBLIC HEALTH ISSUES AND CHALLENGES

During the current rapid expansion, increased availability, and promotion of legalized gambling such as casinos and lotteries (137), the dominant health focus has centered on the emergence and extent of disordered gambling. Also significant are other public health problems related to vulnerable populations, families, and communities, e.g., the high prevalence of youth and underage gambling (e.g., 148, 149, 151, 153), including sports betting at colleges and universities. The notion that gambling interacts with individual psychoeconomics and social determinants to levy a regressive tax on the poor and contribute to upward income redistribution from certain vulnerable groups deserves close study (e.g., 25). The effect of gambling on the quality of life for families is often mentioned, including concerns about dysfunctional relationships, neglect, violence, and abuse (e.g., 29, 86, 153).

There is a public and professional perception that disordered gambling can be "a gateway" to substance abuse, depression, and other mental health maladies (e.g., 29, 45, 72, 93, 132). Observers have juxtaposed suicide and crime with gambling and have attracted considerable attention within the public health community for these concerns. Although some studies have suggested a correlation between gambling and suicide (e.g., 128), a causal link has not been established (e.g., 113). Special conditions associated with an increased risk for problems among seniors, Aboriginal, other minorities, and women are frequently mentioned and need further study. Viewed as worrisome are the introduction of new gaming technologies such as in the wide availability of VLTs and the existence of unregulated offshore and Internet gambling (121).

The implications of expanded gambling for the viability, health, and quality of life for local municipalities have been hotly debated (e.g., 59, 63, 83). This discussion reflects community values and priorities; however, it also echoes planning assumptions surrounding a range of social, economic, and health dimensions of community life. From a social policy perspective, there is a need for comprehensive study of these various aspects of community life to determine which groups gain and which lose when gambling is expanded into a new jurisdiction. Political decisions in the United States and Canada to generate state and provincial revenue through lottery and casino operations rather than new taxes have raised the issue of good governance and the social ramifications of governmental dependence on gambling. To date little scientific attention has been paid to gambling in the financial world of day trading, commodity futures markets, and hedge funds. Although not traditionally thought of as gambling, these activities often meet that definition. High-risk and impulsive financial trading can have profound repercussions for individuals and social institutions.

RECOMMENDATIONS FOR PUBLIC HEALTH POLICY AND PRACTICE

Prevalence research implicitly encourages a clinical, idiographic analysis of gambling disorders—as if understanding individual attributes offered a sufficient explanation. However, public health strategies historically have focused on the interactions among the host, agent, and environment—in this case the gambler, his or her psychological expectations, resistances, and vulnerabilities, and the social setting within which people gamble. This interactive perspective on gambling disorders encourages greater involvement from public health workers and a multilevel integrated approach to interventions.

To encourage this increased involvement, we suggest the following four steps for public health action. First, adoption of strategic goals for gambling to provide a focus for public health action and accountability. These goals can include preventing gambling-related problems among individuals and groups at risk for gambling addiction; promoting balanced and informed attitudes, behaviors, and policies toward gambling and gamblers by both individuals and communities; and protecting vulnerable groups from gambling-related harm.

Second, endorsement of public health principles. Three primary principles can guide and inform decision-making to reduce gambling-related problems: ensuring that prevention is a community priority, with the appropriate allocation of resources to primary, secondary, and tertiary prevention initiatives; incorporating a mental health promotion approach that builds community capacity, incorporates a holistic view of mental health including the emotional and spiritual dimensions, and addresses the needs and aspiration of gamblers, individuals at risk of gambling problems, or those affected by them; and fostering personal and social responsibility for gambling policies and practices.

Third, adoption of harm reduction strategies and tactics (e.g., 174) directed toward minimizing the adverse health, social, and economic consequences of gambling behavior for individuals, families, and communities. At the very least, these initiatives would include healthy-gambling guidelines for the general public (i.e., similar to low-risk drinking guidelines); vehicles for the early identification of gambling problems; nonjudgmental moderation and abstinence goals for problem gamblers; and surveillance and reporting systems to monitor trends in gambling-related participation and the incidence and burden of gambling-related illness.

Fourth, allocation of resources to identify and treat level 2 gamblers. Understanding the behavior of level 2 gamblers could help lower the social costs and harms associated with gambling disorders. "The common risk factors for many diseases are present in a large proportion of the population, and therefore, most of the cases of disease arise from the intermediate- and low-risk groups. Relatively small changes in risk among the middle-risk group can result in a greater overall reduction in disease burden than do greater changes in the high-risk group" (20, p. 736). To illustrate, although level 3 gamblers are characterized by a more intense and potentially destructive relationship with disordered gambling than their level 2 counterparts, their numbers are considerably smaller. In spite of the more moderate and potentially short-lived nature of the problems experienced by level 2 gamblers, their larger numbers produce greater social disruption than their more disordered level 3 counterparts, just as problem drinkers are responsible for more aggregate social disorders than their alcohol-dependent counterparts (e.g., 166). As with research on problem drinkers, future gambling research likely will reveal that level 2 gamblers are more responsive to treatment and social policy interventions than are level 3 gamblers. Consequently, a public health strategy that promotes harm reduction and other secondary prevention objectives needs to concentrate more on level 2 gamblers.

RECOMMENDATIONS FOR PUBLIC HEALTH RESEARCH

Toward Theory Guided Research

Theory guides research; epidemiological prevalence research is no exception to this rule. To advance scientific understanding and the health of the public, new gambling-related research initiatives will require well-developed theoretical maps to guide studies of the distribution and determinants of disordered gambling. In addition, scientific investigators will need to identify where to apply their theoretical maps. For example, epidemiological research focusing on the distribution of gambling has established reliable base rates of gambling-associated disorders across international boundaries. Consequently, future gambling research should follow the recommendations offered previously for psychiatric epidemiology. "After identifying base rates of illness, the ECA study was to identify high-risk subgroups within the population, those with unusually high rates of illness as well as groups with unusually low rates. In addition to providing profiles of individuals at unusually high risk for developing an illness, such a strategy allows testing of causal hypotheses. While it is unlikely that a single cause of mental disorders will be found, just as no single cause explains cancer or heart disease, the eventual aim of epidemiological research is to identify specific components in a causal chain of factors that produce an illness. For those factors that are amenable to change, direct interventions may be designed as a means of reducing rates of illness in a population" (136, p. 3).

As advancing scientific theory enhances our understanding of gambling disorders, a gold standard likely will emerge. Indices that do not rely on the self-reported adverse consequences of gambling will provide a gold standard (e.g., neurobiological or psychosocial indices that accurately identify gambling problems but are not directly related to gambling or its consequences). Ultimately, this development will permit clinicians to improve the diagnostic sensitivity and specificity of screening instruments; in turn, this advance will make available opportunities for more effective treatment matching. Similarly, researchers will become better able to distinguish subtypes of gamblers, match people with the appropriate type and level of preventive and clinical services, and distinguish individuals and groups who do not require intervention. In addition, screening instruments for adolescents, psychiatric patients, inmates, and various ethnic groups will improve as more focused techniques are developed for estimating the consequences of gambling on these population segments.

FUTURE PREVALENCE RESEARCH

To address the variety of problems involved in studying gambling-related disorders, investigators need to focus more on multimethod, multimeasure strategies for prevalence estimation (22). Indices of social desirability are essential, particularly if workers are to establish the needed prospective studies that will help elucidate influences on gambling and its transformation to disordered states. For example, repeated applications of the SOGS can result in lower estimates after respondents have items clarified (91). However, since the original SOGS test-retest reliability indices were only 0.71, and scores tended to lower among inpatients, rather than attribute this shift to the influence of treatment planning, it is possible that social desirability may have influenced respondents' initial responses (6, 101). When seeking treatment, people may either magnify their problems or minimize them. In either event, rather than speculate, investigators need to build devices into their research to protect against such spurious influences.

Much of the prevalence research reveals collinearity (i.e., multiple correlations) between population segments and sample size (151). Studies of the general adult population are large and research on vulnerable populations typically rests upon small sample sizes. Given the consistent prevalence rates obtained across regions and cultures, except for tracking the impact of public policy changes, the era of general population studies is likely near an end (50). We encourage more focus on vulnerable and at-risk populations, where the greatest public health advances are likely to be made. The study of gambling prevalence and any associated mental disorders is a promising young field with enormous potential to advance our understanding of addictive behaviors in general and to protect and improve the health of the public.

CONCLUSION

The recent and dramatic expansion of gambling challenges us to focus on the broad implications for individual and community health. Public health is well suited to address matters of healthy public policy, burden of illness, and lifestyle behaviors. A comprehensive research agenda is needed for the gambling field. By understanding the distribution and determinants of gambling problems in the general population and among subgroups, there is opportunity to develop effective strategies to protect vulnerable people, foster healthy gambling where appropriate, and improve the quality of community life.

ACKNOWLEDGMENTS

This work was supported in part by funding from the National Center for Responsible Gaming and the Institute for the Study of Pathological Gambling and Related Disorders at Harvard Medical School's Division on Addictions. The authors extend special thanks to Chris Freed, Chris Reilly, Gabriel Eber, Joni Vander Bilt, and Matthew Hall for their important contributions to this project. The authors also thank Christine Thurmond, Harvey Skinner, and Richard LaBrie for their advice and thoughtful comments regarding earlier versions of this article.

Visit the Annual Reviews home page at www.annualreviews.org

LITERATURE CITED

1. 1996. *National Gambling Impact Study Commission Act.* PL104-169, 104th Congress
2. Ackerman D. 1999. *Deep Play.* New York: Random House. 235 pp.
3. Am. Acad. Pediatrics. 1998. *Teen Gambling Epidemic Linked To Risky Behavior,* p. 1. http://www.aap.org/
4. Am. Psychiatric Assoc. 1980. *DSM-III: Diagnostic and Statistical Manual of Mental Disorders.* Washington, DC: Am. Psychiatr. Assoc. 886 pp.
5. Am. Psychiatric Assoc. 1994. *DSM-IV: Diagnostic and Statistical Manual of Mental Disorders.* Washington, DC: Am. Psychiatr. Assoc. 886 pp.
6. Am. Psychiatric Assoc. Task Force Handb. Psychiatr. Measures. 2000. *Handbook of Psychiatric Measures.* Washington, DC: Am. Psychiatr. Assoc.
7. Benson H. 1984. *Beyond the Relaxation Response.* New York: Berkley
8. Bergh C, Sodersten EP, Nordin C. 1997. Altered dopamine function in pathological gambling. *Psychol. Med.* 27:473–75

9. Berkson J. 1946. Limitations of the application of fourfold table analysis to hospital data. *Biometrics* 2:47–53

10. Bettencourt BA, Miller N. 1996. Gender differences in aggression as a function of provocation: a meta-analysis. *Psychol. Bull.* 119:422–47

11. Black WB, Moyer T. 1998. Clinical features and psychiatric comorbidity of subjects with pathological gambling behavior. *Psychiatr. Serv.* 49:1434–39

12. Bland RC, Newman SC, Orn H, Stebelsky G. 1993. Epidemiology of pathological gambling in Edmonton. *Can. J. Psychiatry* 38:108–12

13. Blaszczynski A, Farrell E. 1998. A case series of 44 completed gambling-related suicides. *J. Gambl. Stud.* 14:93–109

14. Blaszczynski A, Steel Z. 1998. Personality disorders among pathological gamblers. *J. Gambl. Stud.* 14:51–71

15. Blaszczynski AP, McConaghy N. 1994. Criminal offenses in Gamblers Anonymous and hospital treated pathological gamblers. *J. Gambl. Stud.* 10:99–127

16. Blum K, Braverman ER, Holder MM, Lubar JF, Monastra VJ, et al. 2000. Reward deficiency syndrome: a biogenetic model for the diagnosis and treatment of impulsive, addictive, and compulsive behaviors. *J. Psychoact. Drugs* 32:1–112

17. Boyd JH, Burke JD, Gruenberg E, Holzer CE, Rae DS, et al. 1984. Exclusion criteria of DSM-III: a study of co-occurrence of hierarchy-free syndromes. *Arch. Gen. Psychiatry* 41:983–89

18. Briggs JR, Goodin BJ, Nelson T. 1996. Pathological gamblers and alcoholics: Do they share the same addiction? *Addict. Behav.* 21:515–19

19. Brown RI. 1987. Pathological gambling and associated patterns of crime: comparisons with alcohol and other drug addictions. *J. Gambl. Behav.* 3:98–114

20. Brownson RC, Newschaffer CJ, Ali-Abarghoui F. 1997. Policy research for disease prevention: challenges and practical recommendations. *Am. J. Public Health* 87:735–39

21. Campbell CS, Smith GJ. 1998. Canadian gambling: trends and public policy issues. See Ref. 51a, pp. 22–35

22. Campbell DT, Fiske DW. 1959. Convergent and discriminant validation by the multitrait-multimethod matrix. *Psychol. Bull.* 56:81–105

23. Cent. Dis. Control. 2001. *Compressed Mortality Database* [*world wide web*]. Cent. Dis. Control. http://www.cdc.gov/. Accessed March 9, 2001

24. Christiansen EM. 1998. Gambling and the American economy. See Ref. 51a, pp. 36–52

25. Clotfelter CT, Cook PJ. 1989. *Selling Hope: State Lotteries in America.* Cambridge: Harvard Univ. Press

26. Comings DE. 1998. The molecular genetics of pathological gambling. *CNS Spectr.* 3:20–37

27. Comings DE, Gonzalez N, Wu S, Gade R, Muhleman D, et al. 1999. Studies of the 48 bp repeat polymorphism of the DRD4 gene in impulsive, compulsive, addictive behaviors: Tourette syndrome, ADHD, pathological gambling, and substance abuse. *Am. J. Med. Genet. Neuropsychiatr. Genet.* 88:358–68

28. Costello T. 2001. Gambling's great web of lies. http://www.theage.com.au

29. Crockford DN, el-Guebaly N. 1998. Psychiatric comorbidity in pathological gambling: a critical review. *Can. J. Psychiatry—Rev. Can. Psychiatr.* 43:43–50

30. Cronbach LJ, Meehl PE. 1955. Construct validity in psychological tests. *Psychol. Bull.* 52:281–302

31. Cuadrado M. 1999. A comparison of Hispanic and Anglo calls to a gambling help hotline. *J. Gambl. Stud.* 15:71–81

32. Culleton RP. 1989. The prevalence rates of pathological gambling: a look at methods. *J. Gambl. Stud.* 5:22–41

33. Culleton RP, Lang MH. 1985. *The Prevalence Rate of Pathological Gambling in*

the Delaware Valley in 1984. Forum Policy Res. Public Serv., Rutgers Univ., Camden, NJ

34. Cunningham JA, Sobell LC, Sobell MB, Kapur G. 1995. Resolution from alcohol problems with and without treatment: reasons for change. *J. Subst. Abuse* 7:365–72

35. Cunningham-Williams R, Cottler LB, Compton WM, Spitznagel EL. 1998. Taking chances: problem gamblers and mental health disorders—results from the St. Louis epidemiologic catchment area study. *Am. J. Public Health* 88:1093–96

36. Cunningham-Williams RM, Cottler LB, Compton WM, Spitznagel EL, Ben-Abdallah A. 2000. Problem gambling and comorbid psychiatric and substance use disorders among drug users recruited from drug treatment and community settings. *J. Gambl. Stud.* 16:347–76

37. Curry SJ, Kim EL. 1999. Public health perspective on addictive behavior change interventions: conceptual frameworks and guiding principles. See Ref. 174, pp. 221–50

38. Custer RL, Milt H. 1985. *When Luck Runs Out: Help for Compulsive Gamblers and Their Families*. New York: Warner

39. Daghestani AN. 1987. Impotence associated with compulsive gambling. *J. Clin. Psychiatry* 48:115–16

40. DeCaria CM, Begaz T, Hollander E. 1998. Serotonergic and noradrenergic function in pathological gambling. *CNS Spectr.* 3:38–47

41. Driver BL, Brown PJ, Peterson GL. 1991. *Benefits of Leisure*. State College, PA: Venture

42. Eadington WR, Cornelius JA, eds. 1993. *Gambling Behavior & Problem Gambling*. Reno, NV: Inst. Study Gambl. Commer. Gaming, Coll. Bus. Admin., Univ. Nev., Reno. 678 pp.

43. Eber GB, Shaffer HJ. 2000. Trends in biobehavioral gambling studies research: quantifying citations. *J. Gambl. Stud.* 16:461–67

44. Elia C, Jacobs DF. 1993. The incidence of pathological gambling among Native Americans treated for alcohol dependence. *Int. J. Addict.* 28:659–66

45. Epstein J. 1989. Confessions of a low roller. In *The Best American Essays 1989*, ed. R Atwan, pp. 98–113. New York: Ticknor & Fields

46. Evans RG, Barer ML, Marmor TR, eds. 1994. *Why Are Some People Healthy and Others Not? The Determinants of Health of Populations*. New York: Aldine de Gruyter

47. Faraone SV, Tsuang MT. 1994. Measuring diagnostic accuracy in the absence of a "gold standard." *Am. J. Psychiatry* 151:650–57

48. Feigelman W, Wallisch LS, Lesieur HR. 1998. Problem gamblers, problem substance users, and dual problem individuals: an epidemiological study. *Am. J. Public Health* 88:467–70

49. Fessenden F. 1999. Lottery cost is heaviest on the poor. In *The New York Times*, May 22, p. A12

50. Fisher S. 2000. Measuring the prevalence of sector-specific problem gambling: a study of casino patrons. *J. Gambl. Stud.* 16:25–51

51. Fleming AM. 1978. *Something for Nothing: A History of Gambling*. New York: Delacorte

51a. Frey JH, ed. 1998. *Gambling: Socioeconomic Impacts and Public Policy*. Thousand Oaks, CA: Sage

52. Fromme K, Katz E, D'Amico E. 1997. Effects of alcohol intoxication on the perceived consequences of risk taking. *Exp. Clin. Psychopharmacol.* 5:14–23

53. Fromme K, Katz EC, Rivet K. 1997. Outcome expectancies and risk-taking behavior. *Cogn. Ther. Res.* 21:421–42

54. Galdston I. 1951. The psychodynamics of the triad, alcoholism, gambling, and superstition. *Ment. Hyg.* 35:589–98

55. Gen. Account. Off. 2000. *Impact of Gambling: Economic Effects More Measurable Than Social Effects. Rep. GGD-00-78*. Washington, DC: US GAO

56. Gerstein D, Murphy S, Toce M, Hoffmann J, Palmer A, et al. 1999. *Gambling Impact and Behavior Study: Report to the National Gambling Impact Study Commission.* Chicago: Natl. Opin. Res. Cent.

57. Gerstein D, Murphy S, Toce M, Hoffmann J, Palmer A, et al. 1999. *Gambling Impact and Behavior Study: Final Report to the National Gambling Impact Study Commission.* Chicago: Natl. Opin. Res. Cent.

58. Goldstein JM, Simpson JC. 1995. Validity: definitions and applications to psychiatric research. In *Textbook in Psychiatric Epidemiology,* ed. MT Tsuang, M Tohen, GE Zahner, pp. 229–42. New York: Wiley-Liss

59. Goodman R. 1995. *The Luck Business: The Devastating Consequences and Broken Promises of America's Gambling Explosion.* New York: Free Press. 273 pp.

60. Hays KF. 1999. *Working It Out: Using Exercise in Psychotherapy.* Washington, DC: Am. Psychol. Assoc.

61. Heineman M. 1989. Parents of male compulsive gamblers: clinical issues/treatment approaches. *J. Gambl. Behav.* 5: 321–33

62. Hollander E, Buchalter AJ, DeCaria CM. 2000. Pathological gambling. *Psychiatr. Clin. North Am.* 23(3):629–42

63. Hornblower M. 1996. No dice: the backlash against gambling. In *Time,* pp. 29–33

64. Horvath TA. 1998. *Sex, Drugs, Gambling & Chocolate: A Workbook for Overcoming Addictions.* San Luis Obispo, CA: Impact. 224 pp.

65. Inst. Med. 1990. *Broadening the Base of Treatment for Alcohol Problems: Report of a Study by a Committee of the Institute of Medicine, Division of Mental Health and Behavioral Medicine.* Washington, DC: Natl. Acad. Sci.

66. Jacobs DF. 1989. A general theory of addictions: rationale for and evidence supporting a new approach for understanding and treating addictive behaviors. In *Compulsive Gambling: Theory, Research &* *Practice,* ed. HJ Shaffer, S Stein, B Gambino, TN Cummings, pp. 35–64. Lexington, MA: Lexington

67. Jacobs DF, Marston AR, Singer RD, Widaman K, Little T, Veizades J. 1989. Children of problem gamblers. *J. Gambl. Behav.* 5:261–67

68. Jarrell HR. 1988. Vegas neuropathy. *New Engl. J. Med.* 319:1487

69. Jason JR, Taff ML, Boglioli LR. 1990. Casino-related deaths in Atlantic City, New Jersey: 1982–1986. *Am. J. Forensic Med. Pathol.* 11:112–23

70. Jessor R, Jessor SL. 1977. *Problem Behavior and Psychosocial Development: A Longitudinal Study of Youth.* New York: Academic

71. Kallick M, Suits D, Dielman T, Hybels J. 1979. *A Survey of American Gambling Attitudes and Behavior.* Ann Arbor, MI: Univ. Mich. Press

72. Kandarian P. 1998. Casinos seen as mixed blessing in Conn. In *The Boston Globe,* July 12, p. B9

73. Kaplan GA, Lynch JW. 2001. Is economic policy health policy? *Am. J. Public Health* 91:351–53

74. Karch SB, Graff J, Young S, Ho C. 1988. Response times and outcomes for cardiac arrests in Las Vegas casinos. *Am. J. Emerg. Med.* 16:249–53

75. Kelly J. 1982. *Leisure.* Englewood Cliffs, NJ: Prentice-Hall

76. Deleted in proof

77. Kessler RC, Crum RM, Warner LA, Nelson CB, Schulenberg J, Anthony JC. 1997. Lifetime co-occurrence of DSM-III-R alcohol abuse and dependence with other psychiatric disorders in the National Comorbidity Survey. *Arch. Gen. Psychiatry* 54:313–21

78. Kessler RC, Nelson CB, McGonagle KA, Edlund MJ, Frank RG, Leaf PJ. 1996. The epidemiology of co-occurring addictive and mental disorders: implications for prevention and service utilization. *Am. J. Orthopsychiatry* 66:17–31

79. Khantzian EJ. 1975. Self-selection and

progression in drug dependence. *Psychiatry Dig.* 36:19–22

80. Khantzian EJ. 1985. The self-medication hypothesis of addictive disorders: focus on heroin and cocaine dependence. *Am. J. Psychiatry* 142:1259–64

81. Khantzian EJ. 1997. The self-medication hypothesis of substance use disorders: a reconsideration and recent applications. *Harvard Rev. Psychiatry* 4:231–44

82. Kiesler S, Sproull L. 1985. Pool halls, chips, and war games: women in the culture of computing. *Psychol. Women Q.* 9:451–62

83. Kindt JW. 1994. The economic impacts of legalized gambling activities. *Drake Law Rev.* 43:51–95

84. Kinkead G. 1992. *Chinatown: Portrait of a Closed Society.* New York: Harper Collins

85. Kleinman A. 1987. Culture and clinical reality: commentary on culture-bound syndromes and international disease classifications. *Culture, Medicine and Psychiatry* 11:49–52

86. Knapp TJ, Lech BC. 1987. Pathological gambling: a review with recommendations. *Adv. Behav. Res. Ther.* 9:21–49

87. Korn D, Shaffer HJ. 1999. Gambling and the health of the public: adopting a public health perspective. *J. Gambl. Stud.* 15:289–365

88. Korn DA. 2000. Expansion of gambling in Canada: implications for health and social policy. *Can. Med. Assoc. J.* 163:61–64

89. Korn DA, Skinner HA. 2000. Gambling expansion in Canada: an emerging public health issue. In *CPHA Health Dig.* XXIV:10

90. Ladouceur R, Boisvert JM, Pepin M, Loranger M, Sylvain C. 1994. Social costs of pathological gambling. *J. Gambl. Stud.* 10:399–409

91. Ladouceur R, Bouchard C, Rheaume N, Jacques C, Ferland F, et al. 2000. Is the SOGS an accurate measure of pathological gambling among children, adolescents and adults? *J. Gambl. Stud.* 16:1–24

92. Ladouceur R, Walker M. 1998. The cognitive approach to understanding and treating pathological gambling. In *Comprehensive Clinical Psychology*, ed. M Hersen, pp. 588–601. New York: Pergamon

93. Lakshmanan IAR. 1996. A woman's life lost to gambling: suicide highlights betting's dark side. In *The Boston Globe*, March 9, pp. 13, 20

94. Langenbucher J, Bavly L, Labouvie E, Sanjuan PM, Martin CS. 2001. Clinical features of pathological gambling in an addictions treatment cohort. *Psychol. Addict. Behav.* 15:77–79

95. Lapage C, Ladouceur R, Jacques C. 2000. Prevalence of problem gambling among community service users. *Community Ment. Health J.* 36:597–601

96. Lejoyeux M, Ades J, Tassain V, Solomon J. 1996. Phenomenology and psychopathology of uncontrolled buying. *Am. J. Psychiatry* 153:1524–29

97. Lesieur HR. 1987. Gambling, pathological gambling and crime. In *The Handbook of Pathological Gambling*, ed. T Galski. Springfield IL: Charles C. Thomas

98. Lesieur HR. 1994. Epidemiological surveys of pathological gambling: critique and suggestions for modification. *J. Gambl. Stud.* 10:385–98

99. Lesieur HR. 1998. Costs and treatment of pathological gambling. *Ann. Am. Acad. Polit. Soc. Sci.* 556:153–71

100. Lesieur HR, Blume SB. 1990. Characteristics of pathological gamblers identified among patients on a psychiatric admissions service. *Hosp. Community Psychiatry* 41:1009–12

101. Lesieur HR, Blume SB. 1987. The South Oaks gambling screen (SOGS): A new instrument for the identification of pathological gamblers. *Am. J. Psychiatry* 144:1184–88

102. Lesieur HR, Blume SB, Zoppa RM. 1986. Alcoholism, drug abuse, and gambling. *Alcohol. Clin. Exp. Res.* 10:33–38

103. Lesieur HR, Cross J, Frank M, Welch M,

White CM, et al. 1991. Gambling and pathological gambling among university students. *Addict. Behav.* 16:517–27

104. Lesieur HR, Heineman M. 1988. Pathological gambling among multiple substance abusers in a therapeutic community. *Br. J. Addict.* 83:765–71

105. Lesieur HR, Rosenthal RJ. 1991. Pathological gambling: a review of the literature (prepared for the American Psychiatric Association Task Force on DSM-IV Committee on Disorders of Impulse Control not elsewhere classified). *J. Gambl. Stud.* 7:5–39

106. Lesieur HR, Rothschild J. 1989. Children of Gamblers Anonymous members. *J. Gambl. Behav.* 5:269–81

107. Lillenfield DE. 2000. John Snow: the first hired gun? *Am. J. Epidemiol.* 152:4–12

108. Lopes LL. 1987. Between hope and fear: the psychology of risk. In *Advances in Experimental Social Psychology*, ed. L Berkowitz, vol. 20, pp. 255–95. San Diego: Academic

109. Lorenz VC, Yaffee R. 1988. Pathological gambling: psychosomatic, emotional and marital difficulties as reported by the spouse. *J. Gambl. Behav.* 4:13–26

110. Marlatt GA, ed. 1998. *Harm Reduction: Pragmatic Strategies for Managing High-Risk Behaviors.* New York: Guilford. 390 pp.

111. Marshall K. 1998. The gambling industry: raising the stakes. *Perspect. Labour Income* 10:7–11

112. Martinsen EW. 1990. Benefits of exercise for the treatment of depression. *Sports Med.* 9:380–89

113. McCleary R, Chew K, Feng W, Merrill V, Napolitano C, et al. 1998. *Suicide and Gambling: An Analysis of Suicide Rates in U.S. Counties and Metropolitan Areas.* Irvine, CA: Univ. Calif. Irvine, Sch. Soc. Ecol.

114. McCormick RA, Russo AM, Ramirez LF, Taber JI. 1984. Affective disorders among pathological gamblers seeking treatment. *Am. J. Psychiatry* 141:215–18

115. McGuire WJ. 1964. Inducing resistance to persuasion. In *Advances in Experimental Social Psychology*, ed. L Berkowitz, vol. 1, pp. 191–229. New York: Academic

116. McNeilly DP, Burke WJ. 2000. Late life gambling: the attitudes and behaviors of older adults. *J. Gambl. Stud.* 16:393–415

117. Meehl PE. 1954. *Clinical Versus Statistical Prediction; A Theoretical Analysis and a Review of the Evidence.* Minneapolis: Univ. Minn. Press

118. Meehl PE. 1973. *Psychodiagnosis; Selected Papers.* New York: Norton

119. Moody G. 1989. Parents of young gamblers. *J. Gambl. Behav.* 5:313–20

120. Nadler LB. 1985. The epidemiology of pathological gambling: critique of existing research and alternative strategies. *J. Gambl. Behav.* 1:35–50

121. Natl. Assoc. Atty. Gen. 1996. Executive summary of Internet gambling report. In *NAAG Gaming Developments Bulletin.* Washington, DC: Natl. Assoc. Atty. Gen. 12 pp.

122. Natl. Gambl. Impact Study Comm. 1999. *National Gambling Impact Study Commission Report.* Washington, DC: Natl. Gambl. Impact Study Comm.

123. Natl. Res. Counc. 1999. *Pathological Gambling: A Critical Review.* Washington, DC: Natl. Acad. Press

124. Natl. Steer. Comm. 1999. *First Nations and Inuit Regional Health Survey.* St. Regis, Que.: First Nations Inuit Reg. Health Surv.

125. Off. Public Health. 1999. *Trends in Indian Health.* Rockville, MD: Indian Health Serv.

126. Pasternak AV, Fleming MF. 1999. Prevalence of gambling disorders in a primary care setting. *Arch. Fam. Med.* 8:515–20

127. Petry NM. 2000. Gambling problems in substance abusers are associated with increased sexual risk behaviors. *Addiction* 95:1089–100

128. Phillips DP, Welty WR, Smith MM. 1997. Elevated suicide levels associated

with legalized gambling. *Suicide Life-Threat. Behav.* 27:373–78

129. Politzer RM, Yesalis CE, Hudak CJ. 1992. The epidemiologic model and the risk of legalized gambling: Where are we headed? *Health Values* 16:20–27

130. Poulin C. 2000. Problem gambling among adolescent students in the Atlantic provinces of Canada. *J. Gambl. Stud.* 16:53–78

131. Productivity Commission. 1999. *Australia's Gambling Industries: Final Report. Rep. 10.* Canberra: AusInfo

132. Quinn JP. 1891. *Fools of Fortune.* Chicago: Anti-Gambl. Assoc. 640 pp.

133. Rado S. 1933. The psychoanalysis of pharmacothymia (drug addiction). *Psychoanal. Q.* 2:1–23

134. Raglin JS. 1997. Anxiolytic effects of physical activity. In *Physical Activity and Mental Health*, ed. WP Morgan, pp. 107–26. Washington, DC: Taylor & Francis

135. Regier DA, Farmer ME, Rae DS, Locke BZ, Keith SJ, et al. 1990. Comorbidity of mental disorders with alcohol and other drug abuse. Results from the Epidemiologic Catchment Area (ECA) Study [see comments]. *JAMA* 264:2511–18

136. Regier DA, Robins LN. 1991. *Psychiatric Disorders in America: The Epidemiologic Catchment Area Study*, pp. 1–10. New York: Free Press

137. Rose IN. 1986. *Gambling and the Law.* Hollywood, CA: Gambl. Times

138. Rosecrance J. 1985. Compulsive gambling and the medicalization of deviance. *Soc. Probl.* 32:275–84

139. Rosecrance J. 1988. *Gambling Without Guilt: The Legitimation of an American Pastime.* Pacific Grove: Books/Cole. 174 pp.

140. Rosenhan DL. 1973. On being sane in insane places. *Science* 179:250–58

141. Rugle L, Melamed L. 1993. Neuropsychological assessment of attention problems in pathological gamblers. *J. Nerv. Ment. Disord.* 18:107–12

142. Sebastian JG. 1985. Homelessness: a state

of vulnerability. *Fam. Community Health* 8:11–24

143. Shaffer HJ. 1986. Assessment of addictive disorders: the use of clinical reflection and hypotheses testing. *Psychiatr. Clin. North Am.* 9:385–98

144. Shaffer HJ. 1996. Understanding the means and objects of addiction: technology, the Internet, and gambling. *J. Gambl. Stud.* 12:461–69

145. Shaffer HJ. 1997. The most important unresolved issue in the addictions: conceptual chaos. *Subst. Use Misuse* 32:1573–80

146. Shaffer HJ. 1999. On the nature and meaning of addiction. *Natl. Forum* 79:10–14

147. Shaffer HJ, Freed CR, Healea D. Gambling disorders among a cohort of homeless substance abusing treatment seekers. *Psych. Serv.* In press

148. Shaffer HJ, Hall MN. 1996. Estimating the prevalence of adolescent gambling disorders: a quantitative synthesis and guide toward standard gambling nomenclature. *J. Gambl. Stud.* 12:193–214

149. Shaffer HJ, Hall MN. 2001. Updating and refining meta-analytic prevalence estimates of disordered gambling behavior in the United States and Canada. *Can. J. Public Health* 92:168–72

150. Shaffer HJ, Hall MN. 2002. Longitudinal patterns of gambling and drinking problems among casino employees. *J. Soc. Psychol.* In press

151. Shaffer HJ, Hall MN, Vander Bilt J. 1997. *Estimating the Prevalence of Disordered Gambling Behavior in the United States and Canada: A Meta-analysis.* Boston: Presidents and Fellows of Harvard College

152. Shaffer HJ, Hall MN, Vander Bilt J. 1999. Estimating the prevalence of disordered gambling behavior in the United States and Canada: a research synthesis. *Am. J. Public Health* 89:1369–76

153. Shaffer HJ, Hall MN, Walsh JS, Vander Bilt J. 1995. The psychosocial consequences of gambling. In *Casino Development: How Would Casinos Affect New*

England's Economy? ed. R Tannenwald, pp. 130–41. Boston: Fed. Reserve Bank Boston

154. Shaffer HJ, Jones SB. 1989. *Quitting Cocaine: The Struggle Against Impulse.* Lexington, MA: Lexington. 198 pp.

155. Shaffer HJ, LaBrie R, Scanlan KM, Cummings TN. 1994. Pathological gambling among adolescents: Massachusetts gambling screen (MAGS). *J. Gambl. Stud.* 10:339–62

156. Shaffer HJ, Stein S, Gambino B, Cummings TN, eds. 1989. *Compulsive Gambling: Theory, Research & Practice.* Lexington, MA: Lexington

157. Shaffer HJ, Vander Bilt J, Hall MN. 1999. Gambling, drinking, smoking and other health risk activities among casino employees. *Am. J. Ind. Med.* 36:365–78

158. Single E. 1995. Defining harm reduction. *Drug Alcohol Rev.* 14:287–90

159. Skinner BF. 1969. *Contingencies of Reinforcement: A Theoretical Analysis.* Englewood Cliffs, NJ: Prentice-Hall

160. Skinner HA. 1999. Gambling: achieving the right balance. *J. Gambl. Stud.* 15:285–87

161. Slutske WS, Eisen S, True WR, Lyons MJ, Goldberg J, Tsuang M. 2000. Common genetic vulnerability for pathological gambling and alcohol dependence in men. *Arch. Gen. Psychiatry* 57:666–73

162. Smart RG, Ferris J. 1996. Alcohol, drugs and gambling in the Ontario adult population, 1994. *Can. J. Psychiatry* 41:36–45

163. Smith G, Abt V. 1984. Gambling as play. *Ann. Am. Acad. Polit. Soc. Sci.* 474:122–32

164. Smith GJ, Wynne HJ. 1999. *Gambling and Crime in Western Canada: Exploring Myth and Reality.* Calgary: Canada West Found.

165. Sobell LC, Cunningham JA, Sobell MB. 1996. Recovery from alcohol problems with and without treatment: prevalence in two population surveys. *Am. J. Public Health* 86:966–72

166. Sobell MB, Sobell LC. 1993. Treatment for problem drinkers: a public health priority. In *Addictive Behaviors Across the Life Span: Prevention, Treatment, and Policy Issues,* ed. JS Baer, GA Marlatt, RJ McMahon, pp. 138–57. Newbury Park: Sage

167. Specker SM, Carlson GA, Christenson GA, Marcotte M. 1995. Impulse control disorders and attention deficit disorder in pathological gamblers. *Ann. Clin. Psychiatry* 7:175–79

168. Spunt B, Lesieur H, Hunt D, Cahill L. 1995. Gambling among methadone patients. *Int. J. Addict.* 30:929–62

169. Steinberg M, Kosten T, Rounsaville B. 1992. Cocaine abuse and pathological gambling. *Am. J. Addict.* 1:121–32

170. Stinchfield R, Nadav C, Winter K, Latimer W. 1997. Prevalence of gambling among Minnesota public school students in 1992 and 1995. *J. Gambl. Stud.* 13:25–48

171. Taber JI. 1987. Compulsive gambling: an examination of relevant models. *J. Gambl. Behav.* 3:219–23

172. Taber JI, McCormick RA, Russo AM, Adkins BJ, Ramirez IF. 1987. Follow-up of pathological gamblers after treatment. *Am. J. Psychiatry* 144:757–61

173. Teck-Hong O. 1992. The behavioral characteristics and health conditions of drug abusers: some implications for workers in drug addiction. *Int. Soc. Work* 35:7–17

174. Tucker JA, Donovan DM, Marlatt GA, eds. 1999. *Changing Addictive Behavior.* New York: Guilford. 387 pp.

175. Vaillancourt F, Roy A. 2000. *Gambling and Governments in Canada, 1969–1998: How Much? Who Plays? What Payoff?* Toronto: Can. Tax Found.

176. Vaillant GE. 1983. *The Natural History of Alcoholism: Causes, Patterns, and Paths to Recovery.* Cambridge: Harvard Univ. Press

177. Volberg RA. 1996. *Gambling and Problem Gambling in New York: A 10-Year*

Replication Study, 1986 to 1996. New York: NY Counc. Probl. Gambl.

178. Volberg RA. 1996. Prevalence studies of problem gambling in the United States. *J. Gambl. Stud.* 12:111–28

179. Volberg RA. 1997. *Gambling and Problem Gambling in Colorado: Report to the Colorado Department of Revenue*. Roaring Spring, PA: Gemini Res.

180. Volberg RA. 1997. *Gambling and Problem Gambling in Oregon*. Northampton, MA: Gemini Res.

181. Volberg RA, Abbott MW. 1997. Gambling and problem gambling among indigenous peoples. *Subst. Use Misuse* 32:1525–38

182. Volberg RA, Moore WL. 1999. *Gambling and Problem Gambling in Washington State: A Replication Study, 1992 to 1998*. Northampton, MA: Gemini Res.

183. Waldorf D. 1983. Natural recovery from opiate addiction: some social-psychological processes of untreated recovery. *J. Drug Issues* 13:237–80

184. Walker MB, Dickerson MG. 1996. The prevalence of problem and pathological gambling: a critical analysis. *J. Gambl. Stud.* 12:233–49

185. Wallisch LS. 1993. *Gambling in Texas: 1992 Texas Survey of Adolescent Gambling Behavior*. Austin: TX Comm. Alcohol Drug Abuse

186. Wallisch LS. 1996. *Gambling in Texas: 1992 Texas Survey of Adult and Adolescent Gambling Behavior*. Austin: TX Comm. Alcohol Drug Abuse

187. Wardman D, el-Guebaly N, Hodgins D. 2001. Problem and pathological gambling in North American Aboriginal populations: a review of the empirical literature. *J. Gambl. Stud.* 17:81–100

188. WEFA Group, ICR Surv. Res. Group, Lesieur H, Thompson W. 1997. *A Study Concerning the Effects of Legalized Gambling on the Citizens of the State of Connecticut*. State of Conn. Dep. Revenue Serv., Div. Spec. Revenue

189. Weiss MR. 1995. Children in sport: an educational model. In *Sport Psychology Interventions*, ed. SM Murphy, pp. 39–70. Champaign, IL: Hum. Kinet.

190. Widiger TA, Clark LA. 2000. Toward *DSM-V* and the classification of psychopathology. *Psychol. Bull.* 126:946–63

191. Wildman RW. 1989. Pathological gambling: Marital-familial factors, implications, and treatments. *J. Gambl. Behav.* 5:293–301

192. Wilkinson R, Marmot M, eds. 1998. *Social Determinants of Health: The Solid Facts*. Copenhagen: WHO Reg. Off. Eur.

193. Winick C. 1962. Maturing out of narcotic addiction. *United Nations Bull. Narcotics* 14:1–7

194. Winters KC, Stinchfield RD, Kim LG. 1995. Monitoring adolescent gambling in Minnesota. *J. Gambl. Stud.* 11:165–83

195. Wise RA. 1995. Addictive drugs and brain stimulation reward. *Annu. Rev. Neurosci.* 18:319–40

196. Zane NWS, Huh-Kim J. 1998. Addictive behaviors. In *Handbook of Asian American Psychology*, ed. LC Lee, NWS Zane, pp. 527–54. South Oaks, CA: Sage

197. Zinberg NE. 1974. High states: a beginning study. In *Drug Abuse Counc. Publ. No. SS-3*. Washington, DC: Drug Abuse Counc.

198. Zinberg NE. 1975. Addiction and ego function. *Psychoanal. Stud. Child* 30:567–88

199. Zinberg NE. 1984. *Drug, Set, and Setting: The Basis for Controlled Intoxicant Use*. New Haven: Yale Univ. Press

200. Ziskin J. 1970. *Coping with Psychiatric and Psychological Testimony*. Beverly Hills: Law Psychol. Press. 385 pp.

Annu. Rev. Public Health 2002. 23:213–31

THE PUBLIC HEALTH IMPACT OF ALZHEIMER'S DISEASE, 2000–2050: Potential Implication of Treatment Advances

Philip D. Sloane[1,2], Sheryl Zimmerman[1,3], Chirayath Suchindran[4], Peter Reed[1], Lily Wang[4], Malaz Boustani[5], and S. Sudha[6]

[1]Cecil G. Sheps Center for Health Services Research, [2]Department of Family Medicine, [3]School of Social Work, [4]Department of Biostatistics, [5]Program on Aging, University of North Carolina at Chapel Hill, Chapel Hill, North Carolina 27599; [6]University of North Carolina at Greensboro, PO Box 26170, Greensboro, North Carolina 27402-6170; e-mails:psloane@med.unc.edu, Sheryl_Zimmerman@unc.edu, suchindran@unc.edu, preed@email.unc.edu, liwang@bios.unc.edu, malaz_boustani@med.unc.edu, sudha@email.unc.edu

Key Words public health impact, Alzheimer's disease, Alzheimer's care

■ **Abstract**   Recent developments in basic research suggest that therapeutic breakthroughs may occur in Alzheimer's disease treatment over the coming decades. To model the potential magnitude and nature of the effect of these advances, historical data from congestive heart failure and Parkinson's disease were used. Projections indicate that therapies which delay disease onset will markedly reduce overall disease prevalence, whereas therapies to treat existing disease will alter the proportion of cases that are mild as opposed to moderate/severe. The public health impact of such changes would likely involve both the amount and type of health services needed. Particularly likely to arise are new forms of outpatient services, such as disease-specific clinics and centers. None of our models predicts less than a threefold rise in the total number of persons with Alzheimer's disease between 2000 and 2050. Therefore, Alzheimer's care is likely to remain a major public health problem during the coming decades.

INTRODUCTION

Alzheimer's disease (AD) is a chronic neurodegenerative disease characterized by progressive deterioration of cognitive function. It begins insidiously, with early signs including patchy memory loss and subtle behavioral changes. The illness gradually progresses until, often after a decade or more, the individual is unable to speak or comprehend language, no longer controls his or her bowels, and requires assistance with all aspects of personal care. Persons in the later stages of the illness are often placed in nursing homes, which have become increasingly populated by

0163-7525/02/0510-0213$14.00

older persons with cognitive impairment. Since AD predominantly affects older persons, one outcome of the graying of America during the coming decades is likely to be a tidal wave of persons with AD.

What will be the effect on public health of AD during the coming decades? How many people will have the disease in the future, and what will be their service needs? This paper addresses these questions empirically by presenting and discussing several future scenarios of AD prevalence in the United States between 2000 and 2050. Two of these scenarios have already been published—resulting in high (12) and low (46) estimates of prevalence derived by applying current disease patterns to future population projections. Such projections are likely to be inaccurate, however, because recent developments in AD research suggest that one or more therapeutic breakthroughs is likely in the coming decades (26, 32, 38). Therefore, to project the impact of potential advances in therapy, this paper applies estimates based on historical data from two chronic diseases for which management has changed markedly during the past five decades: congestive heart failure and Parkinson's disease. In this manner, we discuss a fuller range of possibilities facing the public health system, toward the goal of better informing public debate on the needs and priorities of health care for the elderly over the coming decades.

ALZHEIMER'S DISEASE TODAY

Etiology and Clinical Course

The specific cause of AD is unknown, and it may well be a multifactorial syndrome rather than a single disease (41). Age and family history of the disease in a first-degree relative are the strongest epidemiological risk factors for AD. Persons age 85 and older have 14 times the incidence of AD compared with persons age 65 to 69 (16a), and the relative risk of AD for those with at least one first-degree relative with dementia is 3.5 (95% CI 2.6 to 4.6) (46a). Other putative risk factors include head trauma, education level, number of siblings, non-suburban residence, maternal age at birth, hypothyroidism, and apolipoprotein E4 genotype (27a, 46a). In addition, between one and two percent of cases demonstrate an autosomal dominant genetic pattern with nearly complete penetrance (7). During the past decade a number of advances have been made in understanding the biochemical nature of the disease. Current thinking is that several biochemical mechanisms may contribute to neuronal degeneration, with final pathways involving both the cleavage of β amyloid precurser protein to form β amyloid (a major component of senile plaques), and abnormal processing and accumulation of tau protein (a major component of neurofibrillary tangles) (38, 41). In addition, small and large vessel cerebrovascular disease can cause dementia syndromes that often are difficult to distinguish from, and can occur concurrently with, AD (7).

The disease can be characterized by three phases: a prolonged preclinical phase, in which subtle signs are detectable but the diagnosis cannot be established; a mild symptomatic period, where patients suffer memory loss, impaired judgment, and preclinical -[a]-> mild disease -[b]-> advanced disease -[c]-> death

[a]Incidence rate, [b]rate of progression from early disease to advanced disease, [c]mortality rate

Figure 1   General model of the course of Alzheimer's disease and other chronic diseases.

decreasing ability to carry out everyday activities such as shopping, cooking, and grooming [stage 1 on the Clinical Dementia Rating Scale (CDR) (22)]; and a moderate/severe period, in which patients require 24-hour supervision and are increasingly impaired in basic functional areas such as locomotion, speech, ability to maintain continence, feeding, and hydration (23, 33). Figure 1 provides a schematic overview of the course of AD; this schema can be applied to most chronic diseases. The rate of progression of untreated cases of AD varies among individuals. On average, about one quarter of people progress each year from mild (CDR stage 1) to moderate disease (CDR stage 2) (9, 25). In addition, multiple longitudinal studies have identified an average annual decline of 3.5 points on Mini-Mental State Examination (a 30-point scale) and 7–9 points on the Alzheimer's Disease Assessment Scale (a 70-point scale) (43).

Current and Projected Prevalence

Obtaining accurate assessment of the current and projected prevalence of AD is a challenge because there is no definitive diagnostic test and because many of its signs and symptoms are shared by several other forms of cognitive decline and dementia. Other factors that contribute to the difficulty of determining the prevalence of AD include the absence of a formal reporting system for diagnosed cases and misrepresentation of disease prevalence due to unrecognized cases. Therefore, existing prevalence rates vary widely.

A conservative (low) estimate for the current and future prevalence of AD was provided by the U.S. General Accounting Office (GAO) (46). Based on a meta-analysis integrating estimates from 18 studies of Alzheimer's disease prevalence, the GAO published age-specific, five-year prevalence rates for all cases and moderate/severe AD. A more liberal (high) estimate of the current and future prevalence of AD was provided by Evans et al. (12). They estimated prevalence by age, in ten-year intervals, based on a community study of 3623 adults over age 65 in East Boston, MA. While the study provided age-specific rates for Alzheimer's disease, stage-specific rates were provided only for cognitive impairment. Therefore, we estimated stage-specific rates by applying the cognitive impairment staging ratios to the number of estimated cases of AD. This calculation was based on an assumption that, although there are more cases of cognitive impairment than AD, the relative proportions of cases at various disease stages would be equivalent.

These methods estimated that there were between 2.17 and 4.78 million cases of AD in the United States in 2000, of which between 44 (12) and 57 (46) percent had moderate or severe disease. To calculate the possible range of the total number of AD cases over the next 50 years, assuming no significant change in disease epidemiology, we applied both the liberal and conservative rates to the middle series Census estimates for age-specific populations (45). Table 1 displays these projections. They indicate that, if no scientific advances alter the incidence and progression of AD, between 7.98 and 12.95 million people in the United States will be suffering from the illness by the year 2050, a fourfold increase from the current prevalence.

Current Public Health Impact

The clinical symptoms of AD are not limited to memory loss and other cognitive deficits but extend to a wide spectrum of noncognitive secondary features, such as impaired activities of daily living, depression, and challenging behavioral disturbances. Assessment of overall disease impact on quality of life is challenging, but over the last few years several self-report, proxy-report and observational tools have been developed and linked to health outcomes. For example, one proxy-based rating system that assesses behavioral engagement (participation in activities) and subjective states (affective expression) shows increasing decline with dementia severity (1). Another instrument, which evaluates physical condition, mood, interpersonal relationships, ability to participate in meaningful activities, and financial situation, has been associated with depressive symptoms and functional dependence (24a). Given the impact of the disease on function and quality of life, it is not surprising that persons with AD utilize health services at higher rates and experience more accidents and falls than age-matched controls. As their independence continues to decrease, persons with the disease place an increasing physical,

TABLE 1   Three estimates of the prevalence of Alzheimer's disease, by stage, United States, 2000–2050*

	Stage	2000	2005	2010	2015	2020	2025	2030	2035	2040	2045	2050
GAO[a]	Mild	0.93	1.03	1.13	1.26	1.41	1.63	1.93	2.28	2.66	2.99	3.26
	Moderate/severe	1.24	1.38	1.53	1.71	1.94	2.23	2.63	3.13	3.69	4.25	4.72
	All	2.17	2.41	2.67	2.97	3.35	3.86	4.55	5.41	6.35	7.24	7.98
UNC[b]	Mild	0.93	1.21	1.14	1.53	1.55	1.87	2.10	2.56	3.00	3.45	3.75
	Moderate/severe	1.24	1.49	2.00	2.05	2.54	2.83	3.44	4.07	4.88	5.68	6.46
	All	2.17	2.70	3.14	3.58	4.09	4.70	5.54	6.63	7.88	9.12	10.21
Evans[c]	Mild	2.69	2.83	3.10	3.58	4.16	4.83	5.44	5.85	6.13	6.37	6.65
	Moderate/severe	2.08	2.25	2.51	2.86	3.23	3.70	4.24	4.81	5.33	5.85	6.29
	All	4.78	5.07	5.61	6.43	7.39	8.53	9.68	10.66	11.46	12.22	12.95

*Millions of cases.

[a]Source: Reference (46).

[b]Based on applying estimated rates of transition across stages of the disease to U.S. Census projections. See text for details.

[c]Source: Reference (12, pp. 283–399).

psychological, and financial burden on family caregivers. As a result, they are frequently placed in residential care/assisted living facilities, nursing homes, and geropsychiatric hospitals.

There are as many different estimates of the total cost of AD care as there are estimates of disease prevalence. One mid-range estimate, excluding costs of morbidity, premature death, and lost employment income, is $38,000 per patient per year, amounting to $65 billion nationally (1995 dollars), although estimates as much as 50 percent lower and 50 percent higher have been proposed (11). Over time, these costs will increase proportionate to the increase in the total size of the AD population and the proportionate distribution of mild and moderate/severe cases.

Regardless of disease severity, most of the burden of caring for individuals with AD is shouldered by informal caregivers, with unpaid caregiver time constituting one half to two thirds of the total cost of care (11). The average family caregiver spends 16.1 hours per week providing care, with increasing burden as the disease progresses. Thus, the average time spent providing care is 5.9 hours per week for individuals with no impairments in activities in daily living and rises to as much as 35.2 hours per week for those with severe limitations (28).

The largest increase in the cost of care occurs when individuals are institutionalized (11, 17). Nursing home placement is a notable milestone in the progression of AD because it proxies for severe disability and imposes a huge financial burden on our health system. In 1994, the cost to Medicaid of nursing home care for persons with AD is estimated to have exceeded $8 billion. Largely due to the costs of care in nursing homes and other residential long-term care settings, the total cost of caring for persons with severe AD is 2.25 times higher than for patients with mild or moderate disease (21).

Effectiveness of Current Treatment

Until recently, treatment of AD has been entirely supportive. Management has consisted of provision of a safe, "prosthetic" environment, education and support of family caregivers, assistance with daily activities and personal care, and management of behavioral problems using nonpharmacological strategies and psychoactive drugs. Although these treatment strategies remain the mainstay of AD management today (1a), drugs are increasingly being used not just for problem behaviors but also to retard the disease progression. Current pharmacological treatment involves one of four strategies:

- enhancing levels of the brain transmitter acetylcholine by administering cholinesterase inhibitors,
- reducing inflammatory responses that accompany brain injury through the use of nonsteroidal agents such as aspirin or ibuprofen,
- enhancing putative protective factors through strategies such as vitamin E supplementation, and
- treating concomitant cardiovascular risk factors, especially hypertension.

Recent pharmacological advances have been largely limited to the development of cholinesterase inhibitors. Four drugs of this type having been approved by the U.S. Food and Drug Administration during the past decade: tacrine, donepezil, rivastigmine, and galantamine. Numerous randomized clinical trials with thousands of patients have demonstrated small to moderate effects of these agents on cognitive, global, and physical functioning among patients who respond favorably and do not have intolerable side effects (2–4, 35, 37, 44, 47). As many as two thirds of patients fail to respond, however (26). Furthermore, it is unclear whether cholinesterase inhibitors exert only temporary effects on the course of AD, causing patients to improve at best to levels observed six to nine months earlier, or slow long-range progression as well (24).

Other agents for which randomized controlled trials have indicated a possible effect on the course of AD include gingko biloba (31) and vitamin E (38). In addition, the treatment of hypertension has been demonstrated to reduce the incidence of dementia in placebo-controlled trials (13). Although this finding may be largely due to an effect on vascular dementia, AD and vascular dementia coexist often enough to lead to significant treatment interaction effects.

In summary, the current treatment options for AD offer modest but significant benefits for those who already suffer from the disease. Use of cholinesterase inhibitors and vitamin E, treatment of hypertension, and possibly the use of nonsteroidal antiinflammatory agents and gingko biloba may have a stabilizing effect on cognitive and global function of patients with mild to moderate disease and may delay their transition from the community to an institutional setting. Unfortunately, effects are modest, and therefore the public health impact of these treatment advances has been minimal. Recent breakthroughs in basic research suggest, however, that new medications may be introduced during the coming decades that will have an extensive effect on the prevalence and course of AD, which will then result in significant changes in the public health needs of this patient population.

THE LIKELIHOOD OF THERAPEUTIC ADVANCES

The past decade has seen impressive advances in basic research on the etiology of AD, and these advances are likely to lead to more effective treatments in the future. Perhaps the most promising breakthrough has been the elucidation of the biochemical pathways that lead to β-amyloid deposition. Increasingly, amyloid appears to be a central factor in the events leading to neuronal damage in AD. Four autosomal dominant forms of early-onset AD disease have been characterized, each of which involves a defect in some aspect of amyloid metabolism. One is on chromosome 21, where the locus for β-amyloid precurser protein (APP) is located (42). Two are on chromosomes 14 and 1; they involve mutations of presenilin 1 and 2—genes that appear to normally inhibit amyloid formation. The other is on chromosome 12 and involves a mutation on the gene for an α2-macroglobulin that mediates clearance and degradation of β-amyloid (5). Furthermore, the only genetic locus universally accepted to be an important risk factor for late-onset AD, apolipoprotein E on chromosome 19, also appears to be involved in the amyloid pathway, although the mechanism is not yet clear (38). In the late 1990s, two research teams began to zero in on the structure of β-secretase, the enzyme that controls the final step in amyloid production (cleavage of APP to form β-amyloid), and drug companies are already developing compounds that block its activity (32). Similar, less well-developed lines of research involve the tau protein, the key component of neurofibrillary tangles; the tau protein has recently been linked to multiple loci on chromosome 17 that are associated with hereditary frontotemporal dementias (14, 16, 20).

A final area of recent progress is in the development of vaccines. Using a transgenetic mouse model that overexpresses mutant human APP, investigators have demonstrated that immunization with a peptide found in amyloid plaques leads to an effective antibody response. In young mice, immunization prevented the development of β-amyloid formation; in older animals, treatment markedly reduced the progression of neuropathology (29, 40). Another promising line of research involves the use of oral vaccines to generate autoantibodies against the N-methyl-D-aspartate receptor, thereby blocking a key pathway leading to neuronal injury in neurodegenerative diseases (10).

These and other recent discoveries make it increasingly likely that useful treatments will be generated in the years to come (38). In the subsequent sections we provide projections, based on historical data from other treatments for chronic diseases, of the effect that drug development may have on the prevalence and public health needs of persons with AD over the next half-century.

HOW THERAPEUTIC ADVANCES MAY ALTER DISEASE PREVALENCE THROUGH 2050

To model the potential impact of therapeutic advances on the demography of AD during the next 50 years, we applied data based on the observed results of new, effective treatments on the natural history of congestive heart failure (CHF) and Parkinson's disease (PD) over the past half-century. These diseases were chosen as models because they are chronic diseases that commonly affect older persons and lead to gradual, progressive functional decline, and they have both seen significant advances in treatment during the past decades.

Congestive heart failure provides a model of effective delay in the onset of disease. In the 1950s, the mean age of disease onset was 57.3 years; by the 1980s, it was 76.4 years (19). Preventive strategies that have contributed to this change include treatment of hypertension, lower dietary fat intake, and prevention of rheumatic fever. In addition, medications have been developed that slowed the progression of CHF in randomized trials; however, because these new therapies have been associated with adverse effects, comorbid conditions, poor diffusion into common medical practice, noncompliance, and high costs, the prognosis of CHF in the general population has not been altered by these new therapies (8).

Parkinson's disease provides a model of new therapies that slow disease progression. The disease is described in five stages, which had a mean duration ranging from 2 to 5 years in 1949–1954 (18). Subsequently, the introduction of levodopa and other agents, such as selegiline and bromocriptine, has doubled the length of time that patients spend in each stage (34).

Methods

DEVELOPMENT OF UNC ESTIMATES OF DISEASE PREVALENCE, 2000–2050   We estimated the number of individuals in the United States with mild or moderate/severe AD over the next 50 years by using a multistage projection model (30). This method requires the knowledge of a base year population in various stages of AD and age-specific rates of (*a*) disease incidence, (*b*) transition from mild to moderate/severe disease, (*c*) mortality rates for the general population, and (*d*) stage-specific mortality rates for persons with the disease. Our projections considered the U. S. Bureau of Census's middle series estimate of the 2000 U.S. population as the baseline population. We used the prevalence rates of the disease estimated by the GAO (46) to allocate the year 2000 population into various stages of the disease (none, mild, or moderate/severe). Staging by the GAO, and therefore in these analyses as well, was based on the CDR scale, with mild dementia corresponding to CDR stage 1 and moderate/severe dementia corresponding to CDR stages 2 and 3 (22).

Following Brookmeyer et al. (6), we assumed that the age-specific rate of onset of AD increases exponentially with age. Our analyses further assumed that the number of people under age 60 with the disease was negligible, and therefore we modeled disease incidence starting at that age. Specifically, the incidence rate at age greater than 60 is

$$\text{onset incidence rate} = 0.001278 e^{.142(age-60)}. \qquad 1.$$

We assumed the incidence rate at age 60 is 0.001278, which is slightly higher than that of Brookmeyer et al. (6); this change was made so that our number of new cases would be more consistent with the GAO estimates. The age-specific incidence rate of onset was set as constant after age 95, and the incidence rate for transition from mild to moderate/severe was set at a constant of 0.28 for all ages; this value is reasonable under the expectation that on average a person will remain in a mild state for four years (9, 25). The age-specific mortality rates from a disease-free stage were assumed to be the same as for the middle series population projection by the Bureau of Census. Finally, mortality rates were considered to be 10 and 20 percent higher than that of a disease-free state for those who have mild or moderate/severe disease, respectively.

To make the task of projection simple the baseline population was grouped into five-year age groups, with the highest age at 110. These age groupings permitted projections in steps of five years (i.e., 2005, 2010, 2015, . . . 2050). The age-specific incidence rates and mortality rates were assumed to be constant within a five-year age group. The first step in the projection was to convert the single-year incidence rates into a five-year transition matrix. The elements of the five-year transition matrix provided the probability that an individual in a specified state (e.g., normal) at the beginning of the period would be in a specified state (normal, mild, moderate/severe, or dead) at the end of five years. A simple matrix conversion formula was used to convert the incidence matrix into a five-year transition matrix (30). These transition matrices were applied to the population in various stages of the disease at the beginning of a year to obtain the population in the next five-year age class five years later. Repeated applications of the age specific transition rates were used to carry the projection further into the future.

Baseline projections provided estimates of the prevalence of disease, in five-year intervals, by stage and overall. These estimates are provided in Table 1 and displayed graphically in Figure 2 (as the UNC projections); the table compares these results with the GAO report and with the projections of Evans et al. (12). In this baseline projection, the age-specific incidence rates of onset based on the modified Brookmeyer formula remained the same for the years 2000 to 2050. The transition rate from mild to moderate/severe was set at 0.28 for all ages throughout

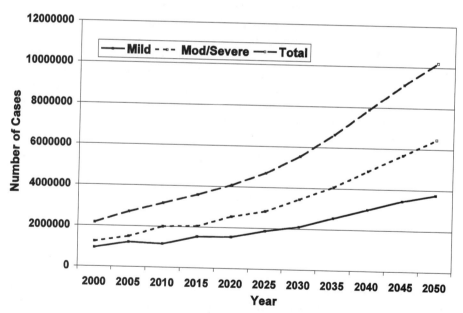

Figure 2   UNC projections of the prevalence of mild, moderate/severe, and total cases of Alzheimer's disease, United States, 2005–2050, assuming no significant change in treatment effectiveness over the next 50 years. Note that the projected total number of cases is projected to more than quadruple between 2000 and 2050, and that the majority of cases will be in the moderate or severe stages throughout that period.

the projection. The age-specific mortality rates were also assumed to be the same as described above.

PROJECTING THE IMPACT OF DRUG DEVELOPMENT ON DISEASE PREVALENCE AND STAGING   We developed modified projections based on three scenarios: delayed disease onset (CHF model), reduced rate of progression (PD model), and combined delayed onset/reduced progression (CHF/PD). Each represented projections based on one or more breakthroughs in therapy being introduced into the general population in 2010.

- The delayed disease onset model projects the impact of effective preventive strategies to delay the age of onset of Alzheimer's disease. Data from the Framingham study indicated that the age of onset of CHF was delayed by 19 years between the 1950s and the 1980s; some of this delay represents aging of the population and some represents true treatment effects (19). Because of the older average age of onset of AD and the incorporation of population aging into our initial projections (Table 1), we assumed that a corresponding breakthrough would be one that increased the median age at disease onset by 6.7 years. This assumption was implemented by altering the rate of increase in the incidence rates in Equation 1 from 0.142 to 0.109, beginning in 2010. All other incidence rates remained the same as in the baseline projections.

- The delayed disease progression model projects the impact of effective treatment strategies that reduce the rate of disease progression. PD patients are severely disabled by stage 3 of the disease, which roughly corresponds in functional status to moderate/severe AD (18); the introduction of levadopa and other agents halved the rate of progression across each of the earlier stages (34). Correspondingly, we modeled a decrease in the rate of transition from mild to moderate/severe AD from 0.28 to 0.10. All other incidence rates remained the same as in the baseline projection.

- The combined model simultaneously applies both delayed onset and reduced progression.

For each model, estimates were generated by a five-year interval of the number of persons aged 65 and older in the U.S. population with mild and moderate/severe AD.

Results

Table 2 displays the projected prevalence of AD based on the three models of treatment advances introduced in 2010. Figures 3–6 provide graphic representation of these results.

Compared with the UNC baseline predictions (Figure 2), the delayed disease onset model projects 35.6 percent fewer cases of Alzheimer's disease by 2050. In this model, a reduction in disease incidence after 2010 leads to a temporary drop in new cases, but within less than two decades the total number of cases is again rising rapidly, owing largely to increases in the numbers of persons over

TABLE 2   Prevalence of Alzheimer's disease, 2005–2050: projections based on three models of the effects of significant treatment advances introduced in 2010

	Delayed disease onset model			Slowed disease progression model			Combined model		
	Number of cases (millions)			Number of cases (millions)			Number of cases (millions)		
Year	Total	Mild	Moderate/ severe	Total	Mild	Moderate/ severe	Total	Mild	Moderate/ severe
2005	2.70	1.21	1.49	2.70	1.21	1.49	2.70	1.21	1.49
2010	3.14	1.14	2.00	3.14	1.14	2.00	3.14	1.14	2.00
2015	2.76	0.56	2.20	3.59	2.05	1.54	2.76	1.26	1.49
2020	2.78	1.09	1.68	4.11	2.49	1.62	2.81	1.50	1.31
2025	3.11	0.96	2.15	4.75	2.89	1.86	3.13	1.78	1.35
2030	3.62	1.34	2.27	5.60	3.39	2.21	3.66	2.11	1.55
2035	4.29	1.44	2.85	6.70	4.04	2.66	4.33	2.49	1.84
2040	5.01	1.75	3.27	7.97	4.78	3.19	5.07	2.89	2.18
2045	5.71	1.91	3.79	9.23	5.49	3.74	5.77	3.27	2.51
2050	6.31	2.10	4.21	10.33	6.08	4.25	6.39	3.58	2.81

age 85. Of cases projected in this model to be present in 2050, the vast majority (66.7%) are in the moderate or late stages. These trends are graphically displayed in Figure 3.

In contrast, the slowed disease progression model projects a slight increase (1.2%) in the number of cases in 2050, when compared with our baseline predictions. This lack of effect on overall prevalence arises because medications that slow disease progression would not reduce disease incidence; instead, they would result in a higher proportion of patients (58.9%) having mild disease, where the mortality rate is lower. This is displayed graphically in Figure 4.

The combined model projects a similar reduction to the delayed onset model (37.4%), since a similar magnitude reduction in incidence rates has been projected. However, because disease progression is also slowed, mild cases predominate (56%). The projected number and distribution of cases in this model are graphically represented in Figure 5.

Figure 6 displays the baseline model and the three projections on a single scale, allowing for comparison of the projected total number of AD patients and the relative proportions of mild and moderate/severe cases across the four models.

IMPLICATIONS ON FUTURE HEALTH SERVICE NEEDS AND COSTS

The estimated number of persons in the U.S. who will have AD in 2050 varies widely. This paper developed estimates that are mid-range between the GAO report (46) and the projections of Evans et al. (12). Our model projects that, if no major

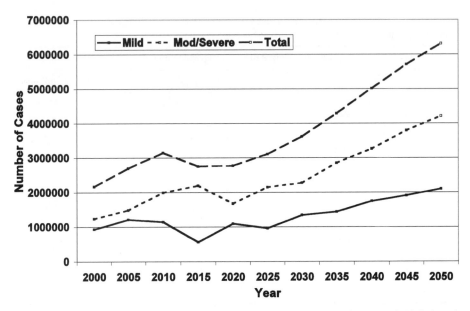

Figure 3 Projected prevalence of mild, moderate/severe, and total cases of Alzheimer's disease, United States, 2005–2050, assuming that a significant breakthrough is introduced into the general population in 2010 that delays disease onset by an average of 6.7 years. An example of such a breakthrough would be the introduction of a vaccine that reduces the rate of accumulation of amyloid in the brain. Note that the overall number of cases would be temporarily reduced but would begin rising by 2025 owing to increases in the elderly population, so that the projected number of cases in 2050 is approximately three times the current number. Also note that moderate/severe disease would constitute the majority of cases.

therapeutic advances occur, 10.2 million persons will have the disease in 2050, of which 3.8 million (37%) will have mild disease and 6.5 million (63%) will have moderate/severe disease. This is a projected increase of 8 million persons with AD over the next half-century, and it represents a more than fourfold increase in the burden of care. The public health impact of this increase would be immense, because of both the absolute increase in numbers and the fact that most cases would have moderate/severe disease and therefore be candidates for institutionalization. At present, the public sector finances only a small proportion of Alzheimer's care (12.5% for community care and 34% for institutional care); however, the roles and responsibilities of the public and private sectors would need to be reassessed in light of this explosive increase in the need for care (36).

It is unlikely, however, that no scientific advances will occur. Already, cholinesterase inhibitors can delay disease progression by six to nine months, and greater advances in treatment are highly probable. For this reason, we developed three alternative scenarios (Table 2 and Figures 3–6), in which we used historical data

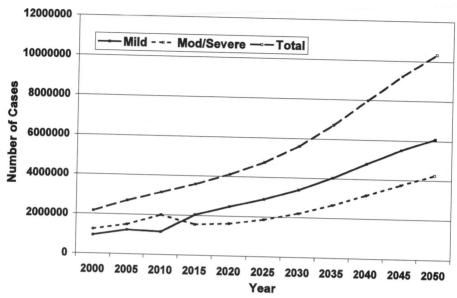

Figure 4 Projected prevalence of mild, moderate/severe, and total cases of Alzheimer's disease, United States, 2005–2050, assuming that a significant breakthrough in treatment is introduced into the general population in 2010 that reduces the rate of progression of mild (CDR 1) to moderate/severe (CDR 2 or 3) disease from 28% to 10% per year. An example of such a breakthrough would be introduction of one or more drugs that blocked the activity of the enzyme β-secretase, thereby reducing the rate of accumulation of amyloid in the brain. Note that such treatment would increase the proportion of mild cases and decrease the proportion of moderate/severe cases while not altering the overall number of cases of the disease.

from treatment for other chronic diseases to model the potential impact of treatment innovations over the next half-century.

If a successful method of delaying the onset of AD were introduced in 2010 (Figure 3), and if treatment compliance and effectiveness were similar to that witnessed for congestive heart failure, the overall projected number of people with AD will be reduced by 38 percent by 2050, becoming 6.31 million, of which 2.10 million (33%) will be mild and 4.21 million (67%) will have moderate/severe disease (Figure 6). The overall burden on the private and public health system would still increase threefold over current estimates; however, the reduction in numbers of persons with the disease would be significant. To put this in an economic perspective, using an estimated cost of $47,000/patient/year (1990 dollars), Brookmeyer et al. estimated that a mere six-month delay in disease onset would save nearly $18 billion annually after 50 years (6). Care systems would not be likely to change under this scenario, however, because the majority of care would remain directed at persons with moderate and advanced disease. Thus, the long-term care industry

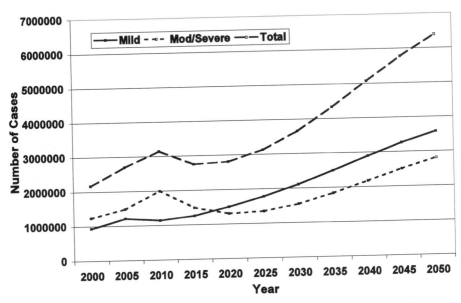

Figure 5 Projected prevalence of mild, moderate/severe, and total cases of Alzheimer's disease, 2005–2050, assuming that in 2010 significant breakthroughs are introduced to delay both disease onset and disease progression. Note that the total number of cases is reduced (as in Figure 2) and that mild cases begin to predominate (as in Figure 3). However, due to growth of the elderly population, the total number of cases is projected to triple during the time period.

would require major expansion, and long-term care quality and financing would be major public health issues. Current innovations, such as certain models in assisted living (48) and the activities of the Pioneer Network to transform institutional culture (27), suggest directions that the long-term care industry may take to better serve this growing population of persons with moderate and severe Alzheimer's disease.

Alternately, if successful treatments to slow disease progression became readily available by 2010 (Figure 4), and assuming that compliance, toxicity, and effectiveness were similar to those of levodopa for Parkinson's disease, then 10.33 million elderly will have AD by 2050 (virtually the same as if there was no change in treatment), but the preponderance of persons with the disease will be mild cases (59%) (Figure 6). This would result in a shift away from institutional care, as has already been modestly demonstrated among patients treated with cholinesterase inhibitors (24). The net effect would be to increase the burden on families by requiring additional years of caregiving. Although many families may want to prolong the time that their relative is able to live at home and, therefore, willingly sacrifice time and energy toward this end, additional outpatient support services would likely be needed. Furthermore, these new treatments would be costly and require medical

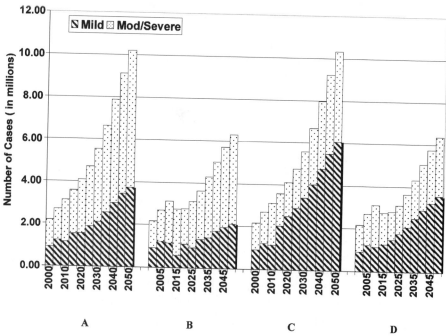

Figure 6   Bar graph comparing the prevalence of mild, moderate/severe, and total cases of Alzheimer's disease in the United States, 2000–2050, based on four projections: no therapeutic advances (*A*), delayed disease onset (*B*), delayed disease progression (*C*), and both delayed disease onset and delayed disease progression (*D*).

monitoring. As a result, this scenario would give rise to whole new service modalities, such as outpatient clinics devoted to Alzheimer's care, expanded dementia day programs and respite care services, and perhaps multipurpose Alzheimer's centers or malls.

The most promising model is one that involves both delayed onset and retarded disease progression (Figure 5). In this model the total number of cases is similar to that for prevention (6.39 compared to 6.31 million), but the majority of cases (56%) are mild. Although the proportionate distribution is skewed toward mild cases, the absolute number of mild cases projected in 2050 is similar to the number had there been no treatment (3.58 compared to 3.75 million with no treatment), whereas the number of moderate/severe cases is markedly less (2.81 compared to 6.46 million). This model would result in continued growth in our systems of care, but that growth would be largely in outpatient services. Long-term care would grow only modestly, as the number of persons with moderate/severe dementia in 2050 would only be twice the current number—not the nearly fourfold rise projected by the no treatment model. Nonetheless, these reductions would allow these same individuals more time to become ill and/or disabled by other costly conditions, such as osteoporosis, osteoarthritis, macular degeneration, heart disease, cancer, and stroke. It is plausible, therefore, that savings in the care required for AD may be less than the costs required to care for other conditions, and that treatment may actually result in societal dissavings (11). On the other hand, the emotional costs of AD may far outweigh the suffering caused by these other conditions, resulting in an overall reduction in the human costs associated with chronic illness.

As the nation enters the twenty-first century, the projected increase in AD will need to be paralleled by efforts to assure the availability and quality of care for persons with the disease. As this chapter outlines, new treatments are likely to occur, altering the epidemiology of the disease and resulting in altered service needs. Such changes in disease patterns could occur over relatively few years (Figures 3–5), so health system responses would need to be rapid in order to meet changing demand. To prepare for these changes, research and planning should address such issues as surveillance and monitoring for the disease, dissemination of new therapies into common practice, the impact of the illness on quality of life, and new models of home, office-based, community-based, and institutional care. Quality-of-life measures developed specifically for AD, in consort with established measures of caregiver burden, will help track the personal impact of the disease and provide direction for future public health efforts.

In conclusion, even if major treatment breakthroughs occur, the management of AD will undoubtedly be a major and growing public health issue during the first half of the twenty-first century. However, the absolute number and the pattern of service needs will vary markedly depending on the timing and the type of treatments that evolve. Also noteworthy is the fact that new treatments would alter disease patterns within a few years after their introduction (Figures 4–6). Thus, our health care system will need to be prepared to rapidly develop new service delivery models. Currently, the focus is on reforming long-term care; as shown here, it is likely that major innovations in outpatient services will be needed as well.

Visit the Annual Reviews home page at www.annualreviews.org

LITERATURE CITED

1. Albert SM, Castillo-Castanada C, Jacobs DM, Sano M, Bell K, et al. 2000. Proxy-reported quality of life in Alzheimer's patients: comparison of clinical and population-based samples. In *Assessing Quality of Life in Alzheimer's Disease*, ed. SM Albert, RG Logsdon. New York: Springer

1a. Barinaga Alzheimer's treatments that work now. *Science* 282:1030–32

2. Birks J, Flicker L. 2000. Selegiline for Alzheimer's disease (Cochrane Review) *Cochrane Database Syst. Rev.* CD 000442

3. Birks J, Grimley Evans J, Iakovidou V, Tsolaki M. 2001. Rivastigmine for Alzheimer's disease. *Cochrane Database Syst. Rev.* Issue 2

4. Birks JS, Melzer D, Beppu H. 2001. Donepezil for mild and moderate Alzheimer's disease. *Cochrane Database Syst. Rev.* Issue 2

5. Blacker D, Wilcox MA, Laird NM, Rodes L, Horvath SM, et al. 1998. Alpha-2 macroglobulin is genetically associated with Alzheimer disease. *Nat. Genet.* 19: 357–60

6. Brookmeyer R, Gray S, Kawas C. 1998. Projections of Alzheimer's disease in the United States and the public health impact of delaying disease onset. *Am. J. Public Health* 88(9):1337–42

7. Clark CM, Trojanowski JQ. 2000. *Neurodegenerative Dementias*. New York: McGraw-Hill

8. Cleland JGF, Clark A. 1999. Has the survival of the heart failure population changed? Lessons from trials. *Am. J. Cardiol.* 83:112D–19D

9. Doody RS, Massman P, Dunn JK. 2001. A method for estimating progression rates in Alzheimer disease. *Arch. Neurol.* 58:449–54

10. During MJ, Symes CW, Lawlor PA, Lin J, Dunning J, et al. 2000. An oral vaccine against NMDAR1 with efficacy in experimental stroke and epilepsy. *Science* 287:1453–59

11. Ernst RL, Hay JW. 1997. Economic research on Alzheimer disease: a review of the literature. *Alzheimer Dis. Assoc. Dis.* 11:135–45

12. Evans DA, Scherr PA, Cook NR, Albert MS, Funkenstein HH, et al. 1992. The impact of Alzheimer's disease in the United States population. In *The Oldest Old*, ed. RM Suzman, DP Willis, KG Manton, pp. 283–399. New York: Oxford Univ. Press

13. Forette F, Seux ML, Straessen JA, Thijs L, Birkenhager WH, et al. 1998. Prevention of dementia in randomized double-blind placebo-controlled Systolic Hypertension in Europe (Syst-Eur) trial. *Lancet* 352:1347–51

14. Forman MS, Lee VM, Trojanowski JQ. 2000. New insights into genetic and molecular mechanisms of brain degeneration in tauopathies. *J. Chem. Neuroanat.* 20:225–44

15. Deleted in proof

16. Goedert M, Ghetti B, Spillantini MG. 2000. Tau gene mutations in frontotemporal dementia and parkinsonism linked to chromosome 17 (FTDP-17). Their relevance for understanding the neurogenerative process. *Ann. NY Acad. Sci.* 920:74–83

16a. Hebert LE, Scherr PA, Beckett LA, Albert MS, Pilgrim DM, et al. 1995. Age-specific incidence of Alzheimer's disease in a community population. *JAMA* 273(17):1354–59

17. Henke CJ, Burchmore MJ. 1997. The economic impact of tacrine in the treatment of Alzheimer's disease. *Clin. Ther.* 19:330–45

18. Hoehn MM, Yahr MD. 1967. Parkinsonism: onset, progression, and mortality. *Neurology* 17:427–42

19. Ho KKL, Anderson KM, Kannel WB, Grossman W, Levy D. 1993. Survival after the onset of congestive heart failure in Framingham Heart Study subjects. *Circulation* 88:107–15

20. Hong M, Zhukareva V, Vogelsberg-Ragaglia V, Wszolek Z, Reed L, et al. 1998. Mutation-specific functional impairments in distinct tau isoforms of hereditary FTDP-17. *Science* 282:1914–17

21. Hu T, Huang L, Cartwright WS. 1986. Evaluation of the costs of caring for the senile demented elderly: a pilot study. *Gerontologist* 26:158–63

22. Hughes CP, Berg L, Danziger WL, Coben LA, Martin RL. 1982. A new clinical scale for the staging of dementia. *Br. J. Psychiatry* 140:566–72

23. Katzman R, Kawas C. 1994. *The Epidemiology of Dementia and Alzheimer's Disease. Alzheimer Disease*, ed. RD Terry, R Katzman, K Bich, pp. 105–22. New York: Raven

24. Knopman D, Schneider L, Davis K, Talwalker S, Smith F, et al. 1996. Long-term tacrine (Cognex) treatment: Effects on nursing home placement and mortality. *Neurology* 47:166–77

24a. Logsdon RG, Gibbons LE, McCurry SM, Teri L. 2000. Quality of life in Alzheimer's Disease: patient and caregiver reports. In *Assessing Quality of Life in*

Alzheimer's Disease, ed. SM Albert, RG Logsdon. New York: Springer

25. Lopez OL, Becker JT, Klunk W, Saxton J, Hamilton RL, et al. 2000. Research evaluation and diagnosis of possible Alzheimer's disease over the last two decades: II. *Neurology* 55:1863–69

26. McCormick WC, Abrass IB. 1998. Shifting thinking about memory impairment. *Lancet* 352:(Suppl. IV):6)

27. Misiorski S. 2001. Building a better life: transforming institutional culture. *Alzheimer's Care Q.* 2(3):5–9

27a. Moceri VM, Kukull WA, Emanuel I, van Belle G, Larson EB. 2000. Early-life risk factors and the development of Alzheimer's disease. *Neurology* 54:415–20

28. Moore MJ, Zhu CW, Clipp EC. 2001. Informal costs of dementia care: estimates from the national longitudinal caregiver study. *J. Gerontol. Soc. Sci.* 56B:S219–28

29. Morgan D, Diamond DM, Gottschall PE, Ugen KE, Dickey C, et al. 2000. A beta peptide vaccination prevents memory loss in an animal model of Alzheimer's disease. *Nature* 408:982–85

30. Namboodiri K, Suchindran CM. 1987. *Life Table Techniques and Their Applications.* Orlando, FL: Academic

31. Oken B, Storzbach D, Kaye J. 1998. The efficacy of Ginkgo biloba on cognitive function in Alzheimer's disease. *Arch. Neurol.* 55:1409–15

32. Pennisi E. 1999. Enzymes point way to potential Alzheimer's therapies. *Science* 286:650–51

33. Peterson RC, Stevens JC, Ganguli M, Tangalos EG, Cummings JL, DeKosky ST. 2001. Practice parameter: early detection of dementia: mild cognitive impairment (an evidence-based review). *Neurology* 56:1133–42

34. Poewe WH, Wenning GK. 1996. The natural history of Parkinson's disease. *Neurology* 47(Suppl. 3):S146–52

35. Raskind MA, Peskind ER, Wessel T, Yuan W. 2000. Galantamine in AD: a 6-month randomized, placebo-controlled trial with a 6-month extension. The Galantamine USA-1 Study Group. *Neurology* 54(12):2261–68

36. Rice DP, Fox PJ, Max W, Webber PA, Lindeman DA, et al. 1993. The economic burden of Alzheimer's disease care. *Health Aff.* Summer 164–76

37. Rosler M, Anand R, Cicin-Sain A, Gauthier S, Agid Y, et al. 1999. Efficacy and safety of rivastigmine in patients with Alzheimer's disease: international randomised controlled trial [see comments]. *BMJ* 318(7184):633–38

38. St. George-Hyslop PH. 2000. Piecing together Alzheimer's. *Sci. Am.* 76–83

39. Sano M, Ernesto C, Thomas RG, Klauber MR, Schafer K, et al. 1997. A controlled trial of selegiline, alpha-tocopherol, or both as treatment for Alzheimer's disease. The Alzheimer's Disease Cooperative Study [see comments]. *New Engl. J. Med.* 336(17):1216–22

40. Schenk D, Barbour R, Dunn W, Gordon G, Grajeda H, et al. 1999. Immunization with amyloid-β attenuates Alzheimer-disease-like pathology in the PDAPP mouse. *Nature* 400:173–77

41. Selkoe DJ. 1999. Translating cell biology into therapeutic advances in Alzheimer's disease. *Nature* 399 (6738):A23–31

42. Shoulson I. 1998. Experimental therapeutics of neurodegenerative disorders: unmet needs. *Science* 282:1072–83

43. Stern RG, Mohs RC, Davidson M, Schmeidler J, Silverman J, et al. 1994. A longitudinal study of Alzheimer's disease: measurement, rate, and predictors of cognitive deterioration. *Am. J. Psychiatr.* 151(3):390–96

44. Tariot PN, Solomon PR, Morris JC, Kershaw P, Lilienfeld S, Ding C. 2000. A 5-month, randomized, placebo-controlled trial of galantamine in AD. The Galantamine USA-10 Study Group. *Neurology* 54(12):2269–76

45. US Census Bur. 2000. National population projections, II. Detailed files: total population by age, sex, race, Hispanic

origin, and nativity. http://www.census.gov/population/www/projections/natdet D1A.html

46. US Gen. Account. Off. 1998. *Alzheimer's Disease: Estimates of Prevalence in the United States*. Washington, DC: GAO/HEHS-98-16

46a. Van Dujin CM, Hofman A. 1992. Risk factors for Alzheimer's disease: the EURODEM collaborative re-analysis of case-control studies. *Neuroepidemiology* 11 (suppl 1):106–13

47. Wilcock GK, Lilienfeld S, Gaens E. 2000. Efficacy and safety of galantamine in patients with mild to moderate Alzheimer's disease: multicentre randomised controlled trial. Galantamine International-1 Study Group. *BMJ* 321(7274): 1445–49

48. Zimmerman S, Sloane PD, Eckert JK, eds. 2002. *Assisted Living: Needs, Practices and Policies in Residential Care for the Elderly*. Baltimore: Johns Hopkins Univ. Press. In press

Annu. Rev. Public Health 2002. 23:233–54

UTILIZATION MANAGEMENT: Issues, Effects, and Future Prospects

Thomas M. Wickizer[1] and Daniel Lessler[2]

[1]Department of Health Services, School of Public Health and Community Medicine, University of Washington, Seattle, Washington 98195-7660, e-mail: tomwick@u.washington.edu
[2]Section of General Internal Medicine, Department of Medicine, Harborview Medical Center and the University of Washington, Box 359704, Harborview Medical Center, Seattle, Washington 98104, e-mail: dlessler@u.washington.edu

Key Words utilization management, managed care, cost containment, utilization review, quality, health economics

■ **Abstract** Utilization management encompasses a diverse set of activities designed to influence the use of health care services and thereby constrain health care resource consumption. Utilization management, which has become one of the most widely used cost-containment approaches, has engendered debate and controversy. Physicians have been outspoken critics of utilization management because it has limited their clinical autonomy and has contributed to an intolerable administrative burden. Insurance carriers, managed care plans, and third-party payers have defended the use of utilization management as an imperfect—but necessary—practice that is needed to reduce consumption of unnecessary or inappropriate health care services. This review examines the operation and effects of three widely used utilization management procedures: prospective utilization review, case management, and physician gatekeeping programs. In addition, it explores the future role of utilization management in the health care system and outlines a set of principles that we believe should be used to guide the development of utilization management strategies in the future.

INTRODUCTION

Utilization management (UM) represents a broad array of techniques designed to influence the consumption of health care services, usually with the objective of promoting cost containment. During the past 20 years, UM has gained acceptance as an approach to cost containment and has become a prominent fixture of the U.S. health care system. Managed care plans, public and private payers of health care services, insurance carriers, and hospitals have used UM in one form or

0163-7525/02/0510-0233$14.00

another to control health care utilization and contain costs (12, 29, 42, 73). Even physician medical groups—often the target of UM—have relied on UM techniques to control the volume of services when they have been placed at financial risk through managed care risk contracts (29). Evaluations of UM have generated mixed findings, with some studies showing reductions in utilization and costs and others showing little effect. Despite its widespread use, UM has engendered debate and controversy. Physicians have been outspoken critics of UM because it has eroded their clinical autonomy. UM has also been criticized for its role in contributing to the mountain of paperwork that now burdens the health care system. Insurance carriers, third-party payers, and health plans have defended the use of UM as an imperfect, but necessary, practice that is needed to reduce consumption of unnecessary or inappropriate health care services and thereby contain health care costs.

The purpose of this review is to: (a) describe the key features and effects of UM; (b) critically examine the process of utilization review, arguably the most controversial and invasive feature of UM; and (c) discuss the future role for UM in the twenty-first century. The health care system is clearly in transition, moving away from restrictive managed care arrangements and toward more flexible consumer-oriented delivery models. The UM program of tomorrow is likely to be quite different from the UM program of today. This review provides an opportunity to consider the purpose of UM and how it might best meet the future needs of the health care system.

BACKGROUND

Definition of UM

No single definition has been developed to date that adequately captures the diverse nature of UM. In its 1989 report on UM, the Institute of Medicine (IOM) adopted a narrow focus on case-by-case preservice review sponsored by purchasers (25). In her study of medical groups, Kerr adopted a broad definition of UM that included the use of physician payment incentives (29). Subsequently, Milstein (41) defined UM in terms of "interventions originating outside the physician/patient relationship with an intent to promote an economical mix of health care services." Milstein's definition highlights two important features of UM: (a) it is a process that is externally imposed upon the physician/patient, and (b) it is directed at containing health care costs for payers.

This review focuses on three widely used UM practices: (a) traditional prospective utilization review (UR), including pre-admission and concurrent review, (b) case management, and (c) physician gatekeeping. Our review touches only peripherally on demand and disease management, which arguably are forms of UM.

Operational Characteristics

The three UM practices examined here, prospective UR, case management and physician gatekeeping, share the common general purpose of promoting health care cost containment, although they vary in their operational characteristics.[1]

UTILIZATION REVIEW   UR typically focuses on hospital care but is also used to review and authorize outpatient care. Most prospective UR programs include pre-admission review to certify the need for hospitalization and assign an initial length of stay, concurrent review to authorize continued hospital stay after expiration of the initial approved stay, and outpatient review to authorize selected diagnostic and surgical procedures, such as magnetic resonance imaging (MRI) or tonsillectomies.

The intent of UR is to constrain health care costs by reducing unnecessary or inappropriate medical care. These two terms generally indicate care that (*a*) provides no significant clinical benefit, or (*b*) could be rendered in a less costly setting. UR is performed on a case-by-case basis, usually by an external review agency, and is offered by health plans and insurance carriers as a benefit design feature. UR is almost always compulsory. If a patient fails to obtain the necessary authorization for an admission, an extended length of stay, or a diagnostic or surgical procedure, he or she may be liable for financial penalties. Alternatively, some form of financial or reimbursement penalty may be levied against the health care organization providing the service. A decision to deny care may not always result from UR but may rather result from coverage limitations included in a patient's health insurance policy. The UR decision is usually made independent of the claims examination process, but confusion sometimes arises in the minds of patients who wrongly assume that any denial of care results from UR.

There are few reliable data on the current use of UR among health insurance carriers, managed care plans, self-insured businesses, or public payers. During the 1980s, the use of UR grew rapidly. In an earlier review paper, Wickizer (73) traced the growth and evolution of UR through the 1980s and noted that by 1985 a substantial majority (>70%) of Blue Cross and Blue Shield plans were using some form of UR to contain costs. More recent data on the use of UR comes from a 1995 physician survey (48), which gathered data on the use of managed care techniques from a national sample of approximately 2000 practicing physicians. Physicians responding to the survey reported that 50% to 60% of their patients were subject to some form of UR (length-of-stay review, site-of-care review, or treatment appropriateness). The number of review organizations provides an indirect measure of the broad reach of UR. In its 2000 Utilization Management Guide (68), URAC, also known as the American Accreditation HealthCare Commission, listed over

---

[1]Some case management programs are focused on patient advocacy and care coordination. These programs may not have cost containment as their primary goal.

300 accredited UR organizations located throughout the country. The number of unaccredited organizations providing UR services is unknown but is surely large.

Although UR is extensively performed, managed care organizations and health plans have begun to question the value of traditional UR approaches. In a widely publicized decision (28), United Health Care abandoned its UR program in late 1999 in favor of programs that emphasized a more consumer-/clinically oriented approach involving demand management and disease management.

CASE MANAGEMENT   Case management, the second form of UM included in this review, represents a highly diverse set of activities. Case management can be grouped into two broad categories that sometimes overlap. Administrative case management provides brokering services to ensure that patients obtain needed services at the lowest available price, assures that available benefits are brought to bear in a coordinated and comprehensive manner, and flexes eligibility so that patients may receive cost-efficient services not included in their original benefit package. On the other hand, clinical case management primarily focuses on optimizing clinical management and often focuses on a specific clinical condition such as diabetes or heart failure. Clinical case managers often work from evidence-based protocols and proactively reach out to patients, assisting them to better manage their illness. Increasingly, such clinical case management occurs as part of a more comprehensive disease management program. Both forms of case management are provided to high-risk patients who may require costly medical care, e.g., patients with spinal cord injuries, serious mental or substance abuse problems, or chronic illnesses. Smith (63) described the diverse nature of case management as follows:

> Case management is a generic term with multiple definitions depending on the profession, client group, context and organizational structure . . .. Despite the large number of definitions, common core tasks, or steps, prevail in all practice settings: client identification, assessment, care planning, implementation, monitoring and reassessment.

Geary & Smeltzer (12) note that despite considerable variation in approach, the goal of most case management programs is to decrease costs by lowering total utilization while maintaining or improving quality and other outcomes of care.

Hospital payment reform enacted by Medicare in the 1980s and managed care developments of the 1990s stimulated the use of case management services. In the 1980s, hospitals began to employ nurses as case managers to perform discharge planning and related tasks. During the 1990s, with the introduction of care maps (treatment guidelines or clinical protocols), the role of the hospital case manager expanded as care coordination became more important (49). Case managers have been used extensively in other clinical settings and treatment systems as well to help coordinate care, including HMOs (1), long-term care facilities (36), and workers' compensation (10).

Published data about the effects of administrative case management on costs and clinical outcomes are sparse, whereas studies about clinical case management are more plentiful. The availability of robust data not withstanding, both forms of case management are now widely used in a variety of settings, including inpatient, outpatient, and long-term care facilities. Often administrative case management is combined with utilization review and provided by private insurance carriers and UR organizations. More recently, there has been a growing trend to combine case management with other forms of UM, in particular demand management or disease management, to establish systems of "integrated care management" (12, 68).[2]

PHYSICIAN GATEKEEPING   Physician gatekeeping, the third type of UM reviewed here, has become a central feature of managed care. In the earlier pre-managed-care era, when fee-for-service reimbursement dominated as the major form of payment, there were few restrictions placed on patients' access to specialty care and often specialty care consumed by patients was not coordinated. As noted by Bodenheimer et al. (3), in 1965 only 40% of the population had a regular physician who was a generalist, 15% had a physician who was a specialist, and 45% had no regular physician. Patients often sought care directly from a specialist, frequently resulting in costly diagnostic or therapeutic care, with some risk for iatrogenic disease. Medical care costs and health risk increased when patients visited physicians in multiple specialties. With no single physician coordinating their care, patients sometimes received duplicative diagnostic tests or medication that adversely reacted with medications they were already taking (3).

The growing problem of duplicative, costly, uncoordinated care gave rise to the concept of the primary care physician (PCP), who could both provide general medical care and coordinate specialty care when it was needed. During the 1980s and 1990s, with the rapid growth of managed care and capitated reimbursement, PCPs took on a new role as physician gatekeeper. In this role, the PCP became responsible for overseeing and authorizing specialty care for managed care patients. The field of primary care, especially family practice, had for some time stressed the need for PCPs to coordinate medical care—and specialty care in particular— but the new emphasis of physician gatekeeping under managed care was on cost containment and limiting, not coordinating, the use of specialty care.

Physician gatekeeping as a form of UM expanded greatly during the 1990s with the growth of managed care. Few reliable data on the use of physician gatekeeping exist, but what data are available suggest this form of UM is widely used.

---

[2]Demand management and case management differ in where they fall on the continuum of care. Demand management is offered en masse to all enrollees of an insurance plan or HMO, or all employees of a business. Case management is offered to patients who have complex clinical needs and focuses on coordination of care and benefits. Disease management focuses on patients with specific clinical conditions, e.g., asthma patients, bringing to bear diverse strategies such as clinical reminders and clinical case management to assure care conforms to evidence-based guidelines.

Survey data indicate that in 1997 almost half of all privately insured patients in major metropolitan regions throughout the United States were in "gatekeeping arrangements in which their primary care physician controlled their access to specialists" (64). The role of managed care gatekeepers became contentious because of the use of economic incentives that financially rewarded primary care physicians for thrifty use of referral and hospital services (17). As managed care expanded, with a corresponding increase in the use of physician gatekeeping, patient and physician dissatisfaction mounted. Patients became increasingly dissatisfied with managed care and its reliance on physician gatekeeping to limit access to specialists (3). Physicians felt that the role of physician gatekeeper often compromised the physician-patient relationship and created conflicting loyalties. Moreover, a national survey found that a quarter of primary care providers felt that they were being asked to provide services that were beyond their clinical skill set (64).

In the late 1990s, patient dissatisfaction with managed care took political expression in the form of the "patient rights movement," which sought to restrict through legal statute the ability of managed care plans to limit patients' access to certain types of hospital and physician care. Over 30 states passed laws either guaranteeing patients the right to secure access to selected forms of medical care without interference from managed care plans or giving them the right to have an independent medical review when their care was denied (46). Although physician gatekeeping continues to be widely used, managed care plans are retreating from their earlier heavy reliance on this form of UM (3, 52). Nonetheless, there continues to be a need for coordination of medical care, especially chronic care (70).

EFFECTS OF UM ON UTILIZATION, COSTS AND QUALITY

Utilization Review

Of the three UM practices reviewed here, utilization review (UR) has the most extensive literature. The early UR literature (prior to 1985), reviewed previously by Wickizer (73), suffered from serious research design flaws, making interpretation of the findings from these studies difficult. Among the more sophisticated early UR studies were evaluations of the Professional Standards Review Organization (PSRO) program conducted by the Health Care Financing Administration (HCFA). These evaluations found modest effects of PSROs on length of stay and on selected admissions subject to pre-admission review (21, 22). Other studies of public and private UR programs showed somewhat larger effects of UR (73), but the usefulness of these studies is limited because of methodological problems.

UR studies conducted after 1985 employed more sophisticated designs and used more rigorous multivariate techniques, and thus yielded more reliable findings. One of the initial series of UR studies published after 1985 was an evaluation of a large private UR program conducted by Wickizer and his colleagues (8, 72, 81, 82). That evaluation found that pre-admission review reduced admissions significantly (approximately 10%) but concurrent review had only a modest effect (2% to 3% reduction) on length of stay. The combined effect of the two UR activities was to reduce hospital inpatient days per 1000 insured persons, on average, by approximately 12%. This estimated effect was dependent upon the baseline level of utilization. Insured groups with higher baseline levels of utilization had substantially greater proportionate reductions in utilization and costs (8). The reduction in inpatient utilization was offset by an increase in outpatient utilization (82); that is, outpatient services were substituted for inpatient services that were constrained under UR. The result was a net decrease in total per capita medical expenditures (including the cost of the UR program) of approximately 5%. Subsequent multivariate analyses of other UR programs operated by Blue Cross and Blue Shield plans (55) and by Aetna Insurance Company (31) generated cost savings estimates similar to those described above.

Left unanswered by these UR studies of the mid- to late-1980s was the effect of UR on access and quality. There was little detailed information regarding the actual frequency of denial among patients, nor was there information about whether denials differed by diagnostic category. Further, almost nothing was known about whether denial of care by UR had any effect on quality as measured by markers such as readmission rates. Wickizer & Lessler conducted a series of studies (33, 77–80, 83) using insurance claims data spanning the period 1989 through 1993 to explore these questions. The data analyzed represent a case series of approximately 60,000 privately insured patients (children and adults) who had been subject to pre-admission review and concurrent review. In addition, the database included approximately 9000 other patients with occupational injuries or diseases who had been subject to UR through workers' compensation.

This series of studies addressed several important gaps in knowledge regarding UR's effect on patterns of care. Contrary to common belief, pre-admission review resulted in few (<2%) denials of hospital treatment (78). Instead, UR more closely managed patients' length of stay through concurrent review after patients were hospitalized. The impact of UR on inpatient care was greatest for mental health patients (78). Whereas mental health patients, including patients with a diagnosis related to substance abuse, represented only 5% of the study population, they accounted for over 50% of the total days saved due to UR. In contrast, obstetric admissions represented almost 40% of the total number of cases reviewed yet they accounted for a trivial (3%) portion of the reduction in hospital days. The fact that obstetric admissions are approved 100% of the time and almost always have short hospital stays, even for cesarean section cases, explains the small proportionate reduction in hospital days. This finding calls into question the common UR approach of using pre-admission review to certify the need for hospitalization when, as in the case of obstetric care, the clinical need for hospitalization is obvious. Further, the volume of such reviews adds significantly to the administrative burden imposed by UR on the health care system.

Length of stay has been declining in the United States, even long after the initiation of hospital payment reform through diagnosis related groups (DRGs), perhaps in part because of UR. Wickizer & Lessler (78) found that UR became more stringent and restrictive over time in approving cases. In a four-year period (1990 through 1993), length-of-stay authorization (total number of hospital days approved) decreased by almost 50% for mental health cases and by almost 25% for medical cases.

As part of this same series of UR studies, Wickizer & Lessler examined the effects of UR on quality, as measured by early readmission rates. Three separate analyses performed on different patient groups, mental health patients (77), pediatric patients (79), and cardiovascular patients (33), generated consistent findings showing that reduction in requested length of stay resulting from UR was associated with increased relative risk of readmission within 60 days. This effect was especially pronounced for cardiovascular patients who had a surgical procedure for which the requested length of stay was reduced by two or more days. Such patients were 2.7 times as likely to be readmitted within 60 days as patients having no reduction in requested length of stay (33). While the increase in absolute risk of readmission associated with UR was small, these findings nevertheless raise questions about the potential effect of UR on quality for some patients.

An additional recent study that contributed to understanding of UR's effects on utilization was conducted by Rosenberg et al. (53). This study examined UR's effect on patterns of care among a sample of New York City municipal employees who were randomly assigned either to a standard UR program or to a "sham" UR program for which all requested procedures and admissions were automatically approved. The "review" group had fewer procedures per 1000 than the "sham" group but otherwise there were few meaningful differences in patterns of hospital or outpatient care.

Case Management

The case management literature is more limited than the UR literature. While the published literature about administrative case management is sparse, several randomized controlled trials have evaluated the impact of clinical case management on clinical outcomes and costs. Despite their theoretical potential, little evidence exists showing a positive effect of either type of case management on health care costs. Some studies, however, have found positive effects of case management on health outcomes and patient satisfaction, although patient follow-up in these studies has been relatively short.

ADMINISTRATIVE CASE MANAGEMENT   We could find only one published randomized trial that evaluated the effects of an administrative case management program, although the literature includes a number of case management studies that lack adequate controls (63). Discharge planning represents a common type of administrative case management that has been widely used. Naylor et al. (44) conducted a randomized trial to investigate the effects of discharge planning on readmissions, hospital days, and medical costs among elderly patients admitted to a major university medical center for selected medical and surgical conditions. The post-discharge follow-up period evaluated was limited to 12 weeks. The researchers reported mixed findings. Discharge planning had little effect on surgical patients but did have a significant effect on utilization among medical patients up to six weeks following discharge. For medical patients who had discharge planning, re-hospitalization rates, total duration of re-hospitalization, and total hospital charges were less relative to medical patients in the control group.

CLINICAL CASE MANAGEMENT   Ferguson & Weinberger (9) provide a useful review of randomized case management trials conducted through 1996 in primary care settings. Of the nine trials included in their review, none affected health care costs but several did improve health outcome and satisfaction measures. Ferguson & Weinberger note that the more successful case management programs targeted patients with specified disease conditions, e.g., congestive heart failure, and had care supervised by a medical subspecialist. Case management programs focusing more generally on post-hospital discharge care or on geriatric care were found to be less successful.

With respect to clinical case management, Rich and colleagues (51) conducted a randomized trial of case management applied to elderly patients treated from 1990 through 1994 for congestive heart failure in a major urban university medical center. Patients were followed for 90 days after discharge. Relative to the control group, patients in the case management group had lower rates of readmission during 90-day follow up (33% versus 46%), but there was no significant difference between the two groups in average length of stay for patients re-hospitalized. In a subsequent report, Rich et al. (50) presented findings for the same study population regarding the effects of case management on patient survival, quality of life indicators, and health care costs assessed at 90 days post hospital discharge. Case management was associated with improved patient survival and with increased quality of life, as measured by indicators such as fatigue, dyspnea, emotional function, and environmental mastery. However, no statistically significant difference in medical costs was found.

In another randomized trial, researchers investigated the effects of a nurse case management program designed to improve health outcomes for diabetic patients (17 type 1 and 121 type 2 patients) enrolled in an HMO (1). The duration of the trial was 12 months. The primary outcome, hemoglobin A_{1c} values at 12 months, decreased significantly for the case management group relative to the controls. Self-reported health status measures also improved for the case management group, but the study found no differences in other outcomes, including blood pressure, body weight, medication type or dose, or lipids.

The Health Care Financing Administration (HCFA) funded three major demonstrations of case management programs established to improve care and contain health care costs for Medicare patients (58). Each of these demonstrations randomly assigned Medicare patients to a case management group or a control group that received standard Medicare services. The conditions targeted for case management varied somewhat among the three demonstration sites. One site focused exclusively on congestive heart failure (CHF), whereas another focused on

CHF or chronic obstructive pulmonary disease (COPD). The third site targeted eight diagnostic groups, including patients with CHF, COPD, ischemic heart disease, stroke, pneumonia and sepsis, and cancer. The number of patients randomized to receive case management in the three sites varied from 209 to 556.

The three demonstration projects differed somewhat in their case management procedures. Although they included elements of administrative case management, they were primarily clinical case management interventions. One demonstration site used a highly structured case management procedure with the frequency and type of communication and interaction between the case manager and the client specified in detail. The other two sites were less structured and allowed individual case managers more flexibility. In addition, the sites differed in their use of client education. One site placed substantial emphasis on client education, the other two sites used it less frequently. The case managers at the three demonstration sites were primarily nurses but also included some social workers.

As reported by Shore et al. (58), none of the three HCFA demonstration sites improved self-care or health or reduced Medicare costs. The researchers suggested that the lack of physician involvement in case management or the lack of specific goals might explain their failure to detect any effects for the demonstrations. Two recent studies, one a randomized trial and the other a cohort study, reported in 2000 also found little evidence of meaningful effects of case management programs (5, 23).

The experience of the Medicare demonstrations may provide insight into why case management has thus far failed to live up to expectations regarding its potential to reduce health care costs. In explaining their failure to detect significant effects of case management, Shore et al. (58) emphasize the lack of cooperation from clients' physicians as a major obstacle hindering successful case management. They also cite the lack of clear goals for case management as a barrier to effective care coordination. The lesson here may be that successful case management requires the active participation and involvement of the patient's physician, and the specification of clear goals toward which case management activities can be directed.

In a recent report of an ongoing quality improvement project, Wickizer et al. (76) describe the Washington State Workers' Compensation Managed Care Pilot (MCP) project, which used case management techniques to coordinate care for injured workers. Case management was provided within each managed care clinic and was closely integrated with other occupational health services, with the specific goals of reducing worker disability and enhancing early return to work. Analysis of disability payments and lost work time suggested that case management, if well integrated into a delivery system and directed at specific goals, can achieve positive results (6, 76).

Physician Gatekeeping

The empirical literature on physician gatekeeping is sparse. One of the more sophisticated studies was a randomized trial reported by Martin et al. (39) of a physician gatekeeper program sponsored by SAFECO Insurance Company of Seattle, Washington. This trial randomized approximately 1100 subscribers (2800 enrollees including insured dependents) to a physician gatekeeper managed care plan or a standard managed care plan. The gatekeeper plan had 6% lower total charges per enrollee compared to the plan without a gatekeeper, primarily due to lower ambulatory care charges associated with reduced use of specialists.

Medicaid established physician gatekeeper programs as part of a larger series of demonstration programs conducted during the 1980s. Evaluations of these programs generally showed little cost-containment effect of gatekeeping (4, 24, 37, 69). Hurley et al. reported that physician gatekeeping programs established through Medicaid programs in California and New Jersey led to decreased use of specialty care but greater concentrated use of primary care services (24). The effect of these particular programs on costs is unclear.

In a subsequent randomized trial of a gatekeeper program established in a large university-affiliated public hospital, Schillinger et al. (56) reported significantly decreased use of specialty care and fewer hospitalizations but slightly increased use of primary care services among patients using physician gatekeeping. This study found no significant differences in patient satisfaction, perceived access to specialists, or use of out-of-network services. The effects of gatekeeping have also been assessed within an international context. Delnoij et al. (7) conducted multivariate analysis of national health care expenditure data for countries (primarily the United States and selected European countries) belonging to the OECD. These analyses found lower expenditure growth on ambulatory care services in countries that adopted gatekeeper programs but no differences in the level or growth in hospital expenditures or total medical expenditures.

Finally, Grembowski et al. (15, 16) recently reported the results of a detailed cohort study designed to assess the effects of managed care activities, including physician gatekeeping, on utilization, satisfaction, and health outcomes among patients with chronic pain and depression. The researchers were unable to isolate the effects of physician gatekeeping from other managed care activities, but they found little effect of "care managedness" (measured empirically as an index that incorporated gatekeeping, provider specialist network limitations, preauthorization, and provider financial risk sharing) on access to specialty services or health outcomes.

The evaluations of physician gatekeeping programs conducted thus far provide limited evidence that this form of UM has a meaningful effect on health care resource consumption. However, we would note that many group or staff model HMOs use a standard physician gatekeeper delivery model that requires patients to obtain a referral from their primary care physician in order to receive specialty care. This model is used at Group Health Cooperative, a large staff model HMO located in Seattle, Washington, which was the HMO site for the RAND Health Insurance Experiment (HIE). A randomized trial, conducted as part of the RAND HIE (38), found that medical expenditures per capita for Group Health Cooperative enrollees were significantly lower than for fee-for-service patients. The reduced expenditure rate resulted primarily from decreased admissions. It is unclear whether, or the extent to which, the observed difference in medical expenses may have been associated with the Group Health Cooperative's physician gatekeeping delivery model as opposed to other organizational or financial factors that affect HMO resource consumption.

SCIENTIFIC BASIS AND APPLICATION OF UTILIZATION REVIEW PROCEDURES

Of the three forms of utilization management reviewed here, utilization review (UR) has been the most closely scrutinized and the most heavily criticized. We therefore turn our attention to an examination of the scientific issues pertaining to UR and to other issues related to its use as a mechanism to review and authorize medical care.

The conduct of utilization review—whether pre-authorization of procedures and/or hospitalizations or concurrent review of hospital care—assumes that inappropriate or unnecessary care can be identified using defined clinical criteria. Utilization criteria may either be embodied in guidelines (e.g., length-of-stay guidelines, appropriateness guidelines), or determined by an algorithm that considers specific clinical attributes (e.g., intensity of clinical need, severity of clinical condition, and diagnosis). Both approaches usually involve an initial screening that compares a patient's clinical characteristics to a set of criteria (explicit review). If care meets established criteria, it is approved. Care that does not meet criteria may be immediately denied, though more commonly, especially in the case of pre-authorization of procedures, a physician is asked to review the request. It is noteworthy that the judgments of physician reviewers, while taking account of explicit criteria or guidelines, are often implicit and based on further discussion with the treating clinician.

Methods for determining appropriateness and necessity must be valid and reliable if they are to promote efficient clinical care and gain the trust of the professional medical community and patients. The ultimate reliability and validity of decisions rendered through utilization review depend on the nature of UR criteria and the process of applying those criteria to the specific clinical circumstances of patients.

Available research findings suggest that current UR decision-making is not always reliable and valid for evaluating the need for hospital admission and/or additional hospital days. In an analysis of three distinct utilization review instruments used to determine necessity of inpatient care for medical conditions, Strumwasser et al. (65) found two approaches to be moderately valid and reliable, and the third to have low reliability and validity. The third approach was based on Intensity-Severity-Discharge criteria (ISD) and was adapted from a well-known and widely utilized UR vendor, InterQual. Subsequent research has also questioned the validity of ISD criteria (13, 14).

The validity of proprietary length-of-stay (LOS) guidelines has also been widely challenged, as has the reliability with which such guidelines are actually applied.

Initially, LOS guidelines were based on historical median LOS data derived from hospital discharge databases. While this approach is still used by several proprietary UR organizations, the most widely used LOS guidelines are produced by Milliman and Robertson (M&R) and reflect goal LOS of stay for uncomplicated patients. These guidelines are either based on published literature, reflect observed "benchmark" LOS performance from hospitals across the country, or both. Several analyses have found a wide variance between actual length of stay data and M&R LOS guidelines (40, 54, 62). These studies raise questions about the generalizability of LOS guidelines based on the performance of selected institutions, as well as their underlying validity.

Anecdotal reports have also raised concerns about the application of LOS guidelines. Many physicians report that such guidelines are sometimes inflexibly applied by managed care organizations and UR firms, and fail to take account of important patient clinical characteristics or limitations of community-based healthcare resources, such as home care. This is particularly the case for M&R guidelines that recommend goal LOS for uncomplicated patients. Consistent with these anecdotal reports, a study of UR psychiatric cases conducted by Wickizer et al. (83) showed a pattern of LOS authorization reflective of a cookie-cutter approach. The study population comprised patients with a wide variety of psychiatric illnesses, including schizophrenia, single-episode depression, recurrent depression, alcohol dependence, drug dependence, and adjustment reaction. Nonetheless, almost all patients were approved initially for six days of inpatient treatment.

Concerns about the validity of proprietary LOS guidelines have led to calls for more evidence-based LOS guideline development, using standards similar to those applied to clinical practice guidelines. In fact, the past decade has seen an increasing number of published evidence-based and prospectively evaluated LOS guidelines for common medical conditions and surgical procedures in peer-reviewed literature (20, 67, 71). These guidelines usually are applied and evaluated among patients who are clinically defined as low risk. Unfortunately, the number of scientifically developed and validated LOS guidelines pales in comparison to the universe of clinical conditions and procedures for which patients are hospitalized. Moreover, clinical and technological innovations can outpace the time needed to undertake such rigorous evaluations, rendering evidence-based LOS guidelines obsolete by the time they are published (61a).

The validity of appropriateness criteria for health procedures and the reliability with which they are applied to individual patients has also generated controversy. The RAND/UCLA method for identifying indications for a procedure is perhaps the best known and widely emulated (61). The RAND/UCLA approach involves convening a panel of experts who review available scientific evidence and independently rank the appropriateness of performing a procedure under a specific set of clinical circumstances. The panel then convenes as a group to discuss and adjust their rankings. This method is most often applied when there is sparse scientific evidence and the indications for a procedure remains uncertain.

A recent evaluation of the reproducibility of the RAND/UCLA method to identify the overuse and underuse of medical procedures found that expert panels differ substantially in their interpretation of available evidence. For example, expert panels using the same methodology to reach consensus on clinical recommendations varied twofold in their categorization of the appropriateness of hysterectomy and coronary-revascularization procedures (61). Thus, it appears that variation in the rates of medical and surgical procedures observed when physicians individually make decisions under conditions of clinical uncertainty can, at best, only be modestly mitigated through the promulgation of appropriateness guidelines by expert consensus panels, because such panels may themselves vary in their recommendations.

Perhaps more troublesome than the consistent promulgation of appropriateness guidelines under conditions of uncertainty is the consistency with which such guidelines, once promulgated, are applied by utilization reviewers. The consistency of UR in rendering authorization decisions is of obvious importance. If a given request for a hospital admission is judged by UR to be clinically unnecessary or medically inappropriate, one would expect the same judgment to be applied to similar cases. Kleinman et al. (32) studied the UR decision-making process for patients with otitis media whose physicians requested pre-certification for the insertion of tympanostomy tubes. Trained nurses compared the clinical characteristics of individual patients to explicit, evidence-based clinical criteria. If a patient's clinical characteristics did not meet appropriateness criteria, then a physician reviewed the case. Kleinman et al. (32) found that physician reviewers often negotiated with the requesting clinician, and that reviewer judgments were often more lenient than explicit appropriateness criteria. Consistent with Kleinman et al.'s (32) findings, in analyzing workers' compensation cases, Wickizer et al. (80) found that initial denials for admission are often reversed when subsequent requests for the same procedure are made on behalf of the same patient. These findings raise questions about the scientific basis of UR and the application of UR criteria to authorize care on an individual case-by-case basis.

Variation in the review styles of utilization review organizations further calls into question the ability of UR to reduce inappropriate practice variation through case-by-case review. A national survey of utilization review organizations found that they varied widely in their denial rates, and that decision-making was significantly influenced by nonclinical considerations, such as financial incentives (57, 84).

Another important question regarding UR concerns the "sentinel effect." Physicians subject to UR may change their clinical practice style knowing that their requests for treatment will be reviewed. Reductions in utilization associated with UR would reflect the combined effect of denials and this sentinel effect. Little direct evidence exists regarding the nature or magnitude of the UR sentinel effect. Wickizer (75) evaluated the effects of a UR program established to review and authorize the use of durable medical equipment for Medicare beneficiaries. This study's findings suggest that the impact of the sentinel effect may be substantial, at least for health care services such as durable medical equipment that are subject to high levels of unnecessary utilization.

In addition to its effects on costs and quality of healthcare, utilization review has had a profound impact on the professional satisfaction of physicians. Recent studies document growing dissatisfaction with the practice of medicine among physicians (18). The growth of managed care with its attendant reliance on utilization management—in particular, utilization review—has significantly contributed to doctor discontent. Both the challenges to physician autonomy (30) and administrative burden inherent in traditional UR are associated with physician dissatisfaction (43). For example, Murray et al. (43) found that 48% of primary care physicians reported spending "an inordinate amount of time seeking plan approval for patient's care." These same physicians reported spending, on average, 2.9 hours per week seeking authorization from plans (43). The potential impact of physician satisfaction on healthcare delivery has not been thoroughly evaluated. However, there is evidence that growing physician dissatisfaction may adversely affect quality of care (18).

Probably the least well understood outcome of utilization review is its effect on overall societal medical costs. As discussed above, UR appears to reduce modestly overall costs of care when analyzed from the perspective of a private payer. However, patients frequently are discharged in need of more intensive and prolonged home or nursing care (34). At some point, the substitution costs associated with caring for sicker, more unstable patients may exceed the cost savings achieved by reducing inpatient utilization (47). Thus it becomes necessary to consider the cost savings generated by utilization management from a social perspective as well as private payer perspective.

FUTURE ROLE FOR UM IN THE HEALTH CARE SYSTEM

For well over a decade, insurance carriers, health plans, employers, and managed care organizations have relied on utilization management to reduce costs and rationalize clinical care. By the mid-1990s, UM was the most widely used cost-containment approach directed at controlling health care utilization. However, UM's rapid and widespread dissemination engendered anger and mistrust among the medical community and patients, causing a backlash that has led to bipartisan support for patient rights legislation at the very moment that managed care organizations are themselves backing away from traditional UM practices.

UM has been disparaged because it was implemented in an uncritical and unregulated manner, was focused on overutilization and cost-containment rather than on quality of care, relied on remote monitoring by sometimes poorly trained personnel, and contributed to the administrative burdens of clinical practice. Yet, health care costs have again begun to climb upward, wide geographical variations in clinical care persist, and there is clear evidence of large gaps in the quality of U.S. healthcare (26, 27).

The pressure to address cost and quality in our healthcare system is, once again, building. With traditional UM on the wane, how will our healthcare system rationalize care and assure its quality? The strengths and weaknesses of traditional UM, along with other evidence-based strategies for managing care and changing physician behavior, provide important insights that can inform the design of new, potentially more effective and acceptable approaches to managing utilization.

Current approaches to utilization management are in large part a response to the nature of our pluralistic and fragmented health care system. At present, UM activities are performed on a case-by-case basis. Moreover, physicians, both in their role as gatekeepers and in response to utilization review inquiries, respond to the individualized requirements of multiple plans. Health plans, for their part, lack robust population-based data on utilization and health outcomes for individual physicians or group practices. Also, because any given plan represents a relatively small proportion of patients for a single physician or group practice, health plans are unable to engage physicians in a systematic and comprehensive approach to utilization management.

Historically, utilization management has not been integrated with quality improvement and outcomes management. Promoting more efficient care will require the integration of UM and quality improvement functions within health plans and delivery systems (2). Moreover, there is a need to find ways to bring together providers, payers, plans, and consumers to foster more collaborative approaches to developing initiatives aimed at enhancing the efficiency and effectiveness of health care delivery. Models for such collaboration exist. For example, in Washington State an ongoing quality improvement initiative was developed through the collaborative efforts of multiple stakeholders to improve the quality and outcomes of occupational health care (76); in Minnesota, health plans have agreed to work collaboratively with the provider community in developing and disseminating a common set of clinical guidelines; and in New England, multiple hospitals worked collaboratively to improve the efficiency and quality of care for patients undergoing coronary artery bypass surgery (45).

In considering future efforts to promote efficient health care through UM, we believe several principles should be followed. These include:

1. UM should be directed at promoting quality of health care, not just containing health care costs. Traditional UM approaches have targeted primarily the overuse of care. But this narrow focus does not address other aspects of care that lead to poor quality. As defined by the IOM (35), quality is "the degree to which health services for individuals and populations increase the likelihood of desired health outcomes and are consistent with current professional knowledge." Schuster et al. (59) emphasize that poor quality can mean too much care, too little care, or the wrong care. UM should provide procedures that can identify, and if possible correct, poor quality for both individual patients and defined populations. Such UM procedures would target not only overuse but also underuse and misuse of care. Further, UM programs should monitor utilization patterns to ensure that efforts to reduce overuse do not lead to adverse health outcomes.

2. UM should be based upon valid and reliable clinical data and/or scientific evidence regarding medical necessity and appropriateness of care. Too often

UM review procedures are based upon inadequate scientific or clinical data. This has created problems for having UM accepted by the medical community and for establishing consistency in review and authorization decisions. To the extent possible, UM should focus attention on those areas of care where the evidence regarding appropriateness and clinical need is most robust. For the areas where evidence is lacking, UM could—and should—play a more active, collaborative role with researchers to advance the state of knowledge. Data gathered by UM programs, if combined with utilization and diagnostic data routinely gathered by health insurance plans, represent a rich source of information that can be used for population-based studies of quality and health outcomes.

3. UM programs and procedures should be designed to minimize administrative burdens on health care providers, health care delivery organizations, and patients. The administrative burden of the U.S. health care system has become intolerable for providers, health care delivery organizations and patients. While much of this burden results from inefficient reimbursement methods used by health insurance plans, UM has contributed significantly to it. As we have previously argued (78, 80), there is little continuing justification for across-the-board review of all patients seeking inpatient hospital care or selected outpatient procedures. Rather, we believe UM should, if conducted on a case-by-case basis, be performed on a targeted basis. Targets for prospective UM review could be defined according to physician utilization profiles, on the basis of patient characteristics, or on the basis of diagnostic criteria, or some combination of these. To the degree that the sentinel effect (75) acts to constrain overuse of care, it is inefficient to perform UM reviews on all cases. Alternatively, UM can be organized to review utilization for some defined population, as is done by disease management programs. The focus here is not on authorizing individual cases for treatment but rather on monitoring a population of patients, e.g., diabetics, to ensure that patients receive needed preventive care and to coordinate acute care.

4. Application of UM procedures should be equitable with regard to ethnicity, income, age, and gender. Relatively little attention to date has been paid to the issue of the equity of UM procedures despite its importance for establishing credibility and acceptance among providers and patients. If providers or patients perceive UM procedures as inequitable, it becomes more difficult to obtain and sustain trust in the review process. The lack of trust can have significant adverse consequences for the operation of UM and creates an atmosphere that invites litigation when disputes over authorization arise.

5. Methods used by UM programs to manage care should be transparent and should uphold the fiduciary responsibility of payers, health plans, and providers toward the patient. UM programs have not been able to secure the trust of patients or providers in part because the review methods and criteria

they use to manage care are not disclosed. In the words of Shapiro & Wenger (60), "The methods of making (utilization management) decisions should be explicit and based on evidence, conflicts of interest should be revealed, and the values of the patients served by the system ... should be addressed."

Ultimately, developing more effective and acceptable strategies for UM will not resolve the fundamental problem our health care system faces. Despite our wealth, we cannot provide all of the health care people want and feel they deserve. The question posed by Victor Fuchs (11) over 25 years ago—"How much care and at what cost?"—remains largely unanswered because so far we have been unwilling to recognize that health and health care, like everything else, involves economic tradeoffs. Improving the efficiency of health care delivery through utilization management, as important as this is, will not solve the dilemma we face. Indeed, this dilemma is likely to become even more difficult in the future as more advanced medical technology and costly pharmaceuticals become available. UM can play an important role in rationalizing care and enhancing efficiency but it cannot, and should not, be asked to do what the public and politicians so far have been unable to do.

ACKNOWLEDGMENTS

The authors wish to thank Anthony Carter and Bert Stover for their assistance in conducting library searches and in organizing the material included in this review article. The research reviewed here that was conducted by Thomas Wickizer was supported by grants from the Robert Wood Johnson Foundation. The opinions and conclusions expressed are those of the authors and do not necessarily represent the views of the Robert Wood Johnson Foundation.

Visit the Annual Reviews home page at www.annualreviews.org

LITERATURE CITED

1. Aubert RE, Herman WH, Waters J, Moore W, Sutton D, et al. 1998. Nurse case management to improve glycemic control in diabetic patients in a health maintenance organization. *Ann. Intern. Med.* 129(8):605–12
2. Audet AM, Scott HD. 1994. The oversight of medical care: a proposal for reform. *Ann. Intern. Med.* 120:423–31
3. Bodenheimer T, Lo B, Casalino L. 1999. Primary care physicians should be coordinators, not gatekeepers. *JAMA* 281(21): 2045–49
4. Bonham GS, Barber GM. 1987. Use of health care before and during Citicare. *Med. Care* 25(2):111–19
5. Boult C, Rassen J, Rassen A, Moore RJ, Robison S. 2000. The effect of case management on the costs of health care for enrollees in Medicare Plus Choice plans: a randomized trial. *J. Am. Geriatr. Soc.* 48(8):996–1001
6. Cheadle A, Wickizer TM, Franklin G, Cain K, Joesch J, et al. 1999. Evaluation of the Washington State Workers' Compensation Managed Care Pilot Project II:

medical and disability costs. *Med. Care* 37(10):982–93

7. Delnoij D, van Merode G, Paulus A, Groenewegen P. 2000. Does general practitioner gatekeeping curb health care expenditure? *J. Health Serv. Res. Policy* 5(1):22–26

8. Feldstein PJ, Wickizer TM, Wheeler JR. 1988. Private cost containment. The effects of utilization review programs on health care use and expenditures. *N. Engl. J. Med.* 318(20):1310–14

9. Ferguson JA, Weinberger M. 1998. Case management programs in primary care. *J. Gen. Intern. Med.* 13(2):123–26

10. Fisher T. 1996. Roles and functions of a case manager. *Am. J. Occup. Ther.* 50(6): 452–54

11. Fuchs VR. 1974. *Who Shall Live? Health, Economics, and Social Choice.* New York: Basic

12. Geary CR, Smeltzer CH. 1997. Case management: past, present, future—the drivers for change. *J. Nurs. Care Qual.* 12(1):9–19

13. Glassman PA, Lopes JH, Witt T. 1997. Using proprietary methods to evaluate acute care admissions to a Veterans Affairs tertiary care center: Are the appropriateness criteria appropriate? *Am. J. Med. Qual.* 12:165–68

14. Goldman RL, Weir CR, Turner CW, Smith CB. 1997. *Am. J. Psychiatry* 154 (3):349–54

15. Grembowski DE, Martin D, Diehr P, Patrick DL, Williams B, et al. 2002. Managed care, access to specialists, and outcomes among primary care patients with pain. *Health Serv. Res.* Submitted

16. Grembowski DE, Martin D, Patrick DL, Diehr P, Katon W, et al. 2002. Managed care, access to mental health specialists, and outcomes among primary care patients with depression symptoms. *J. Gen. Intern. Med.* In press

17. Grumbach K, Selby JV, Damberg C, Bindman AB. 1999. Resolving the gatekeeper conundrum: What patients value in primary care and referrals to specialists. *JAMA* 282(3):261–66

18. Haas JS. 2001. Physician discontent: a barometer of change and need for intervention. *J. Gen. Int. Med.* 16:496–97

19. Halm EA, Causino N, Blumenthal D. 1997. Is gatekeeping better than traditional care? A survey of physicians' attitudes. *JAMA* 278(20):1677–81

20. Hay JA, Maldonado L, Weingarten SR, Ellrodt GA. 1997. Prospective evaluation of a clinical guideline recommending hospital length of stay in upper gastrointestinal tract hemorrhage. *JAMA* 278:2151–56

21. Health Care Financ. Admin. 1979. *Professional Standards Review Organization 1978 Program Evaluation.* Washington, DC: Dep. HEW

22. Health Care Financ. Admin. 1980. *Professional Standards Review Organization 1979 Program Evaluation.* Washington, DC: Dep. HEW

23. Hickey ML, Cook EF, Rossi LP, Connor J, Dutkiewicz C, et al. 2000. Effect of case managers with a general medical patient population. *J. Eval. Clin. Pract.* 6(1):23–29

24. Hurley RE, Freund DA, Gage BJ. 1991. Gatekeeper effects on patterns of physician use. *J. Fam. Pract.* 32(2):167–74

25. Inst. Med. 1989. *Controlling Costs and Changing Patient Care? The Role of Utilization Management.* Washington DC: Natl. Acad. Press

26. Inst. Med. 1999. *To Err Is Human: Building a Safer Health System.* Washington DC: Natl. Acad. Press

27. Inst. Med. 2001. *Crossing the Quality Chasm: A New Health System for the 21st Century.* Washington DC: Natl. Acad. Press

28. Jacob JA. 2000. Physicians still learning about United program. *Am. Med. News,* Sept. 4, p. 23

29. Kerr EA, Mittman BS, Hays RD, Siu AL, Leake B, Brook RH. 1995. Managed care and capitation in California: how do physicians at financial risk control

their own utilization? *Ann. Intern. Med.* 123(7):500–4

30. Kerr EA, Mittman BS, Hays RD, Zemencuk JK, Pitts J, Brook RH. 2000. Associations between primary care physician satisfaction and self-reported aspects of utilization management. *Health Serv. Res.* 35(1):333–49

31. Khandker RK, Manning WG, Ahmed T. 1992. Utilization review savings at the micro level. *Med. Care* 30(11):1043–52

32. Kleinman LC, Boyd EA, Heritage JC. 1997. Adherence to prescribed explicit criteria during utilization review. *JAMA* 278(6):497–501

33. Lessler DS, Wickizer TM. 2000. The impact of utilization management on readmissions among patients with cardiovascular disease. *Health Serv. Res.* 34(6):1315–29

34. LoGerfo JP. 1995. Hospital prospective payment: no skeletons in the closet. *JAMA* 264(15):1995–96

35. Lohr KN, ed. 1990. *Medicare: A Strategy for Quality Assurance.* Washington DC: Natl. Acad. Press

36. Long MJ, Marshall BS. 2000. What price an additional day of life? A cost-effectiveness study of case management. *Am. J. Manage. Care.* 6(8):881–86

37. Long SH, Settle RF. 1988. An evaluation of Utah's primary care case management program for Medicaid recipients. *Med. Care* 26(11):1021–32

38. Manning WG, Leibowitz A, Goldberg GA, Rogers WH, Newhouse JP. 1984. A controlled trial of the effect of a prepaid group practice on use of services. *N. Engl. J. Med.* 310(23):1505–10

39. Martin DP, Diehr P, Price KF, Richardson WC. 1989. Effect of a gatekeeper plan on health services use and charges: a randomized trial. *Am. J. Public Health* 79(12):1628–32

40. Meredith JW, Burney R, Burton S. 1999. Milliman and Robertson length of stay guidelines are not appropriate for trauma

patients: a comparison with the NTDB. *J. Trauma* 47:208

41. Milstein A. 1997. Managing utilization management: a purchaser's view. *Health Aff.* 16(3):87–90

42. Moore SH, Martin DP, Richardson WC. 1983. Does the primary-care gatekeeper control the costs of health care? *N. Engl. J. Med.* 309(22):1400–4

43. Murray A, Montgomery JE, Chang H, Rogers WH, Inui T, Safran DG. 2001. Doctor discontent: A comparison of physician satisfaction in different delivery system settings. *J. Gen. Intern. Med.* 16:451–59

44. Naylor M, Brooten D, Jones R, Lavizzo-Mourey R, Mezey M, Pauly M. 1994. Comprehensive discharge planning for the hospitalized elderly. *Ann. Intern. Med.* 120(12):999–1006

45. O'Connor GT, Plume SK, Olmstead EM, Morton JR, Maloney CT, et al. 1996. A regional intervention to improve the hospital mortality associated with coronary artery bypass graft surgery. The Northern New England Cardiovascular Disease Study Group. *JAMA* 275(11):841–46

46. Pear R. 2001. States dismayed by federal bills on patient rights. *New York Times*, Aug. 13, p. A1

47. Reinhardt UE. 1996. Spending more through 'cost control': our obsessive quest to gut the hospital. *Health Aff. (Millwood)* 15:145–54

48. Remler DK, Donelan K, Blendon RJ, Lundberg GD, Leape LL, et al. 1997. What do managed care plans do to affect care? Results from a survey of physicians. *Inquiry* 34(3):196–204

49. Reynolds S, Smeltzer CH. 1997. Case management: past, present, future—the drivers for change. *J. Nurs. Care Qual.* 12(1):9–19

50. Rich MW, Beckham V, Wittenberg C, Leven CL, Freedland KE, Carney RM. 1995. A multidisciplinary intervention to prevent the readmission of elderly patients

with congestive heart failure. *N. Engl. J. Med.* 333(18):1190–95

51. Rich MW, Vinson JM, Sperry JC, Shah AS, Spinner LR, et al. 1993. Prevention of readmission in elderly patients with congestive heart failure: results of a prospective, randomized pilot study. *J. Gen. Intern. Med.* 8:585–90

52. Robinson JC. 2001. The end of managed care. *JAMA* 285(20):2622–28

53. Rosenberg SN, Allen DR, Handte JS, Jackson TC, Leto L, et al. Effect of utilization review in a fee-for-service health insurance plan. *N. Engl. J. Med.* 333(20): 1326–30

54. Rutledge R. 1998. An analysis of 25 Milliman & Robertson guidelines for surgery: data-driven versus consensus-derived clinical practice guidelines. *Ann. Surg.* 228(4):579–87

55. Scheffler RM, Sullivan SD, Ko TM. 1991. The impact of Blue Cross and Blue Shield Plan utilization management programs, 1980–1988. *Inquiry* 28(3):263–75

56. Schillinger D, Bibbins-Domingo K, Vranizan K, Bacchetti P, Luce JM, Bindman AB. 2000. Effects of primary care coordination on public hospital patients. *J. Gen. Intern. Med.* 15(5):329–36

57. Schlesinger MJ, Gray BH, Perreira KM. 1997. Medical professionalism under managed care: the pros and cons of utilization review. *Health Aff. (Millwood)* 16:106–24

58. Schore JL, Brown RS, Cheh VA. 1999. Case management for high-cost Medicare beneficiaries. *Health Care Financ. Rev.* 20(4):87–101

59. Schuster MA, McGlynn EA, Brook RH. How good is the quality of health care in the United States? *Milbank Q.* 76(4):517–63

60. Shapiro MF, Wenger NS. 1995. Rethinking utilization review. *N. Engl. J. Med.* 333(20):1326–30

61. Shekelle PG, Kahan JP, Bernstein SJ, Leape LL, Kamberg CJ, Park RE. 1998. The reproducibility of a method to identify the overuse and underuse of medical procedures. *N. Engl. J. Med.* 338(26):1888–95

61a. Shekelle PG, Ortiz E, Rhodes S, Morton SC, Eccles MP, et al. 2001. Validity of the Agency for Healthcare Research in Quality clinical practice guidelines: how quickly do guidelines become outdated? *JAMA* 286(12):146–67

62. Sills MR, Huang ZJ, Cheng S, Guagliardo MF, Chamberlain JM, Jill J. 2000. Pediatric Milliman and Robertson length-of-stay criteria: Are they realistic? *Pediatrics* 105(4):733–37

63. Smith JE. 1998. Case management: a literature review. *Can. J. Nurs. Adm.* 11(2):93–108

64. St. Peter RF, Reed MC, Kemper P, Blumenthal D. 1999. Changes in the scope of care provided by primary care physicians. *N. Engl. J. Med.* 341:1980–85

65. Strumwasser I, Paranjpe NV, Ronis DL, Share D, Sell LJ. 1990. Reliability and validity of utilization review criteria. *Med. Care* 28(2):95–111

66. Tischler GL. 1990. Utilization management and the quality of care. *Hosp. Community Psychiatry* 41(10):1099–102

67. Topol EJ, Burek K, O'Neill WW, Kewman DG, Kander NH, Shea MJ. 1988. A randomized controlled trial of hospital discharge three days after myocardial infarction in the era of reperfusion. *N. Engl. J. Med.* 318:1083–88

68. URAC/Am. Accred. HealthCare Comm. 2000. *The Utilization Management Guide.* Washington, DC: Am. Accred. HealthCare Comm. 2nd ed.

69. Vertrees JC, Manton KG, Mitchell KC. 1989. Case-mix adjusted analyses of service utilization for a Medicaid health insuring organization in Philadelphia. *Med. Care* 27(4):397–411

70. Wagner EH, Austin BT, Von Korff M. 1996. Improving outcomes in chronic illness. *Manag. Care Q.* 4(2):12–25

71. Weingarten S, Riedinger MS, Sandhu M, Bowers C, Ellrodt G, et al. 1998. Can

practice guidelines safely reduce hospital length of stay? Results from a multicenter interventional study. *Am. J. Med.* 105:33–40

72. Wheeler JR, Wickizer TM. 1990. Relating health care market characteristics to the effectiveness of utilization review programs. *Inquiry* 27(4):344–51

73. Wickizer TM. 1990. The effect of utilization review on hospital use and expenditures: a review of the literature and an update on recent findings. *Med. Care Rev.* 47(3):327–63

74. Wickizer TM. 1992. The effects of utilization review on hospital use and expenditures: a covariance analysis. *Health Serv. Res.* 27(1):103–21

75. Wickizer TM. 1995. Controlling outpatient medical equipment costs through utilization management. *Med. Care* 33(4):383–91

76. Wickizer TM, Franklin G, Plaeger-Brockway R, Mootz RD. 2001. Improving the quality of workers' compensation health care delivery: the Washington State Occupational Health Services Project. *Milbank Q.* 79(1):5–33

77. Wickizer TM, Lessler D. 1998. Do treatment restrictions imposed by utilization management increase the likelihood of readmission for psychiatric patients? *Med. Care* 36(6):844–50

78. Wickizer TM, Lessler D. 1998. Effects of utilization management on patterns of hospital care among privately insured adult patients. *Med. Care* 36(11):1545–54

79. Wickizer TM, Lessler D, Boyd-Wickizer J. 1999. Effects of health care cost-containment programs on patterns of care and readmissions among children and adolescents. *Am. J. Public Health* 89(9):1353–58

80. Wickizer TM, Lessler D, Franklin G. 1999. Controlling workers' compensation medical care use and costs through utilization management. *JOEM* 41(8):625–31

81. Wickizer TM, Wheeler JR, Feldstein PJ. 1989. Does utilization review reduce unnecessary hospital care and contain costs? *Med. Care* 27(6):632–47

82. Wickizer TM, Wheeler JR, Feldstein PJ. 1991. Have hospital inpatient cost containment programs contributed to the growth in outpatient expenditures? Analysis of the substitution effect associated with hospital utilization review. *Med. Care* 29(5):442–51

83. Wickizer TM, Lessler D, Travis KM. 1996. Controlling inpatient psychiatric utilization through managed care. *Am. J. Psychiatry* 153(3):339–45

84. Wolff N, Schlesinger M. 1998. Risk, motives, and styles of utilization review: a cross-condition comparison. *Soc. Sci. Med.* 47:911–26

Annu. Rev. Public Health 2002. 23:255–86

DIETARY INTERVENTIONS TO PREVENT DISEASE

Deborah J. Bowen[1,2] and Shirley A. A. Beresford[1,2]

[1]*Fred Hutchinson Cancer Research Center, 1100 Fairview Avenue North, MP 900, Seattle, Washington 98109-1024; e-mail: dbowen@fhcrc.org*
[2]*University of Washington, Departments of Health Services (DJB) and Epidemiology (SAAB), Seattle, Washington 98195-7236*

Key Words nutrition intervention, chronic disease prevention

■ **Abstract** Changing dietary behaviors to prevent chronic disease has been an important research focus for the last 25 years. Here we present a review of published articles on the results of research to identify methods to change key dietary habits: fat intake, fiber intake, and consumption of fruits and vegetables. We divided the research reviewed into sections, based on the channel through which the intervention activities were delivered. We conclude that the field is making progress in identifying successful dietary change strategies, but that more can be learned. Particularly, we need to transfer some of the knowledge from the individual-based trials to community-level interventions. Also, more research with rigorous methodology must be done to test current and future intervention options.

INTRODUCTION

Rationale for Changing Dietary Behaviors to Prevent Disease

Differences in people's dietary intake are thought to account for more variation in cancer incidence than any other factor, including cigarette smoking (112, 123). Most of the supporting scientific evidence comes from observational studies, including aggregate population studies (52, 80). Carefully conducted epidemiological observational studies, both prospective and case-control, show repeatedly that dietary factors are associated with several chronic diseases, including coronary heart disease, some types of cancer, stroke, and non-insulin dependent diabetes, and thereby contribute substantially to the burden of preventable illness (31, 36, 41, 48, 49, 54, 59, 67, 79, 86, 89, 94, 101, 111, 118, 122). Although there are exceptions (37, 51, 63, 64, 93, 102, 121), these studies are consistent in pointing to the roles of fat, fruits, and vegetables. However, a recent randomized controlled trial of low-fat, high-fiber dietary intervention failed to find benefit in lowering incidence of recurrent adenomas (88). The scientific consensus remains supportive of the contention that a comprehensive approach to improving dietary lifestyle choices is warranted, and dietary change remains an important behavior

0163-7525/02/0510-0255$14.00

to target for preventing cancer and is a major component of the Healthy People 2010 goals (114). It follows that dietary interventions on a population-wide basis are advisable (71).

Rationale for the Literature Review

Many investigators have designed, implemented, and evaluated dietary change interventions targeting these critical nutrients. Although some changes have been made in the general public, the levels of fat, fruit, and vegetable consumption still fall short of goals in the areas of dietary fat intake and daily servings of fruits and vegetables, for example (55). We must identify successful methods of changing dietary behaviors to prevent disease in order to implement them as part of standard public health and primary care medical practice. Several reviews have been published in the past 15 years on the best methods of intervening in dietary behaviors in several areas of public health activity, such as cholesterol-lowering trials (107), worksites (38), patient education (92), cardiovascular disease prevention trials (23, 113), interventions in whole communities (42), and environmental influences (34). However, this disparate literature has not been pulled together. We have conducted this information synthesis to fill in this gap.

Criteria for the Literature Search

We used an initial electronic search to generate a list of references, followed by the application of a series of criteria that were best applied by hand. The electronic search was done with Medline, using the dates 1966 through April 2001, inclusive. The search terms were: (*a*) at least one key nutrition-related term (diet, dietary, eating, food, food habits, nutrition) as either a key word or an abstract/title inclusion and (*b*) intervention either as a key word or as an abstract/title inclusion. Only English-language articles were reviewed. This search produced 5399 articles. We then applied the following rules of exclusion to the list, using a hand search:

- The study had to report at least one dietary intake or dietary behavior outcome related to fat, fruits and vegetables, or fiber;
- The study had to report the testing of an intervention;
- The participants recruited into the study were healthy free-living adults;
- Weight loss could not be communicated to the participants as the main study goal.

Where studies were reported in more than one article, we chose a single article that presented behavior-related outcome data to report in the review. Taken together, these processes produced 80 studies reviewed for this paper.

Structure of the Review

Here we refer to the "channel" of intervention to describe the place or structure through which the intervention is mainly delivered. Interventions to decrease fat intake are often accompanied by strategies to increase fiber through fruits, vegetables, and whole grains. Some interventions specifically targeted increasing fruit and vegetable intake. In this review, we have not specifically separated studies focusing on only one of these related behaviors (decreasing fat and increasing fruit, vegetables, and whole grains) from those that target all of them. Lack of mention of change in a particular behavior usually means that behavior was not a focus of the intervention and was not assessed. Some studies (e.g., 24, 43) found changes in one dietary behavior and not another, and these discordant results are noted.

We structured the review into sections, grouped by the intervention channel used in the study. First we present a review of individual randomized trials and other individual-level intervention studies that included healthy individuals or individuals at risk for development of disease. Next we present intervention studies focused on family, providers, and community organizations. We then review the evidence for worksite interventions and point-of-purchase interventions. Finally, we review the interventions where entire communities are the channel or unit of focus. We provide somewhat more detail concerning the larger studies that used channels other than the individual. In parallel with this organization, we included the literature in three tables, arranged alphabetically by first author: interventions with individuals (Table 1), interventions using community channels (Table 2), and interventions on whole communities (Table 3). We end with conclusions drawn from our review of the literature and our suggestions for future research in this area.

INDIVIDUAL RANDOMIZED TRIALS

Many individual-randomized studies have been conducted to test the feasibility of making large changes in the dietary habits of healthy individuals. Individuals were recruited who were interested in and able to make large sustained changes in dietary intake in order to test disease-related hypotheses over years of study. The Women's Health Trial found that women aged 55–79 made and maintained large changes, reducing consumption from 39% to 22% daily energy as fat in their dietary fat as a result of a multicomponent group intervention (7, 119), and this finding was consistent with a randomized study in Canada (8). A related study tested the feasibility of dietary fat reduction in a multiethnic, multi-income sample and found large significant changes in dietary fat intake at one-year post randomization (17). A large randomized trial of nutritional counseling in middle-aged men (MRFIT) produced long-term sustained effects in fat and saturated fat intake (40). Smaller-scale studies, with diverse interventions aimed at large changes, have found similar large effects on dietary intake (4, 19, 66).

Other interventions have focused on producing small changes in a more general group of participants, not selected for any ability or interest to change dietary behaviors, through tailoring materials to the personal characteristics of the participants. Lutz et al. tested the effects of tailored versus nontailored newsletters in increasing fruit and vegetable consumption (62). Receipt of a tailored session

TABLE 1 Individual intervention studies to change dietary behaviors

Author	Intervention channel	Model	Study design	Strategies of intervention	Length of intervention/ follow-up[a]	Source of evaluation participants	Demos. of sample	Outcome
Anderson 2001	Individual	None listed	Quasi-experimental (including 2 randomized groups)	Coupon and educational groups	One session/ 2 months	564 WIC participants	49% white female	Coupons and education groups increased fruit and vegetable consumption
Bemelmans 2000	Individual	None listed	Quasi-experimental	Nutritional counseling in Mediterranean diet	2 months/1 year	266 participants within select counties serum cholesterol between 6 and 8 m mol/l and >2 CVD risk factors	Average age 55 years 63% female	Small changes in total and saturated fat intake
Boyd 1997	Individual	None listed	Randomized trial	Nutrition counseling	2 years[a]	220 premenopausal women with high breast densities from mammogram clinics	Female Average age 42 years	Large reductions in fat consumption, relative to control
Brinberg 2000	Individual	Behavioral alternatives model	Randomized trial	Tailored print messages versus general message with and without feedback versus control	Single exposure/ 7 months	168 college students	Adults 56% female	Increases in recommended fiber containing foods and in fiber consumption
Brug 1996	Individual	TTM Others	Randomized trial	Tailored feedback; written materials	2 weeks/6 weeks	347 employees of oil company	Average age 44 years 81% female	Significant reduction in fat for intervention ppts.
Campbell 1994	Individual	TTM Health belief model	Randomized trial of patients	Tailored printed nutrition information	One mailing/ 4 months	558 patients in 4 primary care practices	43% female	Significant changes in fat and saturated fat

Study	Level	Theory	Design	Intervention	Duration	Sample	Population	Results
Coates 1999	Individual	None listed	Randomized trial of women	Group interventions and written materials	18 months[a]	2208 women from 3 cities	Female aged 50–79 years	Large changes in dietary fat intake
Cox 1995	Individual	Health belief model	Quasi-experimental	Cancer prevention lessons (EFNEP)	10–13 lessons/ 6 months	339 women in 3 counties, 1 city	Female aged 20–45 years Low education	Decrease in fat and increase in fiber
Cox 1998	Individual	None	Randomized trial	Nutritional counseling	8 weeks[a]	170 community members from 2 cities eating <5/veg/day	Average age 35 years 74% female	Large changes in F/V intake and in fat intake in individuals with high-fat intake at baseline
Cupples 1999	Individual	None	Randomized trial	Personalized health promotion	2 years/5 years	688 patients under 75 with angina from 18 general practices	Average age 63 years 59% male	Significant improvement in reported diet at 2 years No significant difference at 5 years
Gorder 1997 MRFIT	Individual	None	Randomized trial	Nutrition counseling	6–8 years/6 years	12,866 men at high risk of coronary heart disease in 22 clinical centers	Male aged 35–57 years 8% black	Significant decrease in fat, saturated fat and high-fat foods.
Hartman 1997	Individual	None listed	Randomized trial of educators	Self-help materials Group sessions	10 sessions/ 8 weeks	204 Expanded Food and Nutrition Program participants working with 16 educators	Females EFNEP participants	Significant changes in FFB Nonsignificant changes in 24 h fat intake

(*Continued*)

TABLE 1 (*Continued*)

Author	Intervention channel	Model	Study design	Strategies of intervention	Length of intervention/ follow-up[a]	Source of evaluation participants	Demos. of sample	Outcome
Havas 1998	Individual and small group	TTM	Randomized crossover design of WIC sites	Messages about change Three group sessions Tailored letters	4 months/ 6 months	3122 WIC recipients in 16 sites	Female	Larger increases in fruit and vegetable servings in intervention period then in control period
Heller 1994	Individual	None	Randomized trial	Self-help print materials Referral to physician and checklist for action	Multiple mailed contacts/ 6 months	342 relatives of heart attack survivors	Adult siblings and children of patients	Significant decreases in fat score for self-help materials compared to physician referral and to control
Hjermann 1986 Oslo Study	Individual	None	Randomized trial	Nutrition counseling	5 years/8–5 years	1232 men with high cholesterol	Adult Male aged 40–69 years	Significant decreases in serum cholesterol
King 1999	Individual	None	Quasi-experimental (4 treatment groups)	Nutritional counseling	4 weeks[a]	80 men in primary care clinics	Average age 47 years	Greater decrease in fat consumption in group allowed to eat pre-intervention number of meals
Lawton 1998	Individual	None	Randomized counterbalanced design	Provision of low-fat snacks	3 weeks each	36 community members who snack frequently	50% female Aged 17–44 years	Reductions in fat intake with low-fat snacks
Lutz 1999	Individual	Social cognitive theory TTM	Randomized trial	Newsletters Tailoring Goal setting	4 monthly newsletters/ 6 months	710 HMO participants	65% female Average age 39 years 78% white	Significant increases in F/V intake in all intervention groups
Marcus 1998	Individual	TTM	Randomized trial by day of week	Telephone counseling by CIS specialists	1 telephone call, 2 mailings/ 4 weeks	276 callers to the Cancer Information Service in 5 offices	80% female 89% white	Significant increases in F/V intake

Study	Level	Theory	Design	Intervention	Duration	Sample	Demographics	Results
Mascarene 1999	Individual	None	Randomized trial	Dietary counseling Group meetings	6 months[a]	33 women from ongoing observational study with low F/V intake	Age 35+ years Average age 49 years Female	Significant increase in F/V intake Lower fat (at 3 months only)
Mhurchu 1998	Individual	Motivational interviewing	Randomized trial of 2 interventions	Nutritional counseling	3 months[a]	121 patients with hyperlipidemia	48% female	No significant influence of motivational interviewing on reductions in fat intake
Naslund 1996	Individual	None listed	Randomized factorial trial (exercise, diet)	Nutritional counseling, written materials	2 sessions/ 6 months	158 men with CHD risk factors	Adult male Aged 35–60 years	Changes in fat and fiber intake in smokers and nonsmokers
Nelson 1991	Individual	Behavioral therapy	Case study	Therapeutic sessions	5 months[a]	One patient in therapy	Average age 41 years Female	Changes in fruit and vegetable consumption
Ornish 1998	Individual	None listed	Randomized trial	Prescription dietary plans, classes	5 years[a]	48 patients with CVD risk factors in 2 medical centers	Average age 59 years 9% female	Significant large improvements in dietary fat, compared to control
Reid 1995	Individual	None	Randomized trial of 2 interventions	Community screening, group versus pamphlet intervention	6 months[a]	164 individuals at community health centers and worksites with moderate CVD risk	Average age 40 years 33% female	Improvement in eating fat on meat in group counseling condition, but no differential changes in CVD risk factors

(*Continued*)

TABLE 1 (*Continued*)

Author	Intervention channel	Model	Study design	Strategies of intervention	Length of intervention/ follow-up[a]	Source of evaluation participants	Demos. of sample	Outcome
Reynolds 1997	Individuals at worksites	None	Randomized trial within worksites plus control worksites	Cholesterol screening plus education plus dietary change kit	One screening plus dietary change kit/6 months	635 employees at 6 worksites	Average age 41 years 56% female	Both interventions reduced servings of fat-containing foods compared to control
Rhodes 1996	Individual	Nutritional counseling	Randomized trial	Shopping guide Videotape Dietician consultations	1–7 weeks/3 months	104 outpatients or community residents at risk for CVD	50% female Average age 47 years 94% white	Significant reductions in dietary fat and cholesterol in dietician led arms
Siero 2000	Individual	TTM	Randomized trial	Group nutrition sessions Tailored letters	3 two-hour sessions/ 16 weeks	262 members of public at risk for CVD in 2 counties	55% female 85% low SES	Significant increases in fish, F/V consumption in both intervention groups, compared to control
Simkin-Silverman 1998	Individual	None	Randomized trial	Group meetings	18 months[a]	489 premenopausal women	Female Aged 44–50 years	Significant reductions in fat and saturated fat intake
Steptoe 1999	Individual	TTM	Randomized trial of practices	Individual counseling sessions (nurses) for those with high blood cholesterol	Three sessions/ 12 months	520 patients in 20 primary care practices	55% female Average age 52 years	Significant decreases in dietary fat consumption No change in serum cholesterol
Stockbridge 1989	Individual	None	Post-test only	Educational mailing Cholesterol hotline	1 month[a]	507 individuals from public screening with high cholesterol	Adults	Reports of dietary changes after screening

Study	Level	Theory	Study design	Intervention components	Duration/follow-up	Sample/setting	Demographics	Results
Strychar 1998	Individual	None	Randomized trial of cholesterol results/before-after study	Cholesterol results / Dietician consultations / Booklet	1–7 weeks/ 16–20 weeks	500 maintenance workers at 6 hospitals	34% female / Average age 50 years / 94% white	No significant changes attributable to cholesterol results being given / Significant reductions in dietary fat and cholesterol in both arms
Taylor-Davis 2000	Individual	Adult learning theory / Other	Randomized trial	Newsletters	10 weeks[a], five newsletters	386 Medicare recipients from one medical center	Average age 69 years / 43% female	Significant increases in avoiding fat
Toobert 2000	Individual	None listed	Randomized trial	7-day retreat / Group session	24 months*	28 postmenopausal women with coronary heart disease	Female / Average age 64 years	Significant changes in fat and saturated fat consumption
Wang 1999	Individual	None listed	Before-after design	Cholesterol screening / Education / Physician referral	One visit	1957 employees at 33 worksites with high cholesterol	80% white / 47% female	Self-reported changes in fat consumption in those with baseline high-fat intake
White 1994 WHT	Individual	SLT / Cognitive-behavioral theory / Self-control theory	Randomized trial	Group sessions / Self-monitoring tools / Nutrition and behavioral strategies	5–37 months/ 1 year beyond intervention end	1050 women at increased risk of breast cancer in 3 clinical centers	Female aged 45–69 years / Average age 54 years	No added benefit of physician visit / Significant, large reductions in fat intake, maintained for at least a year after intervention

[a]Length of follow-up is the same as the length of intervention unless specified.

Abbreviations: Demos, demographics; F/V, fruit and vegetable; MRFIT, Multiple Risk Factor Intervention Trial; WHT, Womens Health Trial.

TABLE 2 Channel-level intervention studies to change dietary behavior

Author	Intervention channel	Model	Study design	Strategies of intervention	Length of intervention/ follow-up[a]	Source of evaluation participants	Demos. of sample	Outcome
Anderson 1999	Worksites	No listing	Randomized trial of workers	Sessions and self-help program	12 months[a]	234 employees at 8 worksites with high serum cholesterol	45% female	No differences among intervention conditions
Baer 1993	Worksite	None specified	Individuals Concurrent controls	Screening, counseling	12 months[a]	70 management level employees with high Tg	Male	Reduced calories from fat
Beresford 1997 Eating Patterns Study	Primary care practices	Social learning theory	Randomized trial of practices	Self-help materials Provider encouragement	One brief encounter with reminder letter/ 12 months	2111 Patients in 28 primary care practices	68% female	Significant decreases in fat behaviors, increases in fiber behaviors
Beresford 2001 5-a-Day	Worksites	Trans-theoretical model	Randomized trial of worksites	Environmental and individual level change	12 months/ 24 months	2828 Employees in 28 worksites	51% female Average age 41 years 87% white	Significant increase in fruit and vegetable consumption
Braeckman 1999	Worksites	None	Randomized worksites Individual level analysis	Health risk appraisal Group sessions Environment changes	3 months[a]	770 employees in 4 worksites	Average age 43 years	Significant reductions in fat and calorie intake (ignoring worksite autocorrelation)
Buller 1999 5-a-Day	Small cliques in worksites	None listed	Randomized trial of social networks	Peer educator messages	18 months/ 2 years	997 employees in 92 social networks from 10 public employers	46% white 76% male Average income $16,000	More fruit and vegetable servings
Campbell 1999 5-a-Day	Religious organizations	Ecological	Randomized trial of counties	Church wide activities Tailored bulletins	20 months/ 2 years	2519 members of 50 Black churches in 10 rural counties	98% black	Increased servings fruit and vegetable
Connell 2001	Grocery stores	None listed	Randomized trial of grocery stores	Audiotape and written intervention activities	4 weeks[a]	682 Shopper surveys in 6 stores	81% female Average age 44 years	Increases in fruit and vegetable intake

Study	Setting	Theory/model	Design	Intervention	Duration/follow-up	Sample	Population	Results
Emmons 1999 Working Healthy Project (part of WWT)	Worksites	Participatory strategies model	Randomized trial	Worksite events, Materials, Programs, Contests, Point-of-purchase, Policy	2 and one half years[a]	2055 employees in 26 manufacturing worksites	Adults	Significant increase in fruit/vegetables; No other changes significant
Evans 1996	Physicians	None	Randomized trial	Training in counseling, Cue via finger stick	One visit/10 months	254 patients in 7 primary care practices	68% female, 57% Caucasian	No significant changes in blood cholesterol
Finckenor 2000	Classes of nutrition students	TTM	Quasi-experimental	Group classes	11 weekly sessions/1 year	110 students in 5 sections of nutrition classes	Average age 23 years, 80% female	Significant changes in fat intake at one year
Frack 1997	Classroom setting	None	Quasi-experimental	Nutrition sessions	Unknown/6 months	338 students in ESL classes in 3 adult education centers	50% female, Non-English speaking	Higher fat avoidance in the groups complying with follow-up physical measures
French 1997	Vending machines	None	Before-after study	Increased availability of low-fat snacks through vending machines	3 weeks[a]	9 vending machines in 4 locations in university setting	Unknown	Increases in purchases of low-fat snacks during intervention only
French 2001	Vending machines	None	Randomized trial Factorial design	Decreased relative pricing of low-fat snacks through vending machines, Signs	1 month[a]	75 vending machines in 12 secondary schools and 12 worksites	Unknown	Increases in purchases of low-fat snacks
Fries 1999	Worksite	Community organization	Before-after study	Advisory board, Dietary information, Print materials, Nutrition seminar, Kiosk	9 months/1 year	184 employees of 1 worksite	Average age 42 years, 51% female, 60% African American	Increases in fruit and vegetable consumption
Glasgow 1995 Take Heart program	Worksites	TTM	Randomized trial	Orientation, Events, Feedback, Contests, Changes in offerings	2 years[a]	Two cross-sections of about 2700 employees in 26 worksites	Adults	No significant differences in dietary outcomes using worksite means

(Continued)

TABLE 2 (*Continued*)

Author	Intervention channel	Model	Study design	Strategies of intervention	Length of intervention/ follow-up[a]	Source of evaluation participants	Demos. of sample	Outcome
Howard-Pitney 1997	Vocation training and general education classes	None	Randomized trial of classes	Interactive learning Classes Maintenance sessions	18 weeks/ 5 months	351 participants in 24 classes in 6 community settings	86% female 20% white 63% low income	Significant differences in fat and saturated fat
Jeffery 1982	Supermarkets	None	Randomized trial (supermarkets)	Print materials	6 months[a]	200 shoppers in 8 supermarkets (2 cross-sections)	75% female	No significant differences in dietary behaviors between groups
Kreuter 2000	Primary care providers	None	Randomized trial	Materials Physician advice	1 session/ 3 months	496 adult patients in 4 family medicine clinics	Average age 49 years 76% female 98% white	Changes in dietary fat from dairy sources in groups receiving physician advice
Kristal 1997	Grocery stores	Consumer information processing model	Randomized trial (supermarkets)	Supermarket flyers, store signage, activities in stores	8 months/ 1 year	960 exit interviews and take-home surveys in 8 supermarkets (2 cross-sections)	84% women Age distributed across 18– 65+ years	No significant differences in fruit and vegetable changes
Kumar 1993	Classrooms	Educational theory	Randomized trial	Computer assisted learning sessions in classrooms	1 session/ 7 weeks	92 college students	Age over 18 68% female	Significant differences at posttest in reduction in fat grams and calories
Nader 1992 Family Health Project	Families	Social learning theory, self-management	Randomized trial of families	Group sessions	12 week groups of sessions/ 48 months	206 families	Parents of children Low to middle income	Improved eating habits at 24 months, not present at 48 month follow-up
Oshaug 1995	Worksites	None	Secular change study	Self-help materials	7 years/8 years	530 volunteers in 2 cross-sectional surveys from 3 offshore oil platforms	Male Average age 38 years	Reduced fat consumption, overtime-only part of change attributable to intervention
Resnicow 1998	Schools as worksites	None	Randomized trial of elementary schools	Self-help materials Workshops Campaigns on Teacher Wellness	2 years[a]	2 cross-sectional surveys each of 240 teachers of 32 elementary schools	98% female Average age 38 years 74% white	No differences in dietary behaviors

Study	Setting	Theory	Design	Intervention	Duration/follow-up	Sample	Demographics	Results
Sasaki 1999	Worksites	None	Control group, but not comparable	Nutritional counseling	12 weekly sessions/ 6 months	80 employees at 1 worksite at risk of coronary heart disease and 169 controls	Male Average age 44 years	Significant reductions in fat, and increases in fiber, vegetables at 6 months post randomization
Sorensen 1992 Treatwell	Worksites	None listed	Randomized trial of worksites	Classes, demonstrations Point-of-purchase labeling	1 year[a]	275 employees from each of 16 worksites	53% female Adults	Significant reductions in fat intake
Sorensen 1996 Working Well	Worksites	Individual organizational and community activation	Randomized trial	Cafeteria offering changes Print materials Worksite-wide events Contests	2 years[a]	28,000 employee surveys from 111 worksites	Adults	Significant reductions in fat, and increases in fiber and fruits and vegetables
Sorensen 1999 Treatwell 5 A Day	Worksites	Socio-ecological	Randomized trial of two interventions	Community organizing Discussion series Educational campaigns Learn-at-home materials Family newsletter	2 years[a]	1359 individuals in cohort from 22 community health centers	Adults 17–75 years 84% female 44% college grad	Significant increase in fruit and vegetables
Sorensen 1998 Wellworks	Worksite wide	Multiple	Randomized trial	Worksite-wide activities Family-based intervention	19.5 months/ 2 years	2658 employees in 24 worksites who formed cohort within 2 cross-sections	Adults 24% female	Significant reduction in fat intake, increase in fiber and in fruit/vegetables
Tilley 1999 Next Step Trial	Worksites	TTM Social cognitive theory Social support	Randomized trial of worksites	Self-help materials Classes Tailored feedback	2 years[a]	2765 employees in 28 worksites	4% female 96% white	Significant changes in fat, fruit and vegetable consumption at one year only. Increase fiber at 2 years
Wiesemann 1997	Providers	Three level strategy	Before-after design	Dietary advice Exercise classes Community setting support	4 years[a]	4881 residents in 7 primary care practices in one community	53% female	No significant changes in cholesterol. Reported increases in healthy nutrition

[a]Length of follow-up is the same as the length of intervention unless specified.

Abbreviations: Demos, demographics; F/V, fruit and vegetable; MRFIT, Multiple Risk Factor Intervention Trial; WHT, Women's Health Trial.

TABLE 3 Community intervention studies to change dietary behaviors

Author	Intervention channel	Model	Study design	Strategies of intervention	Length of intervention/ follow-up[a]	Source of evaluation participants	Demos of sample	Outcome
Brownson 1996	Community	SLT, TTM, other	Control group, but not comparable	Coalitions, gatherings, media efforts, classes, clubs, etc	4 years[a]	1510 residents in 6 counties	65% female 92% white	No significant change in % consuming 5+ fruit/vegetables daily
Cheadle 1995	Community	None	Quasi-experimental (9 of 10 were randomized)	Materials Activities Screenings	4 years[a]	500 residents in 11 communities and 15–27 grocery stores per community	Adults	No consistent changes (community means compared)
Farquar 1977 Stanford 3 Community Study	Community	Health education	Quasi-experimental	Mass media Personal counseling of high risk	2 years[a]	Cohort and cross-sectional surveys in 2 intervention and 1 control community	Aged 12–74 years Male	Improved fat consumption
Foerster 1995 5 A Day	Media, grocery stores	Social marketing	Case study	Media activities Point-of-purchase labels	18 months/ 2 years	1000 adults in 2 cross-sectional surveys in California	Adults	Significant increases fruit and vegetables
Fortmann 1995 Stanford 5 City Project	Community	Social learning theory	Quasi-experimental	Mass media Community organization	6 years/4 years and 5 years	22,000 adults in cross-sectional surveys from 5 cities	Aged 12– 74 years	Significantly larger decreases in serum cholesterol
Luepker 1994 Minnesota Heart Health Project	Community	SLT, other	Quasi-experimental	Community organizing, mass media, health professional training, screening, education	6 years[a]	Cohort and cross-sectional surveys from 3 pairs of communities	Adults 25– 74 years	No sustained differential change in total cholesterol

	Neighborhood	Theory	Study design	Intervention	Length	Sample	Demographics	Results
O'Loughlin 1997	Neighborhood	Precede proceed, others	Case study Post measure only	Community events, labeling in shops and restaurants, social activities and contests	18 months[a]	345 households in urban community	Average age 37 years 48% female	About 30% reported trying suggestions for preparing low-fat meals
Osler 1993	Community	SLT	Case study of one community	Mass media	12 months	1010 and 1092 residents in 2 cross-sectional surveys	42% female Adult	Some decrease in eating fat
Reger 2000	Community	None	Quasi-experimental	Public relations Community education vs. paid advertising vs. control	Up to 8 weeks[a]	Cohort of 1232 population-based telephone surveys in 3 cities	66% female 23% college degree	Increased low-fat milk consumption compared to control, with significantly greater increase in the community education city
Sogaard 1992	Country	None	Case study	Mass media TV show Local action	2 weeks/4 weeks	976 randomly sampled telephone surveys	Adults	A percentage reported changes in behaviors to lower fat
Sperber 1996	Kibbutz	None	Case study	Food policy changes in kitchen, health education programs, and counseling	18 months[a]	187 adults in one Kibbutz	Aged 19+ years	Decreased cholesterol (at one year), reduced consumption of red meat, increased consumption of 1% milk
Van Beurden 1993	Region of Australia	Health education	Case study	Community screening, counseling of high risk, monitoring	3 years[a]	14,245 residents with elevated cholesterol who returned for retest	Average age 49 years 42% women	Reduced cholesterol at 3 months, with some recidivism at 1 and 3 years
Van Wechem 1998	Entire country	Social influence Self-efficacy	Case study	Point-of-purchase strategies, mass media, print advertising	1 month/ 6 months	1200 consumers responsible for household purchases in each of 3 years	Adults	Increase in awareness, and intentions to buy low-fat product at one month. No differences in self-rated fat intake at 1 or 6 months

[a]Length of follow-up is the same as the length of intervention unless specified.

Abbreviations: Demos, demographics; F/V, fruit and vegetable; MRFIT, Multiple Risk Factor Intervention Trial; WHT, Womens' Health Trial.

from a nutritionist increased fiber consumption and increased choices of high-fiber recommended foods in college students (10). Receipt of a newsletter produced significant increases, relative to no newsletter controls, but all tested newsletters (tailored versus nontailored) were equal in their effects. Computer-tailored print feedback was found to be ineffective in changing fat consumption among a group of self-selected adults (12). Tailored print feedback to change fat and fruit/vegetable intake was successful, compared to nontailored feedback in a well-designed study (15).

Other generic interventions were aimed at the general population to produce public health changes. A randomized test of a brief educational intervention to increase fruit and vegetable consumption in Cancer Information Service callers found significant increases in fruit/vegetable consumption at the four-week follow-up (65). A randomized trial of two interventions to lower fat versus a control, in relatives of heart attack patients, found that self-help materials were significantly more effective in lowering dietary fat scores than was physician referral alone or control (45). Simple newsletters targeting elderly Medicare recipients in a randomized test produced small changes in avoiding fat as a flavoring (108). In a group of adults, who admitted to snacking between meals, provision of low-fat snacks produced overall decreases in fat consumption in the whole diet, compared with consumption without provision of the low-fat snacks (60). Behavioral therapy produced changes in fruit and vegetable consumption in a single patient (72).

Several studies targeted individuals with risk factors for chronic disease. A randomized trial of dietary change and smoking reduction was conducted in participants with angina, to determine long-term changes in behavior (21, 22). All participants were randomized to receive either standard care or personal health promotion from a trained nurse every four months for two years. At two years the intervention group reported better diet compared to the comparison group, but at five years those differences were not found. Ornish et al., in a randomized test of intensive interventions to reduce coronary arteriosclerosis in patients with coronary artery disease, found long-term changes in fat intake (from 30% of daily energy to 25%), dietary cholesterol, and energy intake (74). In the Netherlands, significant increases in consumption of fish and fruits/vegetables were found in people with one of three risk factors for cardiovascular disease after group intervention sessions and tailored letters (90). In a nonrandomized study of men with hyperlipidemia, allowing participants to continue to eat at their preintervention mean frequency resulted in larger reductions in dietary fat intake than when participants were asked to reduce eating frequency (53). The Oslo Study found that regular dietary counseling produced significant long-term declines in serum cholesterol (interpreted as a marker of dietary fat and saturated fat intakes) compared to control participants (46). Motivational interviewing produced no additional changes in dietary fat intake beyond standard nutritional counseling in subjects with hyperlipidemia (68). Women with coronary heart disease reduced calories from fat and saturated fat consumption by half (net reduction of 12% of energy from fat) in a randomized intervention study (110). An intervention targeting women in menopause reduced fat and saturated fat consumption (from 32% to 23% of energy from fat) compared to the randomized control group (from 32% to 23%) (91). A study using nurses to provide brief behavioral counseling produced significant decreases in dietary fat intake in a randomized test in individuals with coronary risk factors (104). Other studies have found similar changes (70, 103).

Low-income individuals have been the targets of several interventions to improve dietary intake. A nutrition education program targeting low-fat changes in participants in the Expanded Food and Nutrition Education Program found significant changes in overall low-fat eating behaviors, as measured by the Fat and Fiber Behavior Questionnaire, and positive but nonsignificant changes in 24-h recalls (43). This individually randomized intervention trial consisted of 10 group sessions focused on behavioral approaches to eating less fat. A different individual randomized study also found significant changes in EFNEP participants' dietary habits as a result of a 6-month session–based intervention (20). The use of fruit and vegetable coupons and education (nonrandom assignment to either a coupon only, a coupon plus education, an education only, or a no intervention comparison condition) were evaluated in changing the dietary behaviors of WIC and supplemental food program recipients (2). Coupons increased reported change in consumption of fruits and vegetables, but not education, and there were no effects of any intervention on self-reported intake. A one-year intervention to increase fruit and vegetable consumption focused on WIC participants found significant increases in fruit/vegetable servings (44). This individual and group session–based intervention included messages about changing fruit and vegetable consumption and three group sessions for all WIC intervention participants. Another classroom-based program for low-literacy individuals showed no significant changes in percent of calories from fat and saturated fat, compared to control condition (47).

Feedback about risky behaviors has been used to motivate dietary changes. In one instance, blood cholesterol feedback plus an educational session was used to reduce saturated fat intake in normal cholesterol subjects. The study found that feedback produced no larger changes in subjects who received it than in subjects who had not received the feedback (106). In a separate study, physician visits did not add significant benefit to a cholesterol screening visit in changing dietary intake related to cholesterol levels (117). A large proportion (approximately 80%) of individuals screened for blood cholesterol at a public screening reported making changes to their dietary habits, including lowering dietary cholesterol and increasing fiber consumption (105). In another study, adding cholesterol screening to self-help materials did not increase effects on servings of high-fat foods (84).

One randomized trial found that dietician-led interventions produced significant reductions in dietary fat and cholesterol intake compared with material and videotape intervention groups (85). A community-wide screening and follow-up project in low-socioeconomic neighborhoods near Melbourne, Australia, produced significant changes in diet following group interventions compared with pamphlet intervention, but no differences in cardiovascular disease risk (82).

STUDIES BASED IN FAMILIES

Rarely have families been used as the unit of interventions in dietary studies. One study (69) found that 12 weekly sessions in families, including both parents and children, produced consistent significant changes in eating habits to reduce fat, but that the changes were mostly absent at the 4-year follow-up. Explicit strategies to engage families as part of another channel or a full community intervention are reviewed as part of those strategies, in later sections.

INTERVENTIONS DELIVERED THROUGH PROVIDERS

Providers have often served as a source of intervention activities in several studies. A randomized trial of self-help materials delivered through primary care practices found significant decreases in dietary fat-related behaviors and increases in fiber-related behaviors (5). Another study with physician advice and intervention materials found changes in fat from dairy sources at 3 months (56). Two randomized interventions plus a control condition (teaching dietary counseling skills to physicians and a fingerstick before the office visit) resulted in patient's increasing their reports of the likelihood of changing dietary habits, but no long-term changes in cholesterol (25). An entire town in Germany was the target of a provider intervention to improve cardiovascular health (120). Here significant changes were found in reported healthy nutrition, but no significant change in blood cholesterol.

INTERVENTIONS IN OTHER COMMUNITY CHANNELS

Religious organizations have been used to recruit participants for individual interventions to change dietary habits. A well-designed study among rural African American adults in churches in North Carolina found increases over the two-year intervention study of .85 servings (14). In this case, an ecological approach to a 20-month intervention was used, providing church-wide activities and individualized feedback to each member.

Other investigators have worked within adult education settings to change dietary behaviors. One study in undergraduate school classes found significant changes in fat consumption after a session-based intervention during class hours (27). A nutrition session in English as a Second Language classes resulted in changes in fat avoidance behaviors (30). Computer-assisted sessions produced significant posttest changes in fat and calorie consumption of college students (58).

INTERVENTIONS BASED IN WORKSITES

Worksites have been used to deliver dietary change interventions. Baer randomized men within a worksite to receive dietary assessment, monitoring, and counseling (3). The men were followed for one year, and dietary fat, as well as several biological measures, significantly improved over the interventions period compared to the control men within the same worksite. Another within-worksite randomized study found significant changes in total fat (from 24% to 22% of energy from fat), cholesterol, and fiber intake one year after the 12-week intervention (87). Offshore oil installations served as the site of cardiovascular risk–reducing intervention (75). Surveys at baseline and 8 years later indicated reductions in percent of calories from fat (from 44% to 39% of daily energy as fat) and consumption of targeted foods. The Seattle 5 a Day program tested a community-based intervention in worksites to increase fruit and vegetable messages in a randomized trial (6). The interventions consisted of environmental components (cafeteria changes and worksite wide events), and individual strategies (self-help materials, etc.) were used, guided by the Transtheoretical Model over a one-year period. At two-year follow-up, worksite-wide average serving frequency was increased by about one third. A multicomponent intervention in two worksites produced significant reductions in percent energy from fat and total calories compared with two control sites (9). A project in worksites in Colorado in which employees in the intervention worksites selected either a group or self-paced nutrition educational program found no differences in fat consumption or fruit and vegetable consumption at 12 months (1). A single worksite intervention, using community organization strategies, produced changes in fruit and vegetable consumption (35). In another test, peer educators were used to deliver a fruit and vegetable intervention to lower-SES, multicultural adult employees (13). Cliques, or naturally occurring groups of employees, were randomized in a matched pair design, and key members of each intervention clique delivered interpersonal intervention messages to other members. At the 18-month outcome point, interventions cliques were consuming approximately half a serving of fruits and vegetables more compared to control clique members. There was some evidence that this differential change was maintained for at least 6 more months. The Treatwell Program, a randomized worksite-wide program to reduce fat and increase fiber consumption, focused on eating guidelines, classes and food demonstrations, point of choice labeling, and an employee advisory board (96). Results indicated significant changes in fat (net decrease of 1.1% of daily energy as fat), but not fiber consumption, when a cohort of employees was surveyed. A newer randomized controlled, multitheoretical intervention produced significant changes in fruit and vegetable servings (19%) when worksite, family, and employee strategies were combined (97). The Treatwell 5-A-Day further evaluated the extra contribution of family-based intervention to worksite intervention in a randomized trial of community health centers as worksites. Significant increases in fruit and vegetable consumption (approximately half a serving) at two years was found only in the worksite-plus-family intervention condition (98).

A randomized trial of self-help materials and classes in nutrition and screening to reduce colorectal cancer risk targeted to manufacturing worksites (109) found small but significant changes in fat (0.9% energy as fat), fiber, and fruit/vegetable (0.4 servings) consumption after one year of intervention.

A trial with teachers of elementary schools to increase healthy dietary behaviors found no differences in any dietary outcomes after two years of intervention (83). In a study that was one site in a multicenter study (99), a two and one half-year intervention targeting employees in worksites found significant increases in fruit and vegetable consumption at the final survey (24), but no changes in fat consumption, as measured by a food frequency questionnaire. This multiple strategy intervention used sessions, events, contests, materials, and policy changes. However, Take Heart, also using multiple strategies for changing dietary behaviors at worksites, found no significant differences in dietary intake after two years of intervention (39).

The Working Well Trial, targeting decreases in fat and increases in fruits and vegetables, was tested in a randomized trial in four worksite-wide settings in the United States (99). Included were individual-level intervention strategies such as changes in cafeteria offerings, print materials, worksite-wide activities, and contests. The evaluation method consisted of both responses to employee surveys and information gathered from key informant interviews at baseline and at three months post randomization. Consistent changes were found in all nutritional variables, including increased access to fruits and vegetables at work, more access to nutrition information at work, and more endorsement of normative beliefs related to healthy eating. Two years after the main outcome assessment point there were no differences between intervention and comparison worksites in nutrition-related activities (77).

POINT-OF-PURCHASE INTERVENTIONS

Grocery stores were the site of several interventions to change dietary behaviors. In one, a sample of regular shoppers in interventions grocery stores were provided with audiotapes containing skill-building information and nutritional knowledge tests to use at home. Over the four-week duration, public service announcements were played in the store for all shoppers to hear. Average intake of fruit and vegetables, as well as positive beliefs about fruit and vegetable consumption, increased in interventions shoppers by 0.56 servings (8%) over control shoppers (18). An educational intervention in supermarkets found no significant changes in behaviors of surveyed shoppers compared to those in control supermarkets (50). Kristol et al. found no significant differences in fruit and vegetable consumption, but significant shifts in stage of change toward later stages, after a one-year intervention in grocery stores (57). Flyers, point-of-purchase information, and storewide activities were used. Decreasing prices of low-fat snacks in vending machines increased the purchase of these snacks in a university setting (33) and in worksites (32).

COMMUNITY INTERVENTIONS

Finally, entire communities and regions have been targeted in several key studies. Because of the expense and complexities involved, many of these studies have no comparison group. The Five-a-Day campaign (28) was first evaluated in California through efforts by the State Health department to implement a statewide campaign. The interventions consisted of five campaign waves, released over a period of 18 months and including media releases complemented by point-of-purchase information. The evaluation method consisted of questions measuring servings of fruits and vegetables on a random-digit dial survey of 1000 adult residents of California, and other questions measuring awareness, knowledge, beliefs, and attitudes about cancer. Consumption increased by nearly 0.3 servings for white and African Americans, while servings decreased for Latinos by 0.7.

Single communities have been targeted with interventions to change dietary behaviors. One such study provided a low-income neighborhood with a diverse set of interventional activities, including restaurant involvement, point-of-purchase strategies, contests, clubs, workshops, health fairs, and other community events (73). In Israel, a community-wide intervention was implemented in a kibbutz to reduce coronary risk factors in the population living there (100). There were population-based interventions (changes in food service policy in the kibbutz kitchen) and individual-level interventions for high-risk and average-risk individuals (counseling and health education programs) over a one-year period. Individuals reported relevant changes in their food patterns, including decreased consumption of eggs, liquid oil, and red meat, and increased consumption of low-fat milk. The North Coast Cholesterol Check Campaign implemented a coordinated cholesterol-screening and follow-up program for residents of a defined area in Northern Australia (115). The evaluation consisted of cross-sectional surveys of residents measuring food, blood cholesterol, and awareness and attitudes. Significant changes in cholesterol occurred from baseline to three months, with smaller changes remaining at one- and three-year follow-up surveys. Fat Watch, a national campaign to reduce fat, has been conducted annually in the Netherlands, beginning in 1991 (116). The month-long campaign includes mass media activities, cues at food retailers and pharmacies, and print materials. Awareness of the campaign, attitudes, and intentions to buy low-fat products changed in the expected direction, as measured by surveys of the public. A national mass media campaign in Norway found that one quarter of adults surveyed were interested in changing dietary behaviors after viewing the shows on television (95). Another mass media intervention, in Denmark, increased attempts to eat less fat after one year of intervention (76). The Bootheel Heart Health Project, focused on cardiovascular risk reduction in six rural counties, provided community-based activities such as demonstrations, classes, screenings, cooking demonstrations, and other education programs (11). No significant differences were found in fruit and vegetable consumption, but screening increased and prevalence of overweight decreased in the six-county sample, compared to state data. Cheadle et al., in a set of studies evaluating community-based nutrition programs, found that results in each of the three community settings were mixed compared to control communities (16). The interventions were a mixture of print- and activity-based interventions. In a West Virginia program covering three rural counties with similar demographic characteristics, the intervention included both PR- and community-based educational activities in one county, paid advertising only in a second, with the third county acting as the control. In both intervention counties, low-fat milk consumption increased (81).

The Minnesota Heart Health Program was a key research project aimed at reducing cardiovascular risk in three interventions communities, compared to three control communities (61). Community organization strategies, along with mass communications and other models, were used to design the multipronged intervention. Significant gains were recorded in the interventions communities in risk factor variables relevant to cardiovascular disease, although the change in serum cholesterol was small and within chance findings. The Stanford Five–City project (29) and Three Community Study (26) both used mass media and other strategies to change cardiovascular risk behaviors in communities in California. These studies both used dietary recalls as part of multicomponent surveys to assess changes at multiple time points. Significant changes in the intervention communities in dietary fat intake were found in both studies, but design limitations and secular trend make definitive interpretation difficult.

The North Karelia Project (78) was a multicomponent community-based intervention project to reduce high cardiovascular disease rates in an area of Finland. Individual, worksite, point-of-purchase, school-based, and community-wide strategies were combined to produce multiple changes in indicators of diet related to heart disease.

DISCUSSION

By far the most common type of intervention was based on individual or group counseling for dietary change. Most of these studies were successful in changing dietary behaviors, many by large amounts. Most were conducted in individuals with existing risk factors for cardiovascular disease, but some focused on individuals without risk factors. The participants recruited were often motivated and fully resourced, and so there was no attempt to change the dietary behaviors of large segments of the public. Certainly these studies provided support for the idea that changing dietary behaviors in free-living people is possible. Also identified were strategies and models for interventions that could be adapted for use in broader segments of the population.

The most commonly used community channel or intervention setting for dietary change was the worksite. Participants have been recruited through worksites, and the worksite has also been used as the unit of intervention and analysis. Consistent changes were observed in most of the worksite studies, confirming the promise of worksite intervention for dietary change. The size of the effect was often small, and rarely was there long-term follow-up to determine the longevity of the changes. Follow-up and duration of change are topics that need to be addressed in future studies.

Other community settings, such as religious organizations and grocery stores, have mixed records of success. The few published studies in religious organizations indicated a positive finding, but further research is needed to broaden the findings to a more diverse group of religious organizations. The grocery store interventions, by contrast, produced little evidence of efficacy. Point-of-purchase interventions may raise awareness, but the effects on actual behavior in choice of healthy food items are not yet proven. Inasmuch as the influence of advertising of food products by commercial interests on food choice is substantiated, public health researchers have not found the appropriate mechanism for capturing the public's interest and behaviors for healthy choices in places of purchase. More research is needed, with innovative strategies, to enable stores and markets to be used as an effective health-promotion tool.

Community-wide strategies have also shown mixed success in producing changes in dietary intake. Many single-community studies show changes over time in consumption of target nutrients. Ability to attribute this change to an intervention is limited without a control group. Adding control groups provides the opportunity to see changes relative to nonintervention communities. Of the key community studies, only the North Karelia Study reported such clear effects on dietary behavior that statistical evaluation was not necessary (78). However, that study was conducted over 25 years ago. The changes in consumption patterns in many countries over the past 25 years require that statistical evaluation be made current interventions. Taken together, the mixed success of community-wide initiatives to change dietary intake and the need for rigorous statistical evaluation mean that we do not now have proven methods for dietary change at the community level. Future research should test methods of intervention in smaller-scale studies before applying them to large entire sets of communities.

We discussed several topics during the process of reviewing these studies that are worth noting here. First, few individuals report their theoretical basis or model of intervention. When individuals do report and describe their model, they often do not indicate how the theoretical constructs in the model are related to the intervention activities chosen and presented to the target population. This lack of information makes it difficult to group studies according to the model used in the intervention or to understand the usefulness of any particular model. More emphasis should be placed on fully describing the model and intervention activities in future published articles.

In this review, we have summarized studies as if they were asking the question, "Does this strategy work?" or "Is the intervention effective in changing dietary intake of (fat, fruits, or vegetables)?" We included only representative information to answer the question, "How much does this intervention change average intake of (fat, fruits, or vegetables)?" We justify our classical hypothesis testing approach, because relatively few studies have actually been population-based or effectiveness studies of an intervention. More often they have been efficacy studies of a select group of individuals or other channels. Generalizing estimates of efficacy from these studies to the general population is not appropriate because of the highly select nature of the study group. Therefore one cannot compare the size of intervention effects between different studies.

In general, there was a positive relationship between intensity of the goal presented in the intervention and the effect size produced by the intervention. For example, intensive interventions, such as the Women's Health Trial (7, 119) and MRFIT (40), set high goals for their participants and recruited selectively for highly motivated individuals. These studies produced large effects on dietary intake. Studies that targeted worksites (6), religious organizations (14), and entire communities (e.g., 61) produced much smaller effects on average for the people in the worksites, organizations, or communities, yet many more individuals than the more intensive studies.

There is a wide variation in the degree of scientific vigor under which these intervention studies have been conducted. Because it is understood that people respond to interventions of a given type in different ways, a fundamental principle of experimental design is that of replication. Some estimate of the degree of variability in response can be deduced from as few as three units of study (individuals or communities). A second principle is that of a comparison group. Behavior can be influenced by many different factors that have to be accounted for if the observed change is to be attributed to the intervention. A comparison group is assumed to be subject to the same factors, so any change in the intervention group beyond that in the control group can be attributed to the intervention. The best way to incorporate a comparison group is via a randomized controlled trial. Of the individual studies we reviewed, 1 had inadequate replication, 3 had no concurrent comparison group, and 3 did not include a randomized design. For hypothesis testing, the minimum number of units needed in a randomized design to have a defined power (typically 80% or more) to detect a difference or significance at the 5% level can be calculated. All of the individual studies had adequate power to detect small changes in behavioral factors, but 5 of the channel-level intervention studies where the channel was the unit of analysis and 4 of the community-intervention studies had inadequate replication or numbers of units randomized.

It is well known that dietary intake assessment measures lack precision. Precision involves both lack of random error and lack of bias. Some dietary measures have inflated random error because of the large contribution of within-person variability, while others have larger systematic error, yielding biased estimates. These issues and methods to deal with them have been extensively debated in the scientific literature related to epidemiological studies of dietary factors and disease. Ability to measure change in dietary intake attributable to an intervention has these same issues magnified, because change is the difference between baseline and follow-up, and the errors in each component are additive. Some of the dietary assessment measures that are more responsive to change (56a) may also be more subject to intervention bias. It should be noted that the efficacy associated with a particular dietary intervention will be underestimated because of random errors in dietary assessment.

In conclusion, even with widely different approaches to dietary change, using different experimental designs, guided by different theoretical frameworks in different populations, we are definitely making progress in learning about dietary change, but much is left to be learned. We need to determine how best to leverage some of the successes of the individually randomized trials to community and public health settings. We need to be more rigorous in our design and our description of dietary change studies, satisfying the key elements of design to allow wider inferences to be drawn. Finally, we need to develop innovative methods of interventions for those areas where we have not been able to show changes, such as grocery stores and larger communities. Perhaps we can also find ways of increasing dietary change in settings where small changes have been seen to date. Finally, there is the topic of maintenance of dietary change, which we have only addressed in studies of motivated individuals. We must find ways of cementing the changes that we have seen in public health settings, and this will likely prove a challenge.

Visit the Annual Reviews home page at www.annualreviews.org

LITERATURE CITED

1. Anderson J, Dusenbury L. 1999. Worksite cholesterol and nutrition: an intervention project in Colorado. *Amer. Assoc. Occup. Health Nurses J.* 47:99–106

2. Anderson JV, Bybee DI, Brown RM, McLean DF, Garcia EM, et al. 2001. 5 a day fruit and vegetable intervention improves consumption in a low income population. *J. Am. Diet. Assoc.* 101:195–202

3. Baer JT. 1993. Improved plasma cholesterol levels in men after a nutrition education program at the worksite. *J. Am. Diet. Assoc.* 93:658–63

4. Bemelmans WJ, Broer J, de Vries JH, Hulshof KF, May JF, et al. 2000. Impact of Mediterranean diet education versus posted leaflet on dietary habits and serum cholesterol in a high risk population for cardiovascular disease. *Public Health Nutr.* 3:273–83

5. Beresford SA, Curry SJ, Kristal AR, Lazovich D, Feng Z, et al. 1997. A dietary intervention in primary care practice: the Eating Patterns Study. *Am. J. Public Health* 87:610–16

6. Beresford SA, Thompson B, Feng Z, Christianson A, McLerran D, et al. 2001. Seattle 5 a Day worksite program to increase fruit and vegetable consumption. *Prev. Med.* 32:230–38

7. Bowen DJ, Henderson MH, Iverson D, Burrows E, Henry H, Foreyt J. 1994. Reducing dietary fat: Understanding the success of The Women's Health Trial. *Cancer Prev. Int.* 1:21–30

8. Boyd NF, Lockwood GA, Greenberg CV, Martin LJ, Tritchler DL. 1997. Effects of a low-fat high-carbohydrate diet on plasma sex hormones in premenopausal women: results from a randomized controlled trial. Canadian Diet and Breast Cancer Prevention Study Group. *Br. J. Cancer* 76:127–35

9. Braeckman L, De Bacquer D, Maes L, De Backer G. 1999. Effects of a low-intensity worksite-based nutrition intervention. *Occup. Med.* 49:549–55

10. Brinberg D, Axelson ML, Price S. 2000. Changing food knowledge, food choice, and dietary fiber consumption by using tailored messages. *Appetite* 35:35–43

11. Brownson RC, Smith CA, Pratt M, Mack NE, Jackson-Thompson J, et al. 1996. Preventing cardiovascular disease through community-based risk reduction: the Bootheel Heart Health Project. *Am. J. Public Health* 86:206–13

12. Brug J, Steenhuis I, van Assema P, de Vries H. 1996. The impact of a computer-tailored nutrition intervention. *Prev. Med.* 25:236–42

13. Buller DB, Morrill C, Taren D, Aickin M, Sennott-Miller L, et al. 1999. Randomized trial testing the effect of peer education at increasing fruit and vegetable intake. *J. Natl. Cancer Inst.* 91:1491–500

14. Campbell MK, Demark-Wahnefried W, Symons M, Kalsbeek WD, Dodds J, et al. 1999. Fruit and vegetable consumption and prevention of cancer: the Black Churches United for Better Health project. *Am. J. Public Health* 89:1390–96

15. Campbell MK, DeVellis BM, Strecher VJ, Ammerman AS, DeVellis RF, et al. 1994. Improving dietary behavior: the effectiveness of tailored messages in primary care settings. *Am. J. Public Health* 84:783–87

16. Cheadle A, Psaty BM, Diehr P, Koepsell T, Wagner E, et al. 1995. Evaluating community-based nutrition programs: comparing grocery store and individual-level survey measures of program impact. *Prev. Med.* 24:71–79

17. Coates RJ, Bowen DJ, Kristal AR, Feng Z, Oberman A, et al. 1999. The Women's Health Trial Feasibility Study in Minority Populations: changes in dietary intakes. *Am. J. Epidemiol.* 149:1104–12

18. Connell D, Goldberg JP, Folta SC. 2001. An intervention to increase fruit and vegetable consumption using audio communications: in-store public service announcements and audiotapes. *J. Health Commun.* 6:31–43

19. Cox DN, Anderson AS, Reynolds J, McKellar S, Lean ME, et al. 1998. Take Five, a nutrition education intervention to increase fruit and vegetable intakes: impact on consumer choice and nutrient intakes. *Br. J. Nutr.* 80:123–31

20. Cox RH, Parker GG, Watson AC, Robinson SH, Simonson CJ, et al. 1995. Dietary cancer risk of low-income women and change with intervention. *J. Am. Diet. Assoc.* 95:1031–34

21. Cupples ME, McKnight A. 1999. Five year follow up of patients at high cardiovascular risk who took part in randomised controlled trial of health promotion. *Br. Med. J.* 319:687–88

22. Cupples ME, McKnight A. 1994. Randomised controlled trial of health promotion in general practice for patients at high cardiovascular risk. *Br. Med. J.* 309:993–96

23. Ebrahim S, Holloway RG, Benesch CG. 1999. Systematic review of cost-effectiveness research of stroke evaluation and treatment. *Stroke* 30:2759–68

24. Emmons KM, Linnan LA, Shadel WG, Marcus B, Abrams DB. 1999. The Working Healthy Project: a worksite health-promotion trial targeting physical activity, diet, and smoking. *J. Occup. Environ. Med.* 41:545–55

25. Evans AT, Rogers LQ, Peden JG Jr, Seelig CB, Layne RD, et al. 1996. Teaching dietary counseling skills to residents: patient and physician outcomes. The CADRE Study Group. *Am. J. Prev. Med.* 12:259–65

26. Farquhar JW, Maccoby N, Wood PD, Alexander JK, Breitrose H, et al. 1977. Community education for cardiovascular health. *Lancet* 1:1192–95

27. Finckenor M, Byrd-Bredbenner C. 2000. Nutrition intervention group program based on preaction-stage-oriented change processes of the Transtheoretical Model promotes long-term reduction in dietary fat intake. *J. Am. Diet. Assoc.* 100:335–42

28. Foerster SB, Kizer KW, Disogra LK, Bal DG, Krieg BF, et al. 1995. California's "5 a day–for better health!" campaign: an innovative population-based effort to

effect large-scale dietary change. *Am. J. Prev. Med.* 11:124–31

29. Fortmann SP, Flora JA, Winkleby MA, Schooler C, Taylor CB, et al. 1995. Community intervention trials: reflections on the Stanford Five-City Project Experience. *Am. J. Epidemiol.* 142:576–86

30. Frack SA, Woodruff SI, Candelaria J, Elder JP. 1997. Correlates of compliance with measurement protocols in a Latino nutrition-intervention study. *Am. J. Prev. Med.* 13:131–36

31. Fraser GE, Sabate J, Beeson WL, Strahan TM. 1992. A possible protective effect of nut consumption on risk of coronary heart disease. The Adventist Health Study. *Arch. Intern. Med.* 152:1416–24

32. French SA, Jeffery RW, Story M, Breitlow KK, Baxter JS, et al. 2001. Pricing and promotion effects on low-fat vending snack purchases: the CHIPS Study. *Am. J. Public Health* 91:112–17

33. French SA, Jeffery RW, Story M, Hannan P, Snyder MP. 1997. A pricing strategy to promote low-fat snack choices through vending machines. *Am. J. Public Health* 87:849–51

34. French SA, Story M, Jeffery RW. 2001. Environmental influences on eating and physical activity. *Annu. Rev. Public Health* 22:309–35

35. Fries EA, Ripley JS, Figueiredo MI, Thompson B. 1999. Can community organization stategies be used to implement smoking and dietary changes in a rural manufacturing work site? *J. Rural Health* 15:413–20

36. Garcia-Palmieri MR, Sorlie P, Tillotson J, Costas R Jr, Cordero E, et al. 1980. Relationship of dietary intake to subsequent coronary heart disease incidence: The Puerto Rico Heart Health Program. *Am. J. Clin. Nutr.* 33:1818–27

37. Garland C, Shekelle RB, Barrett-Connor E, Criqui MH, Rossof AH, et al. 1985. Dietary vitamin D and calcium and risk of colorectal cancer: a 19-year prospective study in men. *Lancet* 1:307–9

38. Glanz K, Sorensen G, Farmer A. 1996. The health impact of worksite nutrition and cholesterol intervention programs. *Am. J. Health Promot.* 10:453–70

39. Glasgow RE, Terborg JR, Hollis JF, Severson HH, Boles SM. 1995. Take heart: results from the initial phase of a work-site wellness program. *Am. J. Public Health* 85:209–16

40. Gorder DD, Bartsch GE, Tillotson JL, Grandits GA, Stamler J. 1997. Food group and macronutrient intakes, trial years 1–6, in the special intervention and usual care groups in the Multiple Risk Factor Intervention Trial. *Am. J. Clin. Nutr.* 65:258S–271S

41. Graham S, Marshall J, Haughey B, Mittelman A, Swanson M, et al. 1988. Dietary epidemiology of cancer of the colon in western New York. *Am. J. Epidemiol.* 128:490–503

42. Hancock L, Sanson-Fisher RW, Redman S, Burton R, Burton L, et al. 1997. Community action for health promotion: a review of methods and outcomes 1990–1995. *Am. J. Prev. Med.* 13:229–39

43. Hartman TJ, McCarthy PR, Park RJ, Schuster E, Kushi LH. 1997. Results of a community-based low-literacy nutrition education program. *J. Community Health* 22:325–41

44. Havas S, Anliker J, Damron D, Langenberg P, Ballesteros M, et al. 1998. Final results of the Maryland WIC 5-A-Day Promotion Program. *Am. J. Public Health* 88:1161–67

45. Heller RF, Walker RJ, Boyle CA, O'Connell DL, Rusakaniko S, et al. 1994. A randomised controlled trial of a dietary advice program for relatives of heart attack victims. *Med. J. Aust.* 161:529–31

46. Hjermann I, Holme I, Leren P. 1986. Oslo Study Diet and Antismoking Trial. Results after 102 months. *Am. J. Med.* 80:7–11

47. Howard-Pitney B, Winkleby MA, Albright CL, Bruce B, Fortmann SP. 1997. The Stanford Nutrition Action Program:

a dietary fat intervention for low-literacy adults. *Am. J. Public Health* 87:1971–6

48. Howe GR, Friedenreich CM, Jain M, Miller AB. 1991. A cohort study of fat intake and risk of breast cancer. *J. Natl. Cancer Inst.* 83:336–40

49. Howe GR, Hirohata T, Hislop TG, Iscovich JM, Yuan JM, et al. 1990. Dietary factors and risk of breast cancer: combined analysis of 12 case-control studies. *J. Natl. Cancer Inst.* 82:561–9

50. Jeffery RW, Pirie PL, Rosenthal BS, Gerber WM, Murray DM. 1982. Nutrition education in supermarkets: an unsuccessful attempt to influence knowledge and product sales. *J. Behav. Med.* 5:189–200

51. Jones DY, Schatzkin A, Green SB, Block G, Brinton LA, et al. 1987. Dietary fat and breast cancer in the National Health and Nutrition Examination Survey I Epidemiologic Follow-up Study. *J. Natl. Cancer Inst.* 79:465–71

52. Keys A. 1980. *Seven Countries: A Multivariate Analysis of Death and Coronary Heart Disease.* Cambridge, MA: Harvard Univ. Press

53. King S, Gibney M. 1999. Dietary advice to reduce fat intake is more successful when it does not restrict habitual eating patterns. *J. Am. Diet. Assoc.* 99:685–89

54. Knekt P, Albanes D, Seppanen R, Aromaa A, Jarvinen R, et al. 1990. Dietary fat and risk of breast cancer. *Am. J. Clin. Nutr.* 52:903–8

55. Krebs-Smith SM, Cook A, Subar AF, Cleveland L, Friday J. 1995. US adults' fruit and vegetable intakes, 1989 to 1991: a revised baseline for the Healthy People 2000 objective. *Am. J. Public Health* 85:1623–29

56. Kreuter MW, Chheda SG, Bull FC. 2000. How does physician advice influence patient behavior? Evidence for a priming effect. *Arch. Fam. Med.* 9:426–33

56a. Kristal AR, Beresford SAA, Lazovich D. 1994. Assessing change in diet-intervention research. *Am. J. Clin. Nutr.* 59(s):185–89

57. Kristal AR, Goldenhar L, Muldoon J, Morton RF. 1997. Evaluation of a supermarket intervention to increase consumption of fruits and vegetables. *Am. J. Health Promot.* 11:422–25

58. Kumar NB, Bostow DE, Schapira DV, Kritch KM. 1993. Efficacy of interactive, automated programmed instruction in nutrition education for cancer prevention. *J. Cancer Educ.* 8:203–11

59. Kushi LH, Lew RA, Stare FJ, Ellison CR, el Lozy M, et al. 1985. Diet and 20-year mortality from coronary heart disease. The Ireland-Boston Diet-Heart Study. *N. Engl. J. Med.* 312:811–8

60. Lawton CL, Delargy HJ, Smith FC, Hamilton V, Blundell JE. 1998. A medium-term intervention study on the impact of high- and low-fat snacks varying in sweetness and fat content: large shifts in daily fat intake but good compensation for daily energy intake. *Br. J. Nutr.* 80:149–61

61. Luepker RV, Murray DM, Jacobs DR Jr, Mittelmark MB, Bracht N, et al. 1994. Community education for cardiovascular disease prevention: risk factor changes in the Minnesota Heart Health Program. *Am. J. Public Health* 84:1383–93

62. Lutz SF, Ammerman AS, Atwood JR, Campbell MK, DeVellis RF, et al. 1999. Innovative newsletter interventions improve fruit and vegetable consumption in healthy adults. *J. Am. Diet. Assoc.* 99:705–9

63. Lyon JL, Mahoney AW, West DW, Gardner JW, Smith KR, et al. 1987. Energy intake: its relationship to colon cancer risk. *J. Natl. Cancer Inst.* 78:853–61

64. Macquart-Moulin G, Riboli E, Cornee J, Charnay B, Berthezene P, et al. 1986. Case-control study on colorectal cancer and diet in Marseilles. *Int. J. Cancer* 38:183–91

65. Marcus AC, Morra M, Rimer BK, Stricker M, Heimendinger J, et al. 1998. A feasibility test of a brief educational intervention to increase fruit and vegetable

consumption among callers to the Cancer Information Service. *Prev. Med.* 27:250–61

66. Maskarinec G, Chan CLY, Meng L, Franke AA, Cooney RV. 1999. Exploring the feasibility and effects of a high-fruit and -vegetable diet in healthy women. *Cancer Epidemiol. Biomarkers Prev.* 8:919–24

67. McGee DL, Reed DM, Yano K, Kagan A, Tillotson J. 1984. Ten-year incidence of coronary heart disease in the Honolulu Heart Program. Relationship to nutrient intake. *Am. J. Epidemiol.* 119:667–76

68. Mhurchu CN, Margetts BM, Speller V. 1998. Randomized clinical trial comparing the effectiveness of two dietary interventions for patients with hyperlipidaemia. *Clin. Sci.* 95:479–87

69. Nader P, Sallis J, Abramson I, Broyles S, Patterson T, et al. 1992. Family-based cardiovascular risk reduction education among Mexican- and Anglo-Americans. *Fam. Community Health* 15:57–74

70. Naslund GK, Fredrikson M, Hellenius ML, de Faire U. 1996. Effect of diet and physical exercise intervention programmes on coronary heart disease risk in smoking and non-smoking men in Sweden. *J. Epidemiol. Community Health* 50:131–36

71. Natl. Res. Counc. Comm. Diet and Health. 1989. *Diet and Health: Implications for Reducing Chronic Disease Risk.* Washington, DC: Natl. Acad. Press

72. Nelson LJ, Hekmat H. 1991. Promoting healthy nutritional habits by paradigmatic behavior therapy. *J. Behav. Ther. Exp. Psychiatry* 22:291–98

73. O'Loughlin J, Paradis G, Meshefedjian G. 1997. Evaluation of two strategies for heart health promotion by direct mail in a low-income urban community. *Prev. Med.* 26:745–53

74. Ornish D, Scherwitz LW, Billings JH, Brown SE, Gould KL, et al. 1998. Intensive lifestyle changes for reversal of coronary heart disease. *JAMA* 280:2001–7

75. Oshaug A, Helle Bjonnes C, Bugge KH, Bjorge Loken E. 1995. Nutrition promotion and dietary change at off-shore oil installations in the Norwegian sector of the North Sea. *Eur. J. Clin. Nutr.* 49:883–96

76. Osler M, Jespersen NB. 1993. The effect of a community-based cardiovascular disease prevention project in a Danish municipality. *Dan. Med. Bull.* 40:485–89

77. Patterson RE, Kristal AR, Biener L, Varnes J, Feng Z, et al. 1998. Durability and diffusion of the nutrition intervention in the Working Well Trial. *Prev. Med.* 27:668–73

78. Pietinen P, Nissinen A, Vartiainen E, Tuomilehto A, Uusitalo U, et al. 1988. Dietary changes in the North Karelia Project (1972–1982). *Prev. Med.* 17:183–93

79. Potter JD, McMichael AJ. 1986. Diet and cancer of the colon and rectum: a case-control study. *J. Natl. Cancer Inst.* 76:557–69

80. Prentice RL, Sheppard L. 1990. Dietary fat and cancer: consistency of the epidemiologic data, and disease prevention that may follow from a practical reduction in fat consumption. *Cancer Causes Control* 1:81–97; discussion 99–109

81. Reger B, Wootan MG, Booth-Butterfield S. 2000. A comparison of different approaches to promote community-wide dietary change. *Am. J. Prev. Med.* 18:271–75

82. Reid C, McNeil JJ, Williams F, Powles J. 1995. Cardiovascular risk reduction: a randomized trial of two health promotion strategies for lowering risk in a community with low socioeconomic status. *J. Cardiovasc. Risk* 2:155–63

83. Resnicow K, Davis M, Smith M, Baranowski T, Lin LS, et al. 1998. Results of the TeachWell worksite wellness program. *Am. J. Public Health* 88:250–57

84. Reynolds KD, Gillum JL, Hyman DJ, Byers T, Moore SA, et al. 1997. Comparing two strategies to modify dietary behavior and serum cholesterol. *J. Cardiovasc. Risk* 4:1–5

85. Rhodes KS, Bookstein LC, Aaronson LS, Mercer NM, Orringer CE. 1996. Intensive nutrition counseling enhances outcomes of National Cholesterol Education Program dietary therapy. *J. Am. Diet. Assoc.* 96:1003–10; quiz 1011–12

86. Rimm EB, Ascherio A, Giovannucci E, Spiegelman D, Stampfer MJ, et al. 1996. Vegetable, fruit, and cereal fiber intake and risk of coronary heart disease among men. *JAMA* 275:447–51

87. Sasaki S, Ishikawa T, Yanagibori R, Amano K. 2000. Change and 1-year maintenance of nutrient and food group intakes at a 12-week worksite dietary intervention trial for men at high risk of coronary heart disease. *J. Nutr. Sci. Vitaminol.* 46:15–22

88. Schatzkin A, Lanza E, Corle D, Lance P, Iber F, et al. 2000. Lack of effect of a low-fat, high-fiber diet on the recurrence of colorectal adenomas. Polyp Prevention Trial Study Group. *N. Engl. J. Med.* 342:1149–55

89. Shekelle RB, Shryock AM, Paul O, Lepper M, Stamler J, et al. 1981. Diet, serum cholesterol, and death from coronary heart disease. The Western Electric study. *N. Engl. J. Med.* 304:65–70

90. Siero FW, Broer J, Bemelmans WJ, Meyboom-de Jong BM. 2000. Impact of group nutrition education and surplus value of Prochaska-based stage-matched information on health-related cognitions and on Mediterranean nutrition behavior. *Health Educ. Res.* 15:635–47

91. Simkin-Silverman LR, Wing RR, Boraz MA, Meilahn EN, Kuller LH. 1998. Maintenance of cardiovascular risk factor changes among middle-aged women in a lifestyle intervention trial. *Womens Health* 4:255–71

92. Simons-Morton DG, Mullen PD, Mains DA, Tabak ER, Green LW. 1992. Characteristics of controlled studies of patient education and counseling for preventive health behaviors. *Patient Educ. Couns.* 19:175–204

93. Smith-Warner SA, Spiegelman D, Yaun SS, Adami HO, Beeson WL, et al. 2001. Intake of fruits and vegetables and risk of breast cancer: a pooled analysis of cohort studies. *JAMA* 285:769–77

94. Snowdon DA, Phillips RL, Fraser GE. 1984. Meat consumption and fatal ischemic heart disease. *Prev. Med.* 13:490–500

95. Sogaard AJ, Fonnebo V. 1992. Self-reported change in health behaviour after a mass media-based health education campaign. *Scand. J. Psychol.* 33:125–34

96. Sorensen G, Morris DM, Hunt MK, Hebert JR, Harris DR, et al. 1992. Worksite nutrition intervention and employees' dietary habits: the Treatwell program. *Am. J. Public Health* 82:877–80

97. Sorensen G, Stoddard A, Hunt MK, Hebert JR, Ockene JK, et al. 1998. The effects of a health promotion-health protection intervention on behavior change: the WellWorks Study. *Am. J. Public Health* 88:1685–90

98. Sorensen G, Stoddard A, Peterson K, Cohen N, Hunt MK, et al. 1999. Increasing fruit and vegetable consumption through worksites and families in the Treatwell 5-a-day study. *Am. J. Public Health* 89:54–60

99. Sorensen G, Thompson B, Glanz K, Feng Z, Kinne S, et al. 1996. Work site-based cancer prevention: primary results from the Working Well Trial. *Am. J. Public Health* 86:939–47

100. Sperber AD, Galil A, Sarov B, Stahl Z, Shany S. 1996. A combined community strategy to reduce cholesterol and other risk factors. *Am. J. Prev. Med.* 12:123–28

101. Steinmetz KA, Potter JD. 1996. Vegetables, fruit, and cancer prevention: a review. *J. Am. Diet. Assoc.* 96:1027–39

102. Stemmermann GN, Nomura AM, Heilbrun LK. 1984. Dietary fat and the risk of colorectal cancer. *Cancer Res.* 44:4633–37

103. Steptoe A, Doherty S, Kerry S, Rink E, Hilton S. 2000. Sociodemographic and psychological predictors of changes in dietary fat consumption in adults with high blood cholesterol following counseling in primary care. *Health Psychol.* 19:411–19

104. Steptoe A, Doherty S, Rink E, Kerry S, Kendrick T, et al. 1999. Behavioural counselling in general practice for the promotion of healthy behaviour among adults at increased risk of coronary heart disease: randomised trial. *Br. Med. J.* 319:943–47; discussion 947–48

105. Stockbridge H, Hardy RI, Glueck CJ. 1989. Public cholesterol screening: motivation for participation, follow-up outcome, self-knowledge, and coronary heart disease risk factor intervention. *J. Lab. Clin. Med.* 114:142–51

106. Strychar IM, Champagne F, Ghadirian P, Bonin A, Jenicek M, et al. 1998. Impact of receiving blood cholesterol test results on dietary change. *Am. J. Prev. Med.* 14:103–10

107. Tang JL, Armitage JM, Lancaster T, Silagy CA, Fowler GH, et al. 1998. Systematic review of dietary intervention trials to lower blood total cholesterol in free-living subjects. *Br. Med. J.* 316:1213–20

108. Taylor-Davis S, Smiciklas-Wright H, Warland R, Achterberg C, Jensen GL, et al. 2000. Responses of older adults to theory-based nutrition newsletters. *J. Am. Diet. Assoc.* 100:656–64

109. Tilley BC, Vernon SW, Myers R, Glanz K, Lu M, et al. 1999. The Next Step Trial: impact of a worksite colorectal cancer screening promotion program. *Prev. Med.* 28:276–83

110. Toobert DJ, Glasgow RE, Radcliffe JL. 2000. Physiologic and related behavioral outcomes from the Women's Lifestyle Heart Trial. *Ann. Behav. Med.* 22:1–9

111. Trock B, Lanza E, Greenwald P. 1990. Dietary fiber, vegetables, and colon cancer: critical review and meta-analyses of the epidemiologic evidence. *J. Natl. Cancer Inst.* 82:650–61

112. Truswell AS. 1985. ABC of nutrition. Nutritional advice for other chronic diseases. *Br. Med. J. (Clin. Res. Ed.)* 291:197–200

113. Truswell AS. 1994. Review of dietary intervention studies: effect on coronary events and on total mortality. *Aust. NZ J. Med.* 24:98–106

114. U.S. Dep. Health Hum. Serv. 2001. Healthy People 2010: understanding and improving health. http://www.health.gov/healthypeople/Document

115. van Beurden E, James R, Montague D, Christian J, Dunn T. 1993. Community-based cholesterol screening and education to prevent heart disease: five-year results of the North Coast Cholesterol Check Campaign. *Aust. J. Public Health* 17:109–16

116. van Wechem SN, Brug J, van Assema P, Kistemaker C, Riedstra M, et al. 1998. Fat Watch: a nationwide campaign in The Netherlands to reduce fat intake—effect evaluation. *Nutr. Health* 12:119–30

117. Wang JS, Carson EC, Lapane KL, Eaton CB, Gans KM, et al. 1999. The effect of physician office visits on CHD risk factor modification as part of a worksite cholesterol screening program. *Prev. Med.* 28:221–28

118. West DW, Slattery ML, Robison LM, Schuman KL, Ford MH, et al. 1989. Dietary intake and colon cancer: sex- and anatomic site-specific associations. *Am. J. Epidemiol.* 130:883–94

119. White E, Shattuck AL, Kristal AR, Urban N, Prentice RL, et al. 1992. Maintenance of a low-fat diet: follow-up of the Women's Health Trial. *Cancer Epidemiol. Biomarkers Prev.* 1:315–23

120. Wiesemann A, Metz J, Nuessel E, Scheidt R, Scheuermann W. 1997. Four years of practice-based and exercise-supported behavioural medicine in one community of the German CINDI area. Countrywide Integrated Non-Communicable Diseases Intervention. *Int. J. Sports Med.* 18:308–15

121. Willett WC, Hunter DJ, Stampfer MJ,

Colditz G, Manson JE, et al. 1992. Dietary fat and fiber in relation to risk of breast cancer. An 8-year follow-up. *JAMA* 268:2037–44

122. Willett WC, Stampfer MJ, Colditz GA, Rosner BA, Speizer FE. 1990. Relation of meat, fat, and fiber intake to the risk of colon cancer in a prospective study among women. *N. Engl. J. Med.* 323: 1664–72

123. Wynder EL, Gori GB. 1977. Contribution of the environment to cancer incidence: an epidemiologic exercise. *J. Natl. Cancer Inst.* 58:825–32

Annu. Rev. Public Health 2002. 23:287–302

THE MACROECONOMIC DETERMINANTS OF HEALTH

S. V. Subramanian[1], Paolo Belli[2], and Ichiro Kawachi[1]

[1]Department of Health and Social Behavior and [2]Department of Population and International Health, Harvard School of Public Health, Boston, Massachusetts 02115; e-mail: Ichiro.Kawachi@channing.harvard.edu

Key Words economic development, poverty, inequality, health

■ **Abstract** Why are some societies healthier than others? The consensus in development economics is that the health achievement of nations has to do with their levels of economic development. Higher per capita incomes, through steady and stable economic growth, increase a nation's capacity to purchase the necessary economic goods and services that promote health. In this paper, we review the conceptual and empirical linkages between poverty and poor health in both developing and developed countries. The empirical evidence is overwhelming that poverty, measured at the level of societies as well as individuals, is causally related to poor health of societies and individuals, respectively. Recent macroeconomic research has also drawn attention to the role of health as a form of human capital that is vital for achieving economic stability. In particular, attention has been drawn toward the ways in which unhealthy societies impede the process of economic development. However, the reciprocal connection between economic prosperity and improved health is neither automatic nor universal. Other features of society, such as the equality in the distribution of the national wealth, seem to matter as well for improving average population health and especially for reducing inequalities in health. We conclude by arguing for a need to reexamine the way in which health is conceptualized within the macroeconomic development framework.

INTRODUCTION

A child born in 1999 in one of the 24 healthiest countries of the world can expect to live for more than 70 healthy years. By contrast, a child born in one of the 51 least healthy countries can expect to live less than 50 years (11). Why are some societies healthier than others? An obvious starting point for our inquiry is the observation that poorer countries have lower levels of average health achievement. At the individual level, there are cogent grounds for asserting that lack of income is causally linked to poorer health. Higher incomes provide greater command over many of the goods and services that promote health, including better nutrition, access to clean water, sanitation, housing, and good quality health services (10). Although there is little doubt about the effect that individual income has on

0163-7525/02/0510-0287$14.00

287

individual health, the relationship between average national income [measured by per capita Gross Domestic Product (GDP)] to average national life expectancy and other health indicators is by no means universal or automatic. This point is underscored by the existence of "poorer" societies that exhibit unexpectedly high levels of health achievements. For example, the health performance of countries such as Costa Rica (1997 GDP $6650 per capita, life expectancy 76.0 years) or Cuba (GDP $3100 per capita, life expectancy 75.7 years) challenges the notion that economic growth is the sole route to longevity (60). Conversely, the United States is the wealthiest country in the world (GDP $29,010 per capita), yet ranks near the bottom of the most developed countries in terms of health indicators (average life expectancy 76.7 years). The United States is 12th overall on 16 indicators of health status—behind Japan, Sweden, Canada, France, Australia, Spain, Finland, Netherlands, United Kingdom, Denmark, and Belgium (66).

This review traces our current understanding of the macroeconomic determinants of population health. We begin by discussing the conceptual linkages between economic development and health. In particular, we define economic development along two key dimensions: levels of economic poverty and the distributive aspects of economic well-being. We further decompose the notion of economic poverty in terms of its relative and absolute dimensions and more crucially in terms of how these different dimensions can be conceptualized at the individual and contextual levels. Next, we discuss the empirical evidence linking low economic development to poor health. The empirical evidence is drawn from both developed and developing economies. The connection between poverty and health is not simply unidirectional; rather, increasing attention is being paid to the reverse pathway, i.e., how poor aggregate health may pose an obstacle to a country's economic growth and development. We then proceed to discuss the ongoing and contentious debate about the role of economic inequality as a determinant of population health. In the final section, we argue for the need to expand the notion of economic development itself. Drawing on Amartya Sen's capability approach, we discuss the extent to which his approach alters the way we conceptualize health and in turn the implications for macroeconomic policy. We conclude by arguing that the key to answering the question of why are some societies healthier than others hinges on our ability to grasp two issues. First, economic development should not be conceptualized solely in terms of individual poverty reduction; and second, the distributive aspects of economic well-being demand our attention as much as the goal of raising aggregate levels of wealth and income.

ECONOMIC DEVELOPMENT AND HEALTH: A CONCEPTUAL OVERVIEW

Before we outline the several, interrelated yet distinct components of the connection between economic development and health, we clarify the way in which development is typically defined. The view of economic development as increasing the production of goods and services has conventionally informed the assessment of standards of living of people, societies, and countries, and to a large extent continues to do so (2). The informational metric typically used comprises a set of standard economic indicators such as GDP, per capita income, and scale of expenditure on, and consumption of, production-related goods and services. Reducing poverty, at the same time, lies at the heart of development economics (28). A key purpose of economic development, arguably, is to improve the lives of the majority of people, which in economic terms would entail increasing incomes and thereby reducing income-based poverty or economic deprivation. As we argue below, such a narrow definition of economic development seriously truncates the choice of policies available to societies in their pursuit of population health improvement.

Even if one accepts poverty reduction as the major goal of economic development, radically different policy implications emerge depending on the conceptual definition of "poverty" adopted. One commonly adopted definition of poverty draws on Rowntree's classic concept of a "socially acceptable" amount of money required to achieve minimum physical efficiency (48). Based on the nutritional content of various foods and their local prices, a monetary threshold is determined, and the poverty rate is then the proportion of people living below that amount (22). This approach—also termed the *absolute* poverty approach—has been adopted officially by a number of countries, including the United States (14). The World Bank defines poverty according to the lowest level of income that is necessary for purchasing a minimum (subsistence) basket of goods (74). According to this measure, those unable to secure at least that minimum level of income are considered to be poor. For the poorest countries the subsistence level of income is set at a per capita income of $1.00 per day adjusted for purchasing power parity. Absolute notions of poverty thus tend to be prescriptive definitions based on the assessment of experts about people's minimum needs and are usually defined without reference to social contexts or norms (22).

In contrast to the absolute approach to poverty assessment, the relative approach defines poverty in terms of its relation to the standards that exist elsewhere in society. For example, in the Luxembourg Income Study, poverty is measured as a proportion (less than 50%) of the average disposable income per capita (63). Some governments also define poverty in relative terms. In Armenia, for example, the government's poverty line has been fixed at 40% of median per capita expenditure, with 27% of the population living below this line counted as poor. Indeed, "relativeness" of deprivation need not always be made in relation to one reference. For instance, in Nigeria, two poverty lines have been used: those with per capita expenditures below two thirds of the median are defined as poor; those below one third of the median are considered very poor.

Although the two are distinct concepts, they are not unrelated. For instance, if economic growth only helps the non-poor to increase their incomes then the numbers of people in absolute poverty will remain unaffected, but their relative poverty will increase because of the increase in the average per capita income.

Conversely, if economic growth benefits all people across the income distribution, there may be a reduction in the number of people in absolute poverty, but the prevalence of relative poverty will remain unchanged. As is evident, both these approaches are conceptualized at the individual level.

Absolute and relative poverty-based pathways can be conceptualized at a societal or contextual level and often this distinction is not made clear. Indeed, most aggregate analysis develops measures of poverty that are individually based but aggregated at a spatial scale. This can be problematic if appropriate distinctions are not recognized. For instance, there may be different health implications of being poor (an individual characteristic) as opposed to, and/or combined with, living in a poor society (a contextual characteristic). The tendency in the existing literature, as we demonstrate, has been to understate the multilevel nature of connection between economic development and health. Researchers have used the notion of poverty without clearly highlighting the unit at which such a process/phenomenon is being conceptualized.

While it is important to be clear about the unit at which poverty is being observed and understood, it is also necessary to define the evaluation of health in unambiguous terms. In terms of the unit of observation, it is people who die and not places. Measures such as life expectancy or infant and child mortality rate are typical examples of evaluating health at an aggregate level. On the other hand, health data need not always be aggregated to a spatial unit and can be analyzed and evaluated at the individual level. What is critical to the process of evaluating population health, however, is the need to distinguish between the average population health levels of a society, and how equitably is health distributed across different groups within and between societies. Thus, spatially aggregated health measures (such as life expectancy, infant mortality) typically provide average levels of health in a society with no reference to how equally or unequally health is distributed in that society. Meanwhile, health measures evaluated at the individual level have the ability to additionally provide an assessment of the health distribution in a society across various socioeconomic groups of interest. In other words, the framework for addressing the macro effects of poverty on health can take two dimensions: To what extent does poverty (*a*) affect the average health of the populations; (*b*) reduce the between-group health inequalities within a country; and (*c*) reduce the between-country health inequalities?

As can be seen, there are different ways of conceptualizing poverty and its connection to health, and each is important in its own right. The objective of the review, therefore, is twofold; first, to survey the existing evidence between poverty and health; and second, to assess the extent to which existing literature has decomposed this connection. Indeed, most studies on poverty and health tend to conceptualize this connection at an individual level. We draw on evidence from both developing and developed countries to underscore the global dimensions of this important issue. Our focus is essentially on the macroeconomic pathways to aggregate population health and accompanying group inequalities. While there are other important macro-level pathways, such as primary care physician supply

(61, 62), health insurance markets, or the role of state health departments and health systems in general, we focus on income poverty and income inequality, as these are the two key economic indicators that policy makers usually use to evaluate a country's standard of living.

POVERTY AND HEALTH: BETWEEN-COUNTRY AND WITHIN-COUNTRY EVIDENCE FROM DEVELOPING COUNTRIES

Regardless of the diversity of the existing studies in terms of measurement approaches of poverty, study design, and geographical focus, there is a striking consistency in the association between poverty and poor health (77). Beaglehole & Bonita (3) assert that poverty is the most important cause of preventable death, disease, and disability.

For developing countries, the two comprehensive sources of evidence for studying the relationship between poverty and poor health are the Living Standard Measurement Surveys (LSMS) and the Demographic and Health Surveys (DHS). While the LSMS contain very accurate information on households' level of consumption and expenditure, there is less detailed information on different health outcomes in the developing countries. On the other hand, the DHS data are based on very large samples and contain accurate information on health status and health service use, especially for maternal and child health services.

For between-country comparisons, Gwatkin et al. (23) used the DHS data from 40 developing countries to analyze inequalities in (a) infant and under-5 mortality; (b) levels of malnutrition; and (c) incidence of diarrhea and acute respiratory infection. The population in each country was divided in wealth quintiles, according to an index developed by Filmer & Pritchett (18). They showed that disparities between poor and non-poor vary enormously across countries, and across regions. On average, across regions of the world, a child born in a household belonging to the lowest wealth quintile is roughly twice as likely to die as a child born in a household from the highest quintile. An interesting finding of the study was that countries with lower mortality and morbidity rates among children were in general also characterized by wider disparities. This finding seems at odds with the nonlinear relationship between income and health characterized by diminishing returns to scale. For the above relationship to hold, one or a combination of the following must be true:

1. Increase in per capita income is associated with increases in income disparities suggesting that increases in per capita income are not uniform across groups;

2. A potential negative health externality occurs that is associated with being poor in a richer country;

3. Differential rates of diffusion of health-promoting innovations exist across different segments of society, and accessibility and utilization rates are unchanging or very slow for the poor; or

4. Societies experience varying degrees of health disparity because some of them put in place policies that make the health-income relationship more elastic whereas others do not.

An example of within-countries analysis using LSMS data is the study by Wagstaff (68), who compared data on infant and under-5 mortality rates from 9 developing countries. This study also found significant, although less pronounced than Gwatkin et al. (see 23), inequalities in infant and under-5 mortality rates across quintile-expenditure groups in all countries. The focus of both the studies by Gwatkin et al. (23) and Wagstaff (68) is on health inequalities, not aggregate levels of health. Furthermore, these studies, like most, consider health inequalities along "individual" income lines and *not* aggregate poverty or economic inequality.

Turning to the between-country data on poverty and aggregate health, some key findings emerge. The bulk of premature mortality and morbidity affects people living in the developing world. Ninety-eight percent of the deaths between birth and 15 years and 83% of the deaths between 15 and 59 years occur in the developing world (43). At the same time, over 30% (53% in sub-Saharan Africa) of deaths in the developing world occur in children younger than 5 years. That is why in terms of disability-adjusted life-years (DALYs) lost, the three main groups of disease are lower respiratory infections, diarrheal diseases, and perinatal disorders, all of which are prevalent in the developing world, especially in the poorest countries and among the youngest and poorer segments of the population.

During the period 1960–1990, income growth contributed to improvements in under-five mortality rate, adult mortality rate, as well as life expectancy. The contribution was largest in reducing male adult mortality rate (25%) and the least in reducing the under-5 mortality rate (17%) (76). Income growth contributed 20% to the increase in life expectancy (76). At the same time, different countries with similar level of incomes achieve widely disparate results in mortality rates and life expectancies. For example, at a GNP per capita of $600, life expectancy is 69 years in Honduras, whereas it is 51 years in Senegal (76).

Summarizing the literature in developing countries, much of the empirical evidence on poverty and health has focused on documenting the associations at the individual or household level. Few investigators have examined aggregate poverty as an independent contextual influence on the health of individuals and populations. Nor have researchers conceptually distinguished between the effects of absolute versus relative poverty. Although studies have looked at the distribution of health outcomes across different socioeconomic groups, the documented health disparities are consistent with either an effect of absolute poverty or relative poverty, or both. Before we turn to the evidence in developed countries, we turn briefly to discuss the reverse causal pathway, from poor aggregate health to aggregate poverty, and thereby, slower economic development.

IMPROVING HEALTH A NECESSARY CONDITION FOR ECONOMIC DEVELOPMENT

Recent macroeconomic literature on health has drawn heavily on what is referred to as the human capital view (8, 42, 46, 49). Under the human capital approach, substantial attention is given to people's achievements, such as being healthy. Improving human qualities, however, are pursued because of their value as a factor or capital in augmenting the production possibilities of the economy that, in turn, also enhance the income-earning abilities of people. Specifically, investing in people's health is seen to be worthwhile if the rate of return exceeds the cost of the investment in human capital (6).

The instrumental value of health in improving and sustaining economic growth and development has gained increased attention since the 1993 World Development Report publication (75). This is particularly evident in the recent work and deliberation of the WHO Commission on Macroeconomics and Health (CMH). Indeed, this follows the well-established microeconomic evidence; for instance, Leibenstein (4, 36) showed that workers with lower calorie intake tend to be less productive, an observation that was followed by a large volume of research linking education (seen as a form of human capital) to individual economic productivity. In similar vein, the emerging hypothesis is that a healthy population is a critical input into poverty reduction, economic growth, and long-term economic development (64). Specifically, a healthy population, by avoiding premature deaths, chronic disability, and diseases, limits the economic losses to society.

The macroeconomic evidence tells us that countries with the weakest conditions of health have a much harder time in achieving sustained growth than do countries with better conditions of health. According to the CMH preliminary report, the high human development countries (as measured by the Human Development Index of the United Nations Development Program) achieved robust and stable economic growth of 2.3% per year during the years 1990–1998, with 35 of the 36 countries enjoying rising living standards. The growth rate for the same period for the middle human development countries was 1.9%, with 7 of the 34 countries experiencing declines in living standards. The poorest human development countries, meanwhile, experienced a growth close to zero.

Other studies on the contribution of health to economic growth (for example, see 25) show that perhaps 40% of economic growth in developing countries can be ascribed to improved health and nutritional status. These new studies seem to be supported by historical evidence indicating that the initial improvement in health status was one of the leading causes behind the productivity growth observed in Britain during the first phase of the industrial revolution (20). In a more contemporary setting, Gallup et al. (21) provide initial evidence by showing that malaria-affected countries have grown only 0.4% annually in the period 1965–1990, compared with 2.3% annual growth for countries not affected by malaria.

In a recent contribution to the literature on health status and saving behavior (a key macroeconomic variable), Chakraborty (12) shows through an overlapping generation growth model that at low per capita income levels, overall expenditure on health is also low, and so is average life expectancy. This may discourage savings and investment, despite the high returns obtainable, because populations are unwilling to give up present consumption in the context of poor future life prospects. Moreover, low life expectancy discourages human capital investment in education (because populations are uncertain whether they will be able to benefit from those investments), reduces skill accumulation and thus returns to physical capital, which in turn further thwarts growth.

The demographic transition induced by health improvements, referred to as the "demographic gift" in the literature on the East Asian economic miracle [see for example, Bloom & Williamson (9)], can be summarized as follows: Health interventions reduce infant and child mortality and so initially swell the young population. At the same time they induce a decrease in fertility rates. This latter result may also come about because parents decide the size of their family with a concern for the number of surviving children. If health interventions decrease infant mortality rates, they also reduce fertility rates, as parents realize that most of their children will survive. In short, the demographic transition induces a very favorable age structure of the population for a certain period, with few young and old dependents. This favorable age structure may have contributed significantly to the East Asian economic miracle of the 1970s and 1980s.

RELATIVE POVERTY AND HEALTH: EVIDENCE FROM DEVELOPED COUNTRIES

In affluent societies where the majority of the population, even the officially designated poor, do not confront the same level of deprivation as the poor in less developed countries, it is thought that relative poverty plays a correspondingly larger role in the excess burden of ill health associated with lower income [for recent reviews in the United States and the United Kingdom, see House & Williams (24), Marmot & Wilkinson (40)]. A related theme is, therefore, the socioeconomic gradient in health (1). That is, there is a step-wise gradation in poor health associated with progressively lower incomes, such that a person making $20,000 per year (who is not officially poor) nonetheless experiences worse health than someone making $35,000, and so on. Absolute deprivation still occurs within the richest countries, as evidence by the estimated 12 million children who faced hunger in the United States in 1999. The income-health curve is also steepest toward the lowest end of the income distribution.

Most tellingly, despite enjoying much lower rates of average premature mortality and morbidity compared with less developed countries, the magnitude of health disparities in relative terms is just as large within rich countries as in poor countries. The ratio of ill health, comparing the poorest to the most affluent, is twice, three times, or even higher, depending on the health outcome studied. Moreover, these disparities appear to be widening over time in many developed countries (40). The inability of even rich countries to substantially reduce socioeconomic disparities in health poses both a challenge to and riddle for development. Clearly, a society's health achievement is determined by factors beyond income growth alone.

In summary, the existing evidence is strong and conclusive that poverty reduction should be a part of an overall macroeconomic strategy to improve population health. While this is particularly true for developing countries, it is equally relevant for developed countries. The evidence on the contribution of relative poverty to health—demonstrated by the existence of a socioeconomic gradient in health even in rich countries—points to the need to pay attention to the distribution of economic resources as well as the aggregate level of wealth and income. We now turn to this issue.

ECONOMIC INEQUALITY AND HEALTH

In recent years, growing attention has been focused on the distribution of income in a society as an independent determinant of population health. There are sound theoretical reasons for suggesting that inequality in the distribution of income matters for population health. Given the same level of average income, a more unequal society is more likely to have greater numbers of people living in poverty, both in the absolute and relative senses. Because of the concave nature of the relationship between income and life expectancy (i.e., there are diminishing rates of return to health with rising incomes), this implies that a redistribution of income from the rich to the poor will raise average life expectancy (32).

Ecological evidence, at both the cross-country and within-country levels, suggests that the degree of income inequality is indeed related to a society's level of health achievement [see (32) and references therein]. More contentious is whether there is an effect of income inequality per se on population health. To answer this question, it is necessary to distinguish the effects of poverty from the effects of income inequality. This requires multilevel study designs that gather information on income at both the individual and the aggregate levels (67). In other words, studies need to distinguish between the compositional effects of low income within a given society and the contextual effects of income inequality. A growing number of such studies, using some variant of multilevel techniques, have been reported in the literature, although most of them pertain to data from the United States. Different health outcomes have been examined, including mortality (15, 16, 19, 37), self-rated health (7, 35, 41, 65, 67), depressive symptoms (27), and health behaviors (17).

Four of these ten studies have found no effects, or inconsistent effects of income inequality on health (15, 16, 19, 41), whereas the remaining six found a small but independent effect of income inequality even after adjusting for individual-level income (7, 17, 27, 35, 37, 65). The individual studies are not reviewed here, as they have been more extensively discussed by Wagstaff & van Doorslaer (69), Mellor & Milyo (41), and Deaton (16). Rather, we identify and summarize the key areas of debate within this literature.

First, investigators have drawn conflicting conclusions about the effect of income inequality on health depending on what variables were controlled for in statistical models. For the studies examining poor health and income inequality at the state level in the United States, the relationship is independent of poverty status at the individual level. However, investigators disagree when it comes to controlling for additional variables. For example, Mellor & Milyo (41) find no residual effect of state-level income inequality on poor self-rated health once they adjust for individual educational attainment. Some have argued that this procedure represents statistical over-adjustment to the extent that inequalities in public spending on education are theorized to be one of the mechanisms by which state-level inequality in the distribution of income leads to poor health (34). Others have argued that the relationship between metropolitan-level and state-level income inequality and mortality is not robust with respect to control for the percent of the population who are African American (16). In other words, income inequality appears to be correlated with the proportion of black residents in an area, and it is the latter variable that is truly associated with excess black and white mortality rates. Although intriguing, the causal interpretation (or for that matter, the policy implications) of the variable "percent black" is itself unclear. The association of income inequality with mortality is emphatically not confounded by the compositional effect of race, since it has been shown that income inequality is associated with higher rates of mortality for both blacks and whites (16).

A second area of debate concerns whether the United States is unique among countries of the world in terms of exhibiting an association between income inequality and poor health. For example, recent cross-national studies, at least among rich countries, have failed to demonstrate an association between income inequality and adult mortality (16). If an association is found (such as with infant mortality), it seems to have been driven by the outlier status of the United States, which has both high income inequality and high infant mortality (26). In other countries, such as Canada, no relationship between mortality and income inequality has been reported at the province or city level (47). The possibility has therefore been raised that the ecological relationship between income inequality and poor health is not universal, but rather depends on the social policies that governments deploy to mitigate the effects of economic inequalities (39). A useful area for future investigation would be to identify the characteristics of societies in which income inequality is associated with poor health—as in the United States, Britain (5), Brazil (50), Taiwan (13)—and to contrast them to societies in which inequality does not seem to matter.

Yet a third area of debate concerns the relevant geographic level at which income inequality matters for health—whether countries, regions, states, cities, or neighborhoods. Much of the empirical multilevel demonstrations have occurred within the United States at the state level. In ecological analyses, there is some suggestion that income inequality is associated with higher mortality at the metropolitan-area level (38), although the individual-level association with poor self-rated health disappears once the mean income of a city is taken into account (7). No studies have so far demonstrated that income inequality is associated with poor health at the census tract level (65).

The relevant geographic level for testing the association between income inequality and health depends crucially on the postulated mechanism of effect. Thus, states may be relevant if income inequality is hypothesized to affect political participation and patterns of government spending on welfare, public education, and Medicaid (31). On the other hand, smaller geographic units such as communities may be more relevant for examining processes such as the stress induced by invidious social comparisons or competition with affluent neighbors.

Few investigators have attempted to dissect the cross-level interactions between area-level inequality and the health of particular sociodemographic groups. That is, for whom is inequality harmful, and why? Some evidence suggests that living in a high inequality area is beneficial for the health of affluent individuals (27, 67), and other studies suggest that income inequality is particularly detrimental to the health of the poor (35) or near-poor (37). At present, no consensus exists on this issue.

Lastly, much more work remains to be carried out in specifying the mechanisms by which income inequality is postulated to affect health, and testing these pathways against specific data sets. At present, three separate, though not mutually exclusive, mechanisms have been put forward (32). The first is through reduced access to life opportunities, material resources, and opportunity structures (see 29). For instance, in more unequal societies the pooling of resources that could finance public services such as health care systems and education is difficult to achieve. Since the richer segments tend typically to use privately funded and provided services, cross subsidy becomes difficult, thus affecting the accessibility and availability of such services to the poor. This line of argument becomes complex in the case of developing countries where it is usually the non-poor section of the population that ends up using much of the services. The second set of processes is linked to decreasing social capital that manifests through factors such as erosion of social cohesion, increased social exclusion, and conflict (see 30, 33, 44, 45, 70–73). Third, more direct psychosocial pathways such as hopelessness, lack of control, or loss of respect arising as a consequence of inequality have been identified as having a potential effect on individual health (see 71–73).

THE ENDS OF ECONOMIC DEVELOPMENT: A CRITIQUE

The preceding sections traced the major currents that dominate the international literature on the macroeconomic determinants of health. While most of the literature defines poverty in mainly income terms, the notions of poverty and development itself have undergone revisions. As is clear within the conventional economics view of poverty, no direct importance is attached to achievements such as being healthy. Such a view has been responsible for the widely acceptable notion that health is an automatic outcome of improved economic performance of societies. Often improved economic performance of countries is equated with higher economic status of the individuals who live in these countries. Arguably, this view tends to relegate matters to population health as an automatic function of individual opulance. As was shown in the discussion related to the idea of reverse causality between economic poverty and health, this limitation is partly corrected within the human capital view where a direct importance is attached to improving population health. Important as this is, the approach undervalues the direct importance of health and overvalues its indirect importance (58). Thus, while putting people at the center of evaluative procedures, this approach sees human achievements simply as a means to an end. In this final section, we highlight one such perspective that, arguably, alters the way health is positioned in much of the macroeconomics literature. This refers to what is now called the human-capability or capability-poverty view.

Amartya Sen, the noted economist-philosopher, has convincingly argued that the process of development, both in theory and practice, should be conceptualized and assessed as people's ability to do things that they have a reason to value (51–53, 60). According to this view, development does not simply involve the expansion of income. Rather, according to Sen, the view that comes closest to the notion of well-being is one that relates to "what people can do or can be"; what he calls the capability approach.

Critical to the capability argument is the notion of human freedom (54, 55). In this way people are placed at the center of the development agenda. While this is not the first time that the idea of freedom has been invoked, what makes the capability position different is the proposed type of freedom. The concept of capability per se is significantly influenced by the notion of positive freedom ("what a person can actually do") as against the negative view that perceives freedom as the presence or absence of interference from others. The general importance of distinguishing between the ends and the means of development is brought into sharper focus by considering the intrinsic as opposed to the instrumental view of freedom. The intrinsic view values freedom for its own sake whereas the instrumental view considers freedom to be important principally because of its significance for other achievements. In light of this distinction, Sen (54, 55) specifically proposes that assessments be based on the positive-intrinsic type of freedom. Good health, in the sense of freedom from premature mortality and morbidity, is both instrumental to development and constitutive of it (see 56, 57, 59).

As can be seen, while health is viewed as central to development, its treatment varies according to the priority given to the ends versus the means of development. While both have their merits, the capability view is inclusive of the human capital argument. Besides attaching intrinsic importance to health, the capability view also takes a broader view of the instrumental benefits that health could bring about to objectives as broad as social change or as narrow as stabilizing population growth.

Indeed, as we have seen, health status provides an exquisitely sensitive signal of the more general well-being of any given community and society than any macroeconomic measure does. In particular, indicators of population health status sharply bring out the effective well-being of the more vulnerable segments of that community or society as compared to income-related indicators. Since improved health prospects reinforce the potential for economic growth, particularly among the poor, stagnating or even worsening key health indicators convey a serious message of concern, on grounds both of equity as well as long-term efficiency.

CONCLUSION

The evidence is now overwhelming that poverty (whether conceptualized at the country level or at the individual level) is strongly correlated with poorer health outcomes, on average. This applies to both the developing countries of the world (because of absolute poverty), as well as to more developed countries, because of the lingering effects of relative poverty. Moreover, the relationship is likely reciprocal and reinforcing, in that societies burdened with diseases, suffering from endemic diseases, and with lower life expectancies tend to experience low productivity and low and unstable economic growth. At the same time, the connection between economic well-being and improved health status (and reduced health inequalities) is neither automatic nor universal. It seems likely that other factors, such as the degree of equality in the distribution of the national product—especially in the form of government policies that support the living standards of the poor—matter in their own right for health and human development. Most important, improving population health (in terms of increased averages as well as reduced inequalities) and investing in public health in both developed and developing countries should be an intrinsic component of any poverty reduction policy in particular, and macroeconomic policy in general. Finally, further studies need to consider explicitly the complex multilevel nature of the connection between public health and key macroeconomic determinants.

Visit the Annual Reviews home page at www.annualreviews.org

LITERATURE CITED

1. Adler NE, Boyce T, Chesney MA, Cohen S, Folkman S, et al. 1994. Socioeconomic status and health: the challenge of the gradient. *Am. Psychol.* 49:15–24

2. Barro R. 1991. Economic growth in a cross-section of countries. *Q. J. Econ.* 106:404–44

3. Beaglehole R, Bonita R. 1997. *Public Health at the Crossroads.* Cambridge: Cambridge Univ. Press

4. Behrman J. 1996. The impact of health and nutrition on education. *World Bank Res. Obs.* 11:23–37

5. Ben-Shlomo Y, White IR, Marmot M.

1996. Does the variation in socio-economic characteristics of an area affect mortality? *Br. Med. J.* 312:1013–14

6. Bhalla S, Gill I. 1992. *Externalities in the New Growth Theory: The Importance of Female Human Capital.* Washington, DC: World Bank

7. Blakely TA, Lochner K, Kawachi I. 2002. Metropolitan area income inequality and self-rated health—a multilevel study. *Soc. Sci. Med.* In press

8. Blaug M. 1976. The empirical status of human capital theory: a slightly jaundiced survey. *J. Econ. Lit.* 14:827–55

9. Bloom D, Williamson J. 1998. Demographic transitions and economic miracles in emerging Asia. *World Bank Econ. Rev.* 12:419–55

10. Bloom DE, Canning D. 2000. The health and wealth of nations. *Science* 287:1207–9

11. Bloom DE, Canning D. 2001. A new health opportunity. *Development* 44:36–43

12. Chakraborty S. 1999. *Public health, longevity and economic growth.* PhD thesis. Univ. Calif. Los Angeles

13. Chiang T-L. 1999. Economic transition and changing relation between income inequality and mortality in Taiwan: regression analysis. *Br. Med. J.* 319:1162–65

14. Citro CF, Michael RT, eds. 1995. *Measuring Poverty. A New Approach.* Washington, DC: Natl. Acad. Press. 501 pp.

15. Daly MC, Duncan GJ, Kaplan GA, Lynch JW. 1998. Macro to micro links in the relation between income inequality and mortality. *Millbank Q.* 76:315–39

16. Deaton A. 2001. *Health, inequality, and economic development.* Prepared for Work. Group 1 WHO Comm. Macroecon. Health. New Jersey: Princeton Univ.

17. Diez-Roux AV, Link BG, Northridge ME. 2000. A multilevel analysis of income inequality and cardiovascular disease risk factors. *Soc. Sci. Med.* 50:673–87

18. Filmer D, Pritchett L. 1998. Estimating wealth effects without expenditure data— or tears: an application to educational enrollments in the states of India. *World Bank*

Policy Res. Work. Pap., No. 1994. Washington, DC: World Bank

19. Fiscella K, Franks P. 1997. Poverty or income inequality as predictor of mortality: longitudinal cohort study. *Br. Med. J.* 314:1724–27

20. Fogel R. 1997. New findings on secular trends in nutrition and mortality: some implications for population theory. In *Handbook of Population and Family Economics, Vol. 1a,* ed. M Rosenzweig, O Stark, pp. 433–81. Amsterdam: Elsevier

21. Gallup J, Luke J, Sachs J. 1998. The economic impact of malaria: cross-country evidence. In *Health, Health Policy and Economic Outcomes,* Health Dev. Satellite, Geneva: WHO Transit. Team

22. Gordon D, Spicker P, eds. 1999. *The International Glossary of Poverty.* New York: St. Martin's Press. 162 pp.

23. Gwatkin DR, Rutstein S, Johnson K, Pande R, Wagstaff A. 2000. *Socio-economic Differences in Health, Nutrition, and Population in Bangladesh (and comparable publications covering Benin, Bolivia, Brazil, Burkina Faso, Cameroun, Central African Republic, Colombia, Comores, Côte d'Ivoire, Dominican Republic, Ghana, Guatemala, Haiti, India, Indonesia, Kenya, Kyrgyz Republic, Madagascar, Malawi, Mali, Morocco, Mozambique, Namibia, Nepal, Nicaragua, Niger, Nigeria, Pakistan, Paraguay, Peru, Philippines, Senegal, Tanzania, Togo, Turkey, Uganda, Vietnam, Zambia, and Zimbabwe).* Washington, DC: World Bank

24. House JS, Williams DR. 2000. Understanding and reducing socioeconomic and racial/ethnic disparities in health. In *Promoting Health,* ed. BD Smedley, SL Syme, pp. 81–124. Washington, DC: Natl. Acad. Press

25. Jamison D, Lau L, Wang J. 1998. Health's contribution to economic growth, 1965–1990. In *Health, Health Policy and Economic Outcomes.* Health Dev. Satellite. Geneva: WHO Transit. Team

26. Judge K, Mulligan J, Benzeval M. 1997.

Income inequality and population health. *Soc. Sci. Med.* 46:567–79

27. Kahn RS, Wise PH, Kennedy BP, Kawachi I. 2000. State income inequality, household income, and maternal mental and physical health: cross-sectional national survey. *Br. Med. J.* 321:1311–15

28. Kanbur R, Squire L. 1999. *The evolution of thinking about poverty: exploring the interactions.* http://www.worldbank.org/ poverty/wdrpoverty/evolut.htm (accessed on Oct. 6, 2001)

29. Kaplan GA, Pamuk ER, Lynch JM, Cohen RD, Balfour JL. 1996. Inequality in income and mortality in the United States: analysis of mortality and potential pathways. *Br. Med. J.* 312:999–1003

30. Kawachi I, Kennedy BP, Lochner K, Prothrow-Stith D. 1997. Social capital, income inequality, and mortality. *Am. J. Public Health* 87:1491–98

31. Kawachi I, Kennedy BP. 1999. Income inequality and health: pathways and mechanisms. *Health Services Res.* 34(1 Pt.2): 215–27

32. Kawachi I, Kennedy BP, Wilkinson RG, eds. 1999. *The Society and Population Health Reader Volume 1-Income inequality and health.* New York: The New Press, 506 pp.

33. Kawachi I, Berkman LF. Social cohesion, social capital, and health. In *Social Epidemiology*, ed. LF Berkman, I Kawachi, pp. 174–90. New York: Oxford Univ. Press.

34. Kawachi I, Blakely T. 2001. When economists and epidemiologists disagree (commentary). *J. Health Polit. Policy Law* 26:533–41

35. Kennedy BP, Kawachi I, Glass R, Prothrow-Stith D. 1998. Income distribution, socioeconomic status, and self rated health in the United States: multilevel analysis. *Br. Med. J.* 317:917–21

36. Leibenstein H. 1957. *Economic Backwardness and Economic Growth: Studies in the Theory of Economic Development.* New York: Wiley

37. Lochner K, Pamuk E, Makuc D, Kennedy BP, Kawachi I. 2001. State-level income inequality and individual mortality risk: a prospective, multilevel study. *Am. J. Public Health* 91:385–91

38. Lynch JW, Kaplan GA, Pamuk ER. 1998. Income inequality and mortality in metropolitan areas of the United States. *Am. J. Public Health* 88:1074–80

39. Lynch JW, Davey Smith G, Kaplan GA, House JS. 2000. Income inequality and mortality: importance to health of individual income, psychosocial environment, or material conditions. *Br. Med. J.* 320:1200–4

40. Marmot M, Wilkinson RG, eds. 1999. *Social Determinants of Health.* Oxford: Oxford Univ. Press. 291 pp.

41. Mellor JM, Milyo J. 2001. Reexamining the evidence of an ecological association between income inequality and health. *J. Health Polit. Policy Law* 26:487–522

42. Meltzer D. 1995. *Mortality decline, the demographic transition and economic growth.* PhD thesis. Univ. Chicago Sch. Med.

43. Murray C, Lopez A, eds. 1996. *The Global Burden of Disease: A Comprehensive Assessment of Mortality and Disability from Diseases, Injuries and Risk Factors in 1990 and Projected to 2020.* Cambridge, Harvard Sch. Public Health on behalf of the WHO and the World Bank (Global Burden of Disease and Injuries Ser., Vol. 1)

44. Putnam RD. 1993. *Making Democracy Work—Civic Tradition in Modern Italy.* Princeton, NJ: Princeton Univ. Press. 258 pp.

45. Putnam RD. 2000. *Bowling Alone: The Collapse and Revival of American Community.* New York: Simon & Schuster. 541 pp.

46. Rosenzweig M. 1990. Population growth and human capital investment. *J. Polit. Econ.* 98:538–57

47. Ross NA, Wolfson MC, Dunn JR, Berthelot J-M, Kaplan GA, et al. 2000. Relationship between income inequality and mortality in Canada and in the United States:

cross-sectional assessment using census data and vital statistics. *Br. Med. J.* 319: 989–92

48. Rowntree BS. 1910. *Poverty: A Study of Town Life.* London: Macmillan

49. Schultz TW. 1981. *Investing in People: The Economics of Population Quality.* Berkeley, CA: Univ. Calif. Press

50. Szwarcwald CL, Bastos FI, Viavaca F, Andrade CLT. 1999. Income inequality and homicide rates in Rio de Janeiro, Brazil. *Am. J. Public Health* 89:845–50

51. Sen AK. 1973. On the development of basic income indicators to supplement GNP measures. *UN Econ. Bull. Asia Far East* 24:1–11

52. Sen AK. 1985. *Commodities and Capabilities.* Amsterdam: North Holland

53. Sen AK. 1987. *The Standard of Living.* Cambridge: Cambridge Univ. Press

54. Sen AK. 1990. Individual freedom as a social commitment. *NY Rev. Books* 37:49–54

55. Sen AK. 1992. *Inequality Reexamined.* Oxford: Oxford Univ. Press

56. Sen AK. 1993. Economics of life and death. *Sci. Am.* May:18–25

57. Sen AK. 1995. Demography and welfare economics. *Empirica* 22:1–21

58. Sen AK. 1997. Human capital and human capability. *World Dev.* 25:1959–61

59. Sen AK. 1999. Health in development. *Bull. WHO* 77:619–23

60. Sen AK. 1999. *Development as Freedom.* New York: Knopf. 366 pp.

61. Shi L, Starfield B. 2000. Primary care, income inequality, and self rated health in the United States: a mixed-level analysis. *Int. J. Health Ser.* 30:541–55

62. Shi L, Starfield B. 2001. The effect of primary care physician supply and income inequality on mortality among blacks and whites in metropolitan areas. *Am. J. Public Health* 91:1246–50

63. Smeeding T, O'Higgins M, Rainwater L, eds. 1990. *Poverty, Inequality and Income Distribution in Comparative Perspective: The Luxembourg Income Study.* New York: Harvester Wheatsheaf

64. Smith J. 1999. Healthy bodies in thick wallets: the dual relation between health and economic status. *J. Econ. Perspect.* 13:145–66

65. Soobader M-J, LeClere F. 1999. Aggregation and the measurement of income inequality: effects on morbidity. *Soc. Sci. Med.* 48:733–44

66. Starfield B. 2000. Is US health really the best in the world? *JAMA* 284:483–85

67. Subramanian SV, Kawachi I, Kennedy BP. 2001. Does the state you live in make a difference? Multilevel analysis of self-rated health in the U.S. *Soc. Sci. Med.* 53:9–19

68. Wagstaff A. 2000. Socioeconomic inequalities in child mortality: comparisons across nine developing countries. *Bull. WHO* 78:19–29

69. Wagstaff A, van Doorslaer E. 2000. Income inequality and health: What does the literature tell us? *Annu. Rev. Public Health* 21:543–67

70. Wallace R, Wallace D. 1997. Community marginalisation and the diffusion of disease and disorder in the United States. *Br. Med. J.* 314:1341–45

71. Wilkinson RG. 1996. *Unhealthy Societies: The Afflictions of Inequality.* London: Routledge. 255 pp.

72. Wilkinson RG, Kawachi I, Kennedy BP. 1998. Mortality, the social environment, crime and violence. *Sociol. Health Illn.* 20:578–97

73. Wilkinson RG. 2000. *Mind the Gap. Hierarchies, Health and Human Evolution.* London: Weidenfeld & Nicolson

74. World Bank. 1990. *World Development Report 1990: Poverty.* Washington, DC: World Bank

75. World Bank. 1993. *World Development Report: Investing in Health.* Washington, DC: World Bank

76. World Bank. 1999. *Health, Nutrition, and Population Indicators.* Washington, DC: World Bank

77. World Health Organ. 1999. *World Health Report: Making a Difference.* Geneva: WHO

Annu. Rev. Public Health 2002. 23:303–31

SOCIOECONOMIC STATUS AND HEALTH: The Potential Role of Environmental Risk Exposure

Gary W. Evans and Elyse Kantrowitz

Departments of Design and Environmental Analysis and of Human Development, College of Human Ecology, Cornell University, Ithaca, NY 14853-4401; e-mail: gwe1@cornell.edu

Key Words   environmental justice, income, socioeconomic status, poverty, environmental risk

■ **Abstract**   Among several viable explanations for the ubiquitous SES-health gradient is differential exposure to environmental risk. We document evidence of inverse relations between income and other indices of SES with environmental risk factors including hazardous wastes and other toxins, ambient and indoor air pollutants, water quality, ambient noise, residential crowding, housing quality, educational facilities, work environments, and neighborhood conditions. We then briefly overview evidence that such exposures are inimical to health and well-being. We conclude with a discussion of the research and policy implications of environmental justice, arguing that a particularly salient feature of poverty for health consequences is exposure to multiple environmental risk factors.

SOCIOECONOMIC STATUS AND HEALTH: THE POTENTIAL ROLE OF ENVIRONMENTAL RISK EXPOSURE

Satisfactory explanation for the ubiquitous socioeconomic status-health gradient remains elusive, suggesting, in part, that an adequate model of this relation is probably complex and multifaceted (1, 81). In this paper we provide an overview of data indicating that income is inversely correlated with exposure to suboptimal environmental conditions. By environmental conditions we mean the physical properties of the ambient and immediate surroundings of children, youth, and families, including pollutants, toxins, noise, and crowding as well as exposure to settings such as housing, schools, work environments, and neighborhoods. We also briefly cite evidence that each of these environmental factors, in turn, is linked to health.

The implicit conceptual model under discussion is as follows (Figure 1): As can be seen above, what we discuss is evidence for two necessary prerequisites for this model to be valid—namely that socioeconomic status (SES) is associated with environmental quality and, in turn, that environmental quality affects health. This is not equivalent, however, to the conclusion that SES effects on health are caused

0163-7525/02/0510-0303$14.00   **303**

SES ⇒ ENVIRONMENTAL ⇒ HEALTH
QUALITY

Figure 1 Basic underlying conceptual model.

by differential exposure to environmental quality. There are few if any data directly testing this proposition. What is necessary to verify the model shown in Figure 1 is that the SES health link is mediated by environmental quality.

In addition to this fundamental shortcoming in the extant database, results on SES and environmental exposure tend to be restricted to income and, in several cases, are not continuous; instead they compare individuals below and above the poverty line. Furthermore, for certain salient environments, especially work and school settings, scant data are available on income-related differential exposures to hazardous, polluted, or inadequate building conditions. The reader should also bear in mind that for several of the income-related environmental exposure results, the data are confounded with ethnicity. Given that there is also evidence that nonwhite individuals, at least in the United States, are more likely to be exposed to health-threatening environmental conditions than are white individuals, it can be difficult to disentangle associations between income and environmental quality from racism.

There is also a conceptual issue we wish to briefly discuss before overviewing some of the evidence for linkages among SES, environmental quality, and health. Nearly all of the empirical work, and for that matter theoretical discussion about this issue, has examined individual environmental risk factors. Research and discussion tend to be focused on specific pollutants, toxins, or particular ambient conditions such as housing quality and each respective factor's link to income or health. We suspect that the potential of environmental exposure to account for the link between SES and health derives from multiple exposures to a plethora of suboptimal environmental conditions. That is, we would argue that a particularly important and salient aspect of reduced income is exposure to a confluence of multiple, suboptimal environmental conditions. The poor are most likely to be exposed not only to the worst air quality, the most noise, the lowest-quality housing and schools, etc., but of particular consequence, also to lower-quality environments on a wide array of multiple dimensions. We hypothesize that it is the accumulation of exposure to multiple, suboptimal physical conditions rather than any singular environmental exposure that will provide a fruitful explanation for the SES health gradient.

SOCIOECONOMIC STATUS AND ENVIRONMENTAL QUALITY

In this section we overview data on the relations between income or SES and exposure to environmental risks. We examine both individual environmental conditions such as toxic wastes, air pollution, crowding, and noise as well as the physical quality of specific settings such as the home, school, work, and neighborhood.

Hazardous Wastes

The environmental justice movement, launched in the 1980s, called attention to the fact that low-income citizens, and especially low-income, ethnic minority individuals, were much more likely to be exposed to toxic wastes and other forms of health-threatening environmental conditions relative to their more affluent and white fellow citizens (67). An influential book, *Dumping in Dixie* (18), documented the geographic association of toxic waste dumps in the Southeastern region of the United States with low-income, minority neighborhoods. The percentage of families below the federal poverty line in census tracts inclusive of EPA Region IV Hazardous Waste Landfills ranged from 26% (South Carolina) to 42% in Alabama. Twenty-nine percent of families living within one mile of a commercial hazardous waste facility in Detroit are below the poverty line, and 49% of them are non-white. More than 1.5 miles away, 10% are poor and 18% are people of color (89). One hundred percent of U.S. Government uranium mining and 4 of the largest 10 coal strip mines are located on Native American reservations (53). Nearly half of Native Americans live below the federal poverty line. More recent analyses of income and race differentials in hazardous waste exposure reveal similar trends (142). Children's body lead burden is strongly associated with both income and race. For example, in a recent EPA Task Force report, "Environmental Equity: Reducing Risk for All Communities" (136), 68% of urban black children in families with incomes below $6000 had blood lead levels that exceeded safe limits in comparison to 15% of the same population with incomes above $15,000. For white children, the comparable data were 36% and 12%. The National Health and Nutrition Survey conducted in 1980 and 1990 documents elevated blood-lead levels in low-income individuals, particularly among inner-city residents (105).

Air Pollution

Ambient pollutant exposure reveals similar race and income-related trends. Figure 2, for example, depicts factory carcinogen emissions in Britain in relation to income (42a). Analogous data have been found for several other, common ambient air pollutants (e.g., sulfur oxides, fine particulates) with known pathogenic effects in the United States (42). Exposure to ozone, a principal toxic component of photochemical smog, as well as fine particulate matter, in the South Coast Air Basin of California, is inversely related to income levels (15). The World Bank has also become interested in environmental justice, publishing sobering statistical summaries about environmental health threats worldwide. For example, in low-income countries from the 1970s to the late 1980s, the average levels of suspended particulate matter in cities increased from approximately 300 μg per cubic meter of air to 325 μg. The total range of measured particulates for all of these cities at both time periods exceeded even marginal, let alone acceptable, limits from a respiratory health standpoint. Cities in middle-income countries over the same time period witnessed improved air quality (from approximately 180 to 150 μg/cubic meter of air) and wealthy countries improved from ~100 to 75 μg per cubic meter of air. Analogous data are provided by the World Bank for water quality (144).

Factory Pollution and Deprivation
(carcinogen emissions in local wards)

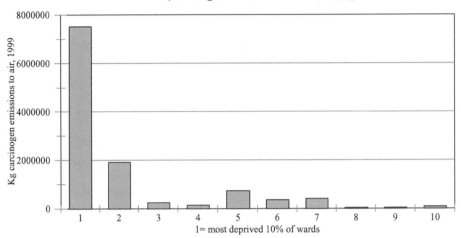

Figure 2   Factory pollution and income in England [reprinted by permission from Friends of the Earth, United Kingdom (42a)].

Today increasing interest is focused on exposure to indoor air quality, which may play an even greater role in the respiratory health and well-being of individuals, particularly young children. Levels of several common airborne toxins are higher indoors, and for young children, the duration of exposure is often greater inside relative to the outdoors. Although there are some suggestive data, with the exception of secondary cigarette smoke, little is known about the association between income levels and exposure to indoor air contaminants.

Parental smoking, which is inversely related to income levels, increases children's exposures to a wide variety of indoor toxins. For example, in the United States, 65% of preschool children living in poverty have been exposed to cigarette smoke at home in comparison to 47% of those not in poverty (94). In both the United States and Britain, mothers who are poorer are also less likely to quit and smoke more than their higher-income counterparts (54, 56). Length of tenure on welfare also predicts maternal smoking prevalence and consumption levels (55). Young children's levels of salivary cotinine increase linearly in relation to lower occupational class (27, 69). Cotinine is a metabolite of nicotine and a valid indicator of exposure to environmental tobacco smoke. Moreover, cumulative risk factors associated with poverty increase smoking prevalence in mothers of newborns. Rental occupied housing, lack of higher education, and single-parenthood status are associated with a ninefold increase in smoking among mothers of newborns in the United Kingdom (121). This association is independent of mother's age, parity, and ethnicity. Smoking during pregnancy is also highly correlated with maternal

TABLE 1   Radon exposure as a function of household income characteristics[a]

Percentage of households exceeding EPA safe limits (4 pCi/L) for radon		
Rental	Owner occupied <$40,000	Owner occupied >$40,000
66	41	36

[a]Adapted from Table 5, in Reference (22).

education. For example, 48% of American women who dropped out of high school smoke during pregnancy compared to 12% going beyond high school and 3% who are college graduates (95).

In rental units in the United States, 10% percent of households with incomes below the poverty line rely primarily upon hot air units without ducts, and 4% use unvented gas heaters as their primary heat source. For rental households with incomes exceeding $30,000, comparable figures are 7% and 1% for ductless hot air heat and unvented gas heaters, respectively (123). Toxic indoor air pollutants, NO_2 and CO, related to combustion processes (stoves, heating, smoking), are substantially higher in low-income, inner-city residences relative to U.S. averages (52, 116). Exposure to radon, a known carcinogen, is related to income levels in rural counties in New York state (see Table 1). Chi & Laquatra (22) suggest that income-related differences in radon exposure are probably related to structural deficiencies that provide more permeable vectors for radon to enter into the residence.

Acute respiratory obstructive diseases such as asthma are associated with serum IgE antibodies to dust mite feces, cats, cockroaches, and certain pollens. Exposure to cockroach allergens as well as antibody sensitivity is associated with socioeconomic status with 0%, 26%, and 46% of high-, middle-, and low-SES, respectively, children exposed (114). Positive skin tests data revealed a parallel SES gradient (114). Rosenstreich et al. (109) also found high levels of allergenic reactions to cockroaches in a general population sample of inner-city children and more than half of low-income asthma patients in several urban, inner-city samples evidenced specific IgE antibodies and positive skin test results to cockroaches (10, 72). Furthermore, dampness in houses, which is inversely associated with household income, is conducive to dust mites as well as molds and fungi, all related to respiratory obstructive disorders (51).

Water Pollution

Although most attention to environmental pollutants and income has been focused on hazardous wastes and air pollution, several case studies suggest higher levels of contaminated water among low-income populations (21). For example, 44% of water supplies for migrant farm workers in North Carolina tested positive for coliform and 26% for fecal coliform. For comparable farm areas in the same region, both levels were at 0% (23). Low-income Chicano populations living along the U.S./Mexico border (Colonias) are plagued by contaminated drinking water. Estimates indicate, for example, that in Texas nearly 50% of the Colonias population lacks safe drinking water, a condition that is largely believed to be the source of the threefold increase in this population's risk for waterborne diseases relative to the overall morbidity rate in Texas (21, pp. 887–88). In 1984, EPA surveyed rural drinking water supplies in the United States and found significantly higher levels of coliform in low-income households (135). Finally, low-SES families are much more likely to swim in polluted beaches (20) as well as consume fish from contaminated waters (141). Statistics on access to safe, clean drinking water do not convey the full picture with respect to public health. For example, in many developing countries people designated as having access to suitable water supplies have to walk long distances to reach them, often averaging 30 minutes or more. Overburdened parents may not have the time or energy to utilize such distant facilities (6).

Ambient Noise

Exposure to ambient noise levels is also associated with income. According to data from the American Housing Survey, low-income residents are nearly twice as likely (9.1%) to report that neighborhood noise is bothersome in comparison to families not in poverty (5.9%) (118). A nationwide survey of major U.S. metropolitan areas found a strong, adverse correlation ($r = -0.61$) between household income and 24-h average sound level exposures (134). Households with incomes below $10,000 had average sound exposure levels more than 10 dBA higher than households above $20,000 annual income. Decibels is a logarithmic scale with an increase of 10 dBA perceived as approximately twice as loud. A recent analysis of airport noise and children's health and cognitive performance around Heathrow Airport documents linkages between income and actual, objective indices of noise exposure. As shown in Table 2, elementary schools with higher levels of aircraft noise exposure have greater percentages of children eligible for free lunches (58). Leq is an index of average intensity of sound exposure, measured in decibels.

Residential Crowding

Residential crowding, which is typically indexed by the ratio of people to number of rooms, is also linked to income. Figure 3 depicts national data from the 1990

TABLE 2 Aircraft noise exposure and elementary school poverty index[a]

	Low noise <57 Leq	Moderate noise 57–63 Leq	High noise 64–72 Leq
% Eligible for free lunch	14	23	28

[a]Adapted from Table 4 in Reference (58).

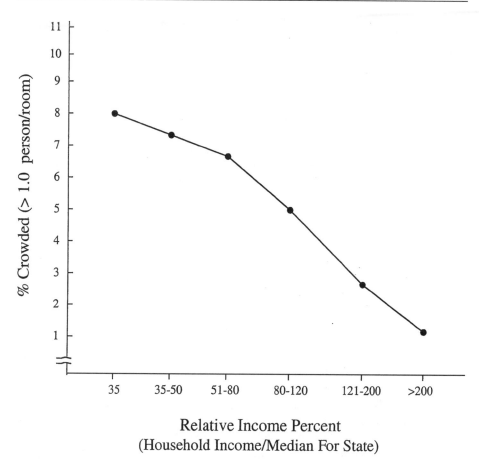

Figure 3 Residential crowding (greater than one person per room) and household income in the United States. Adapted from Table 1 in Reference (92).

census, showing a clear income-related gradient (92). The official U.S. Census definition of a crowded household is greater than one person per room.

Similar trends have been uncovered in economically underdeveloped countries. For example, in 1990 in Monterey, Mexico, 48% of households situated in the lowest income district of the city had one bedroom in comparison to 16% of households in the most affluent district (48). Similar trends have been uncovered in major urban areas in other developing countries (125).

The quantity and quality of space proximate to residences may also bear upon health and quality of life. Low-income neighborhoods in New York City have 17 square yards of park space per child, whereas all other New York City neighborhoods average 40 square yards of park space per child (118). In the United Kingdom, 86% of professionals and supervisors have access to a private garden at home in comparison to 69% of manual laborers (131). Manual laborers are four times more likely (14%) to have a garden or yard at home too small to sit outside in the sun relative to professionals, managers, or supervisors.

Housing Quality

In addition to examining linkages between constituents of environmental quality and SES, one can also look at bundles of environmental quality as embodied in the overall quality of settings such as housing, schools, work, or neighborhoods. In the United States, housing quality is strongly tied to income levels, which in turn are positively associated with home ownership and negatively correlated with residential mobility (40). For example, approximately three quarters of those above the federal poverty line own their own home compared with 40% of those who are poor. Low-income families are five times more likely to be evicted than their non-poor counterparts. Statistics from the American Housing Survey, conducted by the U.S. Census, indicate that the poor are more than three times as likely to have substandard quality housing than the not poor (22% vs. 7%) (118). Thirty-six percent of all American households with a child under the age of 18 report at least one problem with housing compared to 77% of households at or below 50% of the median income for the surrounding geographic area (133). As is evident in Table 3, income is inversely related to various indicators of housing adequacy.

Analogous trends have been uncovered in a representative national sample of households in the United Kingdom (131). We have also found that housing quality is significantly correlated with the income to needs ratios ($r = -0.39$) of rural families in upstate New York. The income to needs ratio is a per capita poverty index formed by taking the ratio of family income to the federally defined poverty index. Thus an income to needs ratio of one equals the poverty line. The federal formula is adjusted annually to the cost of living index. We used a housing composite scale that relied on raters' assessments of cleanliness/clutter, indoor climate quality, privacy, exposure to safety hazards, and structural quality (38).

TABLE 3   Percentage of children living in houses with selected problems from the 1985–1989 American Housing Survey[a]

	Income decile		Income quintile	
	First	**Second**	**Third**	**Fifth**
Incomplete bathroom	2.5	2.2	.7	.6
No sewer/septic system	1.7	.9	.1	.0
No central heat	32.3	34.7	21.4	9.6
Holes in floor	7.0	5.8	1.4	.6
Open cracks (walls, ceiling)	19.9	15.9	6.3	3.2
Leaky roof	11.9	12.5	8.5	7.3
≥1 person/room	19.2	23.4	10.9	5.3

[a]Adapted from Table 4.6 in Reference (87).

Social class differentials in childhood injuries from accidents in the home (e.g., falls) are correlated with hazardous characteristics of residential structures (11).

Poor families in America are also much less likely to have basic amenities such as clothes washers (72%), clothes dryers (50%), air conditioning (50%), or telephone (77%) than the not poor (clothes washer, 93%; clothes dryer, 87%; air conditioning, 72%; telephone, 97%) (40, 87). In the Netherlands, the percentage of persons with one or more housing deficiencies (no refrigerator, no washing machine, no clothes dryer, ≥ 1 person/room) is linearly related to income, ranging from 16% for families in the lowest income sextile to 1% of those in the highest income sextile (126).

Not surprisingly, the situation is even more extreme in the developing world. In Monterey, Mexico, income differences among districts in the city are associated with housing problems such as the absence of a permanent roof, no indoor running water, lack of drainage, and overcrowding (48). Looking at census tracts rather than metropolitan districts, Stephens and colleagues (125) uncovered similar trends in Accra, Ghana, and São Paulo, Brazil. In Accra, 37% of households in the lowest income census tracts have no piped in water, whereas 11% lack this amenity in wealthier areas of the city. In São Paulo, 36% of homes in the lowest income census tracts have no indoor toilets compared to 1% among more affluent tracts in the city.

Developmental psychologists have devised rating instruments to assess dimensions of the home environment of families. These instruments encompass measurements of physical qualities and evaluations of parenting and other aspects of the social environment. Figure 4 depicts a linear relation between the income-to-needs ratio and scores on a common residential environment rating scale, the HOME in the United States (47).

Bradley & Caldwell (13), the principal authors of the HOME scale, reported that the lower the SES, the poorer the HOME scores for infants and two-year-olds in the United States. More recently, Bradley and colleagues (14) examined relations between HOME scores across five biennial waves of a national sample of over 25,000 American children. Parental responsiveness (e.g., answering questions) was lower in poor versus not poor families, and these children had fewer learning resources (e.g., books, tape recorders) in their homes. Low-income homes were also more monotonous, dark, and contained more hazardous conditions. In another analysis using the HOME scale, 6- to 9-year-olds in American families below the poverty line suffered a 34% deficit in overall HOME scores relative to those in families with an income-to-needs ratio above four (88). Moreover, the longer the duration of childhood poverty, the stronger the negative association. Dubow & Ippolito (32) found a correlation of -0.54 between HOME scores and the number of years elementary school-aged children lived below the poverty line.

Sherman (118) provides a sobering statistic that may be indicative of the quality of the home environment available to children in the United States. Fifty-nine percent of children ages 3 to 5 who are poor have 10 or more books at home; 81% of children who are not poor have 10 or more books at home. Sadly, only 38% of low-income parents in the United States read on a daily basis to their preschoolers.

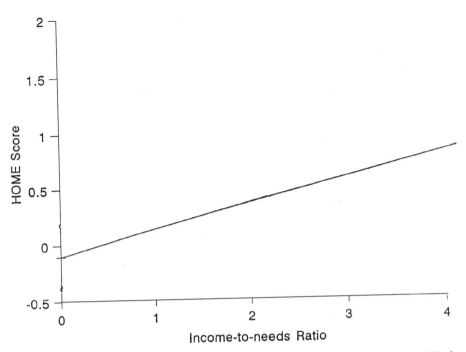

Figure 4 HOME scale values and income. Adapted from Figure 2, Reference (47), by permission from the University of Chicago.

Although substantially higher, the figure for their more affluent counterparts, 58%, is also dismal (133). Not surprisingly, the higher the socioeconomic status of the family, the more time youth spend reading on a daily basis (75). An interesting companion statistic that may interrelate to reading activity is television watching. Numerous studies have documented an inverse relation between household SES and youth TV viewing (75). For example, the percentage of 13-year-olds in the United States who watch more than five hours of television is 18 and 10, respectively, with household heads who did not graduate from high school or are college graduates (133).

In 1998, 94% of American urban children in predominantly low-income neighborhoods (≥40% below poverty line) versus 57% of urban children living in neighborhoods with little poverty (<10% below poverty line) had no Internet access (73). Eighty-four percent of the former households and 35% of the latter had no access to a computer. Across the entire United States, 52% and 15% of elementary and secondary school children, respectively, who are in the bottom income quintile have computer access at home. This contrasts markedly with the 74% and 79% of elementary and secondary children, respectively, in the highest income quintile who have home computer access (133).

Educational Facilities

An important setting for children are schools and daycare environments. The quality of the school environment is tied to income. Per capita school expenditures vary greatly according to community resources given the reliance of many school districts on local property taxes. In 1999, a federal survey of physical facilities in a representative sample of 903 public elementary and secondary schools (93) found that 20% of schools had a building in less than adequate repair, 43% had at least one infrastructure deficiency (e.g., heating, indoor air quality), and about 10% were seriously overcrowded (greater than 125% capacity). Not surprisingly, as shown in Figure 5, predominantly low-income schools suffered a disproportionate burden of inadequate school facilities.

Table 4 provides summary data from the National Center for Education Statistics report on the Condition of America's Public School Facilities: 1999. As is apparent on every dimension, low-income schools fare worst. Moreover, on several indices of facility quality, there appear to be linear gradients in relation to income levels for the school.

Children in schools with a larger proportion of poor children are also more likely to be crowded. Twelve percent of American public schools with more than 70% of their children eligible for subsidized or free lunch programs are above 125% of building capacity in comparison to 6% of schools with less than 20% eligible for lunch programs (93).[1] In terms of health outcomes, low-income children are also more likely to live in seriously overcrowded households, defined as more than one person per room (see Figure 3 above). The adverse impacts of residential crowding are exacerbated among children in more crowded daycare facilities (86).

It is, of course, difficult to disentangle the quality of the physical plant from the social environment of schools. Perhaps the most fundamental resource in a school is the quality of its teachers. Secondary teachers in low-income schools are significantly less likely to have undergraduate majors or minors in the subjects they teach relative to those in more affluent schools. For example, 27% of secondary math teachers in poor school districts majored or minored in mathematics in college compared to 43% in school districts that are not predominantly low income (66). Comparable differences occur in the sciences, whereas the differential in English is smaller.

School safety is associated with income as well. Blue-collar adolescents are twice as likely to report the presence of weapons at school (12%) or fighting in school (32%) as their white-collar counterparts (44).

Recently, several authors have examined the quality of daycare in relation to income levels. The ratio of daycare staff to children as well as expenditure is related to income levels (96, 104). The educational level and pay scales of childcare workers are related to income as well (104). Both of these studies suggest that for

---

[1]The percentage of schools seriously overcrowded in the intermediate ranges of income, 20–39% school lunch eligible and 40–69% school lunch eligible, are 8% and 7%, respectively.

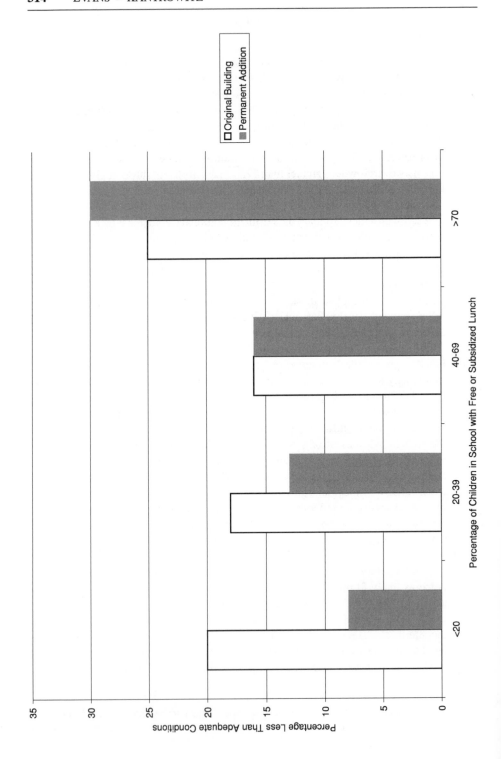

TABLE 4   Percentage of building components inadequate in relation to percentage of children in the school eligible for free or subsidized lunch[a]

Percentage eligible children	Building Features								
	Roof	Plumbing	Heating	Electric power	Lighting	Ventilation	Indoor air quality	Acoustics	Physical security
<20	18	23	28	18	8	24	14	14	17
20–39	21	23	26	20	13	29	20	18	22
40–69	22	23	29	21	10	24	17	15	21
>70	32	32	35	30	19	29	24	25	17

[a]Adapted from Tables 4 and 8 of the National Center for Education Statistics (93).

the very poor, subsidies appear to offset daycare quality relative to the lower middle and working class for institutional daycare center care. For home care, the more typical income-quality gradient is seen, with poorer-quality home daycare associated with reduced family income. Phillips and colleagues have also documented that the quality of childcare provider-child interaction (e.g., sensitivity, harshness, detachment) is also correlated with income levels (104).

Work Environments

Outside of home and school, poorer people may be subject to greater health risks on the job. In a large sample of Swedish workers, Lundberg (80) assessed different environmental and behavioral factors believed to account for SES gradients in health. Of particular interest, the strongest predictor of the gradient was poor working conditions, defined as heavy lifting or tasks with repetitive strain plus daily contact with toxins, fumes, dust, explosives, vibration, and the like. Furthermore, in multiple regression models, poor working conditions were the only independent (i.e., entered last after all other factors) predictor of the SES health gradient. Emerging evidence documents pervasive race differentials in occupational exposure to toxins and physically hazardous, risky working conditions (43, 79, 145). For example, steelworkers located in the most hazardous component of the production process (topside of the coke ovens) are nearly three times more likely to be black than white. Among the most notoriously unhealthy labor sectors are seasonal agricultural work and sweatshop garment production—settings predominated by low-income workers. Moses et al. (91) review several studies suggesting a greater body burden of persistent chlorinated hydrocarbons among low-income, Chicano/Latino, and black agricultural workers. Although these substances are

←

Figure 5   The percentage of inadequate original buildings and permanent additions in relation to the percentage of children in the school eligible for free or subsidized lunches. Adapted from Table 2, in Reference (93).

TABLE 5 DDE (DDT metabolite) serum ppb in relation to SES in Dade County, FL[a]

	Social class (Hollingshead 2 factor index)				
	I	**II**	**III**	**IV**	**V**
White	22.3	25.6	29.9	30.4	33.9
Black	33.1	37.2	29.1	43.8	50.5

[a]Adapted from Table 5 in Reference (30).

now banned in the United States, because they are lipophilic they remain sequestered in fatty tissue for many years. As indicated in Table 5, DDE serum levels are related to SES among blacks and whites in Dade County, Florida (30). DDE is a major metabolite of DDT and more indicative of lifelong exposure. Two aspects of these data are noteworthy. First, the data reveal a nearly perfect linear SES gradient, and second African Americans suffer much higher body-pesticide burdens. DDT concentrations in human breast milk among indigent black women in rural counties in Mississippi and Arkansas averaged 447 ppb. Average levels for middle-class women in Nashville averaged 14 ppb (143). In the National Health and Nutritional Examination Survey II, conducted from 1976–1980, living below the federal poverty line had a significant, independent association with serum DDT (odds ratio = 1.48) and dieldrin (odds ratio = 1.43) levels (124).

Given the robust association of ethnicity and income among American workers, it is reasonable to suspect that differential income-work setting quality relations exist as have been documented with respect to ethnicity. We know with some certainty that work-related injuries are inversely related to wages. Moreover, injury-caused sick days and duration of sick days per injury are both inversely associated with wages (60). Similar trends have been noted in the developing world (106). As shown in Table 6, occupational status in a large, representative sample of workers in the United Kingdom (131) is inversely related to more difficult working conditions.

TABLE 6 Percentage of U.K. men with difficult working conditions as a function of occupational status[a]

	Occupational status			
	Professional	**Managerial**	**Supervisory**	**Manual**
Working conditions				
Mainly outdoors	6	8	14	43
On feet all of the time	2	16	28	79
Work before 8 or at night	15	19	18	50

[a]Adapted from Table 12.2 in Reference (131).

TABLE 7   Age-adjusted mean number of hazard years (males)[a]

	I	II	II Nonmanual	III Manual	IV	V
			British registrar general social class			
Fumes/dust	4.02	12.34	5.36	30.19	19.92	19.10
Arduous labor	.86	11.33	5.45	19.52	20.80	12.58

[a]This table is based on previously unpublished data collected by L. Berney, D. Blane, G. Davey Smith, and P. Holland. This research was funded by the U.K. Economic and Social Research Council grant #L128251003.

Berney and colleagues (9) asked elderly individuals (M = 67.9 years) to retrospectively report the number of years during which they had been exposed to various environmental hazards, including those at work. Exposure to combined occupational hazards (i.e., fumes and dust, physically arduous tasks, lack of job autonomy) was inversely related to class. For example, male manual laborers had more than double the number of years working in hazardous conditions (M = 51.1 years) than nonmanual laborers (M = 20.9 years). Combined occupational hazards are expressed in years, cumulatively across hazards. Thus, for example, an individual exposed to 10 years of dust, 5 years in arduous labor, and 20 years in a job with low autonomy would be assigned a score of 35 hazardous years. Table 7 illustrates some additional analyses of these data, focusing on dust/fumes and arduous task demands as a function of occupational class.

Townsend (131), in his report of occupational class and working conditions in the United Kingdom, developed a composite index of working amenities that included sufficient heat in the winter for those outside, availability of tea/coffee, indoor toilet, facilities for washing/changing clothes, place to buy or eat lunch, secure place to keep coat/spare clothing, lockable personal storage, first-aid kit/facilities, possibility to make at least one call daily, and control over task lighting. He then constructed summary Working Conditions based on the number of amenities available: very poor working conditions, less than four amenities; poor working conditions, between four and six amenities; adequate working conditions, six amenities; and good working conditions, more than six amenities. Table 8 depicts data from this study on men in the United Kingdom working under different levels of overall work quality as a function of occupational status.

Investigation and concern about the plight of child laborers throughout the developing world has largely neglected the environmental conditions these children work in. In addition to long hours and dismal wages, many of these children work in deplorable conditions that are filthy, polluted, hazardous, and unsanitary (115).

Stressful, psychosocial conditions of working settings also appear related to occupational status. Marmot and colleagues (83) have shown among British civil

TABLE 8   Occupational status and percentage of men in the United Kingdom working at different levels of overall work setting quality[a]

	Occupational status			
	Professional	**Manager**	**Supervisory**	**Manual**
Overall work setting quality				
Very poor	0	4	4	13
Poor	2	8	5	17
Adequate	5	22	19	28
Good	93	66	72	42

[a]Adapted from Table A.41 in Reference (131).

servants that grade level is inversely related to autonomy (decision latitude) on the job, monotonous working conditions, and work pace. The trends are linear in relation to civil service grade (1 to 6) and, in turn, are related to sickness absence and incidence of coronary heart disease.

Neighborhood Quality

In addition to school, work, and home, local surroundings may contribute to health and well-being. Low-income urban neighborhoods suffer poorer basic municipal services [e.g., police, fire, sanitation (138)] and experience greater residential mobility (77) relative to more affluent, urban neighborhoods. Nine- to eleven-year-old children in Sydney, Australia, rated their overall neighborhood quality as higher in relation to an objective composite index of neighborhood risk, based upon census data (64). A primary component of this neighborhood risk index was SES. The higher the neighborhood risk index, the more likely it was that children rated their setting as having too much traffic, being dirty and polluted, too much noise, no safe places to play, and having fewer parks and outdoor play spaces. Even within predominantly low-income areas, family income is positively related to the overall quality of neighborhood housing and other amenities (120).

Macintyre and colleagues (82) found that working-class areas of Glasgow, Scotland, in comparison to upper-middle-class sections had fewer shops, paid more for food, had dramatically fewer recreational opportunities, were further from mass transit stops in combination with lower rates of car ownership, and had poorer street cleaning and maintenance. As noted earlier, low-income children have less access to parks and suitable nearby nature (e.g., gardens) (118). Furthermore, as shown by the Sydney study, children seem well aware of this (64). Playgrounds in low-income areas are more hazardous (as assessed by independent, trained raters) relative to those in higher-income neighborhoods (127). Moreover, young children of low-income families are much more likely to have no safe play areas nearby their home (131). Income-related rates of child pedestrian injuries appear to be caused by differential exposure to street traffic. For example, children in Montreal from relatively disadvantaged schools cross 50% more streets a day, on average, than their more affluent schoolmates (82a). Basic housing stock is of significantly lower quality (percentage dilapidated housing) in low-income neighborhoods than in middle- or upper-income areas (71). Abandoned lots and boarded up houses also occur more frequently in low-income areas (128, 139).

Rates of exposure to crime are strongly tied to family income levels as well as neighborhood income composition (113). Children from low-SES neighborhoods are more likely to be exposed to aggressive peers than children from higher-income areas (119). Low-income adolescents perceive their neighborhood as more dangerous, violent, and of poorer overall quality (graffiti, cleanliness, housing quality) than their middle-class counterparts (2). Homel & Burns (64), in their Sydney neighborhood study, also found that neighborhood risk was linearly related to young children's judgments about the presence of unfriendly people. Thus, both the immediate residential environment as well as the neighborhood infrastructure of low-income individuals are likely to be of lower overall quality than the home or surroundings of people with more financial resources.

ENVIRONMENTAL QUALITY AND HEALTH

The section above documents pervasive income-related differences in exposure to environmental risks. The present section provides a much briefer summarization of evidence that the disproportionate burden of suboptimal environmental exposure shared by those who are poorer could have health consequences. The amount and quality of research on environmental effects on health and well-being are substantially greater than evidence of income differentials in exposure to poor environmental quality.

Air Quality

A voluminous literature relying on epidemiological studies as well as human and animal experiments demonstrates that ambient air pollutants cause various respiratory problems including bronchitis, emphysema, and asthma. Less well-documented links exist between certain ambient pollutants and lung cancer. Exposure to carbon monoxide may also be a risk factor for coronary heart disease. In addition, ambient air pollution may increase risk for respiratory infection (63, 78, 98). Exposure to ambient pollutants, principally ozone, a toxic component of photochemical smog, has been linked to psychological distress, negative emotional affect, and behaviors including interpersonal attraction and aggression. The latter function appears to be curvilinear, with moderate levels of irritable pollutants causing increased aggression (33, 110). Although a relatively new area of inquiry, there is already an impressive body of literature linking indoor air quality, including environmental tobacco smoke, with various respiratory problems (5, 68, 112).

Environmental Toxins

Environmental toxins, principally heavy metals (e.g., lead), solvents (e.g., cleaning fluids), and pesticides, occur in hazardous waste-disposal facilities and various manufacturing, mining, and agricultural activities. Toxicological effects include cancer, respiratory morbidity, brain damage, and various neurotoxicological difficulties (70, 98, 117). In utero exposure to several toxins also produces teratological effects. Many of these same toxins in much lower doses produce cognitive and behavioral abnormalities, including attentional and memory disorders, lower IQ, and poorer academic achievement. Behavioral problems including impulse control, frustration intolerance, and aggression have also been associated with several toxins (3, 108). The low-dose behavioral toxicological effects appear to be especially dangerous during the critical period of fetal development.

Ambient Noise

Another aspect of environmental quality, ambient noise levels, also appears to threaten health. Links between chronic noise exposure and hearing damage are well documented (74). Both intensity and duration of exposure are important parameters of noise exposure and health. Suggestive data link noise exposure to coronary heart disease and hypertension, but the evidence is not solid (8, 130). Several community studies have shown that children's blood pressure and possibly neuroendocrine stress hormones are elevated when living or attending schools in the flight paths of major airports (34). There are contradictory findings on ambient noise exposure and prematurity and birth defects, as well as a small number of studies suggesting immunosuppression from noise in animal models (34).

Noise clearly interferes with complex task performance (e.g., dual tasks) but has inconsistent effects on simple tasks (e.g., vigilance) (35). Several studies have uncovered evidence that both acute as well as chronic noise exposure can lead to motivational deficits linked to learned helplessness (25, 34). Glass & Singer (50) found, for example, that immediately following exposure to 20 minutes of noxious noise in the laboratory, subjects were less likely to persist at challenging puzzles. Their data also indicate that it is the uncontrollability of noise, in particular, that is problematic for motivation. A large number of studies have shown that chronic noise exposure is linked to reading deficits in young children. The effects on reading are not due to hearing loss. Moreover, some of this effect is due to problems with speech perception in noise-exposed children (36). Noise also has adverse consequences for interpersonal processes including altruism and aggression (26). Conclusions about an association between ambient noise exposure and mental illness are not well substantiated (122).

Residential Crowding

Crowding, like noise, functions as a stressor, elevating blood pressure and neuroendocrine parameters (34). Several studies have indicated that infectious diseases are more likely in relation to crowding among vulnerable subgroups (e.g., prisoners, refugee camps) and that residential crowding (i.e., people per room) is associated with psychological distress in the general population (34). There is no evidence to substantiate the widespread perception of cultural differences in tolerance for crowding (37). Areal indices of density (e.g., people/acre) appear less important than interior density measures such as people per room for understanding health outcomes associated with crowding. Several studies indicate that a principal pathway linking residential crowding to psychological distress is problems with unwanted social interaction (7, 34). Residents of more crowded homes are more socially withdrawn and perceive lower levels of social support in comparison to individuals living in less crowded settings. Parents in crowded homes are also less responsive to their children and tend to employ harsher, more punitive parenting styles (34). Crowding may also interfere with complex task performance and has been linked to learned helplessness (34, 35). Relations between crowding and aggression are unclear but several studies have indicated reduced altruism and more negative interpersonal interactions in more crowded settings (7).

Housing Quality

Concerns about housing quality and physical health are a longstanding interest within the field of public health. Because of the design of research projects investigating housing and health, it is difficult to draw definitive conclusions; nonetheless, the preponderance of evidence suggests that substandard and more hazardous construction is associated with more unintentional injuries, especially among young children and the elderly. Inadequate heating systems and the presence of dampness, molds, and other allergens are also associated with poor respiratory health (19, 65, 85). Epidemic increases in asthma in inner-city settings may be partially attributable to elevated ambient pollutants along with exposure to allergens in the home. The evidence linking housing and health includes several longitudinal analyses of housing improvements and at least one study with random assignment.

Work investigating a possible link between housing quality and mental health is more controversial. The findings are less numerous and consistent than the physical health research. Evidence suggests that high-rise housing may be linked to elevated psychological distress among low-income women with young children as well as with restricted, outdoor play activities in young children (39, 49, 59).

There is also a good deal of evidence showing relations between the design of public housing and both fear of crime and actual incidence of crime (128). One of the problems with research on mental health and housing is reliance on housing measurements developed originally to assess physical health. Recent work indicates that scales indexing behaviorally relevant aspects of housing may prove more fruitful in research on housing and psychological well-being (38).

The quality of the home environment has also been linked to children's cognitive development. The provision of adequate learning materials and the absence of chaotic conditions predict better achievement, both cross sectionally and longitudinally (12, 84, 137). The role of structure and predictability in family routines has also been implicated in children's socioemotional development (41).

Educational Facilities

The quality of the research on the physical environment of daycare settings and early school environments and children's development is not sufficiently developed to draw definitive conclusions, but trends indicate that the physical environment may play a role directly affecting children's cognitive and social development and indirectly by way of changes in teachers' behaviors (90, 132). Some of the physical characteristics of schools, in addition to noise and crowding, believed to be important to cognitive development include structure and predictability, arrangement and quality of activity areas, degree of openness, privacy, access to nature, availability and variety of age-appropriate toys and learning aids, and play materials for fine and gross motor development that provide graduated challenge, and natural light (101, 140).

Neighborhood Quality

There has been a recent upsurge of interest in neighborhood effects on well-being, focusing on cardiovascular health, crime and violence, and children's development. Some studies look at neighborhood effects, after statistically controlling for individual variation in SES or income levels. Other studies employ hierarchical linear modeling techniques that account for both individual and areal-level variation in SES or income. Low-SES neighborhood characteristics, independent of household SES, are associated with higher all-cause mortality (29, 57); greater cardiovascular risk in men (29, 61), as well as women (29); cardiovascular disease in men and women (29, 76); and with injury mortality (28). As noted earlier, exposure to urban crime is positively associated with both individual income levels and neighborhood income characteristics (113). Interestingly from a psychological health perspective, a key underlying mechanism to explain the linkage between neighborhood poverty and crime is diminished collective efficacy. Residents of low-income, high-crime neighborhoods perceive less social cohesion and diminished social control in their neighborhoods relative to persons living in lower-crime areas (113). Fear of crime in adults, particularly the elderly population, has reached epidemic proportions in low-income, inner-city neighborhoods (103, 139). Finally, exposure to violence has well-documented, adverse consequences on children's socioemotional development (45, 46, 102, 107).

Children growing up in high-SES neighborhoods have a clear advantage in school readiness and perform better academically, independently of familial income or education (77). Mental health in children and youth, particularly externalizing behaviors (acting out, aggression), is associated with residence in low-income neighborhoods. Studies controlling for individual SES as well as multiple level analyses converge on these findings. Adolescents in low-income neighborhoods also appear to become sexually active earlier and are more likely to become teenage parents compared to their peers living in more affluent neighborhoods (77).

CONCLUSIONS

We have reviewed data showing that income is associated with exposure to a wide variety of environmental quality indicators in the ambient environment, at home, in school, on the job, and in one's neighborhood. Differential income and racial exposure to environmental health risks constitute an important and emerging field of scholarship and public policy, frequently termed environmental justice. It would be fair to summarize this body of work as showing that the poor and especially the non-white poor bear a disproportionate burden of exposure to suboptimal, unhealthy environmental conditions in the United States. Moreover, the more researchers scrutinize environmental exposure and health data for racial and income inequalities, the stronger the evidence becomes that grave and widespread environmental injustices have occurred throughout the United States. Such findings moved former President Clinton to establish an Office of Environmental Justice in 1992 within EPA (99, 136) and in 1994, to issue an executive order requiring all federal agencies to identify and address disproportionately high and adverse human health or environmental effects of federal programs and policies on minority and low-income populations (24). [See also the Office on Minority Health (100) within the Department of Health and Human Services and the National Institute for Environmental Health Sciences (97) for further information on U.S. Federal environmental justice programs. Friends of the Earth, United Kingdom, has a research and policy program devoted to environmental justice (42b).]

There are several gaping holes in the current database necessary to critically examine whether the SES health gradient could be partly attributed to environmental exposures. First, data on income or SES and environmental exposure are quite thin for several important settings, especially work, schools, and neighborhood settings. In several instances, a dose-response function is not available; rather, measures of environmental risk for low-income individuals are compared to persons above the poverty line. It would be preferable to have data across the continuum of income or SES and environmental risk exposure. In many instances, the poverty/not poverty comparison is entangled with ethnicity. In the cases of exposure to hazardous waste sites and to occupational risk exposure, respectively, the data on ethnic differentials in exposure are better developed than they are for income. Available data are largely confined to North America and Western Europe. The paucity of data on income and environmental risk for residents of developing countries is particularly troublesome given both the greater population size and more adverse environmental risk exposure in many of these countries.

Second, we hypothesize that the likelihood of singular environmental exposure accounting for the SES health gradient is small. We believe that it is the confluence of suboptimal conditions that is most likely to function as a potent mechanism helping to account for SES-related differences in health. Research on cumulative risk exposure among children offers a useful analogue. This work shows that children exposed to one or perhaps two serious risk factors suffer at most modest decrements in psychological or cognitive functioning. However, the accumulation of multiple risk factors dramatically elevates the probability of adverse socioemotional and cognitive developmental outcomes (16, 111). The gap in our analysis of income, environmental risk, and health is such that few data exist showing the relation between income and multiple sources of environmental risk. We do know with some clarity that income is inversely related to exposure to a higher frequency of social stressors and to more adverse social stressors (4, 17) but parallel data for multiple physical stressor exposure do not exist.

Should this multiple exposure, health, and income hypothesis prove correct, then current estimates of the importance of environmental risk to account for some of the SES health gradient are likely conservative. Nearly all of the available data on environmental risk and income emanate from economically developed countries; whereas the greatest convergence of multiple suboptimal environmental conditions with the severest health consequences likely occurs in the less developed world (62, 115).

The third serious deficiency in the current database for claiming that adverse environmental exposure might account for the SES health gradient is the absence of any data testing for the mediational model depicted in Figure 1. To our knowledge, no data indicate that the effects of poverty or income on health are mediated by exposure to multiple environmental risk factors. Therefore what we have shown herein can be summarized as follows:

■ Income is often directly related to environmental quality, especially when low-income samples are contrasted with samples that are not poor;

■ Environmental quality is inversely related to multiple physical and psychological health outcomes.

Greater progress in addressing the model shown in Figure 1 will require the collection of environmental risk and health data broken down by income or SES levels. Currently, such databases remain the exception. The absence of longitudinal studies also raises the possibility that the relations among income, environmental risk, and health are due to selection factors rather than environmental effects. Such a person-based explanation seems unlikely to account for the wide array of differential, environmental exposure shown herein, but changes in environmental conditions intra-person would provide stronger evidence of an environmentally based mechanism for the SES health gradient than the current preponderance of cross-sectional data. Reliance on cross-sectional data also precludes examination of the temporal course of environmental risk exposure and health in relation to income. Use of hierarchical linear modeling would also enable investigators to tease out nested, ecological niches of environmental exposure (e.g., region, neighborhood, home, work, school) in relation to income, class, or ethnicity (31).

In summary, public health databases need to routinely incorporate information about income and ethnicity. Such databases ideally would be longitudinal, sample across a continuum of income levels, and incorporate whenever possible multiple ecological niches of environmental exposure. Given the income and multiple environmental risk hypothesis, it would also behoove us to construct exposure estimates that include multiple environmental risk factors. This would enable scientists and policy makers to examine whether low-income persons and other disadvantaged individuals are exposed to higher levels of combined environmental risks and, in turn, determine if such multiple risk exposure helps account for their higher levels of morbidity and mortality. Public health professionals should be alert to the reasonable possibility that scrutiny of isolated, distinct physical and/or social risk factors misrepresents the ecology of environmental risk. This misrepresentation might, in turn, lead to underestimation of the contribution of environmental risk exposure to the public's health.

There is clearly consistent evidence that people who are poorer in the United States are more likely to be exposed to multiple, environmental risks that portend adverse health consequences. Exposure to multiple, suboptimal environmental risk factors is one viable mechanism among several that could be a partial explanation for the gradient between SES and multiple health outcomes.

ACKNOWLEDGMENTS

We thank Nancy Adler, Urie Bronfenbrenner, and Judith Stewart for their feedback and support of this work. Preparation of this article was partially supported by the John D. and Catherine T. MacArthur Foundation Network on Socioeconomic Status and Health, and the Cornell University Agricultural Experiment Station, Project Nos. NYC 327404 and NYC 327407.

Visit the Annual Reviews home page at www.annualreviews.org

LITERATURE CITED

1. Adler NE, Boyce T, Chesney M, Folkman S, Syme L. 1993. Socioeconomic inequalities in health: no easy solution. *JAMA* 269:3140–45
2. Aneshensel C, Sucoff C. 1996. The neighborhood context of adolescent mental health. *J. Health Soc. Behav.* 37: 293–310
3. Araki S, ed. 1994. *Neurobehavioral Methods and Effects in Occupational and Environmental Health.* New York: Academic
4. Attar B, Guerra N, Tolan P. 1994. Neighborhood disadvantage, stressful life events, and adjustment in urban elementary school children. *J. Clin. Child Psychol.* 23:391–400
5. Bardana E, Montanaro B, eds. 1997. *Indoor Air Pollution and Health.* New York: Marcel Dekker
6. Bartlett S. 1999. Children's experience of the physical environment in poor urban settlements and the implications for policy, planning, and practice. *Environ. Urban.* 11:63–73
7. Baum A, Paulus PB. 1987. Crowding. See Ref. 125a, pp. 533–70
8. Berglund B, Lindvall T. 1995. Community noise. *Arch. Cent. Sens. Res.* 2:1–195

9. Berney L, Blane D, Davey Smith G, Gunnell D, Holland P, Montgomery S. 2000. Socioeconomic measures in early old age as indicators of previous lifetime exposure to environmental health hazards. *Soc. Health Ill.* 22:415–30

10. Bernton H, McMahon T, Brown H. 1972. Cockroach asthma. *Br. J. Dis. Child.* 66:61

11. Blane D, Barley M, Davey-Smith G. 1997. Disease aetiology and materialist explanations of socioeconomic mortality differentials. *Eur. J. Public Health* 7:385–91

12. Bradley RH. 1999. The home environment. In *Measuring Environment Across the Lifespan*, ed. SL Friedman, TD Wachs, pp. 31–58. Washington, DC: Am. Psychol. Assoc.

13. Bradley RH, Caldwell B. 1984. The HOME inventory and family demographics. *Dev. Psychol.* 20:315–20

14. Bradley RH, Corwyn R, McAdoo H, Garcia C. 2001. The Home environments of children in the United States Part I: variations by age, ethnicity, and poverty status. *Child Dev.* 72:1844–67

15. Brajer V, Hall J. 1992. Recent evidence on the distribution of air pollution effects. *Contemp. Policy Issues* 10:63–71

16. Bronfenbrenner U, Morris P. 1998. The ecology of developmental processes. In *Handbook of Child Psychology*, ed. W Damon, R Lerner, pp. 992–1028. New York: Wiley

17. Brown L, Cowen E, Hightower A, Lotyczewski B. 1986. Demographic differences among children in judging and experiencing specific stressful life events. *J. Spec. Ed.* 20:339–46

18. Bullard RD. 1990. *Dumping in Dixie.* Boulder, CO: Westview

19. Burridge R, Ormandy D, eds. 1993. *Unhealthy Housing*. London: E. F. Spon.

20. Cabelli V, Dufour A. 1983. *Health Effects Criteria for Marine Recreational Waters*. Res. Triangle Park, NC: U.S. EPA, Off. Res. Dev. Res. EPA-600/1-80-031

21. Calderon R, Johnson C, Craun G, Dufour A, Karlin R, et al. Health risks from contaminated water: Do class and race matter? *Toxicol. Ind. Health* 9:879–900

22. Chi P, Laquatra J. 1990. Energy efficiency and radon risks in residential housing. *Energy* 15:81–89

23. Cieselski S, Handzel T, Sobsey M. 1991. The microbiologic quality of drinking water in North Carolina migrant farmer camps. *Am. J. Public Health* 81:762–64

24. Clinton WJ. 1994. Federal actions to address environmental justice in minority populations and low income populations. *Fed. Regist.* 59:7629–33

25. Cohen S. 1980. Aftereffects of stress on human performance and social behavior: a review of research and theory. *Psychol. Bull.* 88:82–108

26. Cohen S, Spacapan S. 1984. The social psychology of noise. In *Noise and Society*, ed. DM Jones, AJ Chapman, pp. 221–45. New York: Wiley

27. Cook D, Whincup P, Jarvis M, Strachan D, Papacosta O, Bryant A. 1994. Passive exposure to cigarette smoke in children aged 5–7 years: individual, family, and community factors. *Br. Med. J.* 308:384–89

28. Cubbin C, LeClere F, Davey Smith G. 2000. Socioeconomic status and injury mortality: individual and neighborhood determinants. *J. Epidemiol. Commun. Health* 54:517–24

29. Davey Smith G, Hart C, Watt G, Hole D, Hawthorne V. 1998. Individual social class, area-based deprivation, cardiovascular disease risk factors, and mortality in Renfrew and Paisley study. *J. Epidemiol. Commun. Health* 52:399–405

30. Davies J, Edmundson W, Raffonelli A, Cassady J, Morgade C. 1972. The role of social class in human pesticide pollution. *Am. J. Epidemiol.* 96:334–41

31. Diez-Roux AV. 2000. Multilevel analysis in public health research. *Annu. Rev. Public Health* 21:171–92

32. Dubow E, Ippolito M. 1994. Effects of poverty and quality of the home environment on changes in the academic and behavioral adjustment of elementary school-age children. *J. Clin. Child Psychol.* 23:401–12

32a. Duncan GJ, Brooks-Gunn J, eds. 1997. *Consequences of Growing Up Poor.* New York: Russell Sage

33. Evans GW. 1994. The psychological costs of chronic exposure to ambient air pollution. In *The Vulnerable Brain and Environmental Risks, Vol. 3: Toxins in Air and Water*, ed. RL Isaacson, KF Jensen, pp. 167–82. New York: Plenum

34. Evans GW. 2001. Environmental stress and health. In *Handbook of Health Psychology*, ed. A Baum, T Revenson, JE Singer, pp. 365–85. Mahwah, NJ: Erlbaum

35. Evans GW, Cohen S. 1987. Environmental stress. See Ref. 125a, pp. 571–610

36. Evans GW, Lepore SJ. 1993. Nonauditory effects of noise on children: a critical review. *Child. Environ.* 10:31–51

37. Evans GW, Lepore SJ, Allen K. 2000. Cross cultural differences in tolerance for crowding: fact or fiction? *J. Pers. Soc. Psychol.* 79:204–10

38. Evans GW, Wells NM, Chan E, Saltzman H. 2000. Housing and mental health. *J. Consult. Clin. Psychol.* 68:526–30

39. Evans GW, Wells NM, Moch A. 2002. Housing and mental health: a review of the evidence and a methodological and conceptual critique. *J. Soc. Issues.* In press

40. Federman M, Garner T, Short K, Cutter W, Levine D, et al. 1996. What does it mean to be poor in America? *Mon. Labor Rev.* May:3–17

41. Fiese B, Kline C. 1993. Development and validation of the family ritual questionnaire: initial reliability and validation studies. *J. Fam. Psychol.* 6:290–99

42. Freeman AM. 1972. The distribution of environmental quality. In *Environmental Quality Analysis*, ed. AV Kness, B Bower, pp. 243–80. Baltimore: Johns Hopkins Press

42a. Friends of the Earth, United Kingdom. 2001. *Pollution and Poverty: Breaking the Link.* London: Friends of the Earth

42b. Friends of the Earth, United Kingdom. 2001. Environmental justice and inequalities. http://www.foe.co.uk/campaigns/sustainable-development/research-progs/env_just_prog.html

43. Frumkin H, Walker D. 1998. Minority workers and communities. In *Maxcy Rosenau Last Public Health and Preventative Medicine*, ed. R Wallace, pp. 682–88. Stamford, Conn: Appleton & Lange. 14th ed.

44. Gallup G. 1993. *America's Youth in the 1990's.* Princeton: Gallup Inst.

45. Garbarino J. 1995. *Raising Children in a Socially Toxic Environment.* San Francisco: Jossey-Bass

46. Garbarino J, Dubrow N, Kostelny K, Pardo C. 1992. *Children in Danger: Coping with the Consequences of Community Violence.* San Francisco: Jossey-Bass

47. Garrett P, Ng'andu N, Ferron J. 1994. Poverty experiences of young children and the quality of their home environments. *Child Dev.* 65:331–45

48. Garza G. 1996. Social and economic imbalances in the metropolitan area of Monterey. *Environ. Urban.* 8:31–42

49. Gifford R. 2002. Satisfaction, health, security and social relations in high rise buildings. In *Social Effects of the Building Environment*, ed. A Seidel, T Heath. London: E. & F. N. Spon. In press

50. Glass DC, Singer JE. 1972. *Urban Stress.* New York: Academic

51. Gold D. 1992. Indoor air pollution. *Clin. Chest Med.* 13:215–29

52. Goldstein I, Andrews L, Hartel D. 1988. Assessment of human exposure to nitrogen dioxide, carbon monoxide and respirable particulates in New York inner

city residents. *Atmos. Environ.* 22:2127–39

53. Goldtooth TBK. 1995. Indigenous nations: summary of sovereignty and its implications for environmental protection. In *Environmental Justice*, ed. B Bryant, pp. 138–48. Washington, DC: Island Press

54. Graham H. 1995. Cigarette smoking: a light on gender and class inequality in Britain? *Int. J. Soc. Policy* 24:509–27

55. Graham H, Blackburn C. 1998. The socioeconomic patterning of health and smoking behavior among mothers with young children on income support. *Sociol. Health Ill.* 20:215–40

56. Groner J, Ahijevych K. Grossman L, Rich L. 1998. Smoking behaviors of women whose children attend an urban pediatric primary care clinic. *Women Health* 8:19–32

57. Haan M, Kaplan G, Camacho T. 1987. Poverty and health. *Am. J. Epidemiol.* 125:898–908

58. Haines M, Stansfeld S, Head J, Job RFS. 2002. Multi-level modeling of aircraft noise on national standardized performance tests in primary schools around Heathrow Airport, London. *J. Epidemiol. Commun. Health.* In press

59. Halpern D. 1995. *More Than Bricks and Mortar?* London: Taylor & Francis

60. Hamermesh D. 1999. Changing inequality in work injuries and work timing. *Mon. Labor Rev.* Oct.: 22–30

61. Harburg E, Erfurt J, Hausentstein L, Chape C, Schull W, Schork M. 1973. Socioecological stress, suppressed hostility, skin color, and black-white male blood pressure: Detroit. *Psychosom. Med.* 35:276–96

62. Hardoy J, Mitlin D, Satterthwaite D. 2001. *Environmental Problems in the Urbanizing World.* London: Earthscan

63. Holgate S, Samet J, Koren H, Maynard R. 1999. *Air Pollution and Health.* New York: Academic

64. Homel R, Burns A. 1987. Is this a good place to grow up in? Neighborhood quality and children's evaluations. *Landscape Urban Plan.* 14:101–16

65. Ineichen B. 1993. *Housing and Health.* London: E & FN Spon

66. Ingersoll RM. 1999. The problem of under qualified teachers in American secondary schools. *Educ. Res.* 28:26–37

67. Inst. Med. 1999. *Environmental Justice.* Washington, DC: Natl. Acad. Press

68. Inst. Med. 2000. *Clearing the Air: Asthma and Indoor Air Exposure.* Washington, DC: Natl. Acad. Press

69. Jarvis M, Strachan D, Feyerbrand C. 1992. Determinants of passive smoking in children in Edinburgh, Scotland. *Am. J. Public Health* 82:1225–29

70. Johnson BL. 1999. *Impact of Hazardous Waste on Human Health.* New York: Lewis

71. Joint Cent. Housing Stud. Harvard Univ. 1999. *The State of the Nation's Housing.* Cambridge, MA: Harvard Univ.

72. Kang B. 1976. Study on cockroach antigen as a probable causative agent in bronchial asthma. *J. Allergy Clin. Immunol.* 58:357–65

73. Kids Count Data Book 2000. 2000. Seattle: Annie Casey Found.

74. Kryter K. 1994. *The Handbook of Hearing and the Effects of Noise.* New York: Academic

75. Larson RW, Verma S. 1999. How children and adolescents spend time around the world: work, play and developmental opportunities. *Psychol. Bull.* 125:701–36

76. Le Clere FB, Rogers R, Peters K. 1998. Neighborhood context and racial differences in women's heart disease. *J. Health Soc. Behav.* 39:91–107

77. Leventhal T, Brooks-Gunn J. 2000. The neighborhoods they live in: the effects of neighborhood residence on child and adolescent outcomes. *Psychol. Bull.* 126:309–37

78. Lippman N. 1992. *Environmental Toxicology.* New York: Van Nostrand

79. Lucas REB. 1974. The distribution of job characteristics. *Rev. Econ. Stat.* 56:530–40

80. Lundberg O. 1991. Causal explanations for class inequality in health—an empirical analysis. *Soc. Sci. Med.* 32:385–93

81. MacArthur Found. 2001. *Network on Socioeconomic Status and Health.* http://www.macses.ucsf.edu

82. Macintyre S, Maciver S, Sooman A. 1993. Area, class and health: Should we be focusing on places or people? *Int. Soc. Policy* 22:213–34

82a. Macpheron A, Roberts I, Press IB. 1998. Children's exposure to traffic and pedestrian injuries. *Am. J. Public Health* 88:1840–45

83. Marmot M, Siegrist J, Theorell T, Feeney A. 1999. Health and the psychosocial environment at work. In *Social Determinants of Health*, ed. M Marmot, RG Wilkinson, pp. 105–31. New York: Oxford Univ. Press

84. Matheny A, Wachs TD, Ludwig J, Phillips E. 1995. Bringing order out of chaos: psychometric characteristics of the confusion, hubbub, and order scale. *J. Appl. Dev. Psychol.* 16:429–44

85. Matte T, Jacobs D. 2000. Housing and health: current issues and implications for research and progress. *J. Urban Health Bull. NY Acad. Med.* 77:7–25

86. Maxwell LM. 1996. Multiple effects of home and day care crowding. *Environ. Behav.* 28:494–511

87. Mayer SE. 1997. Trends in the economic well-being and life chances of America's children. See Ref. 32a, pp. 49–69

88. Miller J, Davis D. 1997. Poverty history, marital history, and quality of children's home environments. *J. Marriage Fam.* 59:996–1007

89. Mohai P, Bryant B. 1992. Environmental racism: reviewing the evidence. In *Race and the Incidence of Environmental Hazards*, ed. B Bryant, P Mohai, pp. 163–76. Boulder, CO: Westview

90. Moore GT, Lackney J. 1993. School design. *Child. Environ.* 10:99–112

91. Moses M, Johnson E, Anger W, Burse V, Horstman S, et al. 1993. Environmental equity and pesticide exposure. *Toxicol. Ind. Health* 9:913–59

92. Myers D, Baer W, Choi S. 1996. The changing problem of overcrowded housing. *J. Am. Plan. Assoc.* 62:66–84

93. Natl. Cent. Educ. Stat. 2000. *Condition of America's Public School Facilities: 1999.* Washington, DC: U.S. Dep. Educ. NCES 2000-032

94. Natl. Cent. Health Stat. 1991. Children's exposure to environmental cigarette smoke. *Advance Data from Vita and Health Statistics*: No. 202. Hyattsville, MD

95. Natl. Cent. Health Stat. 1998. *Socioeconomic Status and Health Chart Book.* Hyattsville, MD: Natl. Cent. Health Stat.

96. Natl. Inst. Child Health Hum. Dev. Early Child Care Res. Network. 1997. Poverty and patterns of child care. See Ref. 32a, pp. 100–31

97. Natl. Inst. Environ. Health Sci. 2001. *Health disparities research.* http://www.niehs.nih.gov/oc/factsheets/disparity/tho me.htm

98. Natl. Res. Counc. 1991. *Environmental Epidemiology*, Vol. 1. Washington, DC: Natl. Acad. Press

99. Off. Environ. Justice. Washington, DC: EPA. http://es.epa.gov/oeca/main/ej/pub lis/html

100. Off. Minority Health. Washington, DC: Dep. Health Hum. Serv. Closing the gap. http://www.omhrc.gov/ctg/ctg-env.htm

101. Olds A. 2000. *Child Care Design Guide.* New York: McGraw-Hill

102. Osofsky J. 1995. The effects of exposure to violence on young children. *Am. Psychol.* 50:782–88

103. Perkins D, Taylor RB. 1996. Ecological assessments of community disorder: their relationship to fear of crime and theoretical implications. *Am. J. Commun. Psychol.* 24:63–107

104. Phillips DA, Voran M, Kisker E, Howes C, Whitebook M. 1994. Childcare for children in poverty: opportunity or inequity? *Child Dev.* 65:472–92

105. Pirkle J, Brody D, Gunter E, Kramer R, Paschal D, et al. 1994. The decline in blood lead levels in the United States. *JAMA* 272:284–91

106. Pryer J. 1993. The impact of adult ill-health on household income and nutrition in Khulna, Bangladesh. *Environ. Urban.* 5:35–49

107. Richters JE, Martinez P. 1993. The NIMH community violence project. *Psychiatry* 56:7–21

108. Riley E, Vorhees C, eds. 1991. *Handbook of Behavioral Teratology.* New York: Plenum

109. Rosenstreich D, Eggleson P, Kattan M, Baker D, Slavin R, et al. 1997. The role of cockroach allergy and exposure to cockroach allergens in causing morbidity among inner-city children with asthma. *N. Engl. J. Med.* 336:1356–63

110. Rotton J. 1983. Affective and cognitive consequences of malodorous pollution. *Basic Appl. Soc. Psychol.* 4:171–91

111. Rutter M. 1981. Protective factors in children's responses to stress and disadvantage. In *Prevention of Psychopathology,* ed. M Kent, J Rold, 1:49–74. Hanover, NH: Univ. Press

112. Samet J, Spengler J, eds. 1991. *Indoor Air Pollution: A Health Perspective.* Baltimore: Johns Hopkins Press

113. Sampson R, Raudenbush S, Earls F. 1997. Neighborhoods and violent crime: a multilevel study of collective efficacy. *Science* 277:918–24

114. Sarpong S, Hamilton R, Eggleston P, Adkinson N. 1996. Socioeconomic status and race as risk factors for cockroach allergen exposure and sensitization in children with asthma. *J. Allergy Clin. Immunol.* 97:1393–401

115. Satterthwaite D, Hart R, Levy C, Mitlin D, Ross D, et al. 1996. *The Environment for Children.* London: Earthscan

116. Schwab M. 1990. An examination of intra-SMSA distribution of carbon monoxide exposure. *J. Air Waste Manag. Assoc.* 40:331–36

117. Scott R. 1990. *Chemical Hazards in the Workplace.* Chelsea, MN: Lewis

118. Sherman A. 1994. *Wasting America's Future.* Boston: Beacon Press

119. Sinclair J, Pettit G, Harrist A, Dodge K, Bates J. 1994. Encounters with aggressive peers in early childhood: frequency, age differences, and correlates of risk for behavior problems. *Int. J. Behav. Dev.* 17:675–96

120. Spencer MB, Mc Dermott P, Burton L, Kochman T. 1997. An alternative approach to assessing neighborhood effects on early adolescent achievement and problem behavior. In *Neighborhood Poverty,* Vol. 2: *Policy Implications in Studying Neighborhoods,* ed. J Brooks-Gunn, GJ Duncan, JL Aber, pp. 145–63. New York: Russell Sage Found.

121. Spencer NJ, Coe C. 2001. *The additive effects of social factors on risk of smoking in households with newborn infants.* Unpubl. Manuscr. Univ. Warwick, UK

122. Stansfeld S. 1993. Noise, noise sensitivity, and psychiatric disorder: epidemiological and psychophysiological studies. *Psychol. Med. Monogr. Suppl.* 22:1–44

123. Statistical Universe. 2000. *Income of families and primary individuals by selected characteristics: renter occupied units, 1999.* http://web.lexis-nexis.com/statuniv/

124. Stehr-Green P. 1989. Demographic and seasonal influences on human serum pesticide residue levels. *J. Toxicol. Environ. Health* 27:405–21

125. Stephens C, Akerman M, Avle S, Maia P, Campanario P, et al. 1997. Urban equity and urban health: Using existing data to understand inequalities in health and environment in Accra, Ghana and Sao Paulo, Brazil. *Environ. Urban.* 9:181–202

125a. Stokols D, Altman I, eds. 1987. *Handbook of Environmental Psychology*. New York: Wiley

126. Stronks K, Dike van de Mheen H, Mackenbach J. 1998. A higher prevalence of health problems in low income groups: Does it reflect relative deprivation. *J. Epidemiol. Commun. Health* 52:548–57

127. Suecoff S, Avner J, Chou K, Drain E. 1999. A comparison of New York City playground hazards in high and low income areas. *Arch. Pediatr. Adolesc. Med.* 153:363–66

128. Taylor RB, Harrell A. 1999. *Physical Environment and Crime*. Washington, DC: Natl. Inst. Justice

129. Deleted in proof

130. Thompson SJ. 1993. Review: extra aural health effects of chronic noise exposure in humans. In *Larm und Krankheit (Noise and disease)*, ed. H Ising, B Kruppa, pp. 107–17. New York: Gustav Fischer Verlag

131. Townsend P. 1979. *Poverty in the United Kingdom*. Berkeley: Univ. Calif. Press

132. Trancik A, Evans GW. 1995. Spaces fit for children: competency in the design of daycare center environments. *Child. Environ.* 12:311–19

133. U.S. Dep. Health Hum. Serv. 2000. *Trends in the Well Being of America's Children and Youth 2000*. Washington, DC: U.S. GPO

134. U.S. Environ. Prot. Agency. 1977. *The Urban Noise Survey*. Washington, DC: EPA 550/9-77-100

135. U.S. Environ. Prot. Agency. 1984. *National Statistical Assessment of Rural Water Conditions*. Washington, DC: EPA 570/9-84-004

136. U.S. Environ. Prot. Agency. 1992. *Environmental Equity: Reducing Risk for All Communities*. Washington, DC: Off. Solid Waste Emerg. Response. EPA 230-R-92-008

137. Wachs TD, Gruen G. 1982. *Early Experience and Development*. New York: Plenum

138. Wallace D, Wallace R. 1998. *A Plague on Your Houses*. London: Verso

139. Wandersman A, Nation M. 1998. Urban neighborhoods and mental health. *Am. Psychol.* 50:647–56

140. Weinstein C, David T. eds. 1987. *Spaces for Children*. New York: Plenum

141. West P, Fly J, Marans R, Larkin F. 1989. *Michigan Sports Anglers Fish Consumption Survey*. Ann Arbor, MI: Univ. Mich. Sch. Nat. Resourc., Nat. Resourc. Sociol. Res. Lab. Tech. Rep. 1

142. White HL. 1998. Race, class, and environmental hazards. In *Environmental Injustices, Political Struggles*, ed. DE Camacho, pp. 61–81. Durham, NC: Duke Univ. Press

143. Woodard B, Ferguson B, Wilson D. 1976. DDT levels in milk of rural indigent blacks. *Am. J. Dis. Child.* 130:400–3

144. World Bank. 1992. *World Development Report*. New York: Oxford Univ. Press

145. Wright BH. 1992. The effects of occupational injury, health, and disease on the health status of Black Americans. See Ref. 89, pp. 114

Annu. Rev. Public Health 2002. 23:333–48

EFFECTS OF SMOKING RESTRICTIONS IN THE WORKPLACE*

Ross C. Brownson,[1] David P. Hopkins,[2] and Melanie A. Wakefield[3]

[1]Department of Community Health and Prevention Research Center, School of Public Health, Saint Louis University, St. Louis, Missouri 63108-3342; e-mail: brownson@slu.edu; [2]Epidemiology Program Office, Centers for Disease Control and Prevention, Atlanta, Georgia 30341; e-mail: dhh4@cdc.gov; and [3]Center for Behavioral Research in Cancer, Anti-Cancer Council of Victoria, Carlton, Victoria, Australia; e-mail: melanie.wakefield@accv.org.au

Key Words attitudes, behavior, public policy, tobacco smoke pollution

■ **Abstract** The health hazards caused by exposure to environmental tobacco smoke (ETS) are well established. Workplace exposure to ETS is strongly influenced by the types of workplace and smoking policy—total bans on smoking have become common in many countries. Blue-collar and service workers are more likely than other types of workers to be exposed to ETS in the workplace. Smokers who are employed in workplaces with smoking bans are likely to consume fewer cigarettes per day, are more likely to be considering quitting, and quit at an increased rate compared with smokers employed in workplaces with no or weaker policies. Despite substantial progress in protecting workers from ETS, additional efforts are needed in areas that include attention to exposure among blue-collar and service workers; policies in workplaces with a limited number of employees; and studies of enforcement, effects on smoking cessation in multiple settings, and cost-effectiveness.

INTRODUCTION

During the past few decades, health hazards related to exposure to environmental tobacco smoke (ETS) have been increasingly recognized. These health effects are summarized in detail elsewhere (10, 40, 41, 55, 59). Among the best-established are lung cancer among healthy adult nonsmokers and childhood respiratory tract ailments (e.g., bronchitis and pneumonia). Other associations have been demonstrated between ETS and low birthweight, sudden infant death syndrome, middle ear infections among children, and nasal sinus cancer (10, 59).

As scientific knowledge of the health risks caused by ETS exposure has increased, public and employer understanding of such risks has also grown. Included in the change in public attitudes toward ETS is the re-framing of smoking as a key social concern beyond a personal behavior. Public policies to eliminate ETS exposure, especially in workplaces, have similarly increased in frequency and scope during the past decade (8). Considerable evidence indicates that these policies reduce the exposure of nonsmokers to ETS (58). However, substantial gaps remain in our understanding of the overall effectiveness of these policies to control ETS, in particular the impact of smoking bans on smoking cessation. Limited systematic research has been done on the extent to which these policies might influence the creation of smoking restrictions in domestic environments, as people come to accept nonexposure to ETS as usual practice. Finally, research is sparse on the effects of enforcement and financial costs and benefits.

The primary purposes of this paper are to describe (a) workplace policy initiatives that have been designed to reduce ETS exposure, (b) effects and effectiveness of such policy measures, and (c) key areas of future influence for health policy development and research. The majority of the studies cited in our review were conducted in the 1990s in the United States. However, we also describe results from high-quality studies from other countries.

SCOPE OF ETS EXPOSURES AND WORKPLACE POLICIES

As described elsewhere (8, 20, 26, 55, 60), multiple reasons exist for restricting smoking in public places:

- ETS causes acute and chronic diseases in otherwise healthy nonsmokers,
- The majority of persons experience annoyance and discomfort from ETS exposure and view ETS as a health hazard,
- Many nonsmokers do not (or are not able to) take personal action to avoid exposure to ETS when smokers light up in their vicinity,
- Employers might realize lower maintenance and repair costs, insurance costs, and higher nonsmoker productivity when smoking is prohibited in the workplace,
- Restricting smoking in work settings might increase the likelihood that smokers in these settings smoke fewer cigarettes or quit smoking entirely,
- Employers might face liability for nonsmokers' health,
- Workplace smoking policies in conjunction with other health policies and regulations challenge the tobacco industry–driven perception of tobacco use as a social norm and might influence change in restrictions in domestic environments and even youth attitudes and behavior regarding tobacco use.

Assessing Workplace ETS Exposure

Investigations of ETS exposure in the workplace and other settings have helped to build the foundation for ETS control policies. In a study of 663 nonsmokers attending a cancer screening (17), 76% of participants reported ETS exposure in the 4 days before the interview. The authors concluded that the workplace and home were the primary sources of ETS exposure among nonsmokers. The best single predictor of urinary cotinine was the number of friends and family members who smoked and were seen regularly by the subject. In a study of 881 nonsmoking volunteers (35), employees in workplaces that allowed smoking in multiple locations were more than 4 times more likely to have detectable saliva cotinine concentrations than those working in workplaces with bans on smoking. Among 186 former and never smokers using a self-reported exposure diary (without biochemical validation), approximately one half of the daily ETS exposure was attributed to the workplace (19). However, for persons who lived with a smoker, more exposure occurred in the home than in the workplace.

Relatively few comprehensive studies have been done regarding the levels of ETS exposure in the workplace. In a 1993 review of existing studies (49), wide variation was noted in ETS concentrations by location, measured by mean levels of nicotine in the ambient air of offices (4.1 μg/m^3), restaurants (6.5 μg/m^3), bars (19.7 μg/m^3), and residences (4.3 μg/m^3) with $\geq$1 smokers. A recently published U.S. study of serum cotinine levels among nonsmokers documented a 75% decrease during 1991 to 1999 (13). Among ethnic groups, non-Hispanic blacks had the highest median cotinine levels. Persons aged $\leq$20 years had higher cotinine levels than those aged $\geq$20 years (13).

Workplace Policy Options and Scope

For employers and policy makers, options exist regarding regulation of ETS in the workplace. Among the options, the least effective is using a designated smoking area without separate ventilation. This option provides only minimal protection to nonsmokers; previous studies have reported substantial exposure to ETS in workplaces with smoking areas without separate ventilation (47). The next most effective option is using separate ventilated smoking lounges; this protects nonsmokers but is costly and can elevate lung cancer risk among smokers (50). Separately ventilated smoking lounges also endanger workers (e.g., waitstaff) who must enter these areas as part of their jobs. Next, an option exists for using separately ventilated smoking lounges with a recommended duration of $\leq$30 min/day, which can minimize health risks among both nonsmokers and smokers (42). Finally, the most effective alternative is a totally smoke-free workplace.

In 1985, approximately 38% of U.S. workers were employed by firms that had policies restricting smoking (23). Since that time, smoking restrictions have become increasingly common. According to the 1999 National Worksite Health Promotion Survey, 79% of workplaces with $\geq$50 employees had formal smoking policies that prohibited smoking or limited it to separately ventilated areas (57). The objective for Healthy People 2010 is 100% (56). U.S. data for 1995–1996 indicate that 64% of indoor workers are covered by a 100% smoking ban in the workplace (9). The proportion of workers who work in a smoke-free workplace varies considerably by state—from 84% in Maryland and Utah to 40% in Nevada.

Limited systematic data exist regarding enforcement of existing policies to restrict workplace smoking, although existing studies indicate that compliance is likely to be high (52, 62). National data also indicate that despite protections, workers in blue-collar and service occupations remain much more likely to be exposed to workplace ETS than other categories of workers (25).

GOVERNMENTAL POLICIES IN THE UNITED STATES   A limited number of federal policies restrict ETS in workplaces, but a key policy is the ban on smoking on airline flights originating from or arriving in the United States, which was strongly supported by flight attendants. Other substantial federal actions have included bans on smoking in federal office buildings, the symbolically critical ban on smoking in the White House, and bans on smoking in day care facilities that receive federal funds (e.g., places providing Women, Infant, and Children services). The Occupational Safety and Health Administration has proposed regulations that would either prohibit smoking or limit it to separately ventilated areas (42). As of 1998, 20 states and the District of Columbia limited smoking in private workplaces (12). However, only one state law (California) met the Healthy People 2000 objective to ban indoor smoking or limit it to areas with separate ventilation.

Clean indoor air ordinances at the local level (i.e., city and county) first appeared in the early 1970s, and have been reported to reduce workplace ETS exposure (38, 46). As of September 2001, approximately 1200 local ordinances in the United States restricted public smoking. Governmental laws and regulations often exclude smaller workplaces (e.g., <50 workers) from coverage. Data are lacking regarding the relative effectiveness of various enforcement mechanisms. Relatively few resources have been dedicated to enforcement of ETS ordinances; probably, policy members assume that substantial regulatory action is self-enforcing.

PRIVATE SECTOR-IMPOSED RESTRICTIONS   In the United States, hospitals are the only industry that has voluntarily implemented a nationwide smoking ban. This ban was announced in November 1991, and full implementation was required by December 31, 1993. Two years after implementation, the policy was judged to be successful, with 96% of hospitals complying with the smoking ban standard (33). Certain firms in other industries have implemented smoking bans without legislation or regulatory actions. For example, bans in certain fast food restaurants (e.g., McDonald's and Taco Bell) are a response to concern for children's health. Another example is the proliferation of nonsmoking rooms in motels and hotels. These changes reflect the firms' responses to substantial consumer demand and potential savings in their housekeeping departments (48). As such, private firm policies not mandated by law serve as a market barometer of public opinion on the desirability of smoke-free indoor air.

GLOBAL SMOKING RESTRICTIONS   A recent overview of legislation restricting smoking at work in different countries has been provided by the American Cancer Society (16) (Table 1). Despite using already published sources and Internet searching, the authors could not locate information for certain countries.

TABLE 1 Variations in workplace smoking policies around the globe[a]

Country	Type of policy[b]				Notes
	B	R	V	X	
Africa					
Benin	x				Certain workplaces only
Botswana	x				Areas accessible to public, common areas
Mali	x				Public service offices
Nigeria	x				Offices
South Africa	x				Designated smoking areas
Uganda			x		
Tanzania			x		
Zambia	x				
Americas					
Argentina		x			
Barbados			x		
Belize			x		Certain private workplaces
Brazil			x		
Canada	x				
Chile	x				Areas accessible to public
Costa Rica	x				
Cuba			x		
Dominican Republic	x				Offices
Ecuador	x				Working areas
El Salvador		x			
Grenada			x		
Guatemala	x				Areas accessible to public
Honduras	x				
Mexico	x				Working areas
Panama	x				Areas accessible to public
Peru	x				
Trinidad and Tobago			x		
United States				x	State and local levels
Venezuela		x			
Eastern Mediterranean					
Cyprus	x				Private and public
Egypt	x				Enclosed public places
Iran					Areas accessible to public
Iraq		x			Administrative measures
Kuwait			x		
Lebanon			x		Upon request by nonsmokers
Morocco	x				Public administration and service offices
Sudan	x				Areas accessible to public
Syria	x				
Tunisia			x		

(Continued)

TABLE 1 (*Continued*)

Country	B	R	V	X	Notes
Europe					
Austria	x				Unless appropriate ventilation exists
Belarus		x			
Belgium	x		x		Areas accessible to public and other areas
Bosnia & Herzegovina		x			
Bulgaria	x				Unless nonsmokers allow smoking in writing
Croatia	x				
Czech Republic	x				During work hours when nonsmokers present
Denmark	x				Voluntary restrictions in private workplaces
Estonia	x				Labor environments
Finland	x				Designated smoking areas
France	x				Except personal offices
Germany			x		
Greece		x			
Hungary	x				Areas accessible to public
Iceland	x				Areas accessible to public
Ireland	x				Areas accessible to public
Israel	x				Except management designated areas
Kyrgyzstan			x		
Latvia		x			
Lithuania	x				Enclosed areas
Netherlands		x			Public and private
Norway	x				With ≥ 2 employees
Poland	x				
Portugal			x		
Moldovia	x				
Romania				x	
Russia	x				
San Marino	x				
Slovakia		x			
Slovenia		x			
Spain		x			
Sweden		x			
Switzerland		x			
Turkey	x				With ≥ 5 employees
Ukraine	x				
United Kingdom			x		

(*Continued*)

TABLE 1 *(Continued)*

Country	Type of policy[b]				Notes
	B	**R**	**V**	**X**	
Southeast Asia					
Bangladesh			X		
India		X			
Nepal		X			
Sri Lanka			X		
Thailand	X				Administrative measures
Western Pacific					
Australia			X		
Cambodia	X				
China	X				Partial ban
Cook Islands		X			Administrative measures
Fiji			X		
Japan			X		
Kiribiti			X		Guideline, Ministry of Labor
Laos			X		
Malaysia	X				
Micronesia		X			Areas accessible to public
Mongolia	X				
New Zealand	X				Designated smoking areas
Niue			X		Common work and public areas
Philippines	X				
Korea		X			
Samoa			X		
Solomon Islands		X			
Tokelau		X			
Tonga			X		

[a]Adapted from Corrao et al. (16); number of additional countries with no information: Africa, 38; Americas, 15; Eastern Mediterranean, 13; Europe, 15; Southeast Asia, 5; Western Pacific, 11.

[b]B: Smoking is prohibited in workplaces according to national legislation or regulation; facilities with a designated smoking area are included in this category if nonsmoking areas must always remain uncontaminated by smoke.

R: Smoking is restricted but not prohibited in workplaces according to national legislation or regulations.

V: Employers voluntarily prohibit or restrict smoking in areas under their management.

X: Different state and county laws apply.

Thus, absence of a law in Table 1 does not imply with certainty that none exists in a country. Conversely, the presence of a law banning or restricting smoking implies nothing regarding enforcement. Apparently, voluntary restrictions under control of the employer are more common in developing countries.

A country that relies on voluntary action to ban or restrict smoking might have high rates of worker protection. For example, although Australia banned smoking in all federal workplaces in 1988, determining their own policies has been left to each workplace. Yet, in 1999, 71% of indoor workers in the state of Victoria reported a total ban on smoking at their workplace; 21% reported certain restrictions on smoking; and 8% reported unrestricted smoking (53). As in other countries, those employed in small Australian workplaces are less likely to report protection, as are workers in certain types of employment (36, 62). For indoor workers, 38% of those employed in a restaurant or hotel, 15% of warehouse/store workers, and 17% of employees in a workshop or factory reported unrestricted smoking where they worked, compared with only 3% of workers in open-plan offices (53). In Britain, workplace restrictions are also voluntary. In 1997, 40% of the workforce was estimated to be working in a totally smoke-free environment (24); 79% of workplaces in Scotland had nonsmoking areas, but only 22% of these had banned smoking completely (28).

Despite the limitations of the data presented in Table 1, the majority of countries have laws that restrict smoking in some form. Yet, considerable need probably exists for improvement in worker protection from ETS in the majority of countries.

EFFECTS AND EFFECTIVENESS OF WORKPLACE SMOKING POLICIES

As previously described, multiple reasons exist for restricting smoking in the workplace. Effects and effectiveness of smoking bans and restrictions have been recently reviewed by the U.S. Task Force on Community Preventive Services (Task Force), published as part of the *Guide to Community Preventive Services* (the *Community Guide*). This review demonstrated the number and variety of published evaluation data regarding workplace smoking policies (29). It identified 54 comparative studies of smoking bans and restrictions published between 1980 and mid-2000, with another 5 papers providing additional information regarding an already included study or study period. Seventeen of these studies evaluated differences or changes in exposure to ETS. Fifty studies evaluated differences or changes in ≥1 tobacco-use behaviors, including consumption, quit attempts, smoking cessation, or smoking prevalence in a workforce or study population.

The methods employed by the Task Force categorize comparative studies of interventions and consider both study design and the quality of the study execution (6, 54). The Task Force recommendations for use are based primarily on the evidence of effectiveness reported in a best-evidence subset of the identified studies.

Evaluations of the effects and effectiveness of workplace smoking policies include study designs and measurements of ETS exposure and tobacco-use behaviors. The majority of published studies are simple assessments conducted before and after adoption of a workplace policy, although more recent (and complex) investigations have employed cross-sectional surveys of workers exposed to different policies. A limited number of studies evaluated and controlled for potential bias and confounding of the observed differences or changes in exposure or tobacco-use behaviors. As a result, the number of studies included in the best-evidence subsets reviewed by the Task Force was small and provide conservative assessments of the effectiveness of workplace smoking policies.

Attitudes and Social Norms

Assessments of attitudes towards workplace smoking policies (typically cross-sectional surveys) have consistently demonstrated support for smoking bans. In a survey of 10 U.S. communities (11), for example, restrictions or bans were favored by a majority of respondents in all locations, including bars, restaurants, hospitals, workplaces, and government buildings. In general, support for workplace smoking policies increases following implementation. Five months post-implementation, 89% of nonsmokers, 86% of ex-smokers, 81% of recent quitters, and 45% of current smokers supported a hospital smoking ban (18).

Nonsmokers' Exposure

The effectiveness of workplace smoking policies has been measured by differences or changes in perceived air quality in the workplace after a ban or restriction, and by differences or changes in active measurements of nicotine vapor, or metabolites, or levels of particulates. Overall, workplace smoking policies have been highly effective in reducing nonsmokers' exposure to ETS. In the "best evidence subset" of studies identified in the *Community Guide* review (see Table 2), workplace smoking policies consistently demonstrated a significant impact on ETS exposures (median relative percentage difference: −60%, range +4% to −97%) regardless of the type of study (e.g., cross-sectional surveys, before and after comparisons), the setting or location (e.g., offices, public sector workplaces, medical centers, workplaces community wide), or the outcome measurement (29). Workplaces with smoking bans tended to show greater reduction in ETS exposure than did workplaces with smoking restrictions in this body of evidence.

Effects on Adult Smoking Behavior

The impact of workplace smoking policies on employee smoking behaviors has been evaluated from multiple perspectives, including measurements of the effect on cigarette consumption, smoking cessation, and overall smoking prevalence within the workplace or study population. Table 3 presents the results from the best evidence subset of studies utilized in the *Community Guide* review. The National Cancer Institute (NCI) review includes recent evidence from cross-sectional surveys of adult indoor workers conducted as part of the 1995/96 Current Population Surveys (CPS) (9).

CIGARETTE CONSUMPTION   Most studies measuring differences or changes in tobacco use in response to the implementation of a workplace smoking policy have observed reductions in daily consumption of tobacco. In the *Community Guide* review, the median decrease was −1.2 cigarettes/day (range: from 0 to −4.3) in follow-up periods of up to 2 years.

In the 1995/96 CPS, the percentage of current smokers reporting smoking 25 or more cigarettes per day differed significantly by workplace smoking policy (9). The percentage of current smokers reporting smoking 25 or more cigarettes per day, for example, was 29.6% in workplaces with no smoking restrictions, and

TABLE 2 Summary of selected studies on the effects of workplace smoking bans on exposure to ETS

First author, year/location	Industry/setting	Sample size	Outcome(s) studied/effect size[a]
Millar 1988 (37)/ Ontario, Canada	Department of Health and Welfare	4200 (12 locations)	Change in mean respirable suspended particulates = $-6\ \mu g/m^3$ to $-22\ \mu g/m^3$ (depending on the floor of the building)
Becker 1989 (1)/ Maryland	Children's Hospital	951 (9 locations)	Change in average nicotine vapor concentrations # $-12.53\ \mu g/m^3$ to $+0.08\ \mu g/m^3$ (depending on the location)
Biener 1989 (2)/ Rhode Island	Hospital	535	Percentage "bothered" by ETS in workplace locations Offices = -20%; lounges = -20%
Gottlieb 1990 (27)/ Texas	Government agency	1158	Percentage "never bothered" by ETS = 38.8%
Mullooly 1990 (39)/ Oregon	Health Maintenance Organization	13,736 1985: pre 764 post 1027 1986: pre 1352 post 1219	Smoke in workplace = -21% (1985 sites); -35% (1986 sites)
Stillman 1990 (52)/ Maryland	Medical Center	8742 (6 locations)	Change in average 7-day nicotine vapor concentrations # minus 7.71 $\mu g/m^3$ to minus 2.08 $\mu g/m^3$ (depending on the location)
Broder 1993 (7)/ Toronto, Canada	Public sector workplaces	179 (3 buildings; 8–12 samples/floor)	Change in the mean measurements (for several ETS components) Volatile organic compounds = $-0.7\ mg/m^3$
Patten 1995 (44)/ California	Statewide workers	8580 (at baseline survey)	% exposed to ETS at work = -56.3% difference between work area ban and no ban
Borland 1992 (4)/ California	Statewide workers	7301	% exposed to ETS at work = -42.1% difference between smoke free policy and no policy
Etter 1999 (21)/ Geneva, Switzerland	University	2,908	Exposure to ETS (score 0–100) = $+2.1$

[a]Values noted are absolute differences from baseline.

16.4% in workplaces with a total ban. The authors note, however, that differences in cross-sectional responses might reflect the difficulty of implementing smoking bans when there are greater numbers of heavy smokers.

Although the average effects on individuals' cigarette consumption summarized previously are relatively limited, the population impact can be significant. In a

TABLE 3 Summary of selected studies on the effects of workplace smoking bans on smoking behavior

First author, year/location	Industry/setting	Sample size	Intervention/ follow-up period	Outcome(s) studied/effect size[a]
Biener, 1989 (2)/ Providence, RI	Hospital	535	12 months	Reduced consumption (RC) = −3.2 cigs/day Smoking prevalence (SP) = −11.4% current smoking
Gottlieb 1990 (27)/ Texas	Government agency	1158	6 months	RC = 12.0% reduction in consumption of 15 or more cigs/day at work; SP = −3.4% current smoking
Mullooly 1990 (39)/ Oregon	Health Maintenance Organization	13,736 1985 sites 1791 1986 sites 2571	12 months	RC = reported as "no significant change" SP = −1.5% smoking (1985 sites); +1.0% smoking (1986 sites)
Stave 1991 (51)/ Durham, NC	University medical center	400 (800)	15 months	RC = −4.3 cigs/day Smoking cessation (SC) = +7.9% quitting
Brigham 1994 (5)/ Baltimore, MD	Hospital	67	4 weeks	RC = −3.4 cigs/shift; SC = 0
Jeffery 1994 (30)/ Minneapolis- St. Paul, MN	Diverse workplaces	32 workplaces	24 months	RC = −2.1 cigs/day; SP = +0.4% smoking
Patten 1995 (43)/ California	Diverse workplaces	1844	15–18 months	RC = −0.96 cigs/day; SP = −1.4% current smoking; SC = +9.6% self-reported quitting
Longo 1996 (32)/ 21 states, US	Representative sample of hospital employees	1469	5 years	RC = −1.1 cigs/day; SC = 1.7-fold difference in quit ratio
Etter 1999 (21)/ Geneva, Switzerland	University	2908	4 months	RC = −0.3 cigs/day; SP = +0.8% current smoking

[a]Values noted are absolute differences from baseline.

summary of existing studies, Chapman et al. (15) estimated the contributions of smoke-free workplaces to recent declines in cigarette consumption in the United States and Australia. In the United States, workplace bans were estimated to be responsible for 12.7% of the 76.5 billion decrease in cigarette consumption during 1988–1994. If workplace bans were universal, the annual number of cigarettes forgone in the United States would increase to 20.9 billion.

CESSATION Five studies in the best evidence subset for the *Community Guide* review measured differences or changes in self-reported cessation (5, 21, 32, 43, 51). The median change or difference in tobacco use cessation in smokers exposed to a workplace smoking ban compared to workers with no or lesser restrictions was a relative increase of 73% (range −3.2% to +272%).

The NCI review conducted an analysis of differences in cessation efforts by workplace smoking policy using multivariate logistic regression that controlled for age, gender, race/ethnicity, education and income levels, number of cigarettes smoked per day, and workplace policies in the state of residence. Responses from a subset of workers in the 1995/96 CPS who reported daily smoking one year prior were compared by workplace smoking policy. Exposure to a total work ban was significantly associated with being a former smoker of 3 or more months' duration (OR = 1.34, 95%CI 1.10–1.63) compared to exposure to no or lesser restrictions. Noting a less consistent impact on self-reported cessation attempts (OR = 1.09, 95%CI 1.00–1.18), the authors concluded that the principal effect of restricting smoking in the workplace appears to be an increase in the success rate of those smokers who are attempting to quit, rather than an increase in the number of smokers who attempt to quit. In addition, a recent prospective study showed that relapse rates were similar among hospital employees in workplaces with smoking bans and other employees where smoking was permitted, even when the quit rate was 2.3 times higher in the hospital group (34).

TOBACCO USE PREVALENCE   Differences in the prevalence of smokers by workplace smoking policy are clearly demonstrated in the 1995/96 CPS (9). The prevalence of current, daily smoking was significantly lower among workers employed in smoke-free workplaces (16%) compared to workers in worksites with no smoking restrictions (26.4%). Never smokers account for much of this difference (59.7% vs 51.9%); however, the prevalence of former smokers was also higher in smoke-free workplaces (20.3% vs 16.9%). Although these results support an association between smoke-free workplaces and the prevalence of tobacco use among workers, the differences in cross-sectional responses may also reflect the movement of smokers to less restrictive workplaces or the greater ease in the implementation of smoke-free workplaces in sites with fewer smokers.

Restrictions in Domestic Environments

Evidence is sparse that more pervasive restrictions on smoking in the workplace might influence the extent to which persons voluntarily restrict smoking in their own homes (i.e., domestic environments). For example, in California, the prevalence of home smoking bans increased markedly during a time when workplace and service industry smoking restrictions became more widespread (45). In Australia, people who work in places where smoking is banned are more likely to ask their visitors at home not to smoke (3), although no relationship existed regarding the practice of smoking outside the home. These relationships might not be strong and might be influenced by concomitant tobacco control strategies (e.g., media campaigns); further research in this area is warranted.

Youth Smoking Behavior

The impact of workplace smoking policies on attitudes and behaviors of youth current and future tobacco use is unclear. The *Community Guide* review identified no studies specifically evaluating this relationship, although a number of studies included variables for state and/or local clean indoor air laws in calculations of youth responsiveness to the price of tobacco products (14, 31, 63). Recently, a large cross-sectional study indicated that smoking restrictions in three settings (i.e., home, schools, and other public places) might reduce teenage smoking (61). Another cross-sectional study determined that adolescents who worked in smoke-free workplaces were substantially less likely to be smokers than were adolescents whose workplaces had no smoking restrictions (22). These intriguing findings require replication and extension using longitudinal and time-series designs.

RECOMMENDATIONS AND CONCLUSIONS

Our review indicates certain areas deserving of future attention as follows:

- Certain subgroups (e.g., service and blue-collar workers) are at highest risk for ETS exposure in the workplace and deserve particular attention.
- In the United States, policies and regulations often exclude workplaces of <50 employees (e.g., bars and restaurants), yet employees in these workplaces represent a substantial workforce.
- Effects of bans on ETS exposure and smoking behavior need to be studied in additional settings (e.g., universities, day care facilities).
- The majority of countries restrict workplace smoking in one form or another, yet because of the variations in the extent of policies, workers' exposure is probably substantial.
- Although bans and other restrictions have become common, sparse information exists regarding the most effective means of enforcing bans at the state and local (i.e., township, county) levels.
- Cost implications to employers with different workplace ETS policies are unclear because little information exists in the literature regarding costs and cost-effectiveness of workplace smoking policies. In a related area, better assessments are needed of the effects of smoking bans on workplace productivity.

During the past few decades, substantial progress has been made in protecting workers from ETS exposure in the workplace. Workplace smoking bans are effective in reducing exposure to ETS. Smokers who are employed in workplaces with smoking bans tend to consume fewer cigarettes per day, are more likely to be considering quitting, and quit at a greater rate than smokers employed in workplaces with no or weaker policies. Overall, the implementation of smoking policies is overwhelmingly supported by nonsmokers, and support for the policy increases with time, even among smokers. The prevalence of tobacco use among employees is lower in workplaces with restrictive smoking policies. Multiple benefits, including the protection of workers, customers, and visitors (including youth) from exposure to ETS, provide a strong incentive for businesses and communities to pursue and maintain smoke-free policies for all workplaces.

Visit the Annual Reviews home page at www.annualreviews.org

LITERATURE CITED

1. Becker DM, Conner HF, Waranch HR, Stillman F, Pennington L, et al. 1989. The impact of a total ban on smoking in the Johns Hopkins Children's Center. *JAMA* 262:799–802

2. Biener L, Abrams DB, Follick MJ, Dean L. 1989. A comparative evaluation of a restrictive smoking policy in a general hospital. *Am. J. Public Health* 79:192–95

3. Borland R, Mullins R, Trotter L, White V. 1999. Trends in environmental tobacco smoke restrictions in the home in Victoria, Australia. *Tob. Control* 8:266–71

4. Borland R, Pierce JP, Burns DM, Gilpin E, Johnson M, Bal D. 1992. Protection from environmental tobacco smoke in California. The case for a smoke-free workplace. *JAMA* 268:749–52

5. Brigham J, Gross J, Stitzer ML, Felch LJ. 1994. Effects of a restricted work-site smoking policy on employees who smoke. *Am. J. Public Health* 84:773–78

6. Briss PA, Zaza S, Pappaioanou M, Fielding J, Wright-De Aguero L, et al. 2000. Developing an evidence-based Guide to Community Preventive Services–methods. The Task Force on Community Preventive Services. *Am. J. Prev. Med.* 18:35–43

7. Broder I, Pilger C, Corey P. 1993. Environment and well-being before and following smoking ban in office buildings. *Can. J. Public Health* 84:254–58

8. Brownson RC, Eriksen MP, Davis RM, Warner KE. 1997. Environmental tobacco smoke: health effects and policies to reduce exposure. *Annu. Rev. Public Health* 18:163–85

9. Burns DM, Shanks TG, Major JM, Gower KB, Shopland DR. 2000. Restrictions on smoking in the workplace. In *Population Based Smoking Cessation: Smoking and Tobacco Control Monograph #12.* Bethesda, MD: US Dep. Health Hum. Serv. Natl. Cancer Inst.

10. Calif. Environ. Prot. Agency. 1997. *Health Effects of Exposure to Environmental Tobacco Smoke.* Sacramento, CA: Calif. Environ. Prot. Agency, Off. Environ. Health Hazard Assess.

11. CDC. 1991. Public attitudes regarding limits on public smoking and regulation of tobacco sales and advertising–10 U.S. communities, 1989. *MMWR* 40:344–5, 51–53

12. CDC. 1998. *State Laws on Tobacco Control–United States, 1998.* Fact Sheet. Atlanta, GA: CDC

13. CDC. 2001. *National Report on Human Exposure to Environmental Chemicals.* Atlanta, GA: Natl. Cent. Environ. Health

14. Chaloupka FJ, Grossman M. 1996. *Price, tobacco control policies and youth smoking. Rep. Work. Pap. No. 5740.* Cambridge, MA: Natl. Bur. Econ. Res.

15. Chapman S, Borland R, Scollo M, Brownson RC, Dominello A, Woodward S. 1999. The impact of smoke-free workplaces on declining cigarette consumption in Australia and the United States. *Am. J. Public Health* 89:1018–23

16. Corrao MA, Guindon GE, Sharma N, Shokoohi DF. 2000. *Tobacco Control Country Profiles.* Atlanta, GA: Am. Cancer Soc.

17. Cummings KM, Markello SJ, Mahoney M, Bhargava AK, McElroy PD, Marshall JR. 1990. Measurement of current exposure to environmental tobacco smoke. *Arch. Environ. Health* 45:74–79

18. Daughton DM, Andrews CE, Orona CP, Patil KD, Rennard SI. 1992. Total indoor smoking ban and smoker behavior. *Prev. Med.* 21:670–76

19. Emmons KM, Abrams DB, Marshall RJ, Etzel RA, Novotny TE, et al. 1992. Exposure to environmental tobacco smoke in naturalistic settings. *Am. J. Public Health* 82:24–28

20. Eriksen MP, LeMaistre CA, Newell GR.

1988. Health hazards of passive smoking. *Annu. Rev. Public Health* 9:47–70

21. Etter JF, Ronchi A, Perneger T. 1999. Short-term impact of a university based smoke free campaign. *J. Epidemiol. Commun. Health* 53:710–15

22. Farkas AJ, Gilpin EA, White MM, Pierce JP. 2000. Association between household and workplace smoking restrictions and adolescent smoking. *JAMA* 284:717–22

23. Farrelly MC, Evans WN, Sfekas AE. 1999. The impact of workplace smoking bans: results from a national survey. *Tob. Control* 8:272–77

24. Freeth S. 1998. *Smoking Related Behaviour and Attitudes*. London: Off. Natl. Stat.

25. Gerlach KK, Shopland DR, Hartman AM, Gibson JT, Pechacek TF. 1997. Workplace smoking policies in the United States: results from a national survey of more than 100,000 workers. *Tob. Control* 6:199–206

26. Glantz SA. 1996. Preventing tobacco use—the youth access trap. *Am. J. Public Health* 86:156–58

27. Gottlieb NH, Eriksen MP, Lovato CY, Weinstein RP, Green LW. 1990. Impact of a restrictive work site smoking policy on smoking behavior, attitudes, and norms. *J. Occup. Med.* 32:16–23

28. Health Educ. Board Scotl. 1997. *Scotland's Health at Work: Baseline Survey Report*. Edinburgh: MVA Consult. Health Educ. Board Scotl.

29. Hopkins DP, Briss PA, Ricard CJ, Husten CG, Carande-Kulis VG, et al. 2001. Reviews of evidence regarding interventions to reduce tobacco use and exposure to environmental tobacco smoke. *Am. J. Prev. Med.* 20:16–66

30. Jeffery RW, Kelder SH, Forster JL, French SA, Lando HA, Baxter JE. 1994. Restrictive smoking policies in the workplace: effects on smoking prevalence and cigarette consumption. *Prev. Med.* 23:78–82

31. Lewit EM, Hyland A, Kerrebrock N, Cummings KM. 1997. Price, public policy, and smoking in young people. *Tob. Control* 6:S17–24

32. Longo DR, Brownson RC, Johnson JC, Hewett JE, Kruse RL, et al. 1996. Hospital smoking bans and employee smoking behavior: Results of a national survey. *JAMA* 275:1252–57

33. Longo DR, Brownson RC, Kruse RL. 1995. Smoking bans in US hospitals. Results of a national survey. *JAMA* 274:488–91

34. Longo DR, Johnson JC, Kruse RL, Brownson RC, Hewett JE. 2001. A prospective investigation of the impact of smoking bans on tobacco cessation and relapse. *Tob. Control* 10:267–72

35. Marcus BH, Emmons KM, Abrams DB, Marshall RJ, Kane M, et al. 1992. Restrictive workplace smoking policies: impact on nonsmokers' tobacco exposure. *J. Public Health Policy* 13:42–51

36. McMaugh K, Rissell C. 2000. Smoking restrictions in small businesses of inner west Sydney: a management perspective. *J. Occup. Health Saf.* 16:37–45

37. Millar WJ. 1988. Evaluation of the impact of smoking restrictions in a government work setting. *Can. J. Public Health* 79:379–82

38. Moskowitz JM, Lin Z, Hudes ES. 1999. The impact of California's smoking ordinances on worksite smoking policy and exposure to environmental tobacco smoke. *Am. J. Health Promot.* 13:278–81

39. Mullooly JP, Schuman KL, Stevens VJ, Glasgow RE, Vogt TM. 1990. Smoking behavior and attitudes of employees of a large HMO before and after a work site ban on cigarette smoking. *Public Health Rep.* 105:623–28

40. Natl. Health and Med. Res. Counc. Aust. 1997. *The Health Effects of Passive Smoking*. Canberra, Aust.: NHMRC

41. Natl. Res. Counc. Board Environ. Stud. Toxicol. Comm. Passive Smok. 1986. *Environmental Tobacco Smoke. Measuring Exposures and Assessing Health Effects*. Washington, DC: Natl. Acad. Press

42. Occup. Saf. Health Admin. 1994. Notice of proposed rulemaking; notice of informal public hearing (29 CFR Parts 1910, 1915,

1926, and 1928). *Fed. Regist* 59:15968–6039

43. Patten CA, Gilpin E, Cavin SW, Pierce JP. 1995. Workplace smoking policy and changes in smoking behavior in California: a suggested association. *Tob. Control* 4:36–41

44. Patten CA, Pierce JP, Cavin SW, Berry C, Kaplan R. 1995. Progress in protecting non-smokers from environmental tobacco smoke in California workplaces. *Tob. Control* 4:139–44

45. Pierce JP, Gilpin EA, Emery SL, Farkas AJ, Zhu SH, et al. 1998. *Tobacco Control in California: Who's Winning the War? An Evaluation of the Tobacco Control Program, 1989–1996.* La Jolla: Univ. Calif., San Diego

46. Pierce JP, Shanks TG, Pertschuk M, Gilpin E, Shopland D, et al. 1994. Do smoking ordinances protect non-smokers from environmental tobacco smoke? *Tob. Control* 3:15–20

47. Repace JL. 1994. Risk management of passive smoking at work and at home. *St Louis Univ. Public Law Rev.* 13:763–85

48. Reuters. 2001. Hotels start smoke-free movement. *Los Angeles Times*, Aug. 31

49. Siegel M. 1993. Involuntary smoking in the restaurant workplace. *JAMA* 270:490–93

50. Siegel M, Husten C, Merritt RK, Giovino GA, Eriksen MP. 1995. Effects of separately ventilated smoking lounges on the health of smokers: Is this an appropriate public health policy? *Tob. Control* 4:22–29

51. Stave GM, Jackson GW. 1991. Effect of a total work-site smoking ban on employee smoking and attitudes. *J. Occup. Med.* 33:884–90

52. Stillman FA, Becker DM, Swank RT, Hantula D, Moses H, et al. 1990. Ending smoking at the Johns Hopkins Medical Institutions. *JAMA* 264:1565–69

53. Trotter L, Letcher T, eds. 2000. *Smoking bans in Victorian workplaces: 1999 update.*

Melbourne, Aust.: Vict. Smok. Heath Program

54. Truman BI, Smith-Akin CK, Hinman AR, Gebbie KM, Brownson R, et al. 2000. Developing the guide to community preventive services—overview and rationale. *Am. J. Prev. Med.* 18:18–26

55. US Dep. Health Hum. Serv. 1986. *The Health Consequences of Involuntary Smoking: A Report of the Surgeon General. Rep. 97–8398.* Washington, DC: US Dep. Health Hum. Serv.

56. US Dep. Health Hum. Serv. 2000. *Healthy People 2010. Vol. 1. Conf. Ed.* Washington, DC: US Dep. Health Hum. Serv.

57. US Dep. Health Hum. Serv. 2000. *National Worksite Health Promotion Survey.* Washington, DC: Off. Dis. Prev. Health Promot.

58. US Dep. Health Hum. Serv. 2000. *Reducing Tobacco Use: A Report of the Surgeon General. Rep. 97–8398.* Atlanta, GA: Cent. Dis. Control Prev.

59. US Environ. Prot. Agency. 1992. *Respiratory Health Effects of Passive Smoking: Lung Cancer and Other Disorders. Rep. EPA/600/6–90/006F.* Washington, DC: US EPA

60. US Environ. Prot. Agency. 1994. *The Costs and Benefits of Smoking Restrictions. An Assessment of the Smoke-Free Environment Act of 1993 (H.R. 3434).* Washington, DC: US EPA. Off. Air Radiat. Indoor Air Div.

61. Wakefield MA, Chaloupka FJ, Kaufman NJ, Orleans CT, Barker DC, Ruel EE. 2000. Effect of restrictions on smoking at home, at school, and in public places on teenage smoking: cross sectional study. *BMJ* 321:333–37

62. Wakefield MA, Roberts L, Owen N. 1996. Trends in prevalence and acceptance of workplace smoking bans among indoor workers in South Australia. *Tob. Control* 5:205–8

63. Wasserman J, Manning WG, Newhouse JP, Winkler JD. 1991. The effects of excise taxes and regulations on cigarette smoking. *J. Health Econ.* 10:43–64

Annu. Rev. Public Health 2002. 23:349–75

SOCIOECONOMIC INEQUALITIES IN INJURY: Critical Issues in Design and Analysis

Catherine Cubbin

Stanford Center for Research in Disease Prevention, Stanford University School of Medicine, 1000 Welch Road, Palo Alto, California 94304-1825; e-mail: ccubbin@stanford.edu

Gordon S. Smith

Center for Safety Research, Liberty Research Center for Safety and Health, 71 Frankland Road, Hopkinton, Massachusetts 01746; e-mail: Gordon.Smith@LibertyMutual.com

Key Words   accidents, morbidity, mortality, socioeconomic factors, residence characteristics

■ **Abstract**   Injuries continue to place a tremendous burden on the public's health and rates vary widely among different groups in the population. Increasing attention has recently been given to the effects of socioeconomic status (SES) as a determinant of health among both individuals and communities. However, relatively few studies have focused on the influence of SES and injuries. Furthermore, those that have, and the other injury studies that have included measures of SES in their analysis, have varying degrees of conceptual and methodological rigor in their use of this measure. Recent advances in data linkage and analytic techniques have, however, provided new and improved methods to assess the relationship between SES and injuries. This review summarizes the relevant literature on SES and injuries, with particular attention to study design, and the measurement and interpretation of SES. We found that increasing SES has a strong inverse association with the risk of both homicide and fatal unintentional injuries, although the results for suicide were mixed. However, the relationship between SES and nonfatal injuries was less consistent than for fatal injuries. We offer potential explanatory mechanisms for the relationship between SES and injuries and make recommendations for future research in this area.

INTRODUCTION

Injury, as a leading cause of morbidity, disability, and premature mortality, represents a tremendous burden to the public's health measured both in years of potential life lost and costs to society (10). However, the injury burden is not shared equally among all groups in society and often disproportionately affects certain groups, including the poor and young populations. The Haddon matrix, a conceptual model developed initially to understand motor vehicle injuries, describes three broad factors involved in injuries: human, agent, and the environment (29).

0163-7525/02/0510-0349$14.00

349

Socioeconomic status (SES) is an important characteristic of both human (people) and environmental factors and is considered to be a fundamental determinant of health (46, 56, 64, 77). However, relatively little attention has been paid to SES in the public health literature focused on injury control and prevention. There are many reasons for this, including data constraints, limited resources devoted to injury research, and the notion that SES is a "fixed" factor (and thus not amenable to intervention). Much of the published research literature on the epidemiology of injuries does not include measures of SES. In the literature that does include SES, it is usually only to adjust for potential confounding and the SES measures used are often inadequate. There are few studies that specifically examine the relationship between SES and injuries as their main research question.

Recently, there has been a resurgence in investigating the role of the community socioeconomic environment in determining health. This is due, in part, to improved analytic techniques such as multilevel modeling, improved data linkage, geographic information systems (GIS) (72), as well as to a general increasing interest in socioeconomic inequalities in health. A central hypothesis that drives this work is that community characteristics represent more than simply the sum of its parts (for example, a high concentration of poverty in an area could affect all residents in the community, regardless of one's own economic standing). In other words, individual socioeconomic position may not protect the health of people who are well off if they live in socioeconomically disadvantaged environments. Socioeconomic characteristics of a community can determine, in part, local access to goods and services, the built environment, the level of residential stability, crime, social norms, and the ability for residents to maintain social controls over individual behavior. Recent reviews of the findings from studies that have examined the effects of community socioeconomic context on individual health concluded that the effects of community context are independent of individual level SES (56, 64, 77). Morbidity and mortality from external causes (i.e., intentional and unintentional injuries) have the most plausible link to the community socioeconomic environment compared to other causes of morbidity and mortality since, by definition, the source of injury is located outside the injured person. However, few studies have investigated the question of whether community context influences individual level injury outcomes independent of the person's SES; most studies have been conducted at one level only (individual or ecological) (16).

The explanatory factors through which SES (characterizing both people and communities) influences the risk of injury are complex. Psychosocial factors are one set of variables that might account for socioeconomic disparities in injuries (e.g., poverty-related stressors and intentional injuries; unemployment-related social isolation and suicide). Access to material resources, such as an adequate income and decent housing, are also believed to explain the relationship between SES and injuries (e.g., use of space heaters and burn/fire injures). The organization of work and occupational exposure is another dominant set of explanatory factors. Alienation, job control, and strain, as well as the physical hazards associated with working conditions, have all been shown to be contributors to occupational injuries

(67). Health behaviors (e.g., seatbelt use, alcohol consumption) may also partly explain the association between SES and injuries. At an area level, favorable community socioeconomic conditions reflect an area's material resources and access to high-quality municipal services, such as fire and police protection, safe roads, and recreational facilities. Affluent neighborhoods have lower crime rates, restrict access to traffic and "undesirable" neighbors, and their residents are less likely to tolerate deviant behavior, each of which may be protective against injury. Multiple explanatory factors are likely to be operating simultaneously to produce an injury occurrence (i.e., the influence of seatbelt use and road conditions on motor vehicle fatalities) and affect an injury outcome (i.e., access to high-quality treatment and rehabilitation). The influence of these factors is likely to vary by cause of injury.

This paper reviews the published epidemiological studies that have investigated the relationship between SES and injuries. Because so few studies have investigated this research question as its main objective, we also included studies that examined various other aspects of the epidemiology of injuries and that included SES as one characteristic (either of the injured persons themselves, or of the areas in which they lived or were injured). Particular attention was paid to the measurement and interpretation of SES and to studies that examined the contribution of SES to the risk of injury at a community or neighborhood level, after accounting for individual level differences. This review is not meant to be exhaustive of all studies that include SES but rather to critically examine the methods used to measure and interpret SES in studies of injury mortality and morbidity. It also suggests promising areas for future study.

METHODS

This review summarizes relevant original research on the subject of SES and injuries published since 1960. It is designed to address injuries and not the extensive literature on social conditions and violence victimization or abusive behavior (61). Studies that examined injuries due to violence were included only if the outcome studied was the resulting injury. English language studies were identified by a librarian via keyword searching (wounds and injuries, accidents, burns, drowning, homicide, poisoning, suicide, violence, socioeconomic factors, residence characteristics, social environment, social context, neighborhood) on the National Library of Medicine's database Medline. Additional studies were also retrieved from reference lists in other articles. Studies from developed countries were included if they examined the relationship between injuries and SES (at an individual or area level).

The results of our review are categorized by severity of outcome (morbidity vs. mortality) and level of analysis (individual, ecological, or multilevel). An individual level of analysis includes those studies where the injury outcome and SES variable(s) are measured for individuals, including studies that used area-based measures, such as neighborhood-level median family income, explicitly to proxy individual-level SES. An ecological level of analysis includes those studies where both the injury outcome and SES variable(s) are measured at the group or area level (e.g. county-level injury rates and per capita income). A multilevel analysis includes those studies where the injury outcome is measured for individuals and the SES variable(s) are examined at both the individual and area levels (e.g., association between the risk of motor vehicle fatalities and neighborhood SES, after adjusting for individual SES). Some studies fall into more than one category (i.e., morbidity and mortality outcomes). Previously published reviews (e.g., 9, 19, 43a, 44, 62), studies of homicide in the criminology or sociology literature (e.g., 55), and studies of violence or collisions rather than injuries themselves (e.g., 1, 53) are not covered in this review. However, original research discussed in these reviews was included if it met the criteria described above.

RESULTS

Tables 1 and 2 present summaries of the fatal and nonfatal injury studies reviewed, grouped according to the level of analysis (i.e., individual level, ecological level, or multilevel). When we refer to a "positive" association, we mean that as SES increases, so does the risk of injury. When we refer to an "inverse" association, we mean that as SES increases, the risk of injury decreases.

Fatal Injuries

INDIVIDUAL LEVEL   Three studies were identified that used nationally representative data sets to investigate the role of SES in overall injury mortality in youth or young adults (see Table 1). Using the U.S. National Longitudinal Mortality Study, Singh & Yu found that low SES was significantly associated with the risk of homicide in both youth (68) and adolescents and young adults (69). The third study investigated childhood mortality from all causes, and its author concluded that the primary source of socioeconomic disparities in overall mortality is due to injuries (49). One study of mortality among young and middle-aged men in New Zealand found that social class, measured using occupation, was strongly associated with all injury mortality and accounted for almost 40% of "excess" deaths (those prevented if everyone experienced the mortality of those in the highest social class) (54).

Two studies were identified that examined the role of SES in homicide in a nationally representative sample from the United States, one among working-age adults (17), and one among youth (31). Both studies found significant inverse associations between SES and homicide after adjusting for potential confounding variables. Two additional studies of homicide in youth also found inverse associations with SES, one using data from Maine (52) and one using data from the city of Boston (76).

Mixed results were found in the five studies that examined the role of SES in suicide. Three studies found that occupation or employment status (proxies for SES) was associated with suicide but the results were inconsistent: higher risk for low-SES workers in Australia (11), a higher risk for those not in the U.S. labor force compared to white-collar workers (17), while a study in England found a higher risk

TABLE 1 Fatal injuries and socioeconomic status: summary of methodological features and results, grouped according to level of analysis

Reference	Sample	Outcome	SES measure(s)	Analysis	Covariates	Results	SES gradient examined? (Yes/No)
Individual Level							
Burnley, 1995	Male deaths between 1986–1989, ages 25–64, New South Wales, Australia	Suicide	Occupation	Stratified SMRs*	Age	Higher SMRs* for manual workers, lower SMRs* for professional, clerical, and service workers	Yes
Cubbin et al., 2000a	NHIS* (1987–1994), ages 18–64, linked to NDI* through 1995, U.S.A.	Homicide, suicide, motor vehicle fatalities, other external causes	Education, income, occupation/ employment	Cox proportional hazards models	Age, gender, race/ethnicity, marital status, SES variables	Low education, income, occupation/ employment status associated with higher risk of homicide, motor vehicle fatalities, other external causes; "not in labor force" associated with higher risk of suicide	Yes
Hussey, 1997	NLMS* (1979–1981), ages 17 and under, linked to NDI through 1989, U.S.A.	Homicide, suicide, unintentional injuries	Household education, income	Cox proportional hazards models	Age, gender, race, household size, household structure, urban/rural, SES variables	Low household education associated with higher risk of homicide, unintentional injuries	Yes
Kellermann et al., 1992	Deaths between 1987–1990 in Shelby Co., TN and King Co., WA	Suicide	Education	Logistic regression	Living alone, alcohol consumption, alcohol-related hospitalization, psychotropic medication, illicit drug use, gun kept in home, education	Low education associated with higher risk of suicide	No

(Continued)

TABLE 1 (Continued)

Reference	Sample	Outcome	SES measure(s)	Analysis	Covariates	Results	SES gradient examined? (Yes/No)
Kelly et al., 1995	Deaths between 1982–1992, ages 16–64, England and Wales	Suicide	Occupation; also husband's occupation for women	Proportional mortality ratios	None	Occupation in social classes I and II at highest risk of suicide	No
Loomis, 1991	Deaths between 1986–1987, ages 15–64, 20 U.S. states	Motor vehicle fatalities	Occupation	Odds ratios	Age	Blue collar occupations had higher than expected numbers of motor vehicle fatalities	Yes
Mare, 1982	Current Population Survey, 1975, ages 20 and under, U.S.A.	Mortality	Maternal education, income	Proportion dead or surviving	None	Primary source of socioeconomic mortality differences is due to injuries	No
Nersesian et al., 1985	Deaths between 1976–1980, ages 19 and under, Maine	Mortality	Income (on public assistance or not)	Bivariate associations	None	Low income at higher risk of homicide and unintentional injuries	No
Pearce et al., 1983	Male deaths between 1975–1977, ages 15–64, New Zealand	Mortality	Social class (based on occupation)	Stratified death rates; relative risks; trend tests	Age	Low social class associated with increased injury mortality	Yes
Singh & Yu, 1996a	NLMS* (1979–1981), ages 1–14, linked to NDI through 1985, U.S.A.	Mortality	Income	Cox proportional hazards	Gender, race/ethnicity, urban/rural status, income	Low income associated with higher risk of external cause mortality	Yes
Singh & Yu, 1996b	NLMS (1979–1981), ages 15–24, linked to NDI through 1985, U.S.A.	Mortality	Education (ages 20–24 only), income	Cox proportional hazards	Gender, race/ethnicity, place of residence, nativity status, marital status, SES variables	Low education and income associated with higher risk of external cause mortality	Yes

Study	Sample	Injury type	SES measure	Analysis	Adjustment	Findings	Gradient
Wise et al., 1985	Deaths between 1972–1979, ages 19 and under, Boston, MA	Mortality	Census tract (income)	Stratified death rates	Age	For ages over 1, income inversely associated with homicide and fire deaths and positively associated with motor vehicle fatalities	Yes
Ecological Level							
Abel, 1986	Deaths between 1972–1984, ages 14 and under, Erie Co., NY	Homicide	Census tract (unemployment, poverty)	Descriptive	None	Number of homicides increased with higher % unemployed and poor	No
Baker et al., 1992, pp. 26–27	Deaths between 1980–1986, U.S.A.	Injury mortality	County (per capita income)	Stratified death rates	None	Unintentional injury and homicide rates higher in low income counties; little relationship between suicide rates and income	Yes
Baker et al., 1987	Deaths between 1979–1981, Fatal Accident Reporting System, U.S.A.	Motor vehicle fatalities	County (per capita income)	Correlations	None	Motor vehicle fatality rates inversely correlated with per capita income	No
Blaser, 1983	Deaths between 1970–1980, ages 15 and under, Atlanta, GA	Homicide	Census tract SES (measurement not included)	Stratified death rates	None	Homicide rates in low SES tracts twice the rates in high SES tracts	No
Burnley, 1995	Male deaths between 1986–1989, ages 25–64, Sydney, Australia	Suicide	Statistical local area (income, education, occupation)	Correlations	Age	Low/moderate correlations between suicide rates and SES found; varied by gender, age, and SES indicator	No
Centerwall, 1984	Deaths between 1971–1972, ages 16 and over, Atlanta, GA	Domestic homicide	Census tract of victim (crowded housing)	Stratified death rates and relative risks	None	Non-significant black/white relative risks at same level of crowded housing	Yes

(Continued)

TABLE 1 *(Continued)*

Reference	Sample	Outcome	SES measure(s)	Analysis	Covariates	Results	SES gradient examined? (Yes/No)
Crawford & Prince, 1999	Male deaths between 1979–1985 and 1986–1992, ages 15–44, England	Suicide	County district (unemployment, car access)	Multiple linear regression	Age	Increasing rates of suicide were associated with decreasing unemployment and increasing car access	Yes
Cubbin et al., 2000c	Black and white male deaths between 1988–1992, U.S.A.	Homicide	Health service area (family income, education, unemployment, crowded housing, relative deprivation)	Hierarchical linear models	Age, region, urban/rural status, % female-headed households, SES variables, and 2 way interactions	Rates higher in areas with low education, high relative deprivation, high income (black men); rates lower in areas with low crowded housing	Yes
Dayal et al., 1986	Deaths between 1974–1980, Philadelphia, PA	Mortality from external causes	Neighborhood SES score (income, education, poverty, rent, house value)	Stratified SMRs*, test of clustering	Age	Significant clustering by SES	Yes
Dougherty et al., 1990	Deaths in 1981, ages 14 and under, urban Canada; deaths between 1979–1983, ages 14 and under, Montreal	Motor vehicle fatalities	Canada: census tract (income); Montreal: health and social services districts (childhood poverty)	Stratified death rates	None	Rates greater in areas of lowest SES compared to areas of highest SES	Yes
Gunnell et al., 1995	Deaths between 1982–1991, ages 11 and over, Bristol, U.K.	Suicide	Postcode (Townsend deprivation index)	Correlations with SMRs*	Age, gender	Strong correlation between deprivation and suicide	No

Kyriacou et al., 1999	Deaths between 1988–1992, Los Angeles, CA	Gang-related homicide	Police divisions (income, employment, education)	Multiple linear regression	Single family households, male, under 20 years, African American, Hispanic, SES variables, interaction between per capita income and employment	Per capita income and employment were inversely associated with the risk of homicide	Yes
Mierley & Baker, 1983	Deaths between 1976–1978, Baltimore, MD	Fire mortality	Census tract (rental value)	Stratified death rates	None	Death rates were highest in areas with lowest rental values	Yes
Whitley et al., 1999	Deaths between 1981–1992, Great Britain	Suicide	Parliamentary constituencies (Townsend deprivation index)	Multiple linear regression	Social fragmentation	Increase in suicide rates associated with increase in deprivation was reduced after adjusting for fragmentation	No
Multilevel							
Cubbin et al., 2000b	NHIS* (1987–1994), ages 18–64, linked to NDI through 1995, U.S.A.	Homicide, suicide, motor vehicle fatalities, other external causes	Census tract (income, poverty, education, occupation, housing value, unemployment)	Cox proportional hazards models	Individual: age, gender, race/ethnicity, marital status, income, education, occupation, employment, tract: one SES variable per model	Tract level low SES generally associated with higher risk of homicide, motor vehicle fatalities, and other external causes, after adjusting for individual variability, but varied according to SES indicator; inconsistent relationships were found between SES and suicide	No

*SMR = standardized mortality ratio; NHIS = National Health Interview Survey; NDI = National Death Index; NLMS = National Longitudinal Mortality Study.

TABLE 2 Nonfatal injuries and socioeconomic status: summary of methodological features and results, grouped according to level of analysis

Reference	Sample	Outcome	SES measure(s)	Analysis	Covariates	Results	SES gradient examined? (Yes/No)
Individual Level							
Anderson et al., 1994	School district, 1990–1991, ages 12–16, Allegheny Co., PA	Injuries requiring medical attention	Township (poverty)	Stratified life-table curves	None	No differences by poverty	Yes
Ballard et al., 1992	Washington Fire Incident Reporting System, 1984–1985, King Co., WA	Residential fire injuries	Household income	Descriptive	None	Income lower for injured persons compared to county	No
Chichester et al., 1998	Emergency department admissions from one hospital, 1996, west coast of Scotland	Motor vehicle injuries	Postcode (deprivation)	Chi-square test for linear trend	Age, gender, victim role, purpose of journey, SES	Positive trend by deprivation	Yes
Cubbin et al., 2000	NHIS* (1987–1994), ages 18–64, U.S.A.	Episodes of nonfatal injuries	Educational attainment, family income/family size, occupation/ employment status	Logistic regression	Age, gender, race/ethnicity, marital status, SES variables	Blue collar workers at increased risk, low education associated with higher risk only for most severe injuries	Yes
Helmkamp & Bone, 1986	Hospitalizations for men enlisted in Navy, 1977–1979, U.S.A.	Unintentional injuries	Seniority measured by pay grade	Injury rates	Age	Higher rates for lower pay grades	Yes

Kelly and Miles-Doan, 1997	NHIS* (1988–1989), ages 18 and over, U.S.A.	Episodes of nonfatal injuries	Education, education of responsible adult, poverty status	Logistic regression	Age, gender, race/ethnicity, health status, family type (children), marital status (adult), urban/rural status, SES variables	Education and poverty not associated with injury in children or adults	Yes
King & Palmisano, 1992	Hospital discharge surveillance data, ages 14 and under, Birmingham, AL	Pedestrian injuries	Insurance status	Odds ratios comparing cases to controls	Age, gender, SES variable	Medicaid/uninsured associated with higher risk of pedestrian injury compared to those with private insurance	No
Kogan et al., 1995	Longitudinal follow-up (1991) to the NMIHS,* ages 3 and under, U.S.A.	Nonfatal injuries requiring medical attention	Maternal education, household income	Relative risks	None	Higher SES associated with higher risk of injury	Yes
Pless et al., 1989a	National Child Development Study, ages 7–16, U.K.	Nonfatal traffic injuries	Father's occupation, crowding, amenities	Logistic regression	Fidgety, in care of local authority, crowding	Crowding associated with higher risk in older girls	Yes
Pless et al., 1989b	Hospital records and police reports, ages 14 and under, Montreal	Pedestrian or bicyclist injuries	Maternal education	Logistic regression	Age, gender, socioeconomic status area of residence	High maternal education associated with lower risk	Yes
Scheidt et al., 1995	Child Health Supplement to the NHIS,* 1988, ages 17 and under, U.S.A.	Nonfatal injuries requiring medical attention	Maternal education, family income, insurance status	Stratified injury rates	None	Higher SES associated with higher injury rates although not significant when adjusted for recall bias	No

(Continued)

TABLE 2 (*Continued*)

Reference	Sample	Outcome	SES measure(s)	Analysis	Covariates	Results	SES gradient examined? (Yes/No)
Sorenson et al., 1996	NSFH* 1987–1988 married adults ages 18 and over, U.S.A.	Injuries among those reporting physical violence in marriage	Education, household income	Logistic regression	Age, gender, race/ethnicity, religion, urban/ rural status, children, marriage duration, SES variables	No association between injuries and SES	Yes
Wagener & Winn, 1991	NHIS* (1983–1987), currently employed ages 18–64, U.S.A.	Episodes of nonfatal injuries	Education, family income, occupation	Stratified injury rates	None	Low income and blue collar occupation associated with higher injury rates	Yes
Ecological Level							
Dougherty et al., 1990	Hospital records and police reports, 1981, ages 14 and under, Montreal	Pedestrian or bicyclist injuries	Health and social services districts (childhood poverty)	Stratified injury rates; rate ratios	None	Rates increased with increasing poverty; rate ratios comparing poorest to least poor quintile significant; inequalities more pronounced for pedestrian vs. bicyclist injuries	Yes
Durkin et al., 1998	Northern Manhattan Injury Surveillance System, 1983–1992, ages 16 and under, New York	Injuries resulting in hospitalization or death	Zip code (poverty)	Rate ratios	None	Rates higher in high poverty zip codes compared to low poverty zip codes	No

Study	Data source	Injury type	SES measure	Statistical method	Adjustment	Findings	Gradient
Durkin et al., 1994	Northern Manhattan Injury Surveillance System, 1983–1991, ages 16 and under, New York	Injuries resulting in hospitalization or death	Census tract (income, poverty, single-headed households, education, crowding, unemployment)	Simple linear regression, rate ratios of incidence rates	None	Low SES generally associated with higher risk of injury, overall and by cause	No
Fife et al., 1986	Hospital admission records, 1979–1980, Rhode Island	Head injuries	Census tract (income)	Stratified injury rates	Age, gender	Rates higher in low income tracts	Yes
Guyer et al., 1989	Hospital records and vital statistics, 1979–1982, ages 19 and under, Massachusetts	Intentional injuries	Community (poverty)	Correlations with rates	None	Rates highly correlated with poverty level	No
Istre et al., 2001	Fire department, hospital, ambulance, medical examiner records, 1991–1997, Dallas, Texas	Fire injuries	Census tract (income)	Stratified injury rates	None	Rates higher in low income tracts	Yes
Jolly et al., 1993	National Injury Surveillance Unit, 1989–1990, ages 14 and under, Brisbane/Melbourne, Australia	Injuries	Postcode (income, unemployment, school dropouts, SES index)	Correlations with rates	None	Rates moderately correlated with low SES	Yes
Kraus et al., 1986	Hospital, medical examiner, vital statistics, nursing home records, 1981, San Diego Co, CA	Serious brain injuries	Census tract (income)	Stratified injury rates	Age, race/ethnicity	Rates higher in low income tracts	No
Locke et al., 1990	New England Regional Burn Program, 1978–1979, 6 New England states, U.S.A.	Burn injuries	Counties or groups of counties (income, poverty, education)	Simple linear regression, correlations	None	Rates inversely associated with SES	Yes

(Continued)

TABLE 2 (*Continued*)

Reference	Sample	Outcome	SES measure(s)	Analysis	Covariates	Results	SES gradient examined? (Yes/No)
Reid et al., 2001	Hospital, vital statistics, 1993, ages 19 and under, Minnesota	Brain injuries	Census block-group (income, education)	Correlations with rates	None	Lower rates correlated with high SES	No
Rivara & Barber, 1985	Police reports, 1982, ages 14 and under, Memphis, TN	Pedestrian injuries	Census tract (income, poverty, crowding)	t-Tests, multiple linear regression	None	Injuries more likely in low SES tracts, strong positive association between injury rates and crowding	No
Roberts et al., 1992	Hospital records, 1982–1987, ages 14 and under, Auckland, New Zealand	Injuries	Census area (unemployment)	Correlations with SMRs	Age	Rates correlated with unemployment	No
Multilevel Reading et al., 1999	Hospital records, 1993–1995, ages 4 and under, Norwich, U.K.	Injuries	Social areas [groups of census enumeration districts] (Townsend material deprivation index)	Hierarchical linear models	Previous live births, maternal age, gender, single parent, distance from hospital, deprivation index (enumeration district), deprivation index (social area)	Social area level deprivation associated with higher risk of injuries after adjusting for individual variability	Yes

*NHIS = National Health Interview Survey; NMIHS = National Maternal and Infant Health Survey; NSFH = National Survey of Families and Households.

for high-SES workers (36). Although these three studies each included working-age adults, they included different adjustment variables. In addition, suicide rates vary widely by country. One study of gun ownership and suicide found that low education was significantly associated with suicide risk in two U.S. counties (35). Another study of suicide among U.S. youth, however, found no relationship between SES and suicide (31).

Five U.S. studies were found that examined SES and unintentional injuries (17, 31, 48, 52, 76). Regardless of the population studied, SES indicator used, or cause of injury examined (i.e., all unintentional injuries, motor vehicle fatalities, fire deaths), all but one study found inverse associations between SES and unintentional injuries. The exception is a study of mortality among youth in Boston that found a positive association between increasing SES and motor vehicle fatalities, possibly reflecting increased access to cars among wealthier city residents (76).

Few of the individual-level studies examined the relationship between SES and injury mortality by gender despite the wide discrepancy in injury rates found in many studies, especially for more serious injuries. One study by Mare of youth mortality in the United States found stronger socioeconomic inequalities in injury mortality among boys compared to girls (49). However, a study of motor vehicle fatalities in the United States found similar effects of SES for adult men and women using occupation as a measure of SES (48). Similarly, a study of suicide in the U.K. found no gender difference by SES (36).

ECOLOGICAL LEVEL   A study of cause-specific mortality rates, including external causes, at the neighborhood level (groups of census tracts) in Philadelphia found significant clustering of injury mortality in low-SES neighborhoods (20). Six U.S. studies investigated the relationship between SES and homicide at an ecological level. Four of the studies used census tracts or other small areas in a single county (2) or city (8, 13, 43) as the unit of analysis. Each study found strong inverse associations between area-level SES and the risk of homicide, regardless of study population or type of homicide (e.g., domestic, gang-related, all homicides). Another study using counties as the unit of analysis also found that homicide rates decreased as per capita income increased (5). The last ecological study identified used health service areas as the unit of analysis and found that homicide rates for both black and white males were significantly inversely associated with SES (18).

The five ecological studies of suicide found inconsistent results, varying from a positive relationship between SES and suicide in Australia and England (11, 15), whereas two other studies in the U.K. found an inverse relationship (27, 74) and a U.S. study found no relationship (5). For unintentional injuries, regardless of whether smaller areas (e.g., census tracts) or larger areas (e.g., counties) are used as the unit of analysis, strong inverse relationships were found between SES and injuries, including motor vehicle fatalities (6, 21), deaths due to fire (51), and other unintentional injuries (5). However, rates for certain very specific injuries such as aircraft crashes may be higher in higher SES groups (5).

Two of the ecological studies examined socioeconomic inequalities in injury mortality by gender. One study found greater inequalities in motor vehicle fatalities among girls compared to boys in Canada (21) and the other study found greater inequalities in suicide among males of all ages compared to females in the U.K. (74).

MULTILEVEL   Only one study was identified that examined the relationship between area-level SES (in this case, census tracts) and injury mortality in working-age adults after adjusting for the effects of individual SES (16). The study found that low census tract level SES was generally associated with higher risk of homicide, motor vehicle fatalities, and other unintentional injuries but, as with other studies, inconsistent relationships were found between SES and suicide. This study did not examine census tract-level SES effects by gender.

Nonfatal Injuries

INDIVIDUAL LEVEL   For nonfatal injuries, unintentional injuries comprise a much larger proportion (the majority) of injuries than for fatal injuries. Four U.S. studies were found that examined all nonfatal injuries among children (see Table 2). No associations were found between SES and the risk of injury among a population of adolescents from one county (3), or among children under 18 years in two different studies using nationally representative data sets (37, 66). However, one study of children ages three and under using a nationally representative data set found a positive relationship between SES and risk of injury (40). Among adults, the results are also inconsistent. Three studies used the National Health Interview Survey (NHIS) to examine the relationship between SES and nonfatal injuries among adults (17, 37, 73). Two found that low SES was associated with higher risk of nonfatal injuries among working-age adults (17, 73), whereas the third study of all adults found no association between SES and nonfatal injuries, possibly reflecting weaker socioeconomic inequalities among the elderly (37). The studies that investigated all unintentional nonfatal injuries as a group or cause-specific unintentional injuries suggest that there is an inverse association with SES, for traffic-related injuries (including motor vehicle, pedestrian, and bicyclist injuries) among youth (38, 57, 58) and at all ages (14). These findings occurred across different cities and countries, although the measures of SES used varied considerably. A study primarily of nonfatal fire injuries occurring in one county in Washington State found that persons who were injured from residential fires were more likely to have lower household incomes compared to the average county household income (7). A study of unintentional injuries resulting in hospitalization among men enlisted in the Navy found higher injury rates among men in the lower ranks, i.e., lower pay grades, a proxy for seniority (30).

Only one individual-level study was identified that investigated intentional nonfatal injuries. This study was among those persons reporting physical violence in their marriage, and it found no association between the resulting injuries and SES, although those reporting violence were more likely to be of lower SES (71).

Two ecological studies of youth examined gender differences in socioeconomic inequalities. One found greater inequalities in pedestrian and bicyclist injuries among girls compared by boys in Canada (21) and the other found similar correlations between SES and injury rates among girls and boys in Australia (33).

ECOLOGICAL LEVEL   Twelve studies were identified that examined the relationship between nonfatal injuries and SES at an ecological level (Table 2). All but one study (47) used small areas (e.g., zip code, census tract, postcode, or an aggregation of small areas) as the unit of analysis. Two studies examined correlations between all nonfatal injury rates among youth and SES, one in Australia (33) and the other in New Zealand (65); both found that injury rates were inversely correlated with measures of area SES. Two studies used the same data source (Northern Manhattan Injury Surveillance System) to examine severe injuries (those resulting in hospitalization or death) but utilized two different levels of analysis: zip code of residence (23) and census tract (22). Both studies found that low SES was associated with higher injury rates among persons ages 16 and under.

For the studies examining cause-specific nonfatal injuries, rates were higher in areas characterized by low SES, or inversely correlated with SES measures for head injuries (24, 41, 60), fire or burn injuries (32, 47), pedestrian or bicyclist injuries (21, 63), and intentional nonfatal injuries (28), regardless of study population and setting, source of data, covariates, or SES measure(s) used. Two of the individual-level studies examined the relationship between SES and nonfatal injuries by gender. Anderson et al. found no differences by gender in injuries requiring medical attention among youth in one U.S. county (3) and Pless et al. found that crowded housing was associated with traffic injuries among girls but not boys in the U.K. (57).

MULTILEVEL   Only one study was identified that examined the influence of area-based SES (in this case, groups of census enumeration districts) on nonfatal injuries among preschool-aged children after adjusting for individual SES using hospital records from Norwich, U.K. (59). Reading et al. found that low area-level SES (measured using a deprivation index) was significantly associated with higher risk of injuries, after adjusting for a range of individual-level variables, including SES. Differences in gender were not examined in this study.

DISCUSSION

Our review of the existing literature examining the relationship between SES (at the individual and/or area levels) and injuries found that the patterns varied according to the cause or intent of injury, level of analysis, population, and/or setting, particularly for nonfatal injuries. To summarize the results for fatal injuries, SES has a strong inverse association with the risk of both homicide and unintentional injuries in all ages; as individual or area SES decreases, the risk of homicide or unintentional injury increases. For suicide, the results for both the individual-level and area-level studies are mixed; some studies found no relationship between SES and the risk of suicide, whereas others found a positive or inverse association, depending upon the population studied and measures of SES used. More than any other injury outcome, there were large variations in the relationship between SES and suicide by country, which may reflect cultural differences or societal stresses that vary by country and among the different SES groups in particular countries.

The only study using multilevel modeling in a nationally representative sample for the United States found evidence of an independent effect of low neighborhood SES on the risk of homicide, motor vehicle fatalities, and other unintentional injuries, after controlling for individual-level demographic characteristics and three measures of SES (16), suggesting that the higher risk of injury mortality associated with low SES residential areas is not due entirely to the aggregation of low-SES individuals living within them. The same study found evidence for independent neighborhood SES effects on suicide, but the results were less consistent than for other fatal injuries.

The findings for nonfatal injuries are less consistent across studies. For all nonfatal injuries combined, some studies found no association and others a positive association with individual measures of SES in youth. For adults, however, there was either no association or an inverse association. For unintentional nonfatal injuries (including fire and traffic injuries) an inverse association was found with individual SES in all ages studied. No association with individual SES was found in the one investigation that examined nonfatal intentional injuries; however, the study used a very select study population (people experiencing physical violence in their marriage) (71). Each ecological study identified found an inverse association between area SES and risk of nonfatal injury, regardless of the injury type, level of aggregation (e.g., census tract, zip code, postcode, county), or study population. Finally, an inverse association between neighborhood SES was found in the one multilevel study of nonfatal injuries among young children in the U.K., after adjusting for an area-based proxy of individual socioeconomic status (59).

Part of the reason for the inconsistency in the relationships between SES and fatal and nonfatal injuries may be that they examine injuries of varying severity. Most nonfatal injuries are minor. Our review found that serious injuries, such as those requiring hospitalization, are similar to fatal injuries in having an inverse relationship to SES. The only studies of nonfatal injuries that found no association or a positive association were those whose injury definition was based on requiring medical attention or a half-day of restricted activity. If access to health care is limited, as has been shown for persons of color and low-SES groups, then minor injuries may be less likely to be reported by those groups. More serious injuries are less likely to be affected by differences in access to care. A positive association between increasing SES and nonfatal injuries may also reflect increasing opportunities for more-hazardous outdoor or recreational activities, such as sports and bicycle riding. This interpretation is supported empirically for certain causes of fatal injuries. Unlike most injury fatalities, airplane fatality rates are higher among high SES individuals because of increased exposure to flying in commercial and personally owned aircraft (5). Swimming pool ownership also increases with SES, and thus the risk of pool drowning in toddlers will be higher in the higher-income groups. Our earlier study of nonfatal injuries using nationally representative data from the United States found that low education was associated with an increased risk of severe nonfatal injuries (those requiring 5 or more days of restricted activity) but the risk was not increased risk for less severe injuries (17).

Although a large number of studies were reviewed, relatively few focused specifically on the relationship between SES and injuries, and of those, most used descriptive epidemiological methods, making it difficult to confirm the influence of SES on the risk of injury in the presence of confounding variables for which there has not been adjustment. Moreover, many of the studies reviewed, whether specifically focused on the SES/injury relationship or not, utilized seemingly arbitrary measures of SES and the measure(s) were often inadequately defined (i.e., how and when they were measured) and/or justified (i.e., why they were selected in relation to a conceptual framework). Furthermore, the interpretation of the role of SES in the risk of injury was lacking in most studies. The use of arbitrary measure(s) of SES is most likely due to data limitations; that is, researchers use what is available to them and, in the United States especially, adequate measures of SES are unavailable in many sources of data (e.g., medical records). However, much of the research reviewed did not adequately define or justify the measures they used; nor did much of the research discuss how inadequate SES measurement may have affected the results. Without adequate measures of SES, it is difficult to assess the role of SES in injury and also its contribution to other associations. For example, race/ethnicity is often considered an "independent" risk factor in health research after adjusting for measures of SES, when considerable residual confounding by SES likely exists (34). In fact, many studies just use race as a proxy for SES with no consideration of true SES factors.

A further issue that deserves attention and applies across all areas of health research is that of SES gradients. Previous research has found that there are socioeconomic effects at all levels of socioeconomic status, and not only at the lowest levels, such as living below the poverty level (2a, 49a). That is, in general, those at each level of SES have better health than those just below them (i.e., there is a dose-response effect). Approximately 60 percent of the studies reviewed in this study examined socioeconomic gradients, either implicitly or explicitly. However, given the heterogeneity in injury outcomes, measures of SES, covariates, study designs, and population studies, it is difficult to draw definitive conclusions regarding the existence or nonexistence (i.e., threshold effects) of socioeconomic gradients in injuries. In addition, few studies examined whether the effects of SES varied by gender.

Based on our review of the existing literature exploring the relationship between SES and injury, the following recommendations emerged, based both on the comments of other papers and our review. Future research on injuries should use multiple measures of SES when possible, and interpret the results accordingly. There has been a great deal of work on the conceptualization and measurement of SES (for example, see 42, 45, 75); this work has confirmed the multidimensional nature of SES, which implies that it can not be completely measured with one variable, i.e., income or educational attainment. Researchers should not simply state that they have "adjusted" for SES when they have adjusted for one measure only.

We recognize that SES is a complex concept that can be measured at multiple levels (e.g., individual, household, neighborhood) and at different time points (e.g., early childhood SES vs. current SES). It is exceedingly difficult to measure it completely, and researchers should acknowledge that residual confounding by SES might exist even when using multiple measures. This issue is particularly important when attempting to examine the relationship of another variable to an injury outcome after controlling for SES, such as in studies of racial/ethnic disparities in injury rates.

In general, we recommend that researchers be more specific in defining and more explicit in justifying the measures of SES used in their studies in order for the audience to interpret the meaning of their findings. Most of the studies identified in this review were fairly complete in defining the measures used but the majority provided little justification for the measures in relation to other possibilities.

Future research needs to consider more carefully the variables chosen to measure SES and to acknowledge their limitations. For example, several studies were identified that used an area-based measure of SES to proxy individual SES (3, 14, 59, 76). Even for small, relatively homogeneous areas, substantial misclassification by SES will exist and may bias the results depending on the direction of misclassification (70). In addition to area-based proxies, other studies used poor measures either to examine the SES/injury relationship or to adjust for SES. For example, one study used public assistance as a measure of low income (52). While it is true that the large majority of persons on public assistance have low incomes, it is not necessarily the case that persons not on public assistance do not have low incomes. Similarly, another study used insurance status as a measure of SES to examine the risk of pedestrian injury, comparing those with Medicaid or no insurance to those with private insurance (38); again, substantial misclassification may exist in that not all persons without insurance are low SES and not all persons with private insurance are high SES. Without paying particular attention to the above issues, the influence of SES on injury, and the influence of other factors on injury after adjusting for SES, cannot be stated with precision.

We offer several suggestions for researchers studying socioeconomic inequalities in injuries or using SES as covariates to study other relationships, e.g., racial/ethnic disparities in injuries. Researchers should acknowledge that SES is a multidimensional construct and that results may vary by the injury outcome, SES measure(s), and/or population studied [for a detailed discussion of the conceptualization and measurement of SES, see (42, 45, 75)]. Investigators should also acknowledge the limitations of the SES measures used in terms of dimensions and specifications (e.g., continuous vs. categorical, individual vs. area based) and in terms of the likelihood of residual confounding by SES. Ideally, it is preferable to measure several dimensions of SES rather than a single measure. Wealth (measured by accumulated assets such as car and home ownership and/or the value of savings and investments) would be preferred in addition to income, particularly because inequalities are much greater by wealth than they are by income, but wealth is very difficult to measure. We also suggest measuring income with many categories so that the full distribution of income in the population can be examined and to allow the assessment of threshold effects. Measuring income as a percentage of the poverty level or dividing by the family size supported on the income (income-to-needs ratio) is also recommended to standardize the resources available by family size (e.g., the resources available to a family of four persons with $50,000 are different than those for a family of one person with the same income). For educational attainment, researchers should use cutpoints that correspond to earned credentials, such as high school graduate and college graduate, since the effect of a year of education will vary along the distribution of educational attainment measured in years (e.g., 10 to 11 years vs. 11 to 12 years). Occupational and employment status should also be considered as potential SES variables, depending upon the population studied. Finally, increasing evidence suggests that area-based measures of SES are correlated with both overall injury rates and with the risk of injury to individuals, after accounting for individual SES. However, there has been little or only limited methodological research on how best to measure area-based socioeconomic characteristics.

Several potential mechanisms have been suggested to explain the general pattern between low SES and increased injury risk. Areas characterized by low SES (which contain, for the most part, low SES individuals) are more likely to expose their residents to increased hazards, such as those related to poor housing, traffic, crime, and work (4, 16, 62). For example, Glik et al. (26) found that low SES had a strong inverse association with observed hazards in homes related to burns, poisonings, and falls. Low SES areas are also often subject to increased traffic density and speed (62) and criminal activity, which may increase its residents' risk of motor vehicle, pedestrian, and bicyclist injuries and intentional injuries (e.g., firearm homicide, injuries resulting from assault), respectively.

Socioeconomic characteristics of residential areas are particularly important to consider in investigations of racial/ethnic disparities in injuries because persons of color are far more likely to live in socioeconomically disadvantaged areas compared to white persons. For example, Cubbin et al. found that the black/white disparity (adjusted for education, income, and employment/occupational status) in homicide was substantially reduced after further adjusting for neighborhood-level (census tract) socioeconomic status in a nationally representative sample of U.S. adults (16). However, differential residential environments for racial/ethnic groups can also present analytical challenges. For instance, Centerwall used census tract-level rates of crowded housing as a measure of socioeconomic conditions to match black and white victims of domestic homicide and categorize each homicide into one of seven socioeconomic strata (13). There were no statistically significant differences in rates of domestic homicide between blacks and whites after matching on crowded housing. However, only three socioeconomic strata were available for analysis since the stratum with the lowest rate of crowded housing contained no black homicides and the three strata with the highest rates of crowded housing contained no white homicides, resulting in the exclusion of two-thirds of the black homicides in the highest risk areas for study.

The goods and services that are available in particular areas depend, to a certain degree, upon their residents' ability to pay for them (16, 39). For instance, a recent MMWR report found that unvented heating appliances and stoves were more likely to be used by low-income households as heating devices compared to higher-income households (12), presumably because they could not afford to use heating from safer sources or to repair the heating equipment in their homes, therefore potentially increasing the risk of poisoning and fire/burn injuries. Certain relationships of goods and services to SES may depend upon location, such as urban/rural status. For example, one study found that motor vehicle injuries were positively associated with census tract–level income in Boston (76), perhaps because of increased access to cars among residents of wealthier urban areas. However, in rural areas, motor vehicle injuries are inversely associated with SES, possibly because of increased access to more crashworthy cars and better roads in wealthier areas. In addition, rural residents have the added risk of increased distances to travel and reduced access to quality trauma care, which may disproportionately affect the poor. Uneven fire and police protection is one example of publicly provided services that may differentially affect persons of low SES.

A third potential mechanism to explain the relationship between SES and injury is that beliefs, access to information, and injury-prevention behaviors vary by SES (25, 39, 50, 62). Without access to information and resources tailored to their needs, low SES individuals are less likely to believe that injuries are preventable, as has been recently found by Girasek (25). As a result, they are also less likely to practice effective injury-prevention measures, demonstrated by Mayer & LeClere (50).

Although the mechanisms discussed above are not mutually exclusive (e.g., inadequate fire protection could be considered a hazardous environment and a service) and often work together to influence an injury outcome (e.g., high crime and access to firearms influencing the risk of homicide), they are useful factors to consider when designing injury-prevention programs or public policies. While modifying the SES of individuals or their communities may be difficult and politically unfeasible, recognition of the factors that mediate the relationship between SES and injuries might lead to effective injury control measures to reduce socioeconomic inequalities in health, such as installing speed bumps or redesigning roads to reduce hazardous traffic conditions for pedestrians, passing gun control legislation to reduce the prevalence of firearms, or organizing workers to hold their employers accountable for safe working environments.

The question that is often asked when looking at SES and health is whether it is causal or simply a proxy for other unmeasured factors. The ultimate test of the causal effects of SES on injury risk can only be determined by intervention trials that are directed at improving SES and determining if it reduces injuries. While such studies are difficult—and potentially unethical—to conduct, insights may be obtained by studying natural experiments such as documenting the effects of social policy changes. One such example is the Moving to Opportunity randomized housing experiments that have been funded by the Department of Housing and Urban Development (HUD) in the United States. For example, moving families from housing projects to census tracts with less than 10 percent poverty reduced arrests for juvenile violent crime by 30 to 50 percent compared to comparison groups

(48a). One study in Boston also found that families moved were less likely to be victims of crime and have their children exposed to risk factors for violence (33a). However, the effect of these studies on injury rates has not yet been specifically examined.

Improved analytic techniques, such as multilevel modeling, GIS, and improved data linkage, have made it possible to simultaneously examine individual and environmental socioeconomic determinants of health. Evidence that injury research is taking advantage of these techniques is encouraging. One promising avenue of investigation in elucidating the causal pathway between socioeconomic disadvantage and injury is whether adverse socioeconomic environments affect all residents equally as opposed to only affecting low SES residents, or, in other words, whether high SES individuals are protected from the adverse environments in which they live. There is a strong need for more theoretical and methodological rigor in research on SES and injury, specifically in conceptualizing, defining, measuring, and interpreting SES, which could be accomplished perhaps through interdisciplinary research. There is also a need for greater understanding of the nature of the relationship between SES and injury, i.e., gradient vs. threshold effects, and whether the gradient or threshold is moderated by gender and/or age. We hope that, through this review, we have clarified the influence of SES on the risk of both fatal and nonfatal injuries and outlined some potential avenues for future work that will contribute to the reduction of socioeconomic inequalities in injury. Only through better study of the role of SES and its component mechanisms can we begin to address the often large disparities in injury risk by socioeconomic status.

ACKNOWLEDGMENTS

We acknowledge the technical assistance of Adeline L. Hwang for literature searching. Support for C. Cubbin was provided by the National Institute of Environmental Health Sciences (1R01HL67731-02) and the Centers for Disease Control and Prevention (TS-521). Support for G.S. Smith was provided by the National Institute of Alcohol Abuse and Alcoholism (R29AA07700) and grants from the Centers for Disease Control and Prevention to the Johns Hopkins Center for Injury Research and Policy (R49/CC R 302486).

Visit the Annual Reviews home page at www.annualreviews.org

LITERATURE CITED

1. Abdalla IM, Raeside R, Barker D, Mc-Guigan DR. 1997. An investigation into the relationships between area social characteristics and road accident casualties. *Accid. Anal. Prev.* 29:583–93

2. Abel EL. 1986. Childhood homicide in Erie County, New York. *Pediatrics* 77:709–13

2a. Adler NE, Boyce T, Chesney MA, Cohen S, Folkman S, et al. 1994. Socioeconomic status and health. The challenge of the gradient. *Am. Psychol.* 49:15–24

3. Anderson R, Dearwater SR, Olsen T, Aaron DJ, Kriska AM, LaPorte RE. 1994. The role of socioeconomic status and injury morbidity risk in adolescents. *Arch. Pediatr. Adolesc. Med.* 148:245–49

4. Baker SP. 1975. Determinants of injury and opportunities for intervention. *Am. J. Epidemiol.* 101:98–102

5. Baker SP. 1992. *The Injury Fact Book.* New York: Oxford Univ. Press. 2nd ed.

6. Baker SP, Whitfield RA, O'Neill B. 1987. Geographic variations in mortality from motor vehicle crashes. *N. Engl. J. Med.* 316:1384–87

7. Ballard JE, Koepsell TD, Rivara FP, Van Belle G. 1992. Descriptive epidemiology of unintentional residential fire injuries in King County, WA, 1984 and 1985. *Public Health Rep.* 107:402–8

8. Blaser MJ. 1983. Epidemiologic characteristics of child homicides in Atlanta, 1970–1980. *Pediatrician* 12:63–67

9. Blumstein AFP, Rivara FP, Rosenfeld R. 2000. The rise and decline of homicide—and why. *Annu. Rev. Public Health* 21:505–41

10. Bonnie RJ, Fulco C, Liverman CT, Inst. Med. (U.S.). Comm. Injury Prev. Control. 1999. *Reducing the Burden of Injury: Advancing Prevention and Treatment.* Washington, DC: Natl. Acad. Press

11. Burnley IH. 1995. Socioeconomic and spatial differentials in mortality and means of committing suicide in New South Wales, Australia, 1985–91. *Soc. Sci. Med.* 41:687–98

12. Cent. Dis. Control. 1997. Use of unvented residential heating appliances–United States, 1988–1994. *MMWR* 46:1221–24

13. Centerwall BS. 1984. Race, socioeconomic status, and domestic homicide, Atlanta, 1971–72. *Am. J. Public Health* 74:813–15

14. Chichester BM, Gregan JA, Anderson DP, Kerr JM. 1998. Associations between road traffic accidents and socio-economic deprivation on Scotland's west coast. *Scott. Med. J.* 43:135–38

15. Crawford MJ, Prince M. 1999. Increasing rates of suicide in young men in England during the 1980s: the importance of social context. *Soc. Sci. Med.* 49:1419–23

16. Cubbin C, LeClere FB, Smith GS. 2000. Socioeconomic status and injury mortality: individual and neighborhood determinants. *J. Epidemiol. Commun. Health* 54:517–24

17. Cubbin C, LeClere FB, Smith GS. 2000. Socioeconomic status and the occurrence of fatal and nonfatal injury in the United States. *Am. J. Public Health* 90:70–77

18. Cubbin C, Pickle LW, Fingerhut L. 2000. Social context and geographic patterns of homicide among US black and white males. *Am. J. Public Health* 90:579–87

19. Cummings P, Koepsell TD, Mueller BA. 1995. Methodological challenges in injury epidemiology and injury prevention research. *Annu. Rev. Public Health* 16:381–400

20. Dayal H, Goldberg-Alberts R, Kinman J, Ramos J, Sharrar R, Shapiro S. 1986. Patterns of mortality from selected causes in an urban population. *J. Chronic Dis.* 39:877–88

21. Dougherty G, Pless IB, Wilkins R. 1990. Social class and the occurrence of traffic injuries and deaths in urban children. *Can. J. Public Health* 81:204–9

22. Durkin MS, Davidson LL, Kuhn L, O'Connor P, Barlow B. 1994. Low-income neighborhoods and the risk of severe pediatric injury: a small-area analysis in northern Manhattan. *Am. J. Public Health* 84:587–92

23. Durkin MS, Olsen S, Barlow B, Virella A, Connolly ES Jr. 1998. The epidemiology of urban pediatric neurological trauma: evaluation of, and implications for, injury prevention programs. *Neurosurgery* 42:300–10

24. Fife D, Faich G, Hollinshead W, Boynton W. 1986. Incidence and outcome of hospital-treated head injury in Rhode Island. *Am. J. Public Health* 76:773–78

25. Girasek DC. 2001. Public beliefs about

the preventability of unintentional injury deaths. *Accid. Anal. Prev.* 33:455–65

26. Glik DC, Greaves PE, Kronenfeld JJ, Jackson KL. 1993. Safety hazards in households with young children. *J. Pediatr. Psychol.* 18:115–31

27. Gunnell DJ, Peters TJ, Kammerling RM, Brooks J. 1995. Relation between parasuicide, suicide, psychiatric admissions, and socioeconomic deprivation. *BMJ* 311: 226–30

28. Guyer B, Lescohier I, Gallagher SS, Hausman A, Azzara CV. 1989. Intentional injuries among children and adolescents in Massachusetts. *N. Engl. J. Med.* 321: 1584–89

29. Haddon W Jr. 1980. Options for the prevention of motor vehicle crash injury. *Isr. J. Med. Sci.* 16:45–65

30. Helmkamp JC, Bone CM. 1986. Hospitalizations for accidents and injuries in the US Navy: environmental and occupational factors. *J. Occup. Med.* 28:269–75

31. Hussey JM. 1997. The effects of race, socioeconomic status, and household structure on injury mortality in children and young adults. *Matern. Child Health J.* 1:217–27

32. Istre GR, McCoy MA, Osborn L, Barnard JJ, Bolton A. 2001. Deaths and injuries from house fires. *N. Engl. J. Med.* 344: 1911–16

33. Jolly DL, Moller JN, Volkmer RE. 1993. The socio-economic context of child injury in Australia. *J. Paediatr. Child Health.* 29:438–44

33a. Katz LF, Kling J, Liebman J. 2001. Moving to opportunity in Boston: early results of a randomized housing mobility study. *Q. J. Economics* (May):607–54

34. Kaufman JS, Cooper RS, McGee DL. 1997. Socioeconomic status and health in blacks and whites: the problem of residual confounding and the resiliency of race. *Epidemiology* 8:621–28

35. Kellermann AL, Rivara FP, Somes G, Reay DT, Francisco J, et al. 1992. Suicide

in the home in relation to gun ownership. *N. Engl. J. Med.* 327:467–72

36. Kelly S, Charlton J, Jenkins R. 1995. Suicide deaths in England and Wales, 1982–92: the contribution of occupation and geography. *Popul. Trends* 80:16–25

37. Kelly SM, Miles-Doan R. 1997. Social inequality and injuries: Do morbidity patterns differ from mortality? *Soc. Sci. Med.* 44:63–70

38. King WD, Palmisano PA. 1992. Racial differences in childhood hospitalized pedestrian injuries. *Pediatr. Emerg. Care.* 8:221–24

39. Klein D. 1980. Societal influences on childhood accidents. *Accid. Anal. Prev.* 12:275–81

40. Kogan MD, Overpeck MD, Fingerhut LA. 1995. Medically attended nonfatal injuries among preschool-age children: national estimates. *Am. J. Prev. Med.* 11:99–104

41. Kraus JF, Fife D, Ramstein K, Conroy C, Cox P. 1986. The relationship of family income to the incidence, external causes, and outcomes of serious brain injury, San Diego County, California. *Am. J. Public Health* 76:1345–47

42. Krieger N, Williams DR, Moss NE. 1997. Measuring social class in US public health research: concepts, methodologies, and guidelines. *Annu. Rev. Public Health* 18:341–78

43. Kyriacou DN, Hutson HR, Anglin D, Peek-Asa C, Kraus JF. 1999. The relationship between socioeconomic factors and gang violence in the City of Los Angeles. *J. Trauma* 46:334–39

43a. Laflamme L. 1998. *Social Inequality in Injury Risks: Knowledge Accumulated and Plans for the Future.* Sweden's Natl. Inst. Public Health

44. Laflamme L, Diderichsen F. 2000. Social differences in traffic injury risks in childhood and youth—a literature review and a research agenda. *Inj. Prev.* 6:293–98

45. Liberatos P, Link BG, Kelsey JL. 1988. The measurement of social class in epidemiology. *Epidemiol. Rev.* 10:87–121

46. Link BG, Phelan J. 1995. Social conditions as fundamental causes of disease. *J. Health Soc. Behav.* (Spec.):80–94

47. Locke JA, Rossignol AM, Burke JF. 1990. Socioeconomic factors and the incidence of hospitalized burn injuries in New England counties, USA. *Burns* 16:273–77

48. Loomis DP. 1991. Occupation, industry, and fatal motor vehicle crashes in 20 states, 1986–1987. *Am. J. Public Health* 81:733–35

48a. Ludwig J, Duncan GJ, Hirschfield P. 2002. Urban poverty and juvenile crime: Evidence from a randomized housing-mobility experiment. *Q. J. Economics.* In press

49. Mare RD. 1982. Socioeconomic effects on child mortality in the United States. *Am. J. Public Health* 72:539–47

49a. Marmot MG, Smith GD, Stansfeld S, Patel C, North F, et al. Health inequalities among British civil servants: the Whitehall study. *Lancet* 337:1387–93

50. Mayer M, LeClere FB. 1994. Injury prevention measures in households with children in the United States, 1990. *Adv. Data* 54:1–16

51. Mierley MC, Baker SP. 1983. Fatal house fires in an urban population. *JAMA* 249:1466–68

52. Nersesian WS, Petit MR, Shaper R, Lemieux D, Naor E. 1985. Childhood death and poverty: a study of all childhood deaths in Maine, 1976 to 1980. *Pediatrics* 75:41–50

53. O'Campo P, Rao RP, Gielen AC, Royalty W, Wilson M. 2000. Injury-producing events among children in low-income communities: the role of community characteristics. *J. Urban Health* 77:34–49

54. Pearce NE, Davis PB, Smith AH, Foster FH. 1983. Mortality and social class in New Zealand II: male mortality by major disease groupings. *NZ Med. J.* 96:711–16

55. Peterson RD, Krivo LJ. 1993. Racial segregation and black urban homicide. *Soc. Forces* 71:1001–26

56. Pickett KE, Pearl M. 2001. Multilevel analyses of neighbourhood socioeconomic context and health outcomes: a critical review. *J. Epidemiol. Commun. Health* 55:111–22

57. Pless IB, Peckham CS, Power C. 1989. Predicting traffic injuries in childhood: a cohort analysis. *J. Pediatr.* 115:932–38

58. Pless IB, Verreault R, Tenina S. 1989. A case-control study of pedestrian and bicyclist injuries in childhood. *Am. J. Public Health* 79:995–98

59. Reading R, Langford IH, Haynes R, Lovett A. 1999. Accidents to preschool children: comparing family and neighborhood risk factors. *Soc. Sci. Med.* 48:321–30

60. Reid SR, Roesler JS, Gaichas AM, Tsai AK. 2001. The epidemiology of pediatric traumatic brain injury in Minnesota. *Arch. Pediatr. Adol. Med.* 155:784–89

61. Reis AJ, Roth JA, eds. 1994. *Understanding and Preventing Violence*: Vol. 3. *Social Influences*. Washington, DC: Natl. Acad. Press

62. Rivara FP. 1995. Developmental and behavioral issues in childhood injury prevention. *J. Dev. Behav. Pediatr.* 16:362–70

63. Rivara FP, Barber M. 1985. Demographic analysis of childhood pedestrian injuries. *Pediatrics* 76:375–81

64. Robert SA. 1999. Socioeconomic position and health: the independent contribution of community socioeconomic context. *Annu. Rev. Sociol.* 25:489–516

65. Roberts I, Marshall R, Norton R, Borman B. 1992. An area analysis of child injury morbidity in Auckland. *J. Paediatr. Child Health.* 28:438–41

66. Scheidt PC, Harel Y, Trumble AC, Jones DH, Overpeck MD, Bijur PE. 1995. The epidemiology of nonfatal injuries among US children and youth. *Am. J. Public Health* 85:932–38

67. Shannon HS, Robson LS, Sale JEM. 2001. Creating safer and healthier workplaces: role of organizational factors and job characteristics. *Am. J. Ind. Med.* 40:319–34

68. Singh GK, Yu SM. 1996. US childhood

mortality, 1950 through 1993: trends and socioeconomic differentials. *Am. J. Public Health* 86:505–12

69. Singh GK, Yu SM. 1996. Trends and differentials in adolescent and young adult mortality in the United States, 1950 through 1993. *Am. J. Public Health* 86:560–64

70. Soobader M, LeClere FB, Hadden W, Maury B. 2001. Using aggregate geographic data to proxy individual socioeconomic status: does size matter? *Am. J. Public Health* 91:632–36

71. Sorenson SB, Upchurch DM, Shen H. 1996. Violence and injury in marital arguments: risk patterns and gender differences. *Am. J. Public Health* 86:35–40

72. Susser M, Susser E. 1996. Choosing a future for epidemiology: II. From black box to Chinese boxes and eco-epidemiology. *Am. J. Public Health* 86:674–77

73. Wagener DK, Winn DW. 1991. Injuries in working populations: black-white differences. *Am. J. Public Health* 81:1408–14

74. Whitley E, Gunnell D, Dorling D, Smith GD. 1999. Ecological study of social fragmentation, poverty, and suicide. *BMJ* 319:1034–37

75. Williams DR, Collins C. 1995. US socioeconomic and racial differences in health: patterns and explanations. *Annu. Rev. Sociol.* 21:349–86

76. Wise PH, Kotelchuck M, Wilson ML, Mills M. 1985. Racial and socioeconomic disparities in childhood mortality in Boston. *N. Engl. J. Med.* 313:360–66

77. Yen IH, Syme SL. 1999. The social environment and health: a discussion of the epidemiologic literature. *Annu. Rev. Public Health* 20:287–308

Annu. Rev. Public Health 2002. 23:377–401

THINKING OUTSIDE THE BOX: Recent Advances in the Analysis and Presentation of Uncertainty in Cost-Effectiveness Studies

Andrew H. Briggs,[1] Bernie J. O'Brien,[2,3] and Gordon Blackhouse[2,3]

[1]Health Economics Research Centre, Department of Public Health, University of Oxford, Oxford OX3 7LF, United Kingdom; e-mail: andrew.briggs@ihs.ox.ac.uk; [2]Centre for Evaluation of Medicines, St. Joseph's Hospital, Hamilton, Ontario L8N 4A6, Canada; and [3]Department of Clinical Epidemiology and Biostatistics, McMaster University, Hamilton L8N 3Z5, Ontario, Canada

Key Words health economics, confidence intervals, net-benefit, power & sample size, acceptability curves

■ **Abstract** As many more clinical trials collect economic information within their study design, so health economics analysts are increasingly working with patient-level data on both costs and effects. In this paper, we review recent advances in the use of statistical methods for economic analysis of information collected alongside clinical trials. In particular, we focus on the handling and presentation of uncertainty, including the importance of estimation rather than hypothesis testing, the use of the net-benefit statistic, and the presentation of cost-effectiveness acceptability curves. We also discuss the appropriate sample size calculations for cost-effectiveness analysis at the design stage of a study. Finally, we outline some of the challenges for future research in this area—particularly in relation to the appropriate use of Bayesian methods and methods for analyzing costs that are typically skewed and often incomplete.

INTRODUCTION

The past decade has seen a rapid increase in the use of clinical trials as a vehicle for collecting economic information and estimating the cost-effectiveness of interventions (43). The existence of patient-level information on both costs and effects from clinical trials has generated interest in statistical methods for cost-effectiveness analysis, with a key focus on the quantification and presentation of uncertainty. This paper reviews recent developments and provides an overview of the state-of-the-art of quantitative methods for cost-effectiveness analysis.

A key structural feature of the paper is the use of a common example to illustrate the various methodological issues and techniques that are discussed. We

0163-7525/02/0510-0377$14.00

have chosen to use our own work on the cost-effectiveness of the implantable cardioverter defibrillator (ICD) versus drug therapy for patients at high risk of sudden cardiac death. This study was chosen for two reasons: First, it illustrates many of the challenging analytical aspects of contemporary trial-based cost-effectiveness analysis, and second, we have the data! A brief summary of the published cost-effectiveness analysis (36) is presented in Box 1. A further published analysis of cost-effectiveness by risk strata (47) is summarized in Box 2.

Box 1

Example: Cost-effectiveness of the implantable cardioverter defibrillator*

Background: In the Canadian Implantable Defibrillator Study (CIDS) we assessed the cost-effectiveness of the implantable cardioverter defibrillator (ICD) in reducing the risk of death in survivors of previous ventricular tachycardia (VT) or fibrillation (VF).

Methods: Health care resource use was collected prospectively on the first 430 patients enrolled in CIDS (n = 212 ICD, n = 218 amiodarone). Mean cost per patient, adjusted for censoring, was computed for each group based on initial therapy assignment. Incremental cost-effectiveness of ICD therapy was computed as the ratio of the difference (ICD–amiodarone) in cost to the difference in life expectancy (both discounted at 3% per year). All costs are in 1999 Canadian dollars; C\$1 ≈ US \$0.65.

Results: Over 6.3 years, mean cost per patient in the ICD group was C\$87,715 versus C\$38,600 in the amiodarone group (difference C\$49,115; 95% CI C\$41,597 to C\$56,593). Life expectancy for the ICD group was 4.58 years versus 4.35 years for amiodarone (difference 0.23, 95% CI −0.12 to 0.57), for incremental cost-effectiveness of ICD therapy of C\$213,543 per life-year gained.

Box 2

Example: Effect of clinical risk stratification on cost-effectiveness of the implantable cardioverter-defibrillator. The Canadian Implantable Defibrillator Study**

Background: Three randomized clinical trials showed that implantable cardioverter-defibrillators (ICDs) reduce the risk of death in survivors of ventricular tachyarrhythmias, but the cost per year of life gained is high. A substudy of the Canadian Implantable Defibrillator Study (CIDS) showed that 3 clinical factors, age ≥70 years, left ventricular ejection fraction ≤35%, and New York Heart Association class III, predicted the risk of death and benefit from the ICD. We estimated the extent to which selecting patients for ICD therapy based on these risk factors makes ICD therapy more economically attractive.

Methods: Patients in CIDS were grouped according to whether they had 2 or more of 3 risk factors. Incremental cost-effectiveness of ICD therapy was computed as the ratio of the difference in mean cost to the difference in life expectancy between the 2 groups.

---

*Source: Abridged abstract from Reference (36).
**Source: Abridged abstract from Reference (47).

Results: Over 6.3 years, the mean cost per patient in the ICD group was Canadian (C) \$87,715 versus \$38,600 in the amiodarone group (C\$1 ≈ US\$0.67). Life expectancy for the ICD group was 4.58 years versus 4.35 years for amiodarone, for an incremental cost-effectiveness of ICD therapy of C\$213,543 per life-year gained. The cost per life-year gained inpatients with ≥2 factors was C\$65,195, compared with C\$916,659 with <2 risk factors.

We begin by introducing the "cost-effectiveness (CE) plane" as a device for presenting and relating the two central parameters of interest in economic evaluation: the difference (treatment minus control) in effectiveness (ΔE) and the difference in cost (ΔC). We show how the CE plane is useful for presenting uncertainty in the location of these two parameters and also uncertainty in the ratio between them, $\Delta C / \Delta E$, known as the incremental cost-effectiveness ratio (ICER). Using the CE plane, we review methods for estimating and presenting the uncertainty that can arise in cost-effectiveness results. Although much research has focused on methods for calculating confidence intervals for cost-effectiveness ratios, this calculation can be problematic with ratio-based statistics. Instead, we advocate plotting the joint density of cost and effect differences on the cost-effectiveness plane, together with cumulative density plots over the cost-effectiveness surface known as cost-effectiveness acceptability curves to summarize the overall value for money of interventions. We also outline the net-benefit formulation of the cost-effectiveness problem and show that it has particular advantages over the standard incremental cost-effectiveness ratio formulation. In the final section of the paper we consider some areas of continuing development of statistical methods for cost-effectiveness analysis such as the use of a Bayesian interpretation of probability, arguing that this is most natural given the decision-making context of cost-effectiveness analysis.

THE COST-EFFECTIVENESS PLANE

In Figure 1 we illustrate the cost-effectiveness (CE) plane, due originally to Black (4). The CE plane is a two-dimensional space with the x-axis being the average difference (treatment minus control) in effectiveness (ΔE) per patient and the y-axis being the average difference in cost (ΔC) per patient. Although costs are in money units such as dollars, the effectiveness units are typically health outcomes such as life-years gained or quality-adjusted life-years (18). In principle, the axes are unbounded from positive to negative infinity, and the origin represents the control group because scales are in difference form. To minimize confusion, we label the four quadrants using the points of the compass.

If we consider the ideal circumstance of knowing our (x, y) coordinates on the CE plane for sure, with no uncertainty, then a number of eventualities can arise. For example, treatment is said to "dominate" control, being less costly and more effective if the (x, y) coordinates are located in the SE quadrant and the

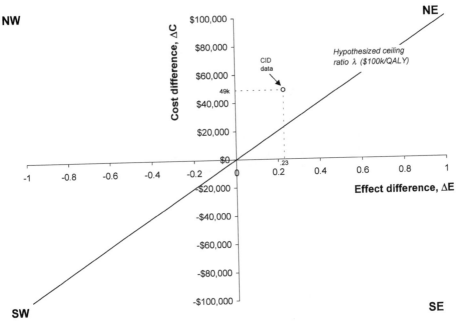

Figure 1 Incremental cost-effectiveness plane showing four quadrants, line representing the ceiling ratio for decision making and the location of the point estimate of incremental costs and effects for the CIDS data example.

mirror image—control dominates treatment—in the NW quadrant. In these two circumstances, the efficiency-based decision to adopt the new therapy or not is self-evident. But most new therapies locate in the NE quadrant where increased effectiveness is achieved at increased cost. In this situation, the decision to adopt the new therapy will depend on where the (x, y) coordinates fall in the NE quadrant and whether this point lies below the acceptable "ceiling ratio" of the decision-maker. As illustrated by the ray extending from the origin, the assumption is that the dollar amount that the decision-maker is willing to pay for a unit of effectiveness is known (call this λ). If the incremental cost-effectiveness ratio (ICER) of the new therapy ($\Delta C / \Delta E$), i.e., the slope of a straight line from the origin that passes through the (ΔE, ΔC) coordinate, is less than the decision-maker's willingness to pay (λ), then the treatment should be adopted.

Using our example, if we assume, for the moment, that our ICD data (Box 1) had no uncertainty, then the true cost difference per patient would be C\$49,100 and the true increase in survival would be 0.23 years for an ICER of C\$214,000 per life-year gained. If we assume that the maximum that society is willing to pay for a year of life is C\$100,000, then ICD therapy should not be adopted. This is shown graphically in Figure 1 by the point estimate of cost-effectiveness falling above and to the left of the line with slope λ = C\$100,000. Of course, the problem is that all the parameters are uncertain, including the amount society is willing to pay for a unit of effect.

ESTIMATION OR HYPOTHESIS TESTING?

In practice, we have only estimates of the cost and effect differences, and it is important that uncertainty in those estimates is also presented. It is straightforward to calculate confidence intervals for each of the cost and effect differences, ΔC and ΔE, using standard methods, and these intervals can also be plotted on the cost-effectiveness plane (38). For example, in the CIDS trial, the 95% confidence intervals for ΔC are (C$41,600 to C$56,600) and for ΔE are (-0.12 to 0.57). These results are represented on the cost-effectiveness plane in Figure 2, which, in addition to a point estimate of the cost and effect difference of ICD therapy, also shows I-bars representing the confidence intervals around those estimates. The horizontal I-bar represents the confidence interval for the effect difference, and the vertical I-bar represents the confidence interval for the cost difference.

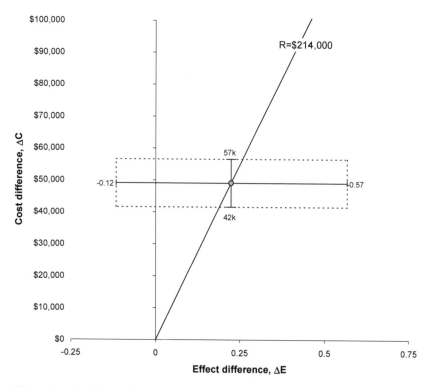

Figure 2 Confidence limits and the confidence box on the cost-effectiveness plane for the ICD data example.

Both have the point estimate of the cost and effect differences at their center and together the intervals define a box on the cost-effectiveness plane. Of note with our ICD example is that the box "straddles" the y-axis but lies completely above the x-axis, reflecting the fact that the difference in survival in the CIDS trial was not significant (p > 0.05) but that the difference in cost was significant (p < 0.05).

Our example in Figure 2 is just one situation that can arise when analyzing the results of an economic analysis conducted alongside a clinical trial with respect to the significance or otherwise of the cost and effect differences. In fact, there are nine possible situations that could arise, and these are illustrated on the cost-effectiveness plane in Figure 3 with multiple "confidence boxes."

In situations 1 and 2, one intervention has been shown to be significantly more effective and significantly cheaper than the other and is therefore clearly the treatment of choice—the new treatment is preferred in the SE quadrant (situation 1) and the control treatment in the NW quadrant (situation 2). In situations 7 and 8, we have one treatment shown to be significantly more costly, but also significantly more effective. It is in these situations that it is clearly appropriate to estimate an ICER and where much research effort has been employed to ascertain the most appropriate method for estimating the ICER confidence interval.

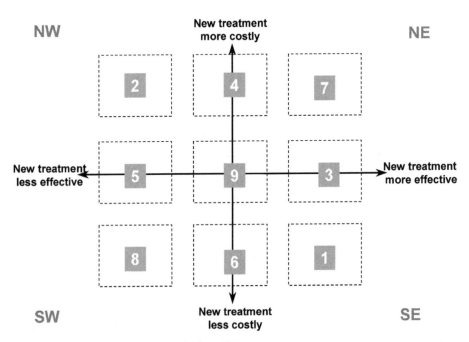

Figure 3   Nine possible situations that can arise concerning the significance (or otherwise) of cost and effect differences illustrated on the cost-effectiveness plane. Boxes indicate the area bounded by the individual confidence limits on cost and effect: statistically significant differences are indicated where the box does not straddle the relevant axis.

A potential problem arises in the situations where either the cost difference (situations 3 and 5) or the effect difference (situations 4 and 6) is not statistically significant. (Note that our ICD example falls into situation 4.) It is common to find analysts in these situations adapting the decision rule to focus only on the dimension where a difference has been shown. For example, it might be tempting in situation 4, our ICD example, to assume that ICD and amiodarone have the same life expectancy and only compare them in terms of cost. This form of analysis, known as cost-minimization analysis, uses the logic that among outcome-equivalent options one should choose the less costly option.

As we have argued elsewhere (10), the problem with this simple approach to decision making in situations where either cost or effect is not statistically significant is that it is based on simple and sequential tests of hypotheses. But the deficiencies of hypothesis testing (in contrast to estimation) are well known and gave rise to the memorable adage, "absence of evidence is not evidence of absence" (2). The concern is that a focus on hypothesis testing leads to an overemphasis on type I errors (the rejection of the null hypothesis of no difference when there is in fact no difference) at the expense of type II errors (the failure to reject the null hypothesis of no difference when in fact a difference does exist). In a review of clinical evaluations, Freiman and colleagues (24) showed how a substantial proportion of studies reporting "negative" results had insufficient power to detect quite important differences in treatment effect. Consistent with these recent debates in the clinical evaluation literature, the goal of economic evaluation should be the estimation of a parameter—incremental cost-effectiveness—with appropriate representation of uncertainty, rather than hypothesis testing.

ESTIMATING UNCERTAINTY: THINKING OUTSIDE THE BOX

The point estimates (means) from the effect and cost distributions provide the best estimate of the treatment and cost effects and should be used in the primary analysis. While confidence intervals for cost-effectiveness ratios are a valid approach to addressing uncertainty in cost-effectiveness analysis for situations 7 and 8, problems arise when uncertainty is such that the ICER could be negative (48). However, these problems can be overcome through either the appropriate representation of uncertainty on the cost-effectiveness plane (6, 51), or the use of the net-benefit statistic that represents a new framework for handling uncertainty in CEA and which does not suffer from the problems associated with the ICER in situations where negative ratios arise (49). In this section we review each of these issues in turn to emphasize how analysts should be estimating and presenting uncertainty in the results of their analyses in the potential situations outlined above.

Confidence Limits for Cost-Effectiveness Ratios

With patient-level information on the costs and effects of treatment interventions, it is natural to consider representing uncertainty in the ICER using confidence intervals. However, as a ratio statistic, the solution to confidence-interval estimation is not straightforward.

The intuition behind this problem is that where there is nonnegligible probability that the denominator of the ratio could take a zero value, the ICER becomes unstable since for a zero denominator the ICER would be infinite. For a positive cost difference (the numerator of the ICER) as the effect difference approaches zero from the positive direction, the ICER tends to positive infinity. As the effect difference approaches zero from the negative direction, the ICER tends to negative infinity. For negative cost differences the ICER signs are reversed. This discontinuity about the zero effect difference causes statistical problems for estimating confidence limits; for example, there is no mathematically tractable formula for the variance of the statistic. Even where the effect difference is significantly different from zero, it would be inappropriate to assume that the ICER's sampling distribution followed a normal distribution.

There have been many proposed solutions to the problem of estimating confidence limits for the ICER, many of which were simply approximations that could perform rather poorly in some situations. However, a general consensus has emerged in support of two main approaches: the parametric method introduced by Fieller (23) half a century ago and the nonparametric approach of bootstrapping (19), both of which have been described in relation to cost-effectiveness analysis (9, 11, 14, 40, 42, 46, 53). We now illustrate each approach in turn, employing the example data from the CIDS trial (Box 1).

FIELLER'S THEOREM CONFIDENCE INTERVALS   In Fieller's approach, it is assumed that the cost and effect differences (represented by ΔC and ΔE, respectively) follow a joint normal distribution. The standard cost-effectiveness ratio calculation of $R = \Delta C / \Delta E$ can be expressed as $R \Delta E - \Delta C = 0$, with known variance $R^2 \operatorname{var}(\Delta E) + \operatorname{var}(\Delta C) - 2R \operatorname{cov}(\Delta E, \Delta C)$. Therefore, we can generate a standard normally distributed variable by dividing the reformulated expression through by its standard error:

$$\frac{R \Delta E - \Delta C}{\sqrt{R^2 \operatorname{var}(\Delta E) + \operatorname{var}(\Delta C) - 2R \operatorname{cov}(\Delta E, \Delta C)}} \sim N(0, 1).$$

Setting this expression equal to the critical point from the standard normal distribution, $z_{\alpha/2}$ for a $(1 - \alpha)$ 100% confidence interval, yields the following quadratic equation in R:

$$R^2 \left[\Delta E^2 - z_{\alpha/2}^2 \operatorname{var}(\Delta E) \right] - 2R \left[\Delta E \cdot \Delta C - z_{\alpha/2}^2 \operatorname{cov}(\Delta E, \Delta C) \right]$$
$$+ \left[\Delta C^2 - z_{\alpha/2}^2 \operatorname{var}(\Delta C) \right] = 0.$$

The roots of this equation give the Fieller confidence limits for the ICER, R. These roots are reproduced in the appendix; while apparently complicated, recall that in order to calculate the roots, only five pieces of information are required: the estimated effect difference, the estimated cost difference, their respective variances

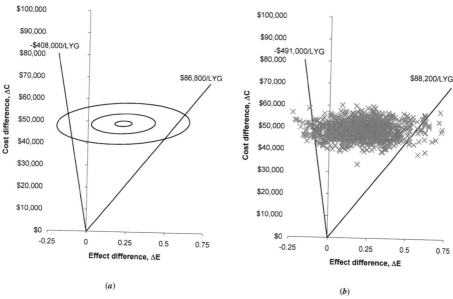

Figure 4   Fieller's theorem (*a*) and bootstrap (*b*) confidence limits on the CE plane for the ICD data example.

and the covariance between them. Figure 4*a* shows the assumption of joint normality on the cost-effectiveness plane for the ICD data of Box 1 by plotting ellipses of equal probability covering 5%, 50%, and 95% of the integrated joint density. Also plotted are the estimated confidence limits using Fieller's theorem (C$86,800 to C$-408,000), represented by the slopes of the lines on the plane passing through the origin. Note that the "wedge" defined by the Fieller confidence limits falls inside the 95% ellipse—taking tangents to the 95% ellipse, as was suggested in an early paper as a possible method for approximating the interval (51), would overestimate the width of the interval since the wedge area covers not only the 95% of the joint density covered by the ellipse but also areas above and below the 95% ellipse. By contrast, Fieller's approach automatically adjusts to ensure that 95% of the integrated joint density falls within the wedge, which makes Fieller's approach an exact method (subject to the parametric assumption of joint normality of costs and effects holding).

BOOTSTRAP CONFIDENCE INTERVALS   The approach of nonparametric bootstrapping has been gaining in popularity with the advent of powerful desktop computing. It is a resampling procedure that employs raw computing power to estimate an empirical sampling distribution for the statistic of interest rather than relying on parametric assumptions. Bootstrap samples of the same size as the original data are drawn with replacement from the original sample and the statistic of interest is calculated. Repeating this process a large number of times generates a vector of

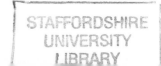

bootstrap replicates of the statistic of interest, which is the empirical estimate of that statistics' sampling distribution.

In terms of the cost-effectiveness application, the approach involves a three-step procedure:

1. Sample with replacement n_C cost/effect pairs from the patients in the control group (where n_C is the number of observed patients in the control group) and calculate the mean cost and effect in this bootstrap resample.

2. Sample with replacement n_T cost/effect pairs from the patients in the treatment group (where n_T is the number of observed patients in the treatment group) and calculate the mean cost and effect in this bootstrap resample.

3. Using the bootstrapped means from the steps above, calculate the difference in effect between the groups, the difference in cost between the two groups, and an estimate of the incremental cost-effectiveness.

This three-step procedure provides one bootstrap replication of the statistic of interest; repeating this process a large number of times (at least 1000 times is recommended for confidence interval calculation) generates the empirical distribution of cost-effectiveness.

Each of 1000 bootstrapped effect and cost differences from step 3 above are plotted on the cost-effectiveness plane in Figure 4b for the ICD data example. Confidence limits can be obtained by selecting the 26th and 975th of the 1000 replicates [which excludes 25 (or 2.5%) of observations from either end of the empirical distribution]; this effectively ensures that 95% of the estimated joint density falls within the wedge on the cost-effectiveness plane defined by the confidence limits. As is clearly apparent from Figure 4b, the bootstrap estimate of the joint density and the bootstrap confidence limits (C\$88,200 to C\$−491,000) are very similar to those generated by Fieller's theorem. This suggests that for this particular example, the assumption of joint normality for the cost and effect differences is reasonable. The Fieller limits are therefore preferred in this case for two main reasons: (a) Parametric methods are commonly more powerful than their nonparametric counterparts when the parametric assumptions hold; and (b) Fieller's approach always generates the same result; two analysts both employing the bootstrap method with the same data will generate slightly different results due to the play of chance.

Beyond the Confidence Interval: Acceptability Curves

Although commentators are now largely agreed on the most appropriate methods for ICER confidence interval estimation, such intervals are not appropriate in all the nine situations outlined above. One important problem concerns negative ratios. In the NW and SE quadrants, the ICER is negative and its magnitude conveys no useful meaning. The problem is that in the positive quadrants low ICERs are preferred to high ICERs (from the point of view of the more costly more effective treatment). However, no such simple arrangement exists in the negative quadrants. Consider the three following points in the SE quadrant: A (1LY, −$2000); B (2LYs, −$2000); C (2LYs, −$1000); giving negative ICERs of −$2000/LY, −$1000/LY and −$500/LY, respectively. Therefore, in terms of magnitude, A has the lowest ICER, with C the highest and B between the two. However, it should be clear that B is preferred to both A and C as it has the highest number of life years saved and the greatest cost-saving. Furthermore, negative ICERs in the NW quadrant of the plane (favoring the existing treatment) are qualitatively different from negative ICERs in the SE quadrant (favoring the new treatment) yet will be grouped together in any naïve rank-ordering exercise (note the treatment of negative ratios in the bootstrapping of the ICD data above; since the negative ratios were in the NE quadrant they were ranked above the highest positive ratios to give a negative upper limit to the ratio).

A solution to this problem can be found by returning to the original decision rule introduced above. If the estimated ICER lies below some ceiling ratio, λ, reflecting the maximum that decision-makers are willing to invest to achieve a unit of effectiveness, then it should be implemented. Therefore, in terms of the bootstrap replications on the cost-effectiveness plane in Figure 4b, we could summarize uncertainty by considering what proportion of the bootstrap replications fall below and to the right of a line with slope equal to λ, lending support to the cost-effectiveness of the intervention. Of course, the appropriate value of λ is itself unknown. However, it can be varied to show how the evidence in favor of cost-effectiveness of the intervention varies with λ. In terms of the bootstrap method, we would simply plot the proportion of bootstrap replications falling on the cost-effective side of the line as λ is varied across its full range from 0 through to ∞. Alternatively, if we are happy with an assumption of joint normality in the distribution of costs and effects, we can consider the proportion of the parametric joint density that falls on the cost-effective surface of the CE plane. We employ this parametric approach and the resulting curve for the ICD example based on the joint normal assumption shown in Figure 4a is presented in Figure 5 and has been termed a cost-effectiveness acceptability curve (51), as it directly summarizes the evidence in support of the intervention being cost-effective for all potential values of the decision rule.

This acceptability curve presents much more information on uncertainty than do confidence intervals. The curve cuts the vertical axis at the p-value (one-sided) for the cost difference (which is p < 0.0001 in our ICD example) since a value of zero for λ implies that only the cost is important in the cost-effectiveness calculation. The curve is tending toward 1 minus the p-value for the effect difference (which in the ICD example is p = 0.10), since an infinite value for λ implies that effect only is important in the cost-effectiveness calculation. The median value (p = 0.5) corresponds to the base-case ICER, which is C$214,000 in our example.

As well as summarizing, for every value of λ, the evidence in favor of the intervention being cost-effective, acceptability curves can also be employed to obtain a confidence interval on cost-effectiveness. For the ICD example, the 95% upper bound is not defined and the 95% lower bound is equal to C$86,800.

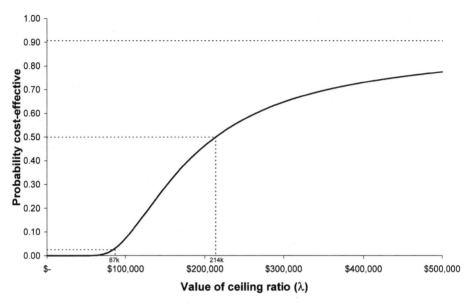

Figure 5 Parametric cost-effectiveness acceptability curve for the ICD data example (assuming joint normality of cost and effect differences).

Acceptability Curves and Stratified Cost-Effectiveness

In addition to the presentation of precision around parameter estimates such as cost-effectiveness, it is important to understand heterogeneity in data. For most (if not all) medical technologies there is variability in response to therapy, and this can often be systematic, identifying subgroups of patients where the treatment effect is larger or smaller. Although the standard cautions regarding the "trawling" for subgroups apply (17, 41), such information is important for presenting cost-effectiveness data to decision-makers. Selective use of therapies in patients where it is more effective and cost-effective requires the analyst to present the decision-maker with data showing both precision and heterogeneity.

The cost-effectiveness acceptability curve is a convenient method for presenting stratified analyses. Consider the ICD example again, based on the summary presented in Box 2 where clinical risk stratification by age (≥70 years), left ventricular ejection fraction (≤35%), and New York Heart Association class (III) indicated patients who were likely to have a higher mortality benefit. In Figure 6a, we show how the presence of 0 through to 3 risk factors impacts on the point estimates of cost-effectiveness, with the cost-effectiveness of treatment being more favorable in persons with more risk factors (i.e., higher prior probability of death). In Figure 6b, the acceptability curves for the same groups are presented so the decision-maker can determine the probability of ICD therapy being cost-effective among subgroups and conditional upon the value of a life-year (λ).

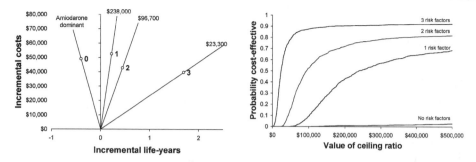

Figure 6   Risk stratified CEA for the ICD data example: (*a*) basecase results on the CE plane, (*b*) risk stratified acceptability curves.

The Net-Benefit Framework

Relatively recently, a number of researchers have employed a simple rearrangement of the cost-effectiveness decision rule to overcome the problems associated with ICERs (15, 16, 49, 50). In particular, Stinnett & Mullahy (49) offer a comprehensive account of the net-benefit framework and make a convincing case for employing the net-benefit statistic to handle uncertainty in stochastic cost-effectiveness analysis. The standard cost-effectiveness decision rule, to implement a new treatment only if $\Delta C/\Delta E < \lambda$, can be rearranged to give two alternative inequalities on either the cost scale (15, 16, 50) or on the effect scale (49). For simplicity, we focus on the cost scale of Net Monetary Benefit (NMB):

$$NMB = \lambda \cdot \Delta E - \Delta C.$$

The advantage of formulating the cost-effectiveness decision rule in this way is that, by using the value of λ to turn the decision rule into a linear expression, the variance for the net-benefit statistics is tractable and the sampling distribution is much better behaved (in that with sufficient sample size net-benefits are normally distributed). The variance expression for net-benefit on the cost scale is given by

$$\text{var}(NMB) = \lambda^2 \cdot \text{var}(\Delta E) + \text{var}(\Delta C) - 2\lambda \cdot \text{cov}(\Delta E, \Delta C).$$

Since the net-benefit statistic relies on the value of the ceiling ratio λ to avoid the problems of ratios statistics when in fact the value of the ceiling ratio is unknown, the net-benefit can be plotted as a function of λ. Figure 7 shows this for the net monetary benefit formulation of net-benefits and includes the 95% confidence intervals on net-benefits using the formula for the variance given above and assuming a normal distribution. The net-benefit curve crosses the horizontal axis at the point estimate of cost-effectiveness of the intervention, which is C$214,000 in our ICD example. Where the confidence limits on net-benefits cross the axis gives the confidence interval on cost-effectiveness. We see from the figure that while

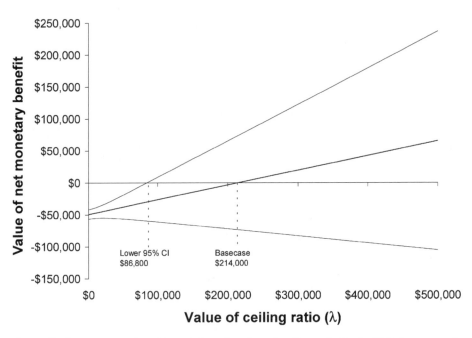

Figure 7   Net monetary benefit statistic as function of ceiling ratio for the ICD data example including 95% CI on net monetary benefit. Where the net benefit curves intersect with the NMB = 0 axis defines the point estimate and 95% confidence interval on cost-effectiveness. Note that the upper 95% limit on cost-effectiveness is not defined in this example.

the lower limit of cost-effectiveness is $86,800, the upper 95% limit of net-benefit does not cross the axis, which indicates that the upper limit on cost-effectiveness is not defined. This is precisely the same result obtained from the analysis of the acceptability curve in Figure 5. Indeed, the net-benefit statistic provides a straight-forward method to estimate the acceptability curve. Each point of the acceptability curve can be calculated from the p-value on the net-benefit being positive. Note that an acceptability curve calculated in this way gives the exact same acceptability curve as the analysis on the CE plane suggested by van Hout and colleagues (51), based on the joint normal distribution of cost and effect differences.

There is much common ground between the net-benefit method and Fieller's theorem. Indeed, the formal equivalence of the confidence limits described from the net-benefit method and from Fieller's theorem (and by extension the limits obtained from the acceptability curve above) have recently been demonstrated (26). Although Fieller's method fails to produce confidence limits for the ICER in some situations at a specified level of alpha, the type I error rate, this reflects a problem not of the method itself, but of the level of uncertainty. While such an interval can be defined for net benefit, that interval, by definition, will include zero at the specified level of confidence.

Since confidence intervals for cost-effectiveness ratios are not always defined, we strongly recommend that analysts plot their results on the cost-effectiveness plane, using either bootstrap replications or ellipses under the assumption of joint normality (see Figure 4a,b). This gives a visual representation of the joint uncertainty that is straightforward to interpret. Further summary can be obtained through the acceptability or net-benefit frameworks. Our own preference is the use of acceptability curves since these curves directly address the question of the study: How likely is it that the new intervention is cost-effective?

Power and Sample Size Calculations for Cost-Effectiveness

Up to this point we have been considering the analysis of cost and effect information generated alongside clinical trials, and we have recommended the reporting of estimated uncertainty in cost-effectiveness results rather than tests of hypothesis due to a concern of low power. These concerns are exacerbated by the fact that cost data are generally considered to have higher variance than effect data and that health economists are rarely invited to contribute to the power calculations at the design stage of a clinical trial. On the rare occasions that economists have been involved, it has tended to be the case that calculations are undertaken on costs and effects separately. However, if the purpose of economic evaluation is to make inference about cost-effectiveness then sample size and power calculations should be directly related to this cost-effectiveness result.

A number of authors have suggested the idea of basing power calculations on the methods used for approximating confidence intervals for cost-effectiveness ratios (7, 45), including the use of simulation techniques (1). However, the introduction of the net-benefit statistic has simplified matters considerably. Sample size calculations can now be derived for cost-effectiveness following exactly the same procedure used for mean effectiveness.

Note that an observed net benefit is significantly positive providing

$$NMB - z_{\alpha/2}\sqrt{\text{var}(NMB)} > 0,$$

where var(NMB) is as given above. Although it is tempting to base the sample size calculation on the numbers of patients required to show an observed difference as significant, in fact sample size calculations should be based on the hypothesized cost and effect differences (denoted $\Delta \tilde{E}$, $\Delta \tilde{C}$, generating a hypothesized net monetary benefit $N\tilde{M}B$) such that the study has the appropriate power to detect the hypothesized net-benefit as different from zero. In algebraic terms:

$$N\tilde{M}B - z_{\beta}\sqrt{\text{var}(N\tilde{M}B)} > z_{\alpha/2}\sqrt{\text{var}(N\tilde{M}B)},$$

where z_{β} is the critical value from the standard normal distribution corresponding to a required power of $1 - \beta$, and the variance expressions for net-benefit are as given above, but based on the hypothesized variance in cost, effect, and their covariance.

Substituting the sample variance calculations into the inequality above allows a straightforward (if rather extensive) rearrangement of the expression to give the sample size requirement (see the derivation given in the appendix). Note that as well as the hypothesized cost and effect differences, their associated variances, and covariance, the sample size also depends on the power and significance levels as well as the ceiling ratio λ. Assuming power and significance are fixed by convention, the sample size calculation can be presented as a function of the remaining unknown value λ; however, at the design stage a single value must be chosen to give the final number of patients to be recruited.

As an example, consider the risk stratification analysis of the CIDS data example as a hypothesis-generating exercise that leads us to suppose that although implantable defibrillators do not seem good value overall, they may be cost-effective for patients with all three of the risk factors specified above. Further suppose that we now wish to design a cost-effectiveness trial to test this hypothesis and we are prepared to use the observed data from the CIDS study as the basis for the sample size calculations for the new study. Figure 8 shows the sample size requirements for such a study for different levels of power to detect a cost-effectiveness ratio significantly below the ceiling ratio at the 5% level as a function of the ceiling ratio. At conventional levels of power and significance (90% and 5%, respectively), we

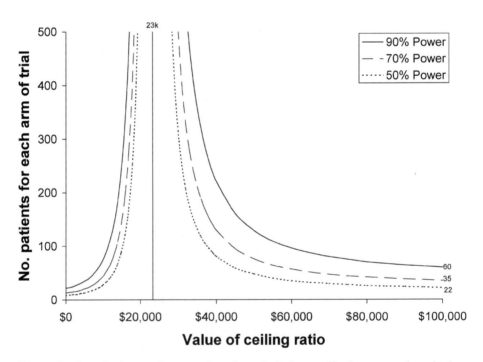

Figure 8 Sample size requirements for a hypothetical cost-effectiveness study to look at the cost-effectiveness of ICDs in patients with three risk factors.

would have to recruit 60 patients with all three risk factors to each arm of the trial, assuming a ceiling ratio of C$100,000 per LYG.

Alternatively, the information in Figure 8 can be used to determine the power of a cost-effectiveness of known study size to show cost-effectiveness significantly below a given ceiling ratio. Note the discontinuity of the figure around the hypothesized point estimate of C$23,300; this occurs when the ceiling ratio used by decision-makers corresponds to the true cost-effectiveness result. In this case then, no study, however large, will be able to show a significant difference. The implications of this are that where interventions are only marginally cost-effective, it is likely to prove very costly to run trials to demonstrate conclusive proof of cost-effectiveness.

FURTHER ISSUES AND FUTURE DIRECTIONS

Statistical methods for economic evaluations running alongside clinical trials is in a state of evolution, and we are likely to see many developments and refinements of the methods in the coming years. We begin by considering the use of Bayesian methods given the decision-making basis of economic evaluation research. We then go on to consider the nature and distribution of cost data and issues relating to their completeness that present particular statistical challenges.

On Being Bayesian with Probability

Although a strict frequentist interpretation of cost-effectiveness acceptability curves is possible through the consideration of the p-value on net benefits (32), the natural way to interpret these curves is as the probability that the intervention is cost-effective. Indeed, this is the way cost-effectiveness acceptability curves have been presented in the literature to date (44, 51). It has also been argued that the widespread mistaken interpretation of traditional p-values by researchers as a probability that the null hypothesis is false may be due to the fact that researchers want to make probability statements about the null hypothesis in this way (5). A number of commentators have stressed that such a view of probability in cost-effectiveness analysis is only possible in a Bayesian framework (27, 33, 39).

Fundamentally, the Bayesian approach includes a learning process whereby beliefs concerning the distributions of parameters (prior distributions) are updated (to posterior distributions), as information becomes available, through the use of Bayes' Theorem. Historically, advocates of the Bayesian approach were seen to inhabit a different scientific paradigm that was at odds with the frequentist paradigm: Frequentists considered Bayes methods as subjective and highly dependent on the prior beliefs employed, whereas frequentist methods were objective and robust. However, the adoption of such an extreme position would be to reject a set of very powerful methods that may be of import, even for frequentists (13). The empirical Bayes methods and Bayesian analysis based on uninformative prior distributions are not subjective and have much to offer the frequentist analyst. Acceptability curves based on observed data, such as those presented in Figures 5 & 6, can be given the Bayesian interpretation assuming an uninformative prior distribution (8). Of course, if there is good prior information available on the cost-effectiveness of an intervention, then analysts may want to use this to formulate the prior in a Bayesian analysis.

At present, and most likely in the immediate future, health economists conducting economic analyses alongside clinical trials will have to work within the sample size constraints imposed by clinical investigators. This is likely to generate the situation where important economic differences cannot be detected at conventional levels of power and significance. A number of commentators have suggested that it may be appropriate for economic analysts to work with "error rates" (in the frequentist sense) that are higher than those employed in clinical evaluation (18, 37). This suggestion indicates the desire of economic analysts to consider the weight of evidence relating to the cost-effectiveness of the intervention under evaluation rather than relying on showing significance at conventional levels. This is most easily achieved through the use of cost-effectiveness acceptability curves, which show the weight of evidence for the intervention being cost-effective for all possible values of the ceiling ratio, λ. Furthermore, a Bayesian view of probability allows analysts to directly address the study question: How likely is it that the intervention is cost-effective?

Work is currently ongoing to reanalyze the cost-effectiveness analysis of the ICD data in a Bayesian framework.

Costing Challenges in Clinical Trials

In the discussion of the previous section on design and analysis issues in cost-effectiveness, we treated the cost data as if it were complete and followed a standard normal distribution. In practice, cost data present particular statistical challenges both in terms of the construct of the cost information and in the expected level of completeness.

The interest of decision-makers is in the mean total cost for a patient group. Patient costs are calculated by observing counts of resources used (e.g., visits to a general practitioner, prescribed medication, outpatient appointments, inpatient procedures, days spent in hospital), weighting these counts by a unit cost related to each resource item and summing across items. When considering this cost stochastically in a clinical trial, it is almost always the case that it is the resource use events that are truly stochastic, but that the unit costs applied are deterministic, with a single fixed value. Hence, total cost is really a weighted mixture of other distributions. Typically, this distribution of cost will be highly skewed with a few patients incurring rare but highly expensive costs (such as inpatient hospital procedures with all the associated costs) and many patients having few or no costs. Where cost data are highly skewed in this way, very large numbers of patients will be required before the assumption of normality (through the central limit theorem) can be applied.

Due to the mixture nature of the cost distribution and the inappropriateness of ordinal methods such as Wilcoxon and ordinal logistic regression for cost data (33a), much recent research has focused on the use of sophisticated statistical models to explain cost distributions. In particular, two-stage (or hurdle) models can be employed to distinguish between groups of patients incurring high and low (often zero) costs (31, 34, 35). However, to prove useful for decision-making these models need to be able to distinguish defining characteristics of patients that make them candidates for high- or low-cost pathways. All too often, it is impossible to predict a priori which patients will turn out to be high cost. Fortunately, however, and as Lumley and colleagues show (33a), standard t-tests and linear regression are robust to nonnormality of the data. Furthermore, that the skew coefficient of the population will be reduced by a factor of $\sqrt{n}$ in the sampling distribution of the mean of that population (where n is the sample size) may guide the analyst as to whether that skew will have an important effect on the sampling distribution of the mean (7a).

Another problem relates to the completeness of the data, both in terms of administrative censoring and missing observations. Decision-makers are interested in the mean cost per patient for the lifetime of the patient. However, clinical trials rarely follow every patient to death. Instead, a cut-off point is specified at which time data collection stops and the analysis of the data begins. Where patients were recruited to the trial over a substantial recruitment period, there can be an administrative censoring problem such that the follow-up time for patients in the trial is different, with some having reached the endpoint of interest and some having been censored.

Of course, censoring is a problem for standard clinical results, not just costs, and the first attempts to handle censoring in cost data employed standard statistical approaches to survival analysis with cost as the survival metric rather than time (21, 22). Unfortunately, this approach is invalid since it can be shown that censoring (which occurs on the time scale) is no longer independent of cost: Patients accruing cost at a slow rate will more likely be censored in a naïve cost censoring analysis leading to a bias upwards in the censor-adjusted cost estimate (25). Instead, a technique has been advocated (known as the Kaplan-Meier sample average estimator) whereby costs are partitioned over time and uncensored costs are aggregated at each time interval and weighted by the probability of survival: Summing across these weighted estimates gives the censor-adjusted total cost estimate (20, 30).

However, this technique too has disadvantages. It is only unbiased in the limit as the partition size tends to zero; it cannot handle covariate adjustment and cannot be used to predict beyond the follow-up of the trial. New techniques are beginning to emerge that address these problems: The inverse probability weighting method is unbiased (3); an extension to the KMSA estimator has been developed that allows for covariate adjustment (29); a two-stage estimator has been developed that when implemented parametrically can be used to predict beyond the study period (12); and the survival analysis problem for costs has been extended to cost-effectiveness through the use of the net benefit statistic (52). Further refinements of these methods are expected to provide a complete solution for analysts wanting to simultaneously handle censored cost and effect data, while adjusting for covariates and predicting beyond the follow-up of the trial.

SUMMARY AND CONCLUSIONS

In this paper, we have been concerned with the emerging quantitative techniques for analyzing the results of cost-effectiveness analyses undertaken alongside clinical trials. In particular, we have emphasized the use of the cost-effectiveness plane as a device to present and explore the implications of uncertainty. As a general rule, we would encourage analysts to make more use of the cost-effectiveness plane because we believe that it gives the clearest intuitive understanding of the implications of uncertainty for the analysis.

We stress the importance of estimation in cost-effectiveness studies rather than hypothesis testing: demonstrating that the application of separate and sequential tests of hypothesis could result in poor inference due to lack of power. Furthermore, any direct test of a cost-effectiveness hypothesis must involve the ceiling ratio for decision-making, λ, which is itself unknown. Therefore, formal tests of hypothesis are unlikely to be useful in economic evaluation studies; however, the use of confidence intervals for representing uncertainty in the ICER is limited. Rather, we advocate the use of acceptability curves that directly address the concern of the decision-maker: How likely is it that the intervention is cost-effective? This interpretation requires a Bayesian view of probability, but a Bayesian approach is the most natural approach for decision-making.

The net-benefit framework provides a very important contribution to the analysis of uncertainty for incremental cost-effectiveness by removing the reliance on ratio statistics, which are inherently problematic from a statistical point of view. In particular, net-benefit methods allow straightforward calculation of acceptability curves, a simple solution to the problem of power calculation, and have recently been employed to directly estimate cost-effectiveness within a regression framework (28). The use of regression for cost-effectiveness is important because it provides both a framework to handle censoring of the data and a mechanism for exploring subgroup analysis. Both these issues are likely to receive increasing attention, and we look forward to continued refinement of the methods in this area.

ACKNOWLEDGMENTS

AB is the recipient of a Public Health Career Scientist Award from the U.K. Department of Health. The Canadian Implantable Defibrillator Study was funded by the Medical Research Council of Canada. However, views expressed in this paper are those of the authors and should not be attributed to any funding bodies.

TECHNICAL APPENDIX

Fieller's theorem for ICER confidence limits

We start from the quadratic equation in R, the limits of which are the Fieller confidence limits:

$$R^2\left[\Delta E^2 - z_{\alpha/2}^2 \operatorname{var}(\Delta E)\right] - 2R\left[\Delta E \cdot \Delta C - z_{\alpha/2}^2 \operatorname{cov}(\Delta E, \Delta C)\right]$$
$$+ \left[\Delta C^2 - z_{\alpha/2}^2 \operatorname{var}(\Delta C)\right] = 0.$$

This equation is solved using the standard quadratic formula

$$\frac{-b \pm \sqrt{b^2 - 4ac}}{2a}$$

where:

$$a = \Delta E^2 - z_{\alpha/2}^2 \operatorname{var}(\Delta E)$$
$$b = -2\left[\Delta E \cdot \Delta C - z_{\alpha/2}^2 \operatorname{cov}(\Delta E, \Delta C)\right]$$
$$c = \Delta C^2 - z_{\alpha/2}^2 \operatorname{var}(\Delta C).$$

Substituting these values into the expression above simplifies only slightly with the 2s cancelling to give

$$\frac{\left[\Delta E \cdot \Delta C - z_{\alpha/2}^2 \operatorname{cov}(\Delta E, \Delta C)\right] \pm \sqrt{\left[\Delta E \cdot \Delta C - z_{\alpha/2}^2 \operatorname{cov}(\Delta E, \Delta C)\right]^2 - \left[\Delta E^2 - z_{\alpha/2}^2 \operatorname{var}(\Delta E)\right] \cdot \left[\Delta C^2 - z_{\alpha/2}^2 \operatorname{var}(\Delta C)\right]}}{\Delta E^2 - z_{\alpha/2}^2 \operatorname{var}(\Delta E)}$$

In order to estimate these limits, only five simple sample statistics require estimation. For a comparison of control and treatment interventions indicated by the subscripts C and T respectively we have:

1. $\Delta E = \bar{E}_T - \bar{E}_C = \dfrac{1}{n_T} \sum\limits_{i=1}^{n_T} E_{Ti} - \dfrac{1}{n_C} \sum\limits_{j=1}^{n_C} E_{Cj}$

2. $\Delta C = \bar{C}_T - \bar{C}_C = \dfrac{1}{n_T} \sum\limits_{i=1}^{n_T} C_{Ti} - \dfrac{1}{n_C} \sum\limits_{j=1}^{n_C} C_{Cj}$

3. $\operatorname{var}(\Delta E) = \operatorname{var}(\bar{E}_T) + \operatorname{var}(\bar{E}_C) = \dfrac{s_{ET}^2}{n_T} + \dfrac{s_{EC}^2}{n_C}$

4. $\operatorname{var}(\Delta C) = \operatorname{var}(\bar{C}_T) + \operatorname{var}(\bar{C}_C) = \dfrac{s_{CT}^2}{n_T} + \dfrac{s_{CC}^2}{n_C}$

5. $\operatorname{cov}(\Delta E, \Delta C) = \operatorname{cov}(\bar{E}_T, \bar{C}_T) + \operatorname{cov}(\bar{E}_C, \bar{C}_C)$
   $\qquad\qquad\qquad = \rho_T \sqrt{\operatorname{var}(\bar{E}_T) \operatorname{var}(\bar{C}_T)} + \rho_C \sqrt{\operatorname{var}(\bar{E}_C) \operatorname{var}(\bar{C}_C)}$

where E and C represent effect and cost respectively, s_{ij}^2 is the sample variance for $i = $ cost or effect in the $j = $ control or treatment groups and ρ_j is the correlation coefficient between costs and effects in each group. Both the sample variance and correlation can be estimated using standard methods and are output by all standard statistical packages.

Sample size calculations

We start from the desire to have the power to show a hypothesized NMB as significant:

$$N\tilde{M}B - z_\beta \sqrt{\mathrm{var}(N\tilde{M}B)} > z_{\alpha/2} \sqrt{\mathrm{var}(N\tilde{M}B)}$$

and rearrange to get

$$N\tilde{M}B > (z_{\alpha/2} + z_\beta) \sqrt{\mathrm{var}(N\tilde{M}B)}.$$

Substituting into the above expression the standard expressions for NMB and its variance gives:

$$\lambda \cdot \Delta\tilde{E} - \Delta\tilde{C} > (z_{\alpha/2} + z_\beta) \sqrt{\lambda^2 \cdot \mathrm{var}(\Delta\tilde{E}) + \mathrm{var}(\Delta\tilde{C}) - 2 \cdot \lambda \cdot \mathrm{cov}(\Delta\tilde{E}, \Delta\tilde{C})}.$$

This gives an expression in the same five statistics as given above. Substituting in the expressions for these five sample statistics and rearranging on n (assuming equal sample sizes in each trial arm) gives

$$n > \frac{(z_{\alpha/2} + z_\beta)^2 \cdot \left\{ \lambda^2 \cdot \left[\tilde{s}_{ET}^2 + \tilde{s}_{EC}^2\right] + \left[\tilde{s}_{CT}^2 + \tilde{s}_{CC}^2\right] - 2 \cdot \lambda \cdot \left[\rho_T \tilde{s}_{ET} \tilde{s}_{CT} + \rho_C \tilde{s}_{EC} \tilde{s}_{CC}\right]\right\}}{[\lambda \cdot (\bar{E}_T - \bar{E}_C) - (\bar{C}_T - \bar{C}_C)]^2}$$

remembering that the variance expressions above relate to the hypothesized variances in the population, not the variances of the estimators.

Visit the Annual Reviews home page at www.annualreviews.org

LITERATURE CITED

1. Al MJ, van Hout BA, Michel BC, Rutten FF. 1998. Sample size calculation in economic evaluations. *Health Econ.* 7(4):327–35

2. Altman DG, Bland JM. 1995. Absence of evidence is not evidence of absence. *Br. Med. J.* 311(7003):485

3. Bang H, Tsiatis AA. 2000. Estimating medical costs with censored data. *Biometrika* 87(2):329–43

4. Black WC. 1990. The CE plane: a graphic representation of cost-effectiveness. *Med. Decis. Mak.* 10:212–14

5. Bland JM, Altman DG. 1998. Bayesians and frequentists. *Br. Med. J.* 317 (7166):1151–60

6. Briggs A, Fenn P. 1998. Confidence intervals or surfaces? Uncertainty on the cost-effectiveness plane. *Health Econ.* 7(8):723–40

7. Briggs A, Gray A. 1998. Power and sample size calculations for stochastic cost-effectiveness analysis. *Med. Decis. Mak.* 18:S81–93

7a. Briggs A, Gray A. 1998. The distribution of health care costs and their statistical analysis for economic evaluation. *J. Health Serv. Res. & Policy* 3(4):233–45

8. Briggs AH. 1999. A Bayesian approach to stochastic cost-effectiveness analysis. *Health Econ.* 8(3):257–61

9. Briggs AH, Mooney CZ, Wonderling DE. 1999. Constructing confidence intervals for cost-effectiveness ratios: an evaluation of parametric and nonparametric techniques using Monte Carlo simulation. *Stat. Med.* 18(23):3245–62

10. Briggs AH, O'Brien BJ. 2001. The death of cost-minimisation analysis? *Health Econ.* 10:179–84

11. Briggs AH, Wonderling DE, Mooney CZ. 1997. Pulling cost-effectiveness analysis up by its bootstraps: a nonparametric approach to confidence interval estimation. *Health Econ.* 6(4):327–40

12. Carides GW, Heyse JF, Iglewicz B. 2000. A regression-based method for estimating mean treatment cost in the presence of right-censoring. *Biostatistics* 1(3):299–313

13. Carlin RP, Louis AT. 1996. *Bayes and Empirical Bayes Methods for Data Analysis*. London: Chapman & Hall

14. Chaudhary MA, Stearns SC. 1996. Estimating confidence intervals for cost-effectiveness ratios: an example from a randomized trial. *Stat. Med.* 15:1447–58

15. Claxton K. 1999. The irrelevance of inference: a decision-making approach to the stochastic evaluation of health care technologies. *J. Health Econ.* 18(3):341–64

16. Claxton K, Posnett J. 1996. An economic approach to clinical trial design and research priority-setting. *Health Econ.* 5(6):513–24

17. Collins R, Gray R, Godwin J, Peto R. 1987. Avoidance of large biases and large random errors in the assessment of moderate treatment effects: the need for systematic overviews. *Stat. Med.* 6(3):245–54

18. Drummond MF, O'Brien B, Stoddart GL, Torrance G. 1997. *Methods for the Economic Evaluation of Health Care Programmes.* Oxford: Oxford Univ. Press. 2nd ed.

19. Efron B, Tibshirani R. 1993. *An Introduction to the Bootstrap.* New York: Chapman & Hall

20. Etzioni RD, Feuer EJ, Sullivan SD, Lin D, Hu C, Ramsey SD. 1999. On the use of survival analysis techniques to estimate medical care costs. *J. Health Econ.* 18(3):365–80

21. Fenn P, McGuire A, Backhouse M, Jones D. 1996. Modelling programme costs in economic evaluation. *J. Health Econ.* 15(1):115–25

22. Fenn P, McGuire A, Phillips V, Backhouse M, Jones D. 1995. The analysis of censored treatment cost data in economic evaluation. *Med. Care* 33(8):851–63

23. Fieller EC. 1954. Some problems in interval estimation. *J. R. Stat. Soc., Ser. B* 16:175–83

24. Freiman JA, Chalmers TC, Smith H Jr, Kuebler RR. 1978. The importance of beta, the type II error and sample size in the design and interpretation of the randomized control trial. Survey of 71 "negative" trials. *N. Engl. J. Med.* 299(13):690–94

25. Hallstrom AP, Sullivan SD. 1998. On estimating costs for economic evaluation in failure time studies. *Med. Care* 36(3):433–36

26. Heitjan DF. 2000. Fieller's method and net health benefits. *Health Econ.* 9(4):327–35

27. Heitjan DF, Moskowitz AJ, Whang W. 1999. Bayesian estimation of cost-effectiveness ratios from clinical trials. *Health Econ.* 8(3):191–201

28. Hoch JS, Briggs AH, Willan A. 2002. Something old, something new, something borrowed, something BLUE: a framework for the marriage of health econometrics and cost-effectiveness analysis. *Health Econ.* In press

29. Lin DY. 2000. Linear regression analysis of censored medical costs. *Biostatistics* 1(1):35–47

30. Lin DY, Feuer EJ, Etzioni R, Wax Y. 1997. Estimating medical costs from incomplete follow-up data. *Biometrics* 53(2):419–34

31. Lipscomb J, Ancukiewicz M, Parmigiani G, Hasselblad V, Samsa G, Matchar DB. 1998. Predicting the cost of illness: a comparison of alternative models applied to stroke. *Med. Decis. Mak.* 18(2 Suppl.):S39–56

32. Lothgren M, Zethraeus N. 2000. Definition, interpretation and calculation of cost-effectiveness acceptability curves. *Health Econ.* 9(7):623–30

33. Luce BR, Claxton K. 1999. Redefining the analytical approach to pharmacoeconomics. *Health Econ.* 8(3):187–89

33a. Lumley T, Diehr P, Emerson S, Chen L. 2002. The importance of the normality assumption in large public health data sets. *Annu. Rev. Public Health* 23:151–69

34. Manning WG, Mullahy J. 2001. Estimating log models: to transform or not to transform? *J. Health Econ.* 20(4):461–94

35. Mullahy J. 1998. Much ado about two: reconsidering retransformation and the two-part model in health econometrics. *J. Health Econ.* 17(3):247–81

36. O'Brien BJ, Connolly SJ, Goeree R, Blackhouse G, Willan A, et al. 2001. Cost-effectiveness of the implantable cardioverter-defibrillator: results from the Canadian Implantable Defibrillator Study (CIDS). *Circulation* 103(10):1416–21

37. O'Brien BJ, Drummond MF. 1994. Statistical versus quantitative significance in the socioeconomic evaluation of medicines. *PharmacoEconomics* 5(5):389–98

38. O'Brien BJ, Drummond MF, Labelle RJ, Willan A. 1994. In search of power and significance: issues in the design and analysis of stochastic cost-effectiveness studies in health care. *Med. Care* 32(2):150–63

39. O'Hagan A, Stevens JW, Montmartin J. 2000. Inference for the cost-effectiveness acceptability curve and cost-effectiveness ratio. *PharmacoEconomics* 17(4):339–49

40. Obenchain RL, Melfi CA, Croghan TW, Buesching DP. 1997. Bootstrap analyses of cost effectiveness in antidepressant pharmacotherapy. *PharmacoEconomics* 11:464–72

41. Oxman AD, Guyatt GH. 1992. A consumer's guide to subgroup analyses. *Ann. Intern. Med.* 116(1):78–84

42. Polsky D, Glick HA, Willke R, Schulman K. 1997. Confidence intervals for cost-effectiveness ratios: a comparison of four methods. *Health Econ.* 6:243–52

43. Pritchard C. 1999. *Trends in Economic Evaluation*. London: Off. Health Econ. OHE Brief. Pap. No. 36

44. Raikou M, Gray A, Briggs A, Stevens R, Cull C, et al. 1998. Cost effectiveness analysis of improved blood pressure control in hypertensive patients with type 2 diabetic patients (HDS7): UKPDS 40. *Br. Med. J.* 317:720–26

45. Ramsey SD, McIntosh M, Sullivan SD. 2001. Design issues for conducting cost-effectiveness analyses alongside clinical trials. *Annu. Rev. Public Health* 22:129–41

46. Severens JL, De Boo TM, Konst EM. 1999. Uncertainty of incremental cost-effectiveness ratios. A comparison of Fieller and bootstrap confidence intervals. *Int. J. Technol. Assess. Health Care* 15(3):608–14

47. Sheldon R, O'Brien BJ, Blackhouse G, Goeree R, Mitchell B, et al. 2001. Effect of clinical risk stratification on cost-effectiveness of the implantable cardioverter-defibrillator: the Canadian implantable defibrillator study. *Circulation* 104(14):1622–26

48. Stinnett AA, Mullahy J. 1997. The negative side of cost-effectiveness analysis. *JAMA* 277(24):1931–32

49. Stinnett AA, Mullahy J. 1998. Net

health benefits: a new framework for the analysis of uncertainty in cost-effectiveness analysis. *Med. Decis. Mak.* 18(2 Suppl.):S68–80

50. Tambour M, Zethraeus N, Johannesson M. 1998. A note on confidence intervals in cost-effectiveness analysis. *Int. J. Technol. Assess. Health Care* 14(3):467–71

51. van Hout BA, Al MJ, Gordon GS, Rutten FF. 1994. Costs, effects and C/E-ratios alongside a clinical trial. *Health Econ.* 3(5):309–19

52. Willan AR, Lin DY. 2001. Incremental net benefit in randomized clinical trials. *Stat. Med.* 20(11):1563–74

53. Willan AR, O'Brien BJ. 1996. Confidence intervals for cost-effectiveness ratios: an application of Fieller's theorem. *Health Econ.* 5:297–305

Annu. Rev. Public Health 2002. 23:403–26

TUBERCULOSIS

Parvathi Tiruviluamala and Lee B. Reichman

New Jersey Medical School, National Tuberculosis Center, Newark, New Jersey 07107-3001; e-mail: tirupa@umdnj.edu

Key Words *Mycobacterium tuberculosis*, nosocomial infection, DOT, MDR TB, TB vaccine

■ **Abstract** Tuberculosis is an infectious disease caused by bacteria in the *Mycobacterium tuberculosis* complex. Of these, the most common species to infect humans is *M. tuberculosis*. The TB bacillus is an extremely successful human pathogen, infecting two billion persons worldwide; an estimated 2 to 3 million people die from tuberculosis each year. In the United States, TB rates decreased steadily at the rate of 5% per year from 1953 until 1985 when the trend reversed, with the number of TB cases peaking in 1992. Outbreaks of multidrug-resistant TB (MDR TB) were reported, and these cases were documented to be transmitted in nosocomial and congregate settings, including hospitals and prisons. AIDS patients infected with *M. tb* developed disease rapidly, and case-fatality rates of >80% were noted in those infected with multidrug-resistant *M. tb*. Intensive intervention, at enormous cost, caused the number of TB cases to decline. This article discusses factors that led to the increase in TB cases, their subsequent decline, and measures needed in the future if TB is to be eliminated in the United States.

INTRODUCTION

Tuberculosis (TB) is an infectious disease caused by bacteria in the *M. tuberculosis* complex, which includes *M. tuberculosis* (*M. tb*), *M. bovis*, *M. africanum*, *M. microti*, and the newly discovered *M. canettii* (5, 87). Ninety-five percent of all TB cases occur in developing countries (5), and TB is a leading cause of disability and death in many parts of the world. Worldwide, an estimated two billion people are infected, 8 million people develop disease, and 2 million die each year from tuberculosis (88), making it the largest single infectious cause of death globally. In countries where the incidence of HIV is increasing (sub-Saharan Africa, Southeast Asia), the incidence of tuberculosis has multiplied severalfold, with devastating effects on already fragile TB control programs (54). In the United States, an estimated 15 million people are infected with *M. tb* (5), and these make up the reservoir from which most new cases arise. As in all developed countries, people affected by TB in the United States are predominantly members of minority groups, foreign born, and poor. Of the total 16,377 cases reported in the United States in 2000, 77% were in non-Hispanic blacks, Hispanics, and Asian/Pacific Islanders; the 25–64-year age group accounted for 66% of all TB cases (36). According to TB-AIDS

0163-7525/02/0510-0403$14.00

403

registry match data, in 1999, at least 20% of TB patients in the 25–44-year age group were coinfected with HIV (33). Both the prevalence of TB and TB-HIV coinfection show geographic differences. Seven states (California, Florida, Georgia, Illinois, New Jersey, New York, and Texas) reported 59% of the total TB cases in 1999. Over one third of persons from five states, in the 25–44-year age range, were coinfected with HIV and TB (District of Columbia, Florida, Georgia, New York City, and South Carolina) (33). HIV-induced immunosuppression probably accounted for a minimum of 30% excess TB cases during the period from 1985 through 1990 (25). A recent study showed that lower socioeconomic status accounted for much of the increased TB risk associated with race/ethnicity in the United States (26).

Humans are the predominant reservoir for *M. tb* and *M. africanum*, and cattle for *M. bovis* (10). Pasteurization of milk and TB control programs in cattle in developed countries (5) have significantly decreased human infection due to *M. bovis*. *M. tb* is transmitted when a person with pulmonary TB coughs or sneezes and aerosolizes the bacteria in droplet nuclei. These droplet nuclei, 1–5 μm in size, are small enough to reach the alveoli and can remain suspended in the air for long periods of time. In contrast, the larger particles deposited on the walls of larger airways are effectively cleared by the mucociliary apparatus of the upper respiratory tract.

M. tb transmission is determined by (*a*) infectiousness of the patient who expels the infectious droplet nuclei, (*b*) the concentration of organisms in the air determined by the volume of the space and ventilation and length of exposure, and (*c*) the immune status of the individual at risk (5). Infection control measures are also targeted to these factors (31). Interestingly, while HIV infection is an extremely important predictor of disease progression [50% in the first year of infection in patients with advanced HIV (52)], the rate of acquiring new infection does not seem to be affected by HIV status (100, 107).

The fate of the *M. tb* in the inhaled droplet nuclei is determined by the virulence of the organism and by the inherent bactericidal property of the resident alveolar macrophage (53). The alveolar macrophage ingests the bacteria, and in a naive host the bacteria multiply uninhibited intracellularly. With no known exotoxins or endotoxins in *M. tb*, there is no immediate host response during the initial period of mycobacterial growth (5), when the organisms are carried via lymphatics throughout the body and settle in various organs. Cellular immune response that is detectable by the positive tuberculin skin test (TST) is elicited in about 2 to 12 weeks. Tuberculous disease in persons with intact cellular immune response is characterized by granuloma formation, where activated lymphocytes and macrophages aggregate and limit the multiplication of *M. tb*.

Tuberculosis is unique in that its latent period can vary from weeks to years. During this time, the organism is presumably dormant, and the infected individual is asymptomatic and not contagious. The lifetime risk of developing active TB is estimated to be 10%, with one half of active cases occurring in the first 2 to 4 years (5). This propensity for latency in *M. tb* causes problems diagnostically because there is no gold standard for diagnosing latent TB infection—the only test currently available is the TST, first developed in the 1880s. Though useful, the test results can vary depending on the reagent used, technique of placement and interpretation, and the immune status of the subject. Both false-negative and false-positive reactions can occur: the former has been noted in about 15–20% of patients with disseminated TB and with immunosuppression from various causes, including HIV infection; the latter, due to infection with non-TB mycobacteria and *M. bovis* BCG. As the prevalence of tuberculosis in the population continues to decrease, these discrepancies will further affect the positive predictive value of the tuberculin test (13). Therapeutically, latent infection is problematic because treatment is prolonged and can have side effects; asymptomatic persons are often reluctant to take medications, particularly when their families and peers erroneously believe that the positive reaction is due to the BCG vaccine received in their native country. This belief often affects adherence to the prescribed therapy (104).

Pulmonary tuberculosis, the most important type of TB from the public health perspective, can be diagnosed on the basis of symptoms, chest radiograph, acid fast smear (AFB) by sputum microscopy, and culture. About 15% of verified TB cases in the United States are not confirmed bacteriologically but rather are diagnosed solely on the basis of high clinical suspicion along with response to anti-TB medicines (41). Chest radiograph may show the characteristic upper lobe cavity; however, in immunosuppressed and HIV-positive patients the radiographic abnormalities may be atypical and mimic other pulmonary conditions. Occasionally, the chest radiograph may appear to be normal in persons infected with HIV. Finding positive AFB smear on sputum microscopy in a patient is considered to be strongly suggestive of TB and is treated as TB until culture results become available. Approximately 10,000 bacilli per ml of sputum are required for a positive sputum smear. Fifty to 80% of patients with untreated pulmonary TB will have a positive smear (5). Molecular techniques allow for rapid identification of *M. tb* from clinical specimens. Specific target sequences in mycobacterial DNA or RNA are amplified and then identified by nucleic acid probes. When the AFB smear is positive, the sensitivity of the amplification method is 95%; when the AFB smear is negative, the sensitivity decreases to as low as 48% (5, 9); the specificity is approximately 95%. A positive nucleic acid amplification test in the setting of a positive AFB smear is indicative of TB (35). An enhanced nucleic acid amplification test (E-MTD), a 3-h test, has been approved by the FDA advisory panel for both smear-positive and -negative patients with clinical suspicion for pulmonary TB (27).

Culture of *M. tb* from a clinical specimen is the diagnostic gold standard for active tuberculosis. At present, culture is also a prerequisite for drug susceptibility tests on *M. tuberculosis*. Culture can detect 100 organism per ml of sputum, compared with 10,000 required for detection by sputum microscopy. Culture of *M. tb* is time-consuming, taking from 3 to 8 weeks; newer techniques using liquid systems have shortened culture time to as early as 1 to 3 weeks. Molecular techniques (nucleic acid hybridization) help in the rapid identification of cultured mycobacteria with very high sensitivity and specificity when there are 10^5 organisms

(5). Cultured specimens can also be rapidly determined by the identification of species-specific cell-wall mycolic acids (41).

Drug susceptibility testing, which takes another 2 to 4 weeks after culture of the organisms, should be performed on initial isolates from all patients to determine or confirm an appropriate and effective anti-TB regimen and then be repeated if the sputum remains persistently positive after 3 months of treatment or if it converts to positive after remaining negative for some time (5). The lengthy process whereby the results of *M. tb* sensitivity tests were reported to clinicians in the late-1980s and early 1990s, the era of lax TB control, is believed to have contributed significantly to the underrecognition and spread of MDR TB in many institutions.

The advances in molecular biology over the past decade have significantly enhanced our understanding of TB (17). Rapid diagnostic tests for clinical diagnosis may prove very cost effective in avoiding unneeded isolation of suspected TB cases. For example, Blumberg et al. showed that only 14% of patients who were isolated were later found to have TB (21).

Fascinating insights have also been gained in the field of TB epidemiology. Current understanding of TB epidemiology was based on the studies dating from the early part of the previous century when only 10% of TB cases were estimated to occur from recent transmission (50). However, recent studies using molecular techniques show that between 20% to 54% of TB is actually from recent transmission (3, 12, 52, 101). Indeed, the decline in TB cases over the past decade is attributable to reduced transmission. DNA fingerprinting, based on the transposon IS6110 (IS stands for insertion sequence, a genetic material), is the standard methodology used in studying TB transmission (108). When the numbers and positions of DNA bands in *M. tb* cultured from two patients match, they are said to be in a cluster, and this is usually considered evidence of recent transmission. When the IS6110 copies are <5 or 6, the specificity for clustering becomes lower and additional tests using secondary markers are recommended to identify clustering (24, 64). These methods require a large quantity of DNA, and pure culture of *M. tb* is therefore a prerequisite (i.e., these tests cannot be performed directly on sputum smears at present) (65).

More recently, spoligotyping, a test based on polymerase chain reaction (PCR), has been used for DNA fingerprinting. Small quantities of DNA are sufficient, and the exciting possibility exists of diagnosing TB and fingerprinting *M. tb* at the same time (71). When standardized, this test should have significant repercussions for TB control, which is still dependent on the definite identification of *M. tb* by culture.

DNA fingerprinting has provided evidence of recent transmission in hospitals (29, 55), prisons (107), restaurants (63), homeless shelters (11), AIDS facilities (52), and neighborhood bars (73). Molecular techniques have also helped in identifying pseudo-outbreaks of TB due to laboratory cross-contamination (14), transmission from smear-negative TB patients (18), and exogenous re-infection in both AIDS patients (102) and non-AIDS (109) patients. Recently, a population-based cross-sectional study using molecular techniques determined the occurrence of a previously undetected outbreak in New Jersey of a highly drug-resistant variant of TB (19). The establishment of a centralized molecular databank should help in early identification of an outbreak (by matching the outbreak with data from existing cases), and thereby allow quick and appropriate action. A National Tuberculosis Genotyping and Surveillance Network has been established by CDC in response to several nosocomial outbreaks in the early 1990s (5).

The serologic tests for TB currently available are expensive, have suboptimal sensitivity, and are unable to distinguish active disease from latent TB infection and *M. tb* from nontuberculous mycobacterial diseases (41). A new in vitro diagnostic test, the ESAT-6 ELISPOT assay, offers promise in diagnosing latent TB infection among symptom-free persons recently exposed to *M. tb*. ESAT-6 is a secreted antigen that is expressed by *M. tb* complex but is absent from all strains of *M. bovis* BCG vaccine (75).

The TST is still the only widely available method to diagnose latent TB infection. In a person infected with *M. tb*, the risk of progression to active disease depends on several factors; treatment for latent TB infection is recommended for those at high risk. Table 1 shows the guidelines for interpreting TST. The three cut points were chosen based on the prevalence of tuberculosis among the different groups. The lowest cut-off point is chosen for those at the greatest risk of developing active tuberculosis when they are infected with *M. tb* (34).

TABLE 1   Criteria for tuberculin test positivity by risk group[a]

Reaction ≥5 mm induration	Reaction ≥10 mm induration	Reaction ≥15 mm induration
HIV-positive status	Recent immigrants (within the last 5 years) from high-prevalence countries	Persons with no risk factors for TB
Recent contacts of TB case patients	Injection drug users	
	Residents and employees of high-risk congregate settings[b]	
Persons with organ transplants and other immunosuppression; persons receiving the equivalent of ≥15 mg/day of prednisone for ≥1 month	Mycobacteriology lab personnel	
	Persons with clinical conditions that place them at high risk of TB reactivation[c]	
	Children ≤ 4 years of age, or infants, children, and adolescents exposed to adults at high risk	

[a]Modified from Reference 34.

[b]Prisons and jails, nursing homes and other long-term facilities for the elderly, hospitals and other health care facilities, homeless shelters, residential facilities for patients with AIDS.

[c]Silicosis, diabetes mellitus, chronic renal failure, some hematological disorders (lymphomas, leukemias), other specific malignancies (e.g., carcinoma of head and neck and lung), weight loss of ≥10% of ideal body weight, gastrectomy, and jejuno-ileal bypass.

Three basic principles govern the treatment of tuberculosis: (*a*) Regimens must contain multiple drugs to which the bacteria are susceptible; (*b*) the drugs must be taken regularly; and (*c*) drug therapy must continue for the requisite period of time (5). In the early days of chemotherapy, the required dosage consisted of isoniazid plus para-amino salicylic acid (PAS), supplemented by streptomycin at least in the first two months, to be given for 18 months. The availability of rifampin in the early 1970s has enabled the duration of chemotherapy to be significantly reduced (6 to 9 months).

Two U.S. studies from the 1980s showed that six-month treatment with regimens containing rifampin achieved high rates of cure (46, 49). Currently, the standard therapy for tuberculosis that is susceptible to all first-line drugs is short-course chemotherapy for six months. A combination of isoniazid (INH), rifampin, pyrazinamide (PZA), and ethambutol or streptomycin is used for the first two months, followed by isoniazid and rifampin for four months. Subsequently, therapy can be given twice weekly, thereby saving time, effort, and money. When therapy is given biweekly, the standard of care for all patients with TB must be by directly observed therapy (DOT), whereby a healthcare worker observes the intake of every dose of medication to ensure completion of treatment and to prevent the emergence of multidrug resistance. This is the only way to ensure that a patient is taking all of his/her medications. A nine-month regimen of INH and rifampin is acceptable for patients who are intolerant of PZA. Treatment of multidrug-resistant TB (MDR TB) (defined as *M. tb* resistant to both isoniazid and rifampin) is difficult, prolonged, time-consuming, and often unsuccessful. Treatment must be individualized in consultation with a clinician with expertise in such management (6).

Treatment should be offered to persons with latent TB infection who are at increased risk for progression to active TB. Isoniazid given for 6 to 12 months used to be the only choice available for treatment of latent TB infection. Recent recommendations by the CDC have expanded the options to alternate, shorter-course regimens, including rifampin as either monotherapy or in combination with pyrazinamide (34). Although shorter courses of therapy are ideal for ensuring treatment completion, close monitoring for side effects is crucial. Several cases of severe hepatotoxicity and deaths were reported recently on a combination therapy using rifampin and pyrazinamide. This regimen has therefore been de-emphasized (37, 37a).

Drug resistance (primary) develops in *M. tb* by random, single-step spontaneous mutations at the gene loci of the chromosome at a low but predictable rate (112). Clinically, it occurs slowly as a result of selection pressure exerted by inadequate therapy. Resistance to one drug is not linked with resistance to another unrelated drug, but cross-resistance among members of similar classes of drugs is common, e.g., rifamycins, fluroquinolines, etc. (68, 112). Mutations in *M. tb* can alter one or more genes, which can eventually affect the primary drug target, its transportation system, or increased synthesis of the drug's target enzyme, thereby rendering the drug ineffective in inhibiting mycobacterial growth (112). The probability of incidence of drug-resistant mutations for INH is 1 in 10^6; for rifampin, 1 in 10^8; for streptomycin (SM), 1 in 10^6; and for ethambutol, 1 in 10^6 (81, 112). When two drugs are considered together, it is the sum of the two resistances, e.g., INH + rifampin = one organism in 10^{14}, with three drugs together, e.g., INH + rifampin + SM, it is one organism in 10^{20}, and so on. Since the average number of organisms in a tuberculous cavity is 10^8–10^9, the chance of finding an organism resistant to all three drugs is very low, and a three-drug combination is therefore adequate for cure (112). However, four drugs are generally used in case there is an unknown, pre-existing resistance to one of the drugs.

The presence of acquired drug-resistance is indicative of poor functioning of a current TB control program, whereas the presence of primary drug-resistance is indicative of a poorly functioning TB program in the past (74). Poor patient compliance is an important cause of drug resistance in TB. Other causes include inadequate therapy, monotherapy, addition of a single drug to a failing regimen, suboptimal drug dosing and poor absorption of drugs; many of these shortcomings are under the treating physician's control (68, 112). Acquired drug resistance is substantially less prevalent in countries in which the national TB control programs have included the successful application of directly observed short-course chemotherapy (DOTS) (72, 74). Epidemiological factors associated with drug resistance in individuals include history of previous therapy, birth/residence in a country with high prevalence of resistant TB, recent exposure to drug-resistant disease, and cavitary disease (68).

Resistance to rifampin is rarely found without resistance to other drugs and, most importantly, predicts resistance to both INH and a poor therapy outcome (48). Mutations in *rpo B* (which encodes for the RNA polymerase subunit β) were found in 97% of over 200 rifampin-resistant clinical isolates of *M. tb* (48). The possibility therefore exists of targeting a single region of the genome for diagnostic purposes, and rifampin resistance could serve as a valid surrogate model for MDR TB. PCR single-stranded conformation polymorphism is a valuable tool for screening for resistance to rifampin (105). Other methods to detect rifampin resistance include PCR amplification of the target sequence and detection by DNA sequencing, line probe assay (5), and luciferase assay (69).

In 1993, the CDC conducted a match between national TB and AIDS registries to compare the rates of drug resistance between AIDS and non-AIDS patients. There was no significant difference in rates of INH resistance (7.8% vs 10%); a significantly higher proportion of patients with AIDS had rifampin monoresistance (3.4% vs 0.5%). A case-control study showed no differences between AIDS and non-AIDS patients with respect to age, sex, race, country of birth, homelessness, history of incarceration, or prior tuberculosis. Cases were more likely to have diarrhea, rifabutin, or antifungal therapy use. All but two of the isolates available for DNA fingerprinting had unique patterns, suggesting that there was no clustering (96).

HISTORIC PERSPECTIVES, FACTORS, AND EVENTS LEADING TO THE INCREASE IN TB CASES IN THE UNITED STATES

Major TB control initiatives began in the United States in the late 1880s, when sanatoria were built to isolate infectious TB patients from the susceptible public. Eventually the patients either died from the disease or became noninfectious. The Division of Tuberculosis Control was established within the U.S. Public Health Service in 1944 to screen residents for TB. After the first curative anti-TB drugs became available in the early 1950s, medical experts at the 1959 Arden House Conference recommended that the U.S. focus should be on community-based outpatient treatment for TB control (106). Specific categorical federal project grants, targeted to state and big city TB control programs, were instituted to meet the logistic and financial demands of the new strategy. Adoption of this policy was followed by a sustained decline in the number of TB cases (94).

From 1970 to 1972, the categorical grants were replaced by block grants to the states, despite warnings from experts that the states would allocate monies to TB only if it was a local priority. As predicted, spending on TB control fell precipitously over the next 20 years (93, 103a).

By the early 1980s, the combined city and state expenditure for the outpatient activities in New York City (NYC) dropped from $18 million to <$2 million. One thousand designated TB beds were eliminated, and diagnosis was left to the private sector in over half of all TB cases. With increasing fiscal crisis, NY State progressively cut back and, in September 1979, entirely terminated its support for TB control activities in NYC. Federal support also decreased from $1.4 million in 1979 to $283,000 in 1980. The number of health department chest clinics fell from 22 to 9. Mandated staff increases had not occurred; therefore there were no home visits by the public health nurses or health aides. The number of contacts identified per TB case dropped, drug treatment centers stopped screening patients for TB, and the incidence of TB increased among drug addicts well before the onset of the AIDS epidemic (23).

The incidence of TB continued to increase in New York City over the next 10 years. Beginning 1980, federal funding for a new pilot project, supervised treatment program or STP (now called directly observed therapy), was approved in response to the increasing number of patients who failed to complete treatment (23, 61). This program mandated daily visits to patients' homes and the administration of medications by DOT; the success rate was excellent, with 90% to 95% of the patients completing treatment. However, as funding was not increased from federal, state, or city sources, the project could not expand beyond its initial pilot stage.

The downward trend in the number of TB cases, which had begun in 1953 and continued at the rate of 5% per year until 1984–85, finally reversed in 1986. Reports were surfacing of outbreaks of MDR TB cases in HIV-infected persons from New York City (16, 57, 60), an upstate New York prison (107), New Jersey, and Florida (29). The median survival of these patients was <16 weeks and the all-cause mortality was >80% (29). Recombinant DNA techniques revealed that these MDR TB cases were being transmitted in hospitals and prisons (60, 107). This upsurge of tuberculosis was multifactorial in origin: the HIV epidemic, immigration from countries with high TB prevalence, drug addiction, homelessness, and most important, the deterioration of the public health system and its infrastructure (23, 90). The phenomenon of removing resources from an improving program with the resultant worsening of the original problem was described as the "U-shaped curve of concern" (90). The increases in incidence were directly attributable to the change from categorical grants to block grants for TB a decade earlier.

Finally, the unprecedented public reaction to the death from MDR TB of a non-HIV-infected prison guard in upstate New York roused the attention of Congress. A multiagency governmental task force was quickly organized to coordinate the effort against TB. Huge increases in congressional appropriations were obtained and major research initiatives were started. New cost-effective strategies including DOT, fixed dose-drug combinations, and educational and training interventions were implemented, and long-term solutions were devised (92). TB rates started coming down the very next year, a trend that has continued through 2000, when 16,377 cases were reported, i.e., 5.8 per 100,000 persons, compared with 10.5 per 100,000 persons in 1992 (36).

By international consensus, a country is deemed to be in the TB elimination phase when its case rates are <3.5 per 100,000 persons, and TB elimination is achieved when the case rate is 1 case per 1 million persons (103). In 2000, 21 states in the United States had TB case rates <3.5 per 100,000 persons. The major lesson learned from these recent events is that funding is the key ingredient in controlling TB (94).

FACTORS THAT CONTRIBUTED TO THE
DECREASE IN TB CASES

Directly Observed Therapy

By the early 1960s, experts involved in TB control in three geographically different locations (Madras, Hong Kong, and London) concluded that effective treatment of TB required direct supervision of therapy to prevent patients from discontinuing their medications when they stopped feeling ill (15). DOT also avoided the necessity of predicting which patients would likely be noncompliant with their medications. A study by Sbarboro et al. showed that 75% of patients treated at Denver General Hospital in the mid- to late-1960s were unreliable in completing therapy (98). Despite the demonstrated efficacy of DOT (78, 98) and recommendations by the American Thoracic Society and CDC (4), most patients with TB were continued to be treated with self-administered therapy. DOT was often thought to be unnecessary and unjustified since most patients completed their TB treatment; it was also considered an infringement on a patient's civil liberties (7, 15).

Faced with the threat of an increasing number of cases and nosocomial outbreaks of MDR TB in the 1990s, the U.S Advisory Council for Elimination of Tuberculosis (ACET) made DOT the standard of care as a matter of federal policy (2). Appropriations to CDC for TB control increased from $25 million to $104 million (15). The change in federal policy resulted in the restructuring of policies at the local level. In Chicago, all newly diagnosed cases in 1993 were placed on DOT, and in Rhode Island 80% of patients were on DOT by the end of 1993 (compared with 34% in the first half of the year) (15). Historically, treatment completion has been the most challenging problem in TB management (1); nonadherence to TB treatment is the chief cause of relapse and drug resistance. Age, sex, religion, education, and socioeconomic status do not predict adherence (also referred to as compliance) (97). Psychiatric disease, drug addiction, alcoholism, homelessness, and substance abuse may predict nonadherence, although it may be difficult to detect (104). Treatment completion may be affected by the complexity and duration of therapy, side effects from medications, cultural and social conditions, access to health care, and costs of medications (44, 56). Measures to overcome failure of treatment completion include shortening the duration of treatment, intermittent drug dosing, monitoring for drug side effects, patient education, free anti-TB medication through public health programs, and enforced hospitalization (44).

From 1958 to 1978, Baltimore maintained one of the highest numbers of pulmonary TB cases in the country (45). In 1978, the Baltimore City Health Department implemented a limited program of supervised therapy for its high-risk patients, targeting the homeless, unemployed, and substance abusers (44). In 1981, as recommended by the CDC, the DOT program was expanded citywide using a community-based strategy of home visitation and treatment. Cases were identified by physician report, lab report, or through a city ordinance (authorized in 1976) that required reporting of anti-TB drugs dispensed by pharmacists.

All patients received standard anti-TB drugs endorsed by ATS/CDC, with an induction phase of 3 to 4 drugs given 5 days a week for 15 to 60 days, followed by biweekly DOT for the remainder of treatment. DOT was provided predominantly (90%) at the patients' home/workplace/school/drug treatment facility/city jail, or nursing home. Patients who regularly missed clinic appointments or were absent for the outreach nurse visit were aggressively pursued by the nurse outreach team and field investigator. If improved compliance was not achieved, legal measures were invoked in the form of commissioner's orders, involuntary hospitalization, or incarceration. As an interesting innovation, clinic staff were recruited from the affected Baltimore community.

From 1978 to 1992, while the rest of the country was experiencing an upsurge in the incidence of TB, Baltimore's rate declined by 64%. In 1981, Baltimore ranked 6th for TB; by 1992, it ranked 28th (44).

Baltimore's DOT program had a consistently high proportion of patients with documented sputum conversion after 3 months of therapy (mean 90.7%), and average annual treatment completion rate of 90% (between 1986 and 1992). Multidrug resistance remained rare, at a rate of 0.57%. Within Baltimore, the sputum conversion rate was significantly higher among DOT-managed cases than among non-DOT managed cases (p<0.05). Disease relapse rates were low, even among patients with HIV infection. Within Maryland, Baltimore accounted for 44.4% of all TB cases in 1978, compared with 28.7% in 1992 (p <0.001). These trends could not be attributed to differentials in AIDS, immigration, poverty, or unemployment (44).

In 1989, less than half the patients in New York City who began TB treatment were cured. As a first step in TB control, DOT was implemented as the standard of TB care. The Department of Health reiterated, "TB can be cured and the epidemic reversed." Treatment completion was emphasized, and a DOT program was established as both the standard of care and the primary means of completing therapy (61).

The public health infrastructure, seriously deteriorated from lack of funding and attrition, had to be rebuilt. The advocacy and leadership of nongovernmental organizations such as the American Lung Association (ALA) were instrumental in eliciting increased funding from federal, state, and local governments. A large-scale DOT program was developed through cooperation between different levels of government. The initial skepticism was overcome by involving key organizations and chiefs of departments at medical schools, and by promoting DOT as a supportive rather than a punitive act. Heavily promoted was the importance of the role of the supervised treatment program (STP) worker, once considered to be a routine, low-status job, even though patients enrolled in STP were much more likely to have continuity of treatment (61). In 1993 the department moved from selective to universal DOT. A staff of 50 to 60 outreach workers supported by 6 supervisors and a public health nurse provided DOT for 350 to 400 patients, at sites chosen by the patient. Patients received incentives in the form of a can of food supplement drink and food coupons, with extra incentive for completion of 80% of treatment every week and every month. Each community-based DOT unit had an experienced supervisor responsible for staff oversight; once a patient was found to be <80% adherent, a senior outreach worker or nurse visited the patient to identify the barriers to adherence. Treatment for latent TB infection was given to infected household contacts concurrently with DOT for the case patient. In 1993, the DOT program was extended to include patients dually infected with HIV/TB. The generous incentives that were built in assured consistent adherence of 95% to 100%.

In April 1993, the NYC health code was amended to allow the commissioner of health to require DOT to proven or suspected TB cases (30, 61); persons could be detained, even if no longer infectious, until cured, if all other alternatives had failed. This provision is in sharp contrast to the earlier STP, where enrollment and medication intake were both voluntary.

Schluger et al. (99) developed a comprehensive TB control program, with clinic-based DOT at Bellevue Hospital in New York City, an establishment serving inner-city patients often suffering from alcoholism, drug use, and HIV infection. Prior to implementation of the program, only 35% of persons discharged with a diagnosis of TB kept their clinic appointment. Patients received clinic-based DOT biweekly, with incentives and enablers. Outreach was used to track patients who missed appointments, and at least 80% of treatment was ensured. Only 11 of the 113 patients enrolled between November 1992 and July 1993 were lost to follow-up. Of the remaining 102 patients, 99% achieved bacteriologic cure. The average cost of DOT per patient was $2080.

As DOT use increased, the number of cases fell rapidly. Between 1992 and 1995, the number of cases dropped by 35% and MDR TB decreased by >75%. In an analysis of the downward trend in TB cases from 1992 to 1994 in NYC, Frieden et al. (59) found that the number of culture-confirmed cases decreased by 44% in children under 10, by 30% in adults in the 20–40-year age group, by 24% in HIV-infected individuals, and by 24% among non-Hispanic blacks. There was a 44% decrease in MDR TB cases. However, TB cases increased by 22% in the foreign born and 4% in individuals over the age of 60 years.

Similarly, in Tarrant County, TX, Weis et al. (111) described the reduction of drug resistance when DOT was implemented in their program (study period between 1980 and 1992). The DOT team consisted of community service aides, public health investigators, and nurses. DOT was provided according to patients' wishes, at their location of choice; noncompliant patients were counseled, received warning letters, and if noncompliance continued, were quarantined or hospitalized. A total of 988 cases occurred: 407 cases in the pre-DOT and 379 in the post-DOT period. Upon establishment of DOT, primary drug resistance decreased from 13% to 6.7%, acquired drug resistance decreased from 14% to 2.1%, and the relapse rate decreased from 20.9% to 5.5%. All relapses on DOT occurred with drug-susceptible organisms, and the number of relapses with multidrug-resistant organisms decreased from 25 to 5. All these differences were statistically highly significant.

In 1998, the Public Health Tuberculosis Guidance Panel published a consensus statement on DOT for TB. The panel concluded that treatment-completion rates for pulmonary tuberculosis are most likely to exceed 90%, as recommended by CDC, when treatment is based on a patient-centered approach using DOT with multiple enablers and enhancers (43).

Case Management

Patient care and public health are two parallel disciplines involved in TB care. Until early 1994, many U.S. clinics operated with the "parallel activity model" in which clinic staff provided clinical services and the department of health staff provided outreach activities. Self-administered therapy was the norm, and DOT was provided when the patient had MDR TB or did not comply with clinic visits. In effect, there was a reactive approach to failure of therapy. Synchronization between clinical and department of health activities was poor, resulting in scheduling conflicts, disruption of clinic services, and a strained relationship between the patients and health-care providers. With improved funding, many cities applied DOT, and TB rates came down.

In Newark, NJ, between 1985 and 1992, only half of the TB cases completed therapy within 12 months. In 1985, Newark ranked the third highest in TB incidence among 20 U.S. cities with a population >250,000 (77). Like the rest of the country, TB control was poor. In 1993, selective DOT was instituted at Newark's Lattimore Clinic, and the adherence rate was 62%. In 1994, 12 public health representatives were hired, and the adherence rate was 73%, a minimal improvement compared to other successful DOT programs (62). In May 1995, the nurse case–management model was implemented, whereby assessment, implementation, planning, coordination, monitoring, referral, collaboration, and evaluation of patient care were provided to ensure optimal outcome. The process of case management, a patient-oriented approach using a multidisciplinary team, allows the effective delivery of health care services to a cohort of patients according to internal organizational policies and external standards of practice. Clear objectives were set, including improved treatment completion rates to place all newly diagnosed active TB cases under DOT and achieve at least 80% DOT compliance (77). The patient's clinical, social, personal, and public health–related problems were addressed on a real-time basis. The team as a functional unit had a comprehensive picture of the patients rather than the fractured understanding within the parallel service model. Patients were educated about TB, and their knowledge was reinforced throughout. DOT was given at a mutually agreed upon time and location—be it clinic, home, workplace, street corner, McDonald's, methadone treatment program, homeless shelter, railroad station, or crack den. After implementation of the case-management model, adherence increased rapidly to 90% in 1995, and 95% in 1997, with the same personnel, interestingly. Length of treatment completion decreased from 11.6 months to 7.8 months in 1996 (77). The most important lesson to emerge from this model was accountability: "management policies should include one person accountable for each patient's treatment outcome, since DOT can work only when there is accountability for the outcome at the most basic level—service delivery" (77).

In the United States in 1996, an estimated 1200 public health outreach workers were administering DOT to TB patients. The level of funding from CDC increased from $5 million in 1986 to $114.9 million in 1995, with monies directed to improvement in lab services, national surveillance, training programs, and outreach workers. In 1996, about 75% of the outreach workers were supported by CDC grants (110).

IMPROVED INFECTION CONTROL IN THE NOSOCOMIAL SETTINGS

A study by Blumberg et al. in a university-affiliated, inner-city hospital (21) evaluated the efficacy of hospital TB infection control measures consisting primarily of administrative controls. In March 1992, the hospital expanded its infection control measures, including an expanded infection control policy. The authors studied (a) the number of TB exposure episodes (the number of patients found to have TB during admission or within 2 weeks of discharge, who were not placed on respiratory isolation on admission), and (b) the number of health-care workers who converted their TST before and after the infection control measures were strengthened (time periods: before: 7/1/91–2/29/92; after: 3/1/92–6/30/94). Measurements in the preimplementation period were taken retrospectively, and in the postimplementation period, prospectively. In the preimplementation period, respiratory isolation rooms were not working properly 16.5% of the time and the number of air exchanges were 4.9 per hour, detected by using tracer gas. Numbers for TB exposure episodes decreased from 4.4 per month in the pre- to 0.6 in the postimplementation period. The cumulative number of days per month on which potentially infectious patients were not on isolation decreased from 35.4 to 3.3 (p <0.001). Of those patients subsequently diagnosed to have TB, 95% were appropriately isolated after implementation of expanded respiratory isolation procedures. Six-month tuberculin test conversion rates among health-care workers decreased steadily from 3.3% between January and June 1992, to 0.4% between January and June 1994 (p <0.001). Patients were over-isolated; only 14% of patients placed on respiratory isolation (1 of 8) had culture-confirmed TB.

TB control efforts in NYC hospitals improved significantly from July 1992 to July 1994; there were 115 cases with epidemiologic evidence of nosocomial transmission of TB in 1991, 103 in 1992, and fewer than 30 cases in 1993 and 1994 (59). Large homeless shelters that had housed over 800 persons in single rooms in the 1980s were phased out. In the early 1990s, homeless AIDS patients were provided with noncongregate housing. This kept TB patients away from the most vulnerable group—individuals with AIDS. The number of homeless persons with tuberculosis in the computerized registry at the shelter system decreased from 748 in 1991 to 293 in 1994. Practices for screening, isolation, and follow-up of persons incarcerated at Rikers Island Correctional Facility were improved. This facility held >120,000 prisoners annually and had a daily census of >15,000, but no effective facilities for isolation. In May 1992, a communicable disease unit with effective respiratory isolation was constructed and inmates with suspected or confirmed active TB were enrolled in the DOT program. An expanded outreach program, along with the use of incentives, increased the proportion of patients who kept their follow-up appointments after their release from <20% to 92%.

Multipronged Approach by Intensification of TB Control Measures

The three priority strategies for TB prevention and control are to (*a*) identify and treat patients with active TB; (*b*) screen their close contacts for TB infection or disease and provide appropriate treatment; and (*c*) screen persons at high risk for TB infection and progression to disease and provide treatment if infected (31).

In January 1991, TB control measures were intensified in San Francisco, with the focus on prevention of transmission and the use of treatment for latent TB infection (70). From January 1991 to December 1997, the authors conducted a population-based study using a DNA fingerprinting method. TB control measures were intensified in five areas beginning in January 1991.

■ Improved contact investigation: Disease control investigators were trained in improved communications techniques with specific at-risk populations (e.g., the homeless, and substance abusers) and the criteria for determining a significant contact were broadened. The median number of contacts per new case increased from 1 in 1991, to 4 in 1995, and 3 in 1996 and 1997 (p <0.001). Approximately 80% of contacts completed a course of INH preventive therapy in each year. The number of TB cases found through contact investigation ranged from 19 to 25 per year during the study period.

■ Expanded use of DOT.

■ Development of an HIV-related TB-prevention program.

■ Screening for TB and use of preventive therapy among patients in residential care facilities, correctional institutions, and single-room occupancy hotels.

■ Improved hospital infection control measures.

The annual TB case rate fell from its peak of 51.2 in 100,000 persons in 1992 to 29.8 in 100,000 persons in 1997. The rate of clustered cases decreased significantly over time in the entire study sample: from 10.4 clustered cases per 100,000 persons in 1991 to 3.8 cases in 1997 (p <0.001). This decline was very pronounced in U.S.-born (p <0.001) and HIV-infected (p <0.003) persons. However, since this was an observational study, cause and effect could not be established, although the data suggested that the decrease in TB cases and clustering was the result of intensification of TB control measures.

McKenna et al. used case count ratios to analyze the factors associated with the decrease in TB cases in the United States in 1993 and 1994 (79). Values for case count ratios were obtained by dividing the number of incident cases reported in 1993–1994 by the number of cases reported in 1991–1992. The smallest case count ratio (i.e., the highest reduction in cases) was observed for areas with the highest AIDS incidence. There was no evidence of a definite trend in the magnitude of the change in case counts with increasing levels of poverty. The largest decreases in U.S.-born cases generally occurred in areas reporting greater increases in treatment completion, sputum conversion, and number of contacts per person. The steep decline in areas with high AIDS rates indicates that measures to control recent transmission were the primary determinants of decreased TB incidence in these areas.

Although these factors have been shown to cause reductions in the number of TB cases, other factors whose significance often cannot be measured are equally important in our opinion. The TB surveillance system implemented and continuously updated by the CDC has led to the early recognition of increased numbers of cases, their geographic locations, the connection between the TB and AIDS epidemics, and the recognition of a higher proportion of TB incidence among minorities and the foreign born. Laboratory services for TB microbiology have improved considerably, and drug-susceptibility tests are now performed routinely on the initial isolates. As of 1993, CDC has also funded three national TB centers to provide intensive training, education, and consultation to TB care providers in the United States and abroad. The TB training initiative, which began in 1989 (89), has led to the publication of *The Core Curriculum for Tuberculosis* available free of cost to health-care providers; it is updated periodically, and its fourth edition was published in the year 2000.

THE FUTURE

The Advisory Council for Elimination of TB (ACET) has proposed the goal of TB elimination in the United States by the year 2010 (28). Elimination of tuberculosis in the United States will require sustained effort to preserve and strengthen current TB control activities (67). As the number of cases decrease, manpower dedicated to TB will be curtailed in states with low TB incidence, risking delay in diagnosis of an outbreak. An outbreak lasting for 8 years was recently reported from Kansas (36), a state with a TB incidence of 2.9 cases/100,000 in 1999 (33). To forestall such occurrences, the CDC and the Institute of Medicine recommend that the states have adequate fallback resources in case of an outbreak. An Outbreak Response Plan was recently implemented by the CDC (38). Improvements in serological and molecular diagnostic techniques may help in the rapid recognition of contacts before an outbreak occurs (71, 75).

Since a growing proportion of cases in the U.S.-born is occurring among the homeless and drug users, contact investigations are increasingly shifting periph-erally from clinics and hospitals to homeless shelters and crack dens (12, 20, 38). The nature and lifestyle of these populations, with their complex social networks, present a challenge to implementing effective TB control activities.

As the number of cases shrinks so too will expertise in diagnosing and manag-ing TB (22). There have been missed opportunities for TB prevention, delays in diagnosis, deficiencies in provider knowledge, and a lack of adherence to published guidelines for TB treatment and infection control (82). A major training-related initiative of the three model TB centers in collaboration with the Division of TB Elimination of the CDC is the Strategic Plan for TB Training and Education. This educational plan targets providers involved in the diagnosis and management of persons at high risk for TB infection and progression to disease once infected with *M. tb*, e.g., HIV-infected persons, homeless persons, injection-drug users, nationals of countries with high TB prevalence, prison/jail inmates, and elderly individu-als in congregate settings (82). Children of foreign-born individuals in whom TB is often missed should also be included in this category (51, 76).

While the number of TB cases has declined overall, the proportion of TB cases in the foreign born continues to increase; approximately 46% of all TB cases in the United States in 2000 were among the foreign born. In 1999, the four states that border Mexico (Arizona, Texas, California, and New Mexico) accounted for almost one third of the total TB cases reported, 50% reported TB cases among the foreign born, and 72% of TB cases reported among those born in Mexico (40). Consequently, tuberculosis elimination in the United States is impossible unless TB can be reduced in those born outside its borders. To this end, both the

ACET and the Institute of Medicine recommend U.S. involvement in global TB control measures to reduce the total reservoir of TB worldwide (28, 32, 67). Sorely needed is development of an effective vaccine against TB. Successful control or elimination of other major infectious diseases such as smallpox, poliomyelitis, and measles was accomplished through effective vaccination. The National Institute of Health developed a blueprint for tuberculosis vaccine development in 1998. Development of the vaccine is estimated to cost $800 million and will likely take up to 20–50 years (9).

Over 90% of TB cases—many of which are MDR TB—occur in developing nations, which lack the resources to assume this financial burden. New classes of anti-TB drugs are urgently needed. Less than 1% of all drugs approved for marketing in the past 20 years are for infectious diseases in developing countries (86); this is due partly to lack of financial incentives (91) and partly to the complexity of clinical development of anti-TB drugs. Because no new anti-TB drugs have been developed since the rifamycins in the late-1960s, there are no well-defined, standardized, regulatory requirements. In February 2000, a global alliance for TB drug development was formed in a partnership between the public and private sectors. The Rockefeller Foundation, WHO, CDC, the World Bank, the NIH, the Wellcome Trust, and the Bill and Melinda Gates Foundation are all participating (86, 95). Recently, the *M. tb* genome was sequenced (47), a breakthrough that it is hoped will promote major advances in the development of a vaccine and new classes of drugs.

The increased penetration of managed care in the United States has had serious consequences for the public sector. In 1995, 50% of patient care received for TB was provided partly or fully by the private sector whereas now almost one fourth of all TB cases are enrolled in managed care programs (80). There is some optimism that the managed care environment could lead to better management practices based on standards of care. On the other hand, because managed care organizations emphasize cost control and assume responsibility only for the enrolled members, crucial but less visible and thus less well-understood TB control activities such as contact investigations and DOT may well be neglected. In addition, the high patient turnover rate in managed care organizations creates the risk of their treatment being interrupted when patients leave and of losing them to follow-up.

Rapid diagnostic tests with better sensitivity and specificity are needed to diagnose TB disease and latent TB infection. Moreover, latency in *M. tb* is poorly understood. What causes *M. tb* to reactivate at a later date and why does the host allow *M. tb* to stay dormant instead of eliminating it? These are topics of intense research interest (58) and their elucidation may help in developing an effective TB vaccine and other therapies to enhance the host immune system. Research is also needed in human behavior, effective communication techniques with hard-to-reach and follow-up patients, and measures to improve patient acceptance of and adherence to medical care and treatment regimens.

Underlying these recommendations is the urgent need for financial and political commitment. Chaulk et al. calculated that without DOT there would have been an excess of 1577 to 2233 TB cases in Baltimore, at a cost of between $18.8 to $27.1 million. They proposed that the savings garnered from the operation of DOT be reinvested to support effective TB control programs (42). Nolan, using the same logic, calculated the savings from averting the need for TB treatment in the United States between 1993–1998 at $1.7 billion. These savings could easily cover the cost of development of a new TB vaccine ($0.8 billion), the endowment of a global TB fund ($0.5 billion), and could fund the annual operation of the International Union Against Tuberculosis (IUALTD) for 45 years! (85). The excess health care cost incurred in controlling the MDR-TB outbreak in New York City alone was estimated at $1 billion.

In centuries past, an estimated 1 in 5 adults died of tuberculosis, and 1 billion deaths between 1850 and 1950 are thought to be attributable to TB (93). The past 100 years, however, have seen significant advances in the concepts, diagnosis, and management of tuberculosis, from Robert Koch's discovery of the tubercle bacillus during the nineteenth century to sequencing its genome during the twentieth. We have enough understanding of the disease and adequate resources in the United States to eliminate tuberculosis. Nevertheless, epidemics of tuberculosis continue to recur. The United States has witnessed a record low number of TB cases in the twenty-first century (39). At the same time as the number of TB cases has fallen, the basic factors underlying its increase in the late 1980s, homelessness, drug addiction, HIV, immigration from foreign countries with high TB prevalence, and most important, deteriorated public health infrastructure, still persist (83). To maintain the downward trend and ultimately achieve TB elimination, these socioeconomic problems must be addressed, and simultaneously, political will and financial commitment must be secured. Our enemy, *M. tuberculosis*, is an extremely successful human pathogen that has been with us for over 3000 years; it will be ready for us, if we lose our guard!

Visit the Annual Reviews home page at www.annualreviews.org

LITERATURE CITED

1. Addington WW. 1979. Patient compliance: the most serious remaining problem in the control of tuberculosis in the United States. *Chest* 76 (Suppl.):741–43

2. Advisory Counc. Elimin. Tuberc. 1993. Initial therapy for tuberculosis in the era of multidrug resistance: recommendations of the Advisory Council for Elimination of Tuberculosis. *MMWR* 42:RR-7

3. Alland D, Kalkut GE, Moss AR, McAdam RA, Hahn JA, et al. 1994. Transmission of tuberculosis in New York City. An analysis by DNA fingerprinting

and conventional epidemiologic methods. *N. Engl. J. Med.* 330:1710–16

4. Am. Thorac. Soc. 1980. Guidelines for short-course tuberculosis chemotherapy. *Am. Rev. Respir. Dis.* 212:611–14

5. Am. Thorac. Soc. 2000. Diagnostic standards and classification of tuberculosis in adults and children. *Am. J. Respir. Crit. Care Med.* 161:1376–95

6. Am. Thorac. Soc. and Cent. Dis. Control. 1994. Treatment of tuberculosis infection in adults and children. *Am. J. Respir. Crit. Care Med.* 149:1359–74

7. Annas GJ. 1993. Control of tuberculosis—the law and the public health. *N. Engl. J. Med.* 328:585–88

8. Anonymous. 1997. Rapid diagnostic tests for tuberculosis. What is the appropriate use? Am. Thorac. Soc. Workshop. *Am. J. Respir. Crit. Care Med.* 155:1804–14

9. Anonymous. 1998. *Blueprint for tuberculosis vaccine development* [Report of a workshop]. Rockville, MD: Natl. Inst. Health, Natl. Inst. Allergy Infect. Dis.

10. Anonymous. 2000. Tuberculosis. In *Control of Communicable Diseases Manual*, ed. J Chin, pp. 521–30. Washington, DC: Am. Public Health Assoc.

11. Barnes PF, El-Hajj H, Preston-Martin S, Cave MD, Jones BE, et al. 1996. Transmission of tuberculosis among the urban homeless. *JAMA* 275:305–7

12. Barnes PF, Yang Z, Preston-Martin S. 1997. Patterns of tuberculosis transmission in central Los Angeles. *JAMA* 278:1159–63

13. Bass JB Jr. 1993. The tuberculin test. In *Tuberculosis: A Comprehensive International Approach*, ed. LB Reichman, ES Hershfield, pp. 139–48. New York: Marcel-Dekker. 1st ed.

14. Bauer J, Thomsen VO, Poulsen S, Anderson AB. 1997. False-positive results from cultures of *Mycobacterium tuberculosis* due to laboratory cross-contamination confirmed by restriction fragment length polymorphism. *J. Clin. Microbiol.* 35:988–91

15. Bayer R, Wilkinson D. 1995. Directly observed therapy for tuberculosis: history of an idea. *Lancet* 345:1545–48

16. Beck-Sague C, Dooley SW, Hutton MD, Otten J, Breeden A, et al. 1992. Hospital outbreak of multidrug-resistant *Mycobacterium tuberculosis* infections: factors in transmission to staff and HIV-infected patients. *JAMA* 268:1280–86

17. Behr MA, Small PM. 1997. Molecular fingerprinting of *Mycobacterium tuberculosis*: How can it help the clinician? *Clin. Infect. Dis.* 25:806–10

18. Behr MA, Warren SA, Salamon H, Hopewell PC, Ponce de Leon A, et al. 1999. Transmission of *Mycobacterium tuberculosis* from patients smear negative for acid fast bacilli. *Lancet* 353:444–49

19. Bifani P, Mathema B, Liu Z, Moghazeh SL, Shopsin B, et al. 1999. Identification of a W variant of *Mycobacterium tuberculosis* via population-based molecular epidemiology. *JAMA* 282:2321–27

20. Bishai WR, Graham NMH, Harrington S, Pope DS, Hooper N, et al. 1998. Molecular and geographic patterns of tuberculosis transmission after 15 years of directly observed therapy. *JAMA* 280:1679–84

21. Blumberg HM, Watkins DL, Berschling JD, Antley A, Moore P, et al. 1995. Preventing the nosocomial transmission of tuberculosis. *Ann. Intern. Med.* 122:658–63

22. Broekmans JF. 2000. Tuberculosis control in low prevalence countries. See Ref. 95a, pp. 75–93

23. Brudney K, Dobkin J. 1991. Resurgent tuberculosis in New York City. *Am. Rev. Respir. Dis.* 144:745–49

24. Burman WJ, Reves RR, Hawkes AP, Rietmeijer CA, Xang Z, et al. 1997. DNA fingerprinting with two probes decreases clustering of *Mycobacterium tuberculosis*. *Am. J. Respir. Crit. Care Med.* 155:1140–46

25. Burwen DR, Bloch AB, Griffin LD, Ciesieleski CA, Stern HA, et al. 1995. National trends in the concurrence of tuberculosis and acquired immunodeficiency syndrome. *Arch. Intern. Med.* 155:1281–86

26. Cantwell MF, McKenna MT, McCray E, Onorato IM. 1998. Tuberculosis and race/ethnicity in the United States: impact of socioeconomic status. *Am. J. Respir. Crit. Care Med.* 157:1016–20

27. Catanzaro A, Perry S, Clarridge JE,

Dunbar S, Goodnight-White S, et al. 2000. The role of clinical suspicion in evaluating a new diagnostic test for active tuberculosis: results of a multicenter prospective trial. *JAMA* 283:639–45

28. Cent. Dis. Control Prev. 1989. A strategic plan for the elimination of tuberculosis in the United States. *MMWR* 38(S-13):1–25

29. Cent. Dis. Control Prev. 1991. Nosocomial transmission of multidrug-resistant tuberculosis among HIV-infected persons—Florida and New York, 1988–1991. *MMWR* 40:585–91

30. Cent. Dis. Control Prev. 1993. Tuberculosis control laws—United States 1993; Recommendations of the Advisory Council for the Elimination of Tuberculosis (ACET). *MMWR* 42 (RR-15): 1–15

31. Cent. Dis. Control Prev. 1995. Essential components of a tuberculosis prevention and control program. Recommendations of the Advisory Council for the Elimination of Tuberculosis. *MMWR* 44 (RR-11):1–16

32. Cent. Dis. Control Prev. 1999. Tuberculosis elimination revisited: obstacles, opportunities, and a renewed commitment: recommendations of the Advisory Council for Elimination of Tuberculosis (ACET). *MMWR* 48 (RR-9):1–13

33. Cent. Dis. Control Prev. 2000. Reported tuberculosis in the United States, 1999. www.cdc.gov/nhstp/tb/surv/surv99/surv99.htm

34. Cent. Dis. Control Prev. 2000. Targeted tuberculin testing and treatment of latent tuberculosis infection. *MMWR* 49 (RR-6):1–43

35. Cent. Dis. Control Prev. 2000. Update: nucleic acid amplification tests for tuberculosis. *MMWR* 49:593–94

36. Cent. Dis. Control Prev. 2001. Cluster of tuberculosis cases among exotic dancers and their close contacts—Kansas, 1994–2000. *MMWR* 50:291–93

37. Cent. Dis. Control Prev. 2001. Fatal and severe hepatitis associated with rifampin and pyrazinamide for the treatment of latent tuberculosis infection—New York and Georgia, 2000. *MMWR* 289–91

37a. Cent. Dis. Control Prev. 2001. Fatal and severe liver injuries associated with rifampin and pyrazinamide for latent tuberculosis infection, and revisions in American Thoracic Society/CDC recommendations—United States. *MMWR* 50(34):733–35

38. Cent. Dis. Control Prev. 2001. *National Center for HIV, STD and TB Prevention. NCHSTP program briefing.* 57–74. www.cdc.gov.nchstp.od/program_brief_2001/default/htm

39. Cent. Dis. Control Prev. 2001. *Reported tuberculosis in the United States, 2000.* www.cdc.gov/nchstp/tb/surv/surv2000/

40. Cent. Dis. Control Prev. Performance Plan. 2001. *Tuberculosis prevention and control.* 107–15. www.cdc.gov/od/perfplan/2001perfplan.pdf

41. Chan ED, Heifets L, Iseman MD. 2000. Immunologic diagnosis of tuberculosis: a review. *Tuberc. Lung. Dis.* 80:131–40

42. Chaulk CP, Friedman M, Dunning R. 2000. Modeling the epidemiology and economics of directly observed therapy in Baltimore. *Int. J. Tuberc. Lung. Dis.* 4: 201–7

43. Chaulk CP, Kazandjian VA. 1998. Directly observed therapy for treatment completion of pulmonary tuberculosis. *JAMA* 279:943–48

44. Chaulk CP, Moore-Rice K, Rizzo R, Chaisson RE. 1995. Eleven years of community-based directly observed therapy for tuberculosis. *JAMA* 274:945–51

45. Chaulk CP, Pope DS. 1997. The Baltimore City Health department program of directly observed therapy for tuberculosis. *Clin. Chest Med.* 18:149–54

46. Cohn DL, Catlin BJ, Peterson KL, Judson FN, Sbarboro JA. 1990. A 52 dose, 6-month therapy for pulmonary and extrapulmonary tuberculosis: a twice weekly,

directly observed, and cost-effective regimen. *Ann. Intern. Med.* 112:407–15

47. Cole ST, Brosch R, Parkhill J, Garnier T, Churcher C, et al. 1998. Deciphering the biology of *Mycobacterium tuberculosis* from the complete genome sequence. *Nature* 393:537–44

48. Cole ST, Telenti A. 1995. Drug resistance in *Mycobacterium tuberculosis.* *Eur. Respir. J.* 8(Suppl. 20):701s–13

49. Combs DL, O'Brien RJ, Geiter LJ. 1990. USPHS Tuberculosis Short-Course Chemotherapy Trial 21: effectiveness, toxicity and acceptability: the report of final results. *Ann. Intern. Med.* 112:397–406

50. Comstock GW. 1974. The prognosis of a positive tuberculin reaction in childhood and adolescence. *Am. J. Epidemiol.* 99:131–38

51. Curtis AB, Rizdon R, Vogel R, McDonough S, Hargreaves J. 1999. Extensive transmission of *Mycobacterium tuberculosis* from a child. *N. Engl. J. Med.* 341:1491–95

52. Daley CL, Small PM, Schecter GF, Schoolnik GK, McAdam RA, et al. 1992. An outbreak of tuberculosis with accelerated progression among persons infected with the human immunodeficiency virus. *N. Engl. J. Med.* 326:231–35

53. Dannenberg AM. 2000. Pathophysiology: basic aspects. In *Tuberculosis and Non-Tuberculous Mycobacterial Infections,* ed. D Schlossberg, pp. 17–47. New York: Saunders

54. De Cock KM, Chaisson RE. 1999. Will DOTS do it? A reappraisal of tuberculosis control in countries with high rates of HIV infection. *Int. J. Tuberc. Lung. Dis.* 3:457–65

55. Diperri G, Cruciani M, Danzi MC, Luzzati R, De Chechni G, et al. 1989. Nosocomial epidemic of active tuberculosis among HIV-infected patients. *Lancet* 2:1502–4

56. Dudley DL. 1979. Why patients don't take pills. *Chest* 76 (Suppl.):744–49

57. Edlin BR, Tokars JI, Grieco MH, Crawford JT, Williams J, et al. 1992. An outbreak of multidrug-resistant tuberculosis among hospitalized patients with the acquired immunodeficiency syndrome. *N. Engl. J. Med.* 326:1514–21

58. Flynn JA, Chan J. 2001. Tuberculosis: latency and reactivation. *Infect. Immun.* 69:4195–201

59. Frieden TR, Fujiwara PI, Washko RM, Hamburg MA. 1995. Tuberculosis in New York City—turning the tide. *N. Engl. J. Med.* 333:229–33

60. Frieden TR, Sherman LF, Maw KL, Fujiwara P, Crawford J, et al. A multi-institutional outbreak of highly drug-resistant tuberculosis: epidemiology and clinical outcomes. *JAMA* 276:1229–35

61. Fujiwara PI, Larkin C, Frieden TR. 1997. Directly observed therapy in New York City: history, implementation, results and challenges. *Clin. Chest Med.* 18:135–48

62. Galanowsky K, Napolitano E, Wolman M, Timmer G, McDonald RJ, et al. 1996. Directly observed therapy (DOT) is not the entire answer. *Am. J. Respir. Crit. Care Med.* 153(4):A491

63. Genewein A, Talenti A, Bernasconi C, Weiss S, Maurer A, et al. 1993. Molecular approaches to identifying route of transmission of tuberculosis in the community. *Lancet* 342:841–44

64. Glynn JR, Bauer J, de Boer AS, Borgdorff MW, Fine PEM, et al. 1999. Interpreting DNA fingerprint clusters of *Mycobacterium tuberculosis.* *Int. J. Tuberc. Lung. Dis.* 3:1055–60

65. Hayward AC, Watson JM. 1998. Typing of mycobacteria using spoligotyping. *Thorax* 53:329–30

66. Deleted in proof

67. Inst. Med. 2000. *Ending Neglect: The Elimination of Tuberculosis in the United States.* Washington, DC: Natl. Acad. Press

68. Iseman MD. 1993. Treatment of multidrug-resistant tuberculosis. *N. Engl. J. Med.* 329:784–91

69. Jacobs WR Jr, Barletta RG, Udani R, Chan J, Kalkut G, et al. 1993. Rapid assessment of drug susceptibilities of *Mycobacterium tuberculosis* by means of a luciferase reporter phage. *Science* 260:819–22

70. Jasmer RM, Hahn JA, Small PM, Daley CL, Behr MA, et al. 1999. A molecular epidemiologic analysis of tuberculosis trends in San Francisco, 1991–1997. *Ann. Intern. Med.* 130:971–78

71. Kamerbeek J, Schouls L, Kolk A, van Agterveld M, van Soolingen D, et al. 1997. Simultaneous detection and strain differentiation of *Mycobacterium tuberculosis* for diagnosis and epidemiology. *J. Clin. Microbiol.* 35:907–14

72. Kim SJ, Hong YP. 1992. Drug resistance of *Mycobacterium tuberculosis* in Korea. *Tuberc. Lung. Dis.* 73:219–22

73. Kline SE, Hedemark LL, Davies SF. 1995. Outbreak of tuberculosis among regular patrons of a neighborhood bar. *N. Engl. J. Med.* 333:222–27

74. Kochi A, Vareldzis B, Styblo K. 1993. Multidrug-resistant tuberculosis and its control. *Res. Microbiol.* 144:104–10

75. Lalvani A, Pathan AA, Durkan H, Wilkinson KA, Whelan A, et al. 2001. Enhanced contact tracing and special tracking of *Mycobacterium tuberculosis* infection by enumeration of antigen-specific T cells. *Lancet* 357:2017–21

76. Lobato MN, Mohle-Boetani JC, Royce SE. 2000. Missed opportunities for preventing tuberculosis among children less than 5 years of age. *Pediatrics* 106(6): PE75

77. Mangura BT, Galanowsky KE. Case Management: 2000. The key to successful tuberculosis control program. See Ref. 95a, pp. 597–606

78. McDonald RJ, Memon AM, Reichman LB. 1982. Successful supervised ambulatory management of tuberculosis treatment failures. *Ann. Intern. Med.* 96:297–303

79. McKenna MT, McCray E, Jones JL, Onorato IM, Castro KG. 1998. The fall after the rise: tuberculosis in the United States, 1991 through 1994. *Am. J. Public Health* 88:1059–63

80. Miller B, Rosenbaum S. 2000. The impact of managed care on tuberculosis control in the United States. See Ref. 95a, pp. 817–27

81. Mitchison DA. 1984. Drug resistance in *Mycobacteria. Br. Med. Bull.* 40:84–90

82. Napolitano EC, Stoller EJ. 2000. Tuberculosis education. See Ref. 95a, pp. 705–25

83. Nardell EA, Brickner PW. 1996. Tuberculosis in New York City: focal transmission of an often fatal disease. *JAMA* 276:1259–60

84. Natl. Tuberc. Assoc. and US Public Health Serv. Tuberc. Progr. 1961. *The Arden House Conference on Tuberculosis 1960.* Washington, DC: US GPO. DHEW Public Health Service Publ. ML 784

85. Nolan CM. 2000. The fruits of the labor: reinvesting the savings from good tuberculosis control in the United States. *Int. J. Tuberc. Lung Dis.* 4:191–92

86. O'Brien RJ, Vernon AA. 1998. New tuberculosis drug development. How can we do better? *Am. J. Respir. Crit. Care Med.* 157:1705–7

87. Pfyffer GE, Auckenthaler R, van Embden JDA, Van Soolingen D. 1998. *Mycobacterium canettii*, the smooth variant of *M. tuberculosis*, isolated from a Swiss patient exposed in Africa. *Emerg. Infect. Dis.* 4:631–34

88. Raviglione MC, Snider DE Jr, Kochi A. 1995. Global epidemiology of tuberculosis. Morbidity and mortality of a worldwide epidemic. *JAMA* 273:220–26

89. Reichman LB. 1989. The National Tuberculosis Training Initiative. *Ann. Intern. Med.* 111:197–98

90. Reichman LB. 1991. The U-shaped

curve of concern. *Am. Rev. Respir. Dis.* 144:741–42

91. Reichman LB. 1996. How to ensure the continued resurgence of tuberculosis. *Lancet* 347:175–77

92. Reichman LB. 1997. Defending the public's health against tuberculosis. *JAMA* 278:865–67

93. Reichman LB. 1997. Tuberculosis elimination—what's to stop us? *J. Tuberc. Lung. Dis.* 1:3–11

94. Reichman LB. 2000. The 2000 Simon Robard Memorial Lecture: Diffusing the Time-bomb. Speech presented at ACCP Convention, San Francisco

95. Reichman LB, Fanning A. 2001. Drug development for TB: the missing ingredient. *Lancet* 357:236

95a. Reichman LB, Hershfield ES, eds. 2000. *Tuberculosis: A Comprehensive International Approach.* New York: Marcel-Dekker. 2nd. ed.

96. Ridzon R, Whitney CG, McKenna MT, Taylor JP, Ashkar SH, et al. 1998. Risk factors for rifampin monoresistant tuberculosis. *Am. J. Respir. Crit. Care Med.* 157:1881–84

97. Sbarboro JA. 1980. Public health aspect of tuberculosis: supervision of therapy. *Clin. Chest Med.* 1:253–63

98. Sbarboro JA, Johnson S. 1968. Tuberculosis chemotherapy for recalcitrant outpatients administered directly twice weekly. *Am. Rev. Respir. Dis.* 97:895–903

99. Schluger N, Ciotoli C, Cohen D, Johnson H, Rom WM. 1995. Comprehensive tuberculosis control for patients at high risk for noncompliance. *Am. J. Respir. Crit. Care Med.* 151:1486–90

100. Selwyn PA, Hartel D, Lewis VA, Schoenbaume EE, Vermund SH, et al. 1989. A prospective study of the risk of tuberculosis among intravenous drug users with Human Immunodeficiency Virus infection. *N. Engl. J. Med.* 320:545–50

101. Small PM, Hopewell PC, Singh SP, Paz A, Parsonnet J, et al. 1994. The epidemiology of tuberculosis in San Francisco: a population based study using conventional and molecular methods. *N. Engl. J. Med.* 330:1703–9

102. Small PM, Shafer RW, Hopewell PC, Singh SP, Murphy MJ, et al. 1999. Exogenous reinfection with multi-drug-resistant tuberculosis in patients with advanced HIV infection. *N. Engl. J. Med.* 328:1137–44

103. Styblo K. 1990. The elimination of tuberculosis in the Netherlands. *Bull. Int. Un. Tuberc.* 65:49–55

103a. Subcomm. Public Health and Gov. Comm. Interstate For. Commerce. 1972. *Hearing on HR 14030.* April 27, pp. 71–75, 89–91. Washington, DC: US GPO

104. Sumartojo E. 1993. When tuberculosis treatment fails: a social behavioral account of patient adherence. *Am. Rev. Respir. Dis.* 147:1311–20

105. Telenti A, Imboden P, Marchesi F, Lowrie D, Cole S, et al. 1993. Detection of rifampicin resistant mutations in *Mycobacterium tuberculosis. Lancet* 341:647–50

106. US Congress, Off. Technol. Assess. 1993. *The Continuing Challenge of Tuberculosis.* OTR H574. Washington, DC: US GPO. 91–106

107. Valway S, Richards SB, Kovacovich J, Greilinger RB, Crawford JT, Dooley SW. 1994. Outbreak of multi-drug-resistant tuberculosis in a New York State prison. *Am. J. Public Health* 140:113–22

108. Van Embden JDA, Cave MD, Crawford JT, Dale JW, Eisenach KD, et al. 1993. Strain identification of *Mycobacterium tuberculosis* by DNA fingerprinting: recommendations for a standardized methodology. *J. Clin. Microbiol.* 31:406–9

109. Van Rie A, Warren R, Richardson M, Victor TC, Gie RP, et al. 1999. Exogenous reinfection as a cause of recurrent tuberculosis after curative treatment. *N. Engl. J. Med.* 341:1174–79

110. Voelker R. 1996. 'Shoe-leather therapy'

is gaining on TB. *JAMA* 275:743–44

111. Weis SE, Slocum PC, Blais FX, King B, Nunn M, et al. 1994. The effect of directly observed therapy on the rates of drug resistance and relapse in tuberculosis. *N. Engl. J. Med.* 330:1179–84

112. Yew WW, Chau CH. 1995. Drug-resistant tuberculosis in the 1990s. *Eur. Respir. J.* 8:1184–92

Annu. Rev. Public Health 2002. 23:427–48

THE FUTURE OF BENEFIT-COST ANALYSES OF THE CLEAN AIR ACT

Alan Krupnick and Richard Morgenstern

Resources for the Future, 1616 P St. NW, Washington, DC 20036;
e-mail: krupnick@rff.org; morgenst@rff.org

Key Words

■ **Abstract** This review examines the first two studies conducted pursuant to a Congressional mandate that the U.S. Environmental Protection Agency analyze the effects of the Clean Air Act on the "public health, economy, and the environment of the United States." While these studies indicate that overall, the nation received good value for the resources it invested in improving air quality over the past three decades, we don't know if even higher value could have been obtained by changing or eliminating certain potentially inefficient elements. The review focuses on the critical policy and technical choices made in the analyses, including the selection of the appropriate baseline and the level of disaggregation for the studies. It is proposed that a potential third analysis focus on potential new policies not yet mandated by law or regulation. It is also proposed that the next study fill in key information gaps, expand the benefit categories, and incorporate new research on topics such as mortality and morbidity benefits, cost uncertainties, and others.

INTRODUCTION

Since the Clean Air Act (CAA) was enacted in 1970, critics have repeatedly questioned whether the health and environmental benefits of air pollution control justify the costs incurred by industry, taxpayers, and consumers. Until Congress added Section 812 to the 1990 CAA Amendments, a requirement that the U.S. Environmental Protection Agency (EPA) conduct periodic, scientifically reviewed studies on the effects of the CAA on the "public health, economy, and the environment of the United States," there was not a specific mandate for the Agency to compare the overall benefits of the CAA with the costs imposed on society. The resulting studies, *The Benefits and Costs of the Clean Air Act: 1970 to 1990* (29) and *The Benefits and Costs of the Clean Air Act, 1990 to 2010* (31), are widely seen as the "gold standard" of benefit-cost studies conducted by government, both in the United States and abroad. Under the auspices of the Advisory Committee for Clean Air Compliance Analysis (ACCACA), operating under the charter of the EPA's Science Advisory Board, both studies were scrutinized throughout the decade-long preparation by at least three expert committees of outside economists, air quality modelers, epidemiologists, and other health experts. They are probably the most intensive and expensive benefit-cost analyses ever conducted at the EPA.

Notwithstanding the many assumptions needed to address such a broad legislative mandate, the results of the analyses are clear: Overall, the nation has received high returns on its investment in improved air quality over the past three decades. For the early years benefits are estimated to exceed costs by an order of magnitude. Prospectively, benefits still exceed costs, although by a smaller margin.

Particularly because the analyses were conducted at such a highly aggregate level, it is possible that the overall results reflect large gains from only a few programs within the CAA. Indeed, the overall finding of large net benefits may be masking ineffective or inefficient programs or regulations carried out under some titles of the CAA. In addition, many of the technical choices made in these studies involve important methodological issues about which experts differ. Understanding these issues is crucial to interpreting the overall findings. Currently, the EPA and one of its expert committees are meeting to consider the need for and the appropriate focus of a second prospective study. In contrast to the first two studies, the EPA has considerably greater latitude in defining the scope of such an analysis. Arguably, little would be gained by simply updating the existing studies with the same focus and methods used previously.

The overall goal of this review is to elucidate the results of the first two studies, including a critical examination of the policy and technical choices made in the analyses, and to highlight areas for improvement in a potential second prospective study. With this, the reader will develop some perspective on the practice and pitfalls of cost-benefit analysis as practiced by the government, as well as a better understanding of the net benefits to society of the CAA.

This review emphasizes the disaggregation issue and areas where specific methodological choices could make a significant difference to the outcome. One additional attractive option discussed involves focusing the next study on a set of specific policy issues that have the potential to increase the net benefits of the CAA in the decades to come.

The next section describes the basic methods and results of both the prospective and the retrospective studies. Particular attention is paid to the baseline and aggregation issues. The third section considers alternative foci for a new prospective study, including the option of focusing on the key policy challenges likely to be considered in coming years. The fourth section considers a wide range of technical and methodological issues including the need to fill in key information gaps, expand the benefit categories, and incorporate new research on topics such as mortality and morbidity benefits, cost uncertainties, and others. The last section draws overall conclusions and recommendations.

METHODS AND RESULTS OF RETROSPECTIVE
AND PROSPECTIVE STUDIES

The EPA's retrospective and prospective studies were designed to examine a specific set of policies that had been enacted by Congress since 1970 and implemented by the EPA. The retrospective analysis focused on air quality policies and regulations put in place from 1970–1990, and the prospective study addressed provisions added in the 1990 CAA Amendments. Both studies were conducted at a highly aggregate, economy-wide level. The retrospective study did not estimate either the benefits or the costs of individual regulations, pollutants, or any subcategories (e.g., stationary versus mobile sources) of the federal air pollution program. The prospective study estimated costs but not benefits by title of the CAA Amendments.

From a policy perspective, an analysis of total benefits and total costs represents a very simple approach to a complex issue. Arguably, few propose abandoning all federal air pollution control. The more policy-relevant question concerns the benefits and costs of individual regulations and, even more relevant, the benefits and costs of marginal changes to individual regulations. The principal rationale offered by the EPA for this highly aggregate analysis is that whereas costs can be reliably attributed to individual regulations or programs, the broad-scale methodology used for the benefits analysis precludes reliable estimation of the benefits by regulation or program, especially because some pollutants, e.g., nitrogen oxides (NO_x), show up in multiple titles. This has been a highly controversial issue throughout these studies and remains so in the design of any new analysis. Indeed, the EPA's own Regulatory Impact Analyses for Ozone and Particulate Matter disaggregates the benefits of controlling these pollutants, although not by CAA Title.[1]

In both the retrospective and the prospective studies the EPA analyzed air pollution programs by comparing specific policy and baseline scenarios. The retrospective study contrasted a scenario reflecting historical economic and environmental conditions observed with the CAA in place with a hypothetical scenario that projects the economic and environmental conditions that would have existed assuming that the stringency and effectiveness of air pollution control technologies were frozen at their 1970 levels. In the prospective study all rules promulgated or expected to be promulgated pursuant to the 1990 CAA were contrasted to a scenario that essentially freezes federal, state, and local air pollution controls at the levels of stringency and effectiveness prevailing in 1990. Both studies hold constant the geographic distributions of populations and economic activities across the scenarios.[2]

---

[1] In addition, work by Smith & Ross (27) contains an analysis in which the Section 812 study results and other information is processed into a title by pollutant cost-benefit analysis.

[2] Although the scenarios do reflect the basic trends in population and economic growth across the country over the relevant time periods, they do not allow for the possibility that people would respond to pollution by moving away from the dirtiest areas.

The frozen technology assumption—an obvious simplification—is central to the overall results. Arguably, in the absence of new federal regulation, one would expect to see some air pollution abatement activity, owing to state or local regulation or, possibly, on a voluntary basis. As Davies (9) has reported, nonfederal air pollution efforts date back to 1881 when the city of Chicago adopted an ordinance that declared that "the emission of dense smoke from the smokestack of any boat or locomotive or from any chimney anywhere within the city shall be . . . a public nuisance." More recently, some states have imposed particularly stringent controls in some areas, e.g., California. If one assumed that state and local regulations would have been equivalent to federal regulations, then a benefit-cost analysis of the federal CAA would be a meaningless exercise: Both benefits and costs would equal zero. For both studies, the EPA and the outside experts wrestled with the possibility of developing more realistic baseline scenarios. In the end they decided that any attempt to predict how states' and localities' regulations or voluntary efforts would have differed from the CAA is too speculative.

Each of the two (aggregate) scenarios is evaluated by a sequence of economic, emissions, air quality, physical effect, economic valuation, and uncertainty models to measure the differences between the scenarios in economic, human health, and environmental outcomes. Both studies examine the benefits and costs of reducing volatile organic compounds, nitrogen oxides (NO_x), sulphur dioxide (SO_2), carbon monoxide (CO), coarse particulate matter (PM_{10}), and fine particulate matter ($PM_{2.5}$).[3] The retrospective analysis assessed the effect of CAA provisions governing lead in the environment. However, because the 1990 Amendments do not include new provisions for the control of lead, it is not considered in the prospective analysis.

Although both studies attempt broad coverage, there are some notable omissions, largely because of data or modeling limitations. Emissions of hazardous air pollutants are not extensively considered in either study.[4] Recent revisions to the particulate matter and ozone ambient standards are also omitted from the prospective study, although the EPA analysis indicates that because of similarities in the baseline assumptions, the benefits and costs reported in the Regulatory Impact

---

[3]Although the incremental effects of the CAA Amendments on primary particulate matter emissions are relatively small, particulate matter in the atmosphere is comprised of both directly emitted primary particles and particles that form in the atmosphere through secondary processes as a result of emissions of SO_2, NO_x, and organic compounds. These particulate matter species, formed by the conversion of gaseous pollutants emissions, are referred to collectively as secondary particulate matter. Because the CAA, especially the 1990 Amendments, achieved substantial reductions in these gaseous precursor emissions, it has a much larger effect on PM_{10} and $PM_{2.5}$ than might be apparent if only the changes in directly emitted particles are considered.

[4]Some pilot analyses of hazardous air pollutants were conducted but it was determined that the poor quality of the available information precluded comprehensive quantification of the effects.

Analyses for these pollutants can be considered incremental to the results of the prospective analysis. Estimates for that part of the CAA Amendments regarding stratospheric ozone depletion (Title VI) are developed in the prospective study but they are not fully integrated into the main analysis.

Emissions estimates reflect the expected growth in population, transportation, electric power generation, and other economic activity over the relevant time periods. Different estimation procedures are used for stationary, mobile, and area sources, although the benefit and cost estimates are not disaggregated in that manner. Costs are estimated as increases in expenditures by different entities to meet the additional control requirements of the CAA, including operation and maintenance expenditures plus amortized capital costs (i.e., depreciation plus interest costs associated with the existing capital stock). Changes in employment and prices as well as impacts that might be experienced among customers of the firms that must incur these costs were partially examined in the retrospective analysis but omitted in the prospective study. In limiting consideration of these so-called general equilibrium effects, the EPA reports effectively preclude analysis of the economy-wide costs of imposing additional environmental regulations in the context of existing labor and other (distortionary) taxes.[5]

Although the air quality modeling efforts focused on the full range of pollutants, both studies found that the majority of the total benefits are attributable to changes in particulate matter concentrations. Consistent with current scientific understandings, neither the specific source categories nor the chemical composition of the particles were considered. Thus, secondary particles formed from SO_2, NO_x, and volatile organic compounds were all treated (uniformly) as fine particles. The retrospective study found significant benefits associated with the reductions in lead—principally the phase-down of lead in gasoline. The monetary benefits of air quality improvement include reduced incidence of premature mortality and other human health effects, as well as improvements in visibility and avoided damage to agricultural crops. Despite efforts to characterize the impacts of air pollution on natural systems, the inability to quantify and/or place a monetary value on the damages precluded the development of benefits estimates for ecosystem impacts (except for a supplementary calculation for avoided costs of nitrate reductions; see below). A similar story applies to potential carcinogenic and certain other health effects associated with criteria pollutants.

The monetary benefits reflect interpretations of the available science and economic literature made by the EPA in consultation with its outside experts. As a form of sensitivity analysis, a number of alternative interpretations of the literature were also examined. The quantitatively most important concern the valuation of premature mortality. In both the retrospective and prospective analyses, the EPA developed an alternative scenario based on the loss of life-years approach to reflect

---

[5]Costs for meeting Title IV through the SO_2 trading program were estimated by a model that allocates emissions reductions cost-effectively in a context of responding to market signals in the electric power and tradable allowance markets.

the greater susceptibility of older individuals to air pollution–induced mortality. In both studies this scenario yielded significantly lower benefits. The prospective study also examined alternative assumptions about the incidence of mortality and the incidence and valuation of chronic bronchitis, as well as certain other effects. Sensitivity analysis was used to examine alternative behavioral responses to stratospheric ozone depletion (Title VI), such as remaining indoors or increasing use of sunscreen or hats.

Table 1 displays the present value of monetary benefits of the CAA by endpoint category, along with comparisons to estimated costs, for 1970–1990. An array of benefit estimates is presented, reflecting the underlying uncertainties. Overall, the present value of total benefits is estimated to range from $3.5 trillion (5th percentile of the underlying probability distribution) to $56.3 trillion (95th percentile) over the 20-year period. Comparing the mean benefit estimate ($22.2 trillion) with the present value point estimate of costs ($.5 trillion), benefits are seen to dwarf costs

TABLE 1   Present value of 1970–1990 costs and monetized benefits by endpoint category for population of continental United States (billions of 1990 dollars, discounted to 1990 at 5%) [from Reference (29)]

Endpoint	Pollutant(s)[a]	5th percentile	Mean	95th percentile
Mortality	PM	$2,369	$16,632	$40,597
Mortality	Pb	$121	$1,339	$3,910
Chronic bronchitis	PM	$409	$3,313	$10,401
IQ (lost IQ pts. + children w/IQ <70)	Pb	$271	$399	$551
Hypertension	Pb	$77	$98	$120
Hospital admissions	PM, O3, Pb, CO	$27	$57	$120
Respiratory-related symptoms, restricted activity, decreased productivity	PM, O3, NO$_2$, SO$_2$	$123	$182	$261
Soiling damage	PM	$6	$74	$192
Visibility	particulates	$38	$54	$71
Agriculture (net surplus)	O3	$11	$23	$35
Total benefits		$3,452	$22,171	$56,258
Total costs			$523	
Net benefits (total benefits − total costs)			$21,648	

[a]PM, particulate matter; Pb, lead.

TABLE 2   Alternative mortality benefits' mean estimates for 1970–1990 (in trillions of 1990 dollars, discounted at 5%) [from Reference (29)]

Benefit estimation method	Benefits particulate matter	Total
Statistical life method ($4.8 million/life)	16.6	18.0
Life-years lost method ($293,000/year)	9.1	10.1

by a factor of 42:1.[6] Net benefits amount to $21.6 trillion. Note that according to the mean estimates particulate matter mortality is estimated to account for 75% of total benefits, followed by chronic bronchitis (15%) and lead mortality (6%). The remaining eight categories comprise the residual 4% of benefits.

Table 2 presents alternative particulate matter mortality benefits when the life-years lost method as opposed to the statistical life approach is used in the calculations. Although the latter approach has historically been used by the EPA in conducting its benefit-cost analyses, some short-term particulate matter exposure studies suggest that a disproportionate share of particulate matter–related premature mortality occurs among persons 65 years of age or older. Thus, at the urging of the outside review committee, the EPA combined standard life expectancy tables with the limited available data on age-specific incidence to develop (crude) approximations of the number of life-years lost by those who die prematurely as a result of exposure to particulate matter. These were presented as alternative estimates. As shown in Table 2, the particulate matter mortality benefits, the largest single benefit category overall, fall by 45% when this alternative valuation method is used. Although use of the life-years lost method does not change the basic conclusion of the retrospective study that the monetized benefits greatly exceed costs over the period 1970–1990, the magnitude of the change demonstrates the importance of answering the question of valuation with greater clarity. As discussed in Updating The Information, below, the life-years lost method is but one of several current issues in the valuation literature.

Table 3, drawn from the prospective study, summarizes the central estimates on a present value basis of the costs and benefits of the Clean Air Act (CAA) for 1990–2010. About 90% of the benefits are associated with avoided mortality, a slightly higher proportion than in the retrospective study. The remainder of the benefits are associated with avoided morbidity and ecological and welfare benefits. On the cost side, the prospective analysis finds that Title I [National Ambient Air Quality Standards (NAAQS)] accounts for almost half of the total cost of the first five titles. Title II (mobile sources) accounts for another third, with the balance distributed among Title III (toxic emissions), Title IV (SO_2 and NO_x from power plants), and Title V (permitting). Because of the long-term nature of the

---

[6]Note that the costs were treated as if they were certain, when in fact there is much uncertainty about such costs (see Updating The Information, below).

TABLE 3 Summary of quantified primary central estimate benefits and costs of Clean Air Act amendments, 1990–2010 (estimates in millions of 1990 dollars) [from Reference (31)][a]

Cost or benefit category	Annual estimates		
	2000	**2010**	**Present value**
Costs:			
Title I	$8,600	$14,500	$85,000
Title II	$7,400	$9,000	$65,000
Title III	$780	$840	$6,600
Title IV	$2,300	$2,000	$18,000
Title V	$300	$300	$2,500
Total costs, Title I-V	$19,000	$27,000	$180,000
Title VI	$1,400*		$27,000*
Monetized benefits:			
Avoided mortality	$63,000	$100,000	$610,000
Avoided morbidity	$5,100	$7,900	$49,000
Ecological and welfare effects	$3,000	$4,800	$29,000
Total benefits, Title I-V	$71,000	$110,000	$690,000
Stratospheric ozone	$25,000*		$530,000*

[a]Annual estimates for Title VI stratospheric ozone protection provisions are annualized equivalents of the net present value of costs from 1990 to 2075 (for costs) or 1990 to 2165 (for benefits). The difference in time scales for costs and benefits reflects the persistence of ozone depleting substances in the atmosphere, the slow processes of ozone formation and depletion, and the accumulation of physical effects in response to elevated UV-b radiation levels.

benefits of Title VI (stratospheric ozone), its results are not fully integrated into the overall findings. However, the present value benefits of this title exceed costs by a factor of twenty. Overall, while the monetized benefits of the CAA Amendments over the period 1990–2010 still exceed the costs, the ratio of benefits to costs (about 4:1 for Titles I–V) is considerably lower than in the retrospective analysis, suggesting that the "truly low hanging fruit" may have been picked in the early years.[7]

Overall, as the EPA has noted in the prospective study, the conclusion of the Section 812 analysis is clear:

> While alternative choices for data, models, modeling assumptions, and valuation paradigms may yield results outside the range projected in our primary analysis, we believe based on the magnitude of the difference between the estimated benefits and costs that it is unlikely that eliminating uncertainties or adopting reasonable alternative assumptions would change the fundamental

[7]In one of the scenarios presented in the prospective study (low benefits), costs actually exceed benefits by $1 billion per year.

conclusion of ... [the] study: the Clean Air Act(s') ... total benefits to society exceed its costs. (31, page v)

Although the findings of these studies have been discussed in the media and, to some extent, on Capitol Hill, it is fair to say they have played only a modest role in the policymaking process. In our judgment, the EPA needs to disaggregate the benefits and costs into those applicable to specific titles, sectors, or regulations in order to have a significant impact on policy decisions. Although the EPA did not do this in the Section 812 study, others have done so for specific titles of the CAA, taking the EPA's aggregate benefit estimate (and cost estimates by title) as given (27). Extensive analysis has also been conducted on the electricity generation sector (Title IV) alone (7, 5). In addition, the EPA was able to develop separate benefit estimates for their new ozone and fine particulate National Ambient Air Quality Standards (30). The findings from these studies are presented in Table 4. This table shows that some titles deliver more net benefits than others and that the new fine particulate NAAQS is likely to be a much better buy for society than the new ambient ozone standard.

TABLE 4 Summary of cost-benefit studies of the 1990 Clean Air Act Amendments for 2010 (estimates in millions of 1990 dollars)

Study	Benefits	Costs
Title IV		
Burtraw et al. (5)[a]	$25,000	$800
Chestnut (7)	$35,277	NA
New NAAQS (30)[b]		
Ozone (8-h), partial attainment	$400–$2,100	$1,100
Ozone (8-h), full attainment	$1,500–$8,500	$9,600
Fine particulates, partial attainment	$19,000–$104,000	$8,600
Fine particulates, full attainment	$20,000–$110,000	$37,000
Clean Air Act Amendments (27)[c]		
Title I	$26,564	$14,500
Title II	$14,968	$9,000
Title III	$1,925	$840
Title IV	$69,297	$2,000

[a]While this estimate is specific to the eastern United States, these benefits are expected to account for 98% of total U.S. benefits.

[b]Partial attainment costs are incremental to partial attainment of current standards and reflect partial attainment of promulgated standards. The EPA estimates 17 potential residual nonattainment areas for ozone and 30 potential residual nonattainment areas for fine particulates as of 2010. Full attainment costs, however, are incremental to full attainment of current standards.

[c]Total CAA Amendments benefit estimate ($110 billion; see Table 2) and cost estimates by title (see Table 2) are from Reference (31).

DESIGN OF A NEW PROSPECTIVE STUDY

The scope of the first two studies was clearly established by Congress based on policies and regulations implemented prior to 1990 or, in the case of the prospective analysis, based on the new provisions of the 1990 CAA Amendments. In contrast, the framework for a second prospective study is less well defined. There have been no revisions to the Act since 1990. Thus, there is not a clear set of Congressionally mandated policies to examine. We believe this absence of specific Congressional direction creates an opportunity for the EPA to establish its own agenda for the second prospective study that enhances the opportunity to further incorporate economic considerations in future policies.

How should the EPA best approach a new Section 812 study? Some might argue for a simple updating of the first prospective study, with the addition of new data and research results. In our judgment, it would be unwise to proceed with such an approach, because the new information generated is unlikely to justify the considerable resource costs involved. Further, the results of such a study would likely have only marginal policy impacts, as most of the regulations considered in such an analysis would have been implemented by the time the study was completed. We believe the new study should focus on critical policy issues likely to be considered by the EPA over the next decade. Specifically, we propose that the EPA use a new Section 812 study as a vehicle for considering how it can improve the net benefits of the CAA in the coming decades. The net benefits framework assures that potential opportunities to increase total benefits as well as those that would decrease total costs are examined. Because the study would likely be completed prior to Congressional and EPA action on these new policies (or alterations of existing policies), there would be a clear opportunity for the analysis to influence policy decisions. If conducted in a timely way, such a study would represent a departure from the first two Section 812 studies, which were conducted after the bulk of the policy decisions were made. Indeed, using the new prospective study in this planning function would show Congress that the EPA is serious about using benefit-cost analysis to inform its regulatory agenda and decision-making.

In contrast to the first two studies, in which the focus was largely on aggregate analyses, a new study aimed at improving the design and implementation of the CAA requires an understanding of how specific elements of the Act are performing. To make decisions on the efficacy and efficiency of specific elements of the CAA requires costs and benefits disaggregated in a useful manner. The disaggregations could include the stringency of air quality standards for ozone and particulate matter (Title I); their implementation through the State Implementation Plan process, including various requirements for mobile source controls (Title II); the provisions for SO_2 allowance trading and reductions in NO_x from power plants (Title IV); and provisions for control of toxic emissions (Title III) and permitting (Title V).

Overall, we believe that the new Section 812 study should also focus on potential new policies not yet part of EPA policy or regulation. The so-called multi-pollutant bills, which focus on SO_2, NO_x, mercury, and possibly CO_2, would be strong candidates for consideration. It would be particularly useful to consider the benefits and costs of alternative stringency levels for each of the pollutants, as well as the interaction among them. For example, how do the marginal costs (and benefits) of controlling CO_2 vary with alternative stringency levels of SO_x, NO_x, and mercury? The tradeoffs being contemplated between tightening down on these pollutants and loosening or eliminating New Source Review requirements would be particularly illuminating. It would also be useful to examine other initiatives that might be considered to meet new or anticipated NAAQS requirements, e.g., new regulations whose primary goal is to reduce ground-level ozone or those primarily designed to reduce fine particles. When doing this kind of analysis it will be important to note how some regulations (e.g., those dealing with nitrogen oxides and volatile organic compounds in particular) provide benefits in terms of tropospheric ozone, as well as fine particle reductions. Other possible areas of interest include new policies to reduce emissions of hazardous air pollutants, possibly including so-called residual risk standards. For all these policies it would be appropriate to analyze a number of different scenarios that attempted to encompass the bounds of possible new policies.

Consistent with the goal of illuminating issues likely to have particular policy relevance over the next decade, the most important policies to analyze would be those with potentially high costs, whose benefits are uncertain. Examples would be the currently mandated bans on episodic controls currently in the CAA, the current New Source Review process, the Inspection and Maintenance Program, and even the State Implementation Plan conformity process. These represent existing parts of the Act in which alternative approaches may yield significant environmental benefits relative to the costs incurred. It is also possible that selected regulations mandated over the past several years but not yet implemented could be reconsidered in the Section 812 context.

In general, the appropriate level of aggregation depends on the use to which the analysis is to be put. The EPA's review committee has previously urged the EPA to pursue a title-by-title approach (ACCACA 1999). To a limited extent the EPA has done so in the first prospective analysis by estimating the costs of the 1990 amendments on a title-by-title basis. However, because of the difficulty of uniquely attributing individual pollutants to specific titles, it is difficult to break out benefits by title. In the case of SO_2 and NO_x reductions from power plants (Title IV), this is relatively straightforward. However, NO_x controls show up in three separate titles. For future analyses it may be more appropriate from both a methodological and a policy standpoint to distinguish regulations on a broad sectoral basis, e.g., stationary, mobile, and area sources. To the extent feasible, it would also be desirable to seek finer distinctions within these categories, e.g., regulations on electric utilities, petroleum refineries, and other large sources. Individual as opposed to groups of policies should be examined to provide the maximum amount of information to decision makers. Benefits and costs computed by sector can indicate the relative efficiency of controls or other emissions management options aimed at different pollution source categories. For example, in such a framework it would be possible to compare the net benefits of ozone strategies focusing on emission reductions from stationary sources (e.g., NO_x controls on the electric power industry) with motor vehicle strategies (e.g., enhanced inspection and maintenance programs).

UPDATING THE INFORMATION

The EPA's prospective study was published in 1999, but most of the analyses were completed in 1998. Since then, progress has been made in a number of research areas, including the valuation of health effects and cost analysis. In this section we focus on the new economic research that we believe could and should be incorporated into a second prospective study, and by extension, any cost-benefit analysis of this type of pollution. At the outset, however, we note new developments in the areas of air pollution modeling and in the epidemiological studies used to estimate health effects.

The first prospective study relied on one air quality model to convert SO_2 and NO_x emissions into particulate air pollution and another to convert NO_x and volatile organic compound emissions into ozone. Unfortunately, this approach did not allow the air chemistry underlying these conversions to be addressed in a unified fashion. The newest generation of air quality models addresses both secondary particulate and ozone formation in a single, comprehensive and internally consistent model. Examples of these models include EPA's MODELS3 (32) and the Georgia Tech Model (37). These models are very complex and expensive to set up, so the new analysis probably cannot depend entirely on them. Nevertheless, there is for the first time a capability to examine how the use of a unified air quality model alters the benefit estimates relative to the framework previously used.

Recent epidemiological evidence has led to some new questions and an understanding of the effects of particulate pollution on mortality in adults. Similarly, there is growing evidence of the effect of elevated concentrations of particulate matter on infants—a category that was excluded from both the retrospective and the prospective studies. In the Health Effects Institute-led re-analysis of the long-term study by Pope et al. (24), which was the primary study used by the EPA to estimate mortality effects in their prospective analysis, Krewski et al. (13) clearly reaffirmed the qualitative relationships but found several interesting anomalies.[8] Other recent studies, both long-term and short-term, came to similar conclusions.

Considering the short-term studies, Samet et al. (25), in their 20 and 90 cities studies, found an aggregate coarse particulate matter (PM_{10}) effect of about half of that estimated by earlier short-term studies. They also found evidence of region-specific variation in mortality effects, most notably in the northeastern United

---

[8]Long-term studies involve following a cohort of individuals in many cities for years, relating their pollution exposures to the probability of death. Short-term studies involve examining how daily death rates in a given city vary with daily pollution exposures.

States, where mortality effects were estimated to be twice as high as those for the 90 cities overall. Zanobetti & Schwartz (38), in examining potential socioeconomic modifiers of PM_{10} effects, found the mortality effect for females to be approximately one third larger than that for males. Interestingly, adding sulfates (SO_4) and some heavy metals to such models significantly lowers the fine particulate matter ($PM_{2.5}$) effect (4), whereas adding gaseous pollutants generally does not affect the particulate matter coefficients (25). Wichmann et al. (35) finds that the ultra-fine particles (PM_1 or lower) are a significant predictor of mortality, until other pollutants are added.

With respect to the long-term studies, Krewski et al. (13) found slightly larger effects of $PM_{2.5}$ on mortality than that found by Pope et al. (24), but these effects fall dramatically and even become insignificant under some specifications, while SO_2 effects become large and significant. In addition, the mortality effects of fine particles ($PM_{2.5}$) varied with education level, the estimated effect being higher for individuals without a high school education than for those with higher levels of education. Furthermore, Abbey et al. (1) found no relationship of $PM_{2.5}$ for females, and Lipfert et al. (18) in a major study of veterans' mortality and pollution, found no PM effects, whereas they found ozone and NO_2 to be significant predictors of mortality.

At the same time that these new analyses are introducing new questions about mortality effects in adults, several studies around the world have strengthened the case for infant mortality being caused by exposure to particulates. Woodruff et al. (36) found mortality for respiratory causes and sudden infant death syndrome to be positively associated with high PM_{10} exposure for normal birth weight infants but no significant relationship for low birth weight infants. Lipfert et al. (19) replicated the findings of Woodruff et al., though they did not observe differences among categories of birth weights. Also, Bobak & Leon (3), who conducted a matched population-based case-control study covering all births registered in the Czech Republic from 1989 to 1991, found that only particulate matter showed a consistent association with death when all pollutants were entered in one model; these effects were strongest in the postneonatal (rather than the neonatal) period and were specific for respiratory causes.

Filling in Valuation Gaps

A number of key linkages between pollution and endpoints that people value were missing from the prospective study. These include visibility, ecosystem damage, negative benefits (i.e., increased risks of melanomas) to ozone control from added exposure to ultraviolet radiation (UV-B), and effects of toxic exposure. Many of these benefit categories have been examined in recently published literature reviews [e.g., Cropper (8)]. The ACCACA (2) questioned the quality of all the visibility benefits studies, either because of methodological problems or because they had not been peer reviewed. Although the academic interest in valuing visibility benefits may have waned, perhaps from a lack of recent research support, the available studies suggest that such benefits could comprise a significant fraction of total benefits. In addition, the methods for eliciting values for visibility in a recreational context and in the western United States appear to be reasonably reliable. So few studies are available to set a value for urban visibility benefits that this area must be considered more speculative.

Ecosystem damages were largely ignored in both the retrospective and the prospective EPA studies, for the good reasons that there are no studies suitable for estimating physical ecosystem level benefits from air pollution reduction at the broad regional level (except in very specialized areas, such as the Adirondacks). Also, there are no studies providing a firm basis for valuing such improvements at this broad level, even in places where physical damage might be estimated.

The prospective study attempts to capture some ecosystem damage by counting foregone cleanup costs as a reasonable proxy for losses from nitrification of Chesapeake Bay and other waters associated with NO_x emissions. The expert review committee was adamant that this approach was an unreliable estimate of benefits because, except in special cases, there is no necessary relationship between foregone cleanup costs and the benefits of cleanup.

Finally, both studies were silent on the possible increase in skin cancers associated with increased UV-B radiation, itself associated with ozone reductions. Lutter & Wolz (20) and others have estimated these effects and find them to be nontrivial. The EPA ignored these effects, as it did in the regulatory impact analysis for its recently promulgated new ozone standard. This action was rejected by the Supreme Court (33) and the EPA agreed to consider this effect. Thus, there is no reason why future cost-benefit analyses of the CAA should omit what could be an important perverse effect of reducing ozone air pollution.

Using Better Methods/Newer Studies

The most important valuation number in the report is the value of a statistical life (VSL), which is the average willingness to pay for a given (small) reduction in risk of death divided by that risk reduction. The product of the VSL and the expected number of deaths avoided by the CAA yields an estimate of benefits that represents almost 90% of all benefits calculated in the Section 812 studies. The EPA's VSL estimate of $6 million was based on a review of 26 of the studies in the literature—21 labor market studies and 5 contingent valuation studies. The analytical methods applied to this review were ad hoc at best, and the reason for choosing the 26 studies was never entirely clear.

We believe that improvements in these estimates could come from two distinct elements of the health valuation literature. The first is a systematic evaluation of this literature. Mrozek & Taylor (22) have performed a meta-analysis of 38 studies contributing 203 VSL estimates. They found that the EPA's best estimate for the VSL ($6 million in 1998 dollars) is three times too large, i.e., Mrozek & Taylor's best estimate is $2 million, owing to a number of factors. The most important of these is a false attribution of wage rate differentials to mortality rate differences, when in fact much of this variation is due to interindustry differences in wage rates that occur for other reasons—a point first raised by Leigh (17).

Just as importantly, there are some new studies in the mortality risk valuation literature [e.g., Hammitt & Graham (11), Krupnick et al. (15), Strand (28), Johannesson & Johansson (16)] that are specifically designed to reflect the mortality risks associated with air pollution, but using contingent valuation and conjoint analysis approaches. Much of this literature also suggests that the EPA's $6 million estimate for the VSL is too high, with the appropriate adjustment being quite uncertain, as this literature needs to mature. Nevertheless, some of the literature suggests that the consideration of dread (e.g., with cancer-causing pollution exposures) and altruism (the willingness to pay for health improvements for others) could significantly increase the VSL.

The second most important valuation number in these studies is the value of a case of chronic disease. This is the analogue of the VSL, but for the reduced risk of getting chronic lung or heart disease. The estimate used in the EPA reports ($266,000) was derived from two small (300 person) pilot conjoint analysis studies (34, 14) that scarcely can support the weight placed upon them. Conjoint analyses and other stated preference techniques have evolved since these studies were done. Unfortunately, no new numbers are available for improving on this estimate. Clearly, this is an important area for future research, if only to do the same studies with a larger sample size.

Estimating Costs

The EPA has a long history of conducting its analyses of the costs of regulations based on engineering abatement cost estimates that are generally "on the shelf." This approach has the advantage of being transparent and easy to defend. One chooses technologies to abate a pollutant from a set of agreed upon technologies, the most cost-effective first.

Unfortunately, this approach is likely to lead to overestimation of control costs for two reasons. First, it does not account for future technological advances that may bring down such costs (or raise effectiveness). This is a particularly important failing when time horizons are long. Second, it often ignores options for reducing costs that are not classified as engineering approaches or do not show up in the approved list of technologies. This applies, in particular, to market or economic incentive approaches to pollution control, which may involve changes in input mix, process changes, product redesign, or others that respond to the need to minimize abatement costs. Recent work by Harrington et al. (12) has found empirical support for the notion that *ex ante* cost estimates tend to overstate true costs. In examining *ex post* information, Morgenstern et al. (21) found that reported environmental expenditures are generally not overstated, although considerable variation exists at the plant level.

The EPA's prospective study, while generally ignoring the cost consequences of incentive approaches, did consider them in the one place where they would be particularly important, namely for reducing SO_2 from power plants. Title IV of the CAA Amendments of 1990 set up an SO_2 allowance trading system for utilities to substantially reduce their SO_2 emissions through a trading program. The benefits of such a program (forecast out to 2010 estimated from the Integrated Planning Model for the EPA), which accounted for fuel switching, use of lower sulfur coal, new and retiring plants, demand reductions in reaction to higher electricity prices and generation load reallocations as ways of meeting the standard. Several other studies (5, 6, 10) also estimated costs and generally corroborate the EPA's estimates.

An omission in the report, albeit one whose inclusion would significantly raise costs, is the cost to society of imposing environmental regulations in the context of the existing tax structure—the so-called tax interaction effect (23). The tax interaction effect refers to the economy-wide economic losses associated with the imposition of additional environmental (or any other) regulation—losses that tend to be exacerbated by existing labor and other taxes. Aggregate losses are potentially quite large because there are so many people affected.[9] The tax interaction effect was extensively discussed by the expert review committee and the EPA and is mentioned in the prospective study, but it is not incorporated quantitatively. Clearly, future prospective studies could and should take this effect into account.

Inclusion of Other CBA Studies

Although the EPA studies are quite thorough in referencing the literature underlying key elements of the analysis, they generally omit references to other integrating studies similar in nature to the Section 812 reports. This is in marked contrast to benefit-cost studies in the academic literature, in which one can often find commentary on estimates from similar studies and an attempt at reconciliation of any differences that arise [e.g., Burtraw et al. (5)]. One good example pertains to the EPA's Regulatory Impact Analysis of the Proposed Ozone Standard (30), which is a benefit-cost analysis. The American Petroleum Institute sponsored a study of the costs of meeting the EPA's proposed ozone standard in a multi-state area around the Great Lakes (26). Their estimate was as large as the EPA's estimate for the entire country. No reference was made to the study, nor was any attempt made to reconcile the results. One would hope that future studies would attempt to acquire, analyze, and reconcile results of other major studies addressing relevant parts of future EPA benefit-cost analyses of air quality improvements.

Peer Review

Currently, peer review of the Section 812 studies is performed through unpaid review committees, mostly made up of academics, who meet and participate in conference calls periodically to consider issues that come up in the design,

---

[9]One committee member estimated that costs of the implemented CAA Amendments could be 30% higher than shown in the report.

implementation, and writing of the review. Because of the necessarily limited attention that such reports can be given by unpaid committees, we recommend that their resources be supplemented by some paid reviewers with expertise in specific areas. This is an approach used by the EPA to do other reviews of agency work under the CAA, such as the reviews conducted of the voluminous *Criteria Documents*, issued periodically to survey the literature relevant to setting new National Ambient Air Quality Standards, under Title I of the Act.

REPRESENTING UNCERTAINTIES ABOUT COSTS AND BENEFITS

Over the years, benefit-cost analyses at the EPA have been getting more sophisticated in terms of their representation of the benefits of environmental improvements. Early analyses either ignored uncertainties, focusing on a best estimate for each of the parameters in the analysis, or identified rather arbitrary "low" and "high" estimates around a "best" estimate and used all the low or high estimates of parameters to create a "super low" and a "super high" benefit estimate, respectively. More recently, as exemplified in both the retrospective and the prospective studies, Monte Carlo simulation techniques were used. Such techniques apply a more logical and rigorous approach to propagating uncertainties in parameters through the various steps of the benefit analysis.[10]

No one doubts that costs are uncertain. In fact, costs may be just as uncertain as benefits. However, costs are routinely considered at if they were certain. The same techniques used to analyze uncertainties in benefit estimates should be used to estimate uncertainties in costs. This will not be easy to do. For one thing, the databases containing the engineering data used to estimate costs of reducing air emissions typically offer only "best estimates," with no information provided on the dispersion of such costs across plants. Second, because the cost estimates are engineering-derived rather than statistically based, they come from analyses that do not generate the kind of error distributions found in the statistically based epidemiological and valuation literature.

These points lead to two research strategies. One would be to comb the economics literature for abatement cost functions estimated for various pollutants and sectors and use these instead of the engineering data. Another would be to comb the engineering literature for references to cost distributions across plants and use such information to develop cost ranges.

---

[10]This approach involves first defining probability distributions for each parameter—often based on confidence intervals around estimated regression coefficients—e.g., from the effect of a change in pollution concentration on a health effect. Then simulations are run to draw parameter values from these distributions, computing benefits for each set of trial values drawn. The result is a benefit distribution that truly represents the underlying uncertainties in the parameters.

USE OF COST-EFFECTIVENESS RATHER THAN BENEFIT-COST TECHNIQUES

Up to now we have assumed that future Section 812 studies need to be benefit-cost studies. Yet, under certain reasonable conditions, cost-effectiveness analysis—dividing the cost of a particular regulation by a measure of the effectiveness of that regulation and then comparing various regulations (or regulatory options) according to this cost-per-unit effectiveness measure—may be almost as useful as benefit-cost analysis.

The rationale for this strategy begins by noting that attaching monetary values to health effects is highly controversial, so avoiding doing so has an obvious attraction. Arguably, in the analysis of air pollution policies, in which such a large portion of the benefits are mortality-related and the morbidity benefits tend to move proportionally with changes in mortality, a physical measure of mortality benefits, such as "lives saved" or "life-years saved" may be a good proxy for all health effects. In this case, a cost-per-life-saved measure may be a useful basis for discriminating among various policy initiatives.

There are drawbacks to this approach, however. First, and most importantly, only with benefit-cost analysis can any normative claim be made, i.e., whether the contemplated or already implemented policy makes economic sense. When a benefit-cost analysis of a contemplated action yields negative net benefits, one can make the statement that, on efficiency grounds (and subject to many caveats), society would be made worse off by advancing that particular option. If option A has greater (positive) net benefits than option B, then one can say that both options increase social welfare, but that A is the better option, again, solely from the criterion of efficiency. With only a cost-effectiveness analysis, in contrast, if one finds that option A is more cost-effective than option B (cost per life saved is lower for A than B), one can only conclude that A is preferred to B, not that A is socially beneficial on net.

Second, for a cost-effectiveness analysis to be a reasonable substitute for benefit-cost analysis, one category of benefits (e.g., the mortality benefits) needs to be a large fraction of all benefits. In the context of the CAA, we have argued above that there is some reason to expect that the VSL estimates will be coming down. This means that morbidity benefits may assume a greater share of the total and that, as a consequence, the cost-effectiveness strategy may be less attractive. Further, to the extent that ecological benefits are involved, human mortality benefits may be a poor proxy for them. Certainly, once these as yet poorly understood benefit areas are better understood, the cost-effectiveness strategy will be less compelling as applied to the CAA.

CONDUCT VALUE OF INFORMATION ANALYSIS

Finally, many benefit-cost analyses, including the Section 812 studies, are also useful in helping to set a research agenda. Once one goes to the trouble and expense of conducting such a study, it is not much more complicated to estimate whether a reduction in the uncertainty of various parameters would materially affect the ultimate conclusions of the analysis. In other words, one can determine which parameters contribute the most to benefit (or cost) uncertainty and would, therefore, be the most important for reducing uncertainty. Implicitly at least, the EPA conducted such a thought process in developing a list of key areas of future research to improve future Section 812 studies. It might be appropriate to formalize that process to get a deeper understanding of the value of proposed new research.

CONCLUDING THOUGHTS

The EPA's Section 812 studies are unique in government. To our knowledge, no other agency provides broad-scope benefit-cost analyses for statutes it implements that are as carefully developed or reviewed. Whereas benefit-cost analyses are now required for all major regulations, the Section 812 analysis serves to integrate such analyses while taking a national and forward-looking perspective on air pollution control.

Subject to some methodological qualifications, the two Section 812 studies already completed indicate that the aggregate benefits of past and ongoing policies to improve air quality have clearly exceeded the costs incurred by industry, taxpayers, and consumers. Whether benefits exceed costs by a factor of 40 or 4 or less, the professional consensus is that, overall, the nation received good value for the resources it invested in improving air quality over the past three decades. Yet we don't know if that value could have been far higher by changing or eliminating certain inefficient elements of the CAA. One of the challenges of a second prospective study is to answer that question.

Another challenge in conducting a new Section 812 study, which is less constrained by Congressional mandate than the first two, is to develop the analysis in such a way as to have the maximum impact on the design and implementation of future air pollution control policies. Specifically, we have recommended the goal of increasing the net benefits of future air quality regulations. We believe the best way to accomplish this is to focus the study on already mandated but not fully implemented polices where significant future costs are anticipated and, particularly, to focus on potential new policies not yet mandated by law or regulation. We have recommended specific candidates for study, but clearly a fuller debate on the issue is appropriate.

We also believe the EPA faces a number of key challenges in incorporating the most recent research in a new Section 812 study and in making the Section 812 study effort a model of how good benefit-cost analyses are designed, performed, and reviewed. The EPA should resist the temptation to sit on its laurels with respect to the positive outcome of the Section 812 studies, recognize the possibility that the CAA can do a better job of delivering benefits to residents of the United States, and endeavor to keep the analysis at the forefront of the rapidly changing social and physical sciences it must draw upon.

Finally, the EPA should take the opportunity afforded by the new Section 812 study to do something it has rarely done before: actually use benefit-cost analysis prospectively as a planning tool to establish priorities for its regulatory and legislative agenda with respect to air pollution issues. Such an action would demonstrate to Congress that the EPA is serious about delivering efficient regulations and other policy initiatives to the American public.

Visit the Annual Reviews home page at www.annualreviews.org

LITERATURE CITED

1. Abbey DE, Nishino N, McDonnell WF, Burchette RJ, Knutsen SF, et al. 1999. Long-term inhalable particles and other air pollutants related to mortality in non-smokers. *Am. J. Respir. Crit. Care Med.* 159:373–82

2. Advisory Committee on Clean Air Compliance Analysis (ACCACA). 1999. Final Advisory Letter from the committee to Carol Browner, Administrator, US EPA, Nov. 19 and various other letters to the Administrator

3. Bobak M, Leon DA. 1999. The effect of air pollution on infant mortality appears specific for respiratory causes in the post-neonatal period. *Epidemiology* 10(6):666–70

4. Burnett RT, Brook J, Dann T, Delocla C, Philips O, et al. 2000. Association between particulate- and gas-phase components of urban air pollution and daily mortality in eight Canadian cities. *Inhal. Toxicol.* 12(suppl. 4):15–39. Special issue on Particulate Matter and Health

5. Burtraw D, Krupnick A, Mansur E, Austin D, Farrell D. 1998. Costs and benefits of reducing air pollutants related to acid rain. *Contemp. Econ. Policy* XVI:379–400

6. Carlson C, Burtraw D, Cropper M, Palmer K. 2000. SO2 control by electric utilities: What are the gains from trade? *J. Polit. Econ.* 108(6):1292–326

7. Chestnut L. 1995. *Human health bene-fits assessment of the acid rain provisions of the 1990 Clean Air Act Amendments*, final report prepared by Hagler Bailly Consulting, Inc. for the USEPA, Acid Rain Div.

8. Cropper ML. 2000. Has research answered the needs of environmental policy? *J. Environ. Econ. Manag.* 39:328–50

9. Davies JC. 1970. *The Politics of Pollution.* New York: Pegasus

10. Ellerman AD, Montero J-P. 1998. Why are allowance prices so low? An analysis of the SO2 Emissions Trading Program. *J. Environ. Econ. Manag.*

11. Hammitt JK, Graham JD. 1999. Willingness to pay for health protection: inadequate sensitivity to probability? *J. Risk Uncertain.* 18(1):33–62

12. Harrington W, Morgenstern R, Nelson P. 2000. On the accuracy of regulatory cost estimates. *J. Policy Anal. Manag.* 19(2):297–322

13. Krewski D, Burnett RT, Goldberg MS, Hoover K, Siemiatycki J, et al. 2000. Reanalysis of the Harvard Six Cities Study and the American Cancer Society Study of Particulate Air Pollution and Mortality. A special report of the institute's Particle Epidemiology Reanalysis Project. Cambridge, MA: Health Effects Inst.

14. Krupnick AJ, Cropper M. 1992. The effect of information on health risk valuation. *J. Risk Uncertain.* 5:29–48

15. Krupnick AJ, Cropper M, Alberini A, Simon N, O'Brien B, Goeree R. 2002. Age,

health and the willingness to pay for mortality risk reductions: a contingent valuation survey of Ontario residents. *J. Risk Uncertain.* In press

16. Johannesson M, Johansson P-O. 1996. To be or not to be: That is the question: an empirical study of the WTP for an increased life expectancy at an advanced age. *J. Risk Uncertain.* 13:163–74

17. Leigh JP. 1995. Compensating wages, value of a statistical life, and inter-industry differentials. *J. Environ. Econ. Manag.* 28(1):83–97

18. Lipfert FW, Morris SC, Wyzga RE. 2000a. Daily mortality in the Philadelphia metropolitan area and size-classified particulate matter. *J. Air Waste Manag. Assoc.* 1501–13

19. Lipfert FW, Zhang J, Wyzga RE. 2000b. Infant mortality and air pollution: a comprehensive analysis of U.S. data for 1990. *J. Air Waste Manag. Assoc.* 50:1350–66

20. Lutter R, Wolz C. 1997. UV-B screening by tropospheric ozone: implications for the National Ambient Air Quality Standard. *Environ. Sci. Technol.* 31:142A–146A

21. Morgenstern RD, Pizer W, Shih J-S. 2001. The cost of environmental protection. *Rev. Econ. Stat.* 83(4):732–38

22. Mrozek JR, Taylor LO. 2002. What determines the value of a life? A meta-analysis. *J. Policy Anal. Manag.* In press

23. Parry I, Oates WE. 2000. Policy analysis in the presence of distorting taxes. *J. Policy Anal. Manag.* 19(4)

24. Pope CA, Thun MJ, Namboodiri MM, Dockery DD, Evans JS, et al. 1995. Particulate air pollution as a predictor of mortality in a prospective study of U.S. adults. *Am. J. Respir. Crit. Care Med.* 151:669–74

25. Samet JM, Zeger SL, Dominici F, Curriero F, Coursac I, et al. 2000. *The National Morbidity, Mortality, and Air Pollution Study. Part II. Morbidity and Mortality from Air Pollution in the United States.*

Cambridge, MA: Health Effects Inst. Res. Rep. 94

26. Sierra Research. 1996. *Socio-economic study of possible eight-hour ozone standard, Rep. No. SR96-06-01.* Prepared for the Am. Petroleum Inst.

27. Smith A, Ross M. 1999. *Benefit-cost ratios of the CAAA by CAAA Title: an assessment based on EPA's Prospective Study,* prepared for General Motors Corporation by Charles Rivers Assoc., CRA D2050-00

28. Strand J. 2001. *Public and private-good values of statistical lives: results from a combined choice experiment and contingent valuation survey.* Univ. Oslo Working Paper

29. US Environ. Prot. Agency (EPA). 1997a. *The Benefits and Costs of the Clean Air Act: 1970 to 1990.* Washington, DC: Office of Air and Radiation/Office of Policy

30. US Environ. Prot. Agency (EPA). 1997b. *Regulatory Impact Analysis for Ozone and Particulate National Ambient Air Quality Standards.* Washington, DC: EPA

31. US Environ. Prot. Agency (EPA). 1999. *The Benefits and Costs of the Clean Air Act, 1990 to 2010.* Washington, DC: Office of Air and Radiation/Office of Policy

32. US Environ. Prot. Agency (EPA). 2001. *Models 3 Documentation.* http://www.epa.gov/asmdnerl/models3/doc/

33. US Supreme Court. 2001. *Ruling on Whitman v American Trucking Association.* February 27

34. Viscusi WK, Magat W, Huber J. 1991. Pricing environmental health risks: a survey assessment of risk-risk and risk-dollar trade-offs for chronic bronchitis. *J. Environ. Econ. Manag.* 21:32–51

35. Wichmann H-E, Spix C, Tuch T, Wolke G, Peters A, et al. 2000. *Daily mortality and fine and ultrafine particles in Erfurt, Germany. Part I. Role of particle number and particle mass. Res. Rep. no. 98.* Cambridge, MA: Health Effects Inst.

36. Woodruff TJ, Grillo J, Schoendorf KC. 1997. The relationship between selected

causes of post-neonatal infant mortality and particulate air pollution in the United States. *Environ. Health Perspect.* 105:608–12

37. Yang Y-J, Wilkinson JG, Russell AG. 1997. Fast, direct sensitivity analysis of multidimensional photochemical models. *Environ. Sci. Technol.* 31:2859–68

38. Zanobetti A, Schwartz J. 2000. Race, gender, and social status as modifiers of the effects of PM10 on mortality. *J. Occup. Environ. Med.* 42:469–74

SUBJECT INDEX

CUMULATIVE INDEXES

CONTRIBUTING AUTHORS, VOLUMES 14–23

CHAPTER TITLES, VOLUMES 14–23

Environmental and Occupational Health

Mini-Symposium on Managed Care

Public Health Practice

Social Environment and Behavior

Symposium: Cancers of Special Importance to Women

Symposium on Eating-Related Disorders

Symposium: Public Health Aspects of Ophthalmic Disease

Symposium: Public Health Genetics

Symposium: Public Health in the Twentieth Century

04625925